MEDICAL DISCOVERIES

WHO and WHEN

MEDICAL DISCOVERIES

WHO and WHEN

A dictionary listing thousands of medical and related scientific discoveries in alphabetical order, giving in each case the name of the discoverer, his profession, nationality, and floruit, and the date of the discovery.

By

J. E. SCHMIDT, Ph.B.S., M.D., Litt.D.

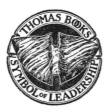

CHARLES C THOMAS • PUBLISHER

Springfield · Illinois · U.S.A.

CHARLES C THOMAS · PUBLISHER
BANNERSTONE HOUSE
301-327 East Lawrence Avenue, Springfield, Illinois, U.S.A.

Published simultaneously in the British Commonwealth of Nations by
BLACKWELL SCIENTIFIC PUBLICATIONS, LTD., OXFORD, ENGLAND

Published simultaneously in Canada by
THE RYERSON PRESS, TORONTO

Library of Congress Catalog Card Number: 58-14086

With THOMAS BOOKS *careful attention is given to all details of manufacturing and design. It is the Publisher's desire to present books that are satisfactory as to their physical qualities and artistic possibilities and appropriate for their particular use.* THOMAS BOOKS *will be true to those laws of quality that assure a good name and good will.*

Printed in the United States of America

THIS BOOK

is respectfully dedicated to a man whose unceasing stream of encouragement, unending patience, and monumental understanding of the author's point of view made the exhausting work upon this book not only possible but even enjoyable

to

PAYNE E. L. THOMAS

INTRODUCTION

This work, a dictionary of MEDICAL DISCOVERIES, is the fruition of a lifelong curiosity with regard to the "Who and When" of medical discoveries and inventions.

When and by whom were rubber gloves introduced in surgery? When was sodium citrate first recognized as an anticoagulant, and by whom? Who was the first to use plaster of Paris in bandaging? Who introduced the wool skein test for color vision? Who was the first to use cordotomy for the relief of pain in the lower part of the body? Such questions, and thousands like them, formed the titillating stimulus to which the dictionary of MEDICAL DISCOVERIES is the quenching reaction.

The title MEDICAL DISCOVERIES: WHO and WHEN is, in a sense, an understatement, for among the more than 6,000 entries the reader will find numerous items relating to methods, tests, operations, diseases, deformities, terms, eponyms, original texts, "fathers" and founders, doctrines, theories, concepts, refutations, etc., which are not "discoveries" at all. Also, while the dictionary concerns itself mainly with medical subjects, the reader will discover that an imposing number of entries are from fields other than medicine, such as dentistry, pharmacy, nursing, opticianry, midwifery, chemistry, and physics. Of course, only those subjects which have a bearing on medical science, at least indirectly, were included. Besides, the dictionary gives considerably more information than the phrase "WHO and WHEN" implies, such as the floruit, nationality, profession, and other pertinent data.

The basic formula of information with regard to every entry in this book consists of the following: the name of the discoverer or inventor, the nationality, the occupation or profession, the dates of birth and death, and the date of the discovery. Explanatory remarks, as well as eponyms and synonyms, are frequently added to this basic formula.

With regard to the names of the discoverers, inventors, etc., I have scrupulously avoided presenting mere surnames — a common practice among compilers of reference works — but spared no effort to secure the proper given name or names, or at least the initials. This task proved extremely difficult and time-consuming in some instances, but it was also exceedingly gratifying. The matter of occupation or profession was also carefully weighed and sifted, and this search paid off with its own brand of surprises, for not infrequently the inventor or discoverer turns out to be one quite different from the expected bacteriologist, orthopedist, biochemist, or, for that matter, even physician. Thus, for example, the first satisfactory laryngoscope was devised by a Spanish singing teacher, the undesirable effects of mouth-breathing were first recognized by an American ethnologist and painter, and the first attempt to catheterize the auditory tube was made by a French postmaster! Similarly, the intermaxillary bone was discovered by a German poet, the use of cocaine was suggested by a psychiatrist, the first accurate account of the tsetse fly was supplied by a Scottish explorer, while the first successful myringotomy was performed by a French quack named "Eli."

The dates of nativity and death, of the discoverers, were often hard to come by, as might be expected. In spite of all efforts, many such dates remained unknown, or only partly known. In every case where a date is not available, the fact is clearly stated. In the case of incomplete dates, question marks are used to indicate the missing components, as 17??-184?. On the other hand, the search for the hitherto unlisted dates was by no means unrewarding, and hence this dictionary contains hundreds of complete birthdates and mortidates not found in standard books of reference.

The securing of reliable dates for the discoveries, inventions, operations, methods, etc., involved its own brand of hardship. Many such dates, while listed, are often in dispute; others are covered by an impenetrable, centuries-old patina of obscurity. But here, too, the effort of search was rewarded by the discovery of hundreds of previously occult dates. In the case of discoveries for which only approximate dates could be found or deduced, the figures are presented with the usual *"circa."*

A look at the text of the dictionary of MEDICAL DISCOVERIES will show the reader that it is composed of standardized units or entries. Each entry is composed of two distinct parts, the heading and the body. The headings, which are in substance the titles of the discoveries, are arranged in an alphabetical order. This method enables the user of the dictionary to locate the particular discovery and the desired information almost as readily as he would find a word and its definition in the conventional word dictionary.

Suppose, for example, that the reader wishes to find the entries dealing with rubber gloves in surgery, a salt-free diet in hypertension, the "safe period" in sexual intercourse, bifocal lenses in spectacles, mal-occlusion of teeth, etc. Since the titles are arranged alphabetically, the reader would look under "Rubber," "Salt-free," "Safe period," etc.

In some cases the finding of an entry is somewhat more complicated. For example, if the reader wishes to find who was the first to describe mottled enamel due to fluorosis, he would have to look under "Enamel, mottled . . ." rather than "Mottled enamel . . ." Similarly, in trying to find the discoverer of animal emanations as a cause of asthma, one would look under "Asthma, animal emanations as cause of" rather than under "Animal emanations." On the other hand, the title dealing with the popularization of the concept of animal magnetism is listed under "Animal magnetism, popularization of concept of" but not under "Magnetism, animal, etc." The reason for this lies in the fact that "animal magnetism" is an established thought concept, but "mottled enamel" is not. In the example dealing with asthma, the term *asthma* is deemed the dominant word, rather than *animal* or *emanations*. It will thus be seen that in the matter of word arrangement in the titles, this dictionary follows the pattern of rhetorical "common sense," rather than any arbitrary and inflexible formula. I may also state here that in determining what constitutes the most useful word order for these titles, I have been guided by the results of experiments with prospective users of this work. The reader will gain a clearer understanding of the principles involved by merely examining a few pages of the text. In doing this, the reader will also note that a comfortable number of cross references were included as an additional aid.

MEDICAL DISCOVERIES

WHO and WHEN

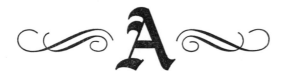

Abasia and astasia, first recorded investigation of

PAUL OSCAR BLOCQ, French physician, 1860-1896, described a condition in which the subject is unable to walk or even stand because of some mental trauma or conflict, without organic lesion or paralysis. Published in 1888. Known as *Blocq's disease, astasia-abasia,* and as *hysterical ataxia.*

Abdomen, planes used as landmarks in topography of

CHRISTOPHER ADDISON, English anatomist, 1869-1951, described several planes, lines, and points used as landmarks in the topography of the thorax and abdomen. Some of these were described in a paper published in 1899. See also under name of particular plane, line, etc.

Abdominal aorta, first successful ligation of

GEORGE TULLY VAUGHAN, American surgeon, 1859-19??, performed the first successful ligation of the abdominal aorta. Recorded in 1921.

Abdominal distention in early stages of rickets

RICHARD CLEMENT LUCAS, English surgeon, 1846-1915, is credited with being the first to describe the abdominal distention observed in most cases of early rickets. Recorded in 1887. Known as *Lucas' sign.*

Abdominal hernia, original research in

JULES GERMAIN CLOQUET, French anatomist, 1790-1883, investigated the causes of abdominal or ventral hernia. Earliest report published in 1817.

Abdominal puncture in diagnosis of abdominal fluid

BERNARD SOLOMON DENZER, American pediatrician, 1886-19??, used abdominal puncture for the diagnosis of peritoneal exudates and transudates in infants. Recorded in 1922.

Abdominal surgery, founder of modern

CHRISTIAN ALBERT THEODOR BILLROTH, Austrian surgeon, 1829-1894, is considered the founder of modern abdominal surgery.

Abscess in right iliac fossa, early description of

GUILLAUME DUPUYTREN, French surgeon, 1777-1835, described a case involving an abscess in the right iliac fossa. Reported in 1829. Known as *Dupuytren's abscess.*

Acanthosis nigricans, early description of—1890

SIGMUND POLLITZER, New York dermatologist, 1859-1937, described acanthosis nigricans (keratosis nigricans), a condition marked by hyperpigmentation of the skin and, sometimes, internal cancer, in 1890.

Acanthosis nigricans, early description of—1893

JEAN F. DARIER, French dermatologist, 1856-1938, gave a good description of acanthosis nigricans, in 1893.

Accelerator nerves of heart, discovery of

ALBERT VON BEZOLD, German physiologist, 1836-1868, discovered the accelerator nerve fibers of the heart and showed that their origin is in the spinal cord. Reported in 1863.

Accessory lacrimal glands, eponymic description of

EMILIJ FRANZEVIC VON WOLFRING, Polish ophthalmologist, 1832-1906, described the small glands in the subconjunctival tissue on the posterior aspect of the tarsal plates of the eyelids. Published in 1868. Known as *Wolfring's glands*; also as *accessory lacrimal glands*.

Accessory nerve, original description of

THOMAS WILLIS, English physician and anatomist, 1621-1675, was the first to describe the spinal accessory nerve. Published in 1664.

Accommodation due to change in curvature of lens—1637

RENÉ DESCARTES, French scientist and philosopher, 1596-1650, explained accommodation of the eye on the basis of changes in the shape of the crystalline lens. He compared the eye to a camera obscura. Recorded in 1637.

Accommodation due to change in curvature of lens—1793

THOMAS YOUNG, English physician, 1773-1829, described the mechanism of accommodation, pointing out that accommodation is accomplished by a change in the curvature of the lens. Recorded in 1793.

Accommodation, Helmholtz's theory of

HERMANN L. F. VON HELMHOLTZ, German physiologist and physicist, 1821-1894, developed a theory of accommodation according to which the lens assumes a more spherical form by its own elasticity when the suspensory ligaments are relaxed, and becomes less convex when the suspensory ligaments are tense. Reported *circa* 1856.

Accommodation, intracapsular mechanism of

ALLVAR GULLSTRAND, Swedish ophthalmologist, 1862-1930, discovered the so-called intracapsular mechanism of accommodation. Reported in 1911.

Acetabulum, osteoarthritic protrusion of

ADOLPH WILHELM OTTO, German surgeon, 1786-1845, described osteoarthritic protrusion of the acetabulum into the pelvis, *circa* 1820. Known as *Otto's disease*.

Acetarsone in treatment of amebiasis

EMILE MARCHOUX, French physician, 1862-1943, introduced acetarsone or stovarsol in the treatment of amebiasis. Recorded in 1923.

Acetone in diabetic urine, discovery of

WILHELM PETTERS, Prague physician, 1824-1889, is credited with being the first to demonstrate the presence of acetone in the urine of diabetics. Recorded in 1857.

Acetonitril test for hyperthyroidism

REID HUNT, American pharmacologist, 1870-19??, introduced the acetonitril test for hyperthyroidism. The blood of hyperthyroid patients increases the resistance of test animals to poisoning by acetonitril. First published in 1905. Modification recorded in 1923.

Acetylcholine, hypotensive effect of

REID HUNT, American pharmacologist, 1870-19??, demonstrated the hypotensive action of acetylcholine. Published in 1906.

Acetylcholine in ergot, finding of

ARTHUR JAMES EWINS, English physician, 1882-   , discovered acetylcholine in ergot. Reported in 1914.

Acetylcholine, inhibitory action of, on heart

HENRY H. DALE, English physiologist, 1875-   , demonstrated the inhibitory action of acetylcholine on the heart, in 1914.

Acetylcholine is liberated when vagus is stimulated

OTTO LOEWI, German pharmacologist in the United States, 1873-19??, demonstrated that a substance identical with acetylcholine is liberated when the vagus is stimulated and that this substance affects the rate of the heart. Recorded in 1921.

Acetylcholine is produced at parasympathetic synapses

HENRY H. DALE, English physiologist, 1875-   , and WILHELM FELDBERG (English physiologist, 1900-   ) demonstrated that acetylcholine is produced at the synapses of parasympathetic nerves. Reported in 1933.

Acetylcholine, isolation of, from spleens of animals

HENRY H. DALE, English physiologist, 1875-   , with HAROLD W. DUDLEY (English physiologist and biochemist, 1887-1935), isolated acetylcholine from the spleens of animals, in 1929.

Acetylcholine, release of, at voluntary motor nerve endings

HENRY H. DALE, English physiologist, 1875-   , with W. FELDBERG and M. VOGT, demonstrated that acetylcholine is released at the endings of voluntary motor nerves. Reported in 1936.

Acetylcholine stimulates parasympathetic nerves, demonstration that

HENRY H. DALE, English physiologist, 1875-   , showed that injection of acetylcholine into the blood stream produces stimulation of the parasympathetic nerves. Reported in 1914.

Achard-Thiers syndrome, original description of

EMILE CHARLES ACHARD, French

physician, 1860-1941, with JOSEPH
THIERS, described a syndrome of
hirsutism in the female associated
with diabetes. Recorded in 1921.

Achilles tendon, subcutaneous section of, in clubfoot

JACQUES M. DELPECH, French orthopedist, 1777-1832, devised an
operation in which the Achilles tendon is cut subcutaneously in the
treatment of clubfoot. Performed
in May, 1816.

Achillodynia or painful heel, original description of

EDUARD ALBERT, Austrian surgeon,
1841-1900, described the condition
known as achillodynia or painful
heel. Published in 1893. Known
also as *Albert's disease* and *Swediaur's disease.*

Achlorhydric anemia, original description of

KNUD H. FABER, Danish physician,
1862-1941, described achlorhydric
anemia, a form of hypochromic anemia associated with achlorhydria.
Reported in 1909.

Achondroplasia, cartilage changes in

EDUARD KAUFMANN, German physician, 1860-1931, was the first to
study and record the cartilage
changes in achondroplasia. Published in 1892.

Achondroplasia, classic description of

MORITZ HEINRICH ROMBERG, German neurologist, 1795-1873, gave
a classic description of achondroplasia (his graduation thesis), in
1817.

Achondroplasia, first description of

SAMUEL THOMAS SOEMMERRING,
German anatomist, 1755-1830, is
credited with being the first to describe achondroplasia. Recorded in
1791.

Achromacyte, early description of

A decolorized red blood cell, due to
loss of hemoglobin, was described
at about the same time, *circa* 1882,
by GIULIO BIZZOZERO (Italian physician, 1846-1901), EMIL PONFICK
(German pathologist, 1844-1913),
and GEORGES HAYEM (French
physician, 1841-1933). Known as
*Bizzozero's blood platelet, Pon-
fick's shadow,* and *Hayem's corpuscle.*

Achromatic lens, microscope having a; first construction

GIOVANNI BATTISTA AMICI, Italian
physicist and astronomer, 1784-
1863, is believed to have been the
first to construct a microscope provided with an achromatic lens. Recorded in 1818.

Achromatic lenses, improved

JOSEPH JACKSON LISTER, English
optician, 1786-1869, made fundamental improvements in achromatic
microscope lenses. Report published in 1830.

Achylia gastrica, etiologic relationship of, to pernicious anemia

WILLIAM BOSWORTH CASTLE,
American physician, 1897-   ,
demonstrated that pernicious anemia is due to the inability of the
stomach to secrete an anti-pernicious-anemia factor. Reported in
1928.

Achylia gastrica, recognition of

MAX EINHORN, American physician, 1862-1953, described the condition achylia gastrica, marked by the absence of rennin and hydrochloric acid from the gastric juice, in 1892.

Acid cells of gastric mucosa

ALEXANDER ROLLET, Austrian physiologist, 1834-1903, described large cells in the fundic glands of the gastric mucosa, about 1878. Known as *Rollet's cells* and *parietal cells*. These cells are believed to secrete hydrochloric acid.

Acid, isobutyric, discovery of

EMIL ERLENMEYER, German chemist, 1825-1909, discovered isobutyric acid in 1866. Isobutyric acid is found in putrefying proteins of the urine.

Acid, lactic, structure of

EMIL ERLENMEYER, German chemist, 1825-1909, discovered the structure of lactic acid, in 1866.

Acid

. . . See also under the name of the particular acid.

Acidosis, introduction of term

BERNARD NAUNYN, Strassburg physician, 1839-1925, is credited with introducing the term *acidosis,* in a treatise on diabetes, in 1898.

Acini, application of name, to lobules of liver

MARCELLO MALPIGHI, Italian anatomist, 1628-1694, introduced the term *acini* to describe the lobules of the liver. Recorded in 1666.

Acne bacillus, first cultivation of

RAYMOND JACQUES ADRIEN SA-

BOURAUD, French dermatologist, 1864-1938, is credited with being first to cultivate the acne bacillus, in 1897.

Acne bacillus, first description of

PAUL GERSON UNNA, German dermatologist, 1850 - 1929, was the first to describe the acne bacillus, in 1894.

Acne varioliformis, early description of—1851

ANTOINE P. E. BAZIN, French dermatologist, 1807-1878, gave a complete account of acne varioliformis in a monograph published in 1851.

Acne varioliformis early description of—1889

CAESAR PETER MOELER BOECK, Norwegian pathologist, 1845-1917, described acne varioliformis. Published in 1889.

Acoustic apparatus, end-organ of, description of

ALFONSO CORTI, Italian anatomist, 1822 - 1888, described the end-organ of hearing within the scala media, including the rods of Corti, the auditory cells, etc. Reported in 1851. Known as *organ of Corti.*

Acquired characteristics, hypothesis relating to the hereditary transmission of

. . . See under *Heredity, hypothesis for explanation of.*

Acquired characteristics, theory of non-inheritance of

AUGUST FRIEDRICH LEOPOLD WEISMANN, German biologist, 1834-1914, propounded a theory that changes in the somatoplasm of the body do not affect the germ plasm, hence acquired characteristics cannot be inherited. Published in 1875. Known as *Weismann's theory.*

Acquired hemolytic jaundice with anemia—1898

GEORGES HAYEM, French physician, 1841-1933, described acquired hemolytic jaundice with anemia, in 1898. The disease was described later, in 1907, perhaps more classically, by Widal and Abrami. Known as *Hayem-Widal disease* and as *Widal-Abrami disease.*

Acquired hemolytic jaundice with anemia—1907

GEORGES F. I. WIDAL, French physician, 1862 - 1929, with PIERRE ABRAMI, French physician, 1879-1945, gave a classic description of acquired hemolytic jaundice with anemia. Recorded in 1907. Known as *Widal-Abrami disease*; also as *Hayem-Widal disease.*

Acrocyanosis, early description of

JEAN B. CROCQ, Belgian physician, 1868-1925, described acrocyanosis in 1896.

Acrocyanosis, vascular mechanism of

THOMAS LEWIS, English physician, 1881-1945, with E. M. LANDIS, described the vascular mechanism involved in acrocyanosis. Recorded in 1930.

Acrodermatitis chronica atrophicans

KARL HERXHEIMER, German dermatologist, 1861-1944, with KUNO HARTMANN, described an idiopathic localized atrophy of the skin and named it *acrodermatitis chronica*

atrophicans. Published in 1902. The same condition was described by ROBERT WILLIAM TAYLOR in 1875. He did not, however, name it.

Acrodermatitis chronica atrophicans, introduction of term

KARL HERXHEIMER, German dermatologist, 1861-1944, with KUNO HARTMANN, introduced the term *acrodermatitis chronica atrophicans,* in 1902.

Acromegaly, classic description of

PIERRE MARIE, French neurologist, 1853-1940, gave a classic description of acromegaly in 1886. Known as *Marie's syndrome.*

Acromegaly, enlargement of pituitary in relation to

OSKAR MINKOWSKI, Russian pathologist in Germany, 1858 - 1931, noted the relation between pituitary enlargement and acromegaly, in 1887.

Acromegaly, first clinical description of

NICOLAS SAUCEROTTE, French physician, 1741-1814, described a condition which is now known to have been acromegaly, in 1772. Published in 1801.

Acromegaly, first use of x-rays to study bone in

GEORGES MARINESCO, Rumanian pathologist, 1864-1938, is credited with being first to use x-rays to study bone changes in cases of acromegaly, *circa* 1909.

Acromegaly, increase in growth hormone in

LAURANCE WILKIE KINSELL, American endocrinologist, 1907-

, with G. D. MICHAELS, C. H. LI, and W. E. LARSEN, noted an increase in pituitary growth factor and growth-promoting androgens in acromegaly. Published in 1948.

Acromegaly, introduction of term

PIERRE MARIE, French neurologist, 1853-1940, is credited with introducing the term *acromegaly*. Published in 1886.

Acrylic prosthesis of femoral head

. . . See under *Femoral head,* etc.

ACTH in treatment of rheumatoid arthritis

PHILIP S. HENCH, American physician, 1896-   , with E. C. KENDALL, C. H. SLOCUMB, and H. F. POLLEY, introduced the use of ACTH and cortisone in the treatment of rheumatoid arthritis. Published in 1949.

ACTH

. . . See also under *Adrenocorticotropic hormone.*

Actinic rays, therapeutic value of, early recognition of

NIELS R. FINSEN, Danish physician, 1860-1904, is credited with proving the therapeutic value of actinic rays, in 1896.

Actinobacillus, discovery of

JOSEPH LÉON MARAL LIGNIÈRES, Argentinian physician, 1868-1933, with J. SPITZ, discovered the actinobacillus. Recorded in 1902.

Actinomyces bovis, isolation of

MAX WOLFF, German pathologist, 1844-1923, with JAMES ADOLF ISRAEL, German surgeon, 1848-1926, isolated *Actinomyces bovis.* Recorded in 1891.

Actinomyces graminis, isolation of, from human case

EUGEN BOSTROEM, German physician, 1850-1928, isolated *Actinomyces graminis* from a case of human actionmycosis. Recorded in 1890. He also devised a method for staining *Actinomyces.*

Actinomycosis, causative agent of

OTTO BOLLINGER, German pathologist, 1843-1909, demonstrated that the disease of cattle known as "lumpy jaw" was caused by a vegetable parasite called *actinomyces bovis.* Reported in 1877.

Actinomycosis in man, early observation of—1878

JAMES ADOLF ISRAEL, German surgeon, 1848-1926, proved the presence of *Actinomyces* in man. Reported in 1878.

Actinomycosis in man is same as in cattle, demonstration that

EMIL PONFICK, German physician, 1844 - 1913, established that the fungus causing actinomycosis in man is the same as that causing the disease in cattle. Recorded in 1882.

Action currents of heart, early studies of

JOHN SCOTT BURDON-SANDERSON, English physiologist, 1828-1905, with F. J. M. Page, did early research on the action currents of the heart of the frog. Reported in 1879.

Action of poisons in living body, first book in English on

THOMAS ADDISON, English physician, 1793-1860, wrote the first book in English on the action of poisons in the living body, in collaboration with JOHN MORGAN,

English physician, 1797-1847. The book is dated 1829.

Actomyosin, contractility of

ALBERT SZENT-GYÖRGYI, Hungarian biochemist, 1893-   , was instrumental in the discovery that actomyosin is contractile, *circa* 1935.

Acute superior hemorrhagic polioencephalitis

CHARLES JULES ALPHONSE GAYET, French physician, 1833-1904, was the first to describe acute superior hemorrhagic polioencephalitis, a condition occurring mainly in chronic alcoholics. Published in 1875. The same condition was described later, in 1881, by CARL WERNICKE. Known as *Wernicke's disease.*

Acute yellow atrophy of liver, original report on

RICHARD BRIGHT, English physician, 1789-1858, made original observations on acute yellow atrophy of the liver. Reported in 1836.

Acute yellow atrophy of liver

. . . See also under *Liver, acute yellow atrophy of.*

Adaptation syndrome to stress

HANS SELYE, Canadian endocrinologist, 1907-   , introduced a theory that animals react to stress with a sequence of physiological manifestations, which he called the "general adaptation syndrome." Published in 1950.

Addison's disease, first description of

. . . See under *Adrenal cortical hypofunction.*

Addison's disease, hypoglycemia in

OTTO PORGES, Austrian physician, 1879-   , was first to note and describe hypoglycemia in patients with Addison's disease. Published in 1909.

Addison's disease, introduction of term

ARMAND TROUSSEAU, French physician, 1801-1867, is credited with the advocacy and perpetuation of the term *Addison's disease, circa* 1855.

Adenoid cystic epithelioma of skin

HENRY A. G. BROOKE, English dermatologist, 1854-1919, described an adenoid cystic epithelioma (epithelioma adenoides cysticum), a rare form of epidermoid carcinoma, in 1892.

Adenoid hypertrophy, first clinical description of

HANS WILHELM MEYER, Danish physician, 1825-1895, is credited with giving the first clinical description of hypertrophy of the adenoids. Recorded in 1868.

Adenoids, forceps for removal of

BENJAMIN BENNO LOEWENBERG, German surgeon, 1836-18??, invented a special forceps for removing adenoid growths from the nasopharynx. Reported in 1879.

Adenoma sebaceum, first description of

PIERRE FRANÇOIS OLIVE RAYER, French dermatologist, 1793-1867, was the first to describe adenoma sebaceum, in 1826.

Adiposis dolorosa, first description of

FRANCIS XAVIER DERCUM, American neurologist, 1856 - 1931, described the condition known as adiposis dolorosa, marked by painful, localized deposits of fat and by nerve lesions. Reported in 1888. Known also as *Dercum's disease.*

Adiposogenital dystrophy, eponymic description of

ALFRED FRÖHLICH, Austrian neurologist in the United States, 1871-1953, gave the first classic description of adiposogenital dystrophy, pointing out the genital hypoplasia, the feminine - type adiposity, the changes in the secondary sex characteristics, the metabolic disturbances, etc. Recorded in 1901. Known as *Fröhlich's syndrome.*

Adiposogenital hystrophy, first description of

JOSEPH F. F. BABINSKI, Polish neurologist in France, 1857-1932, was the first to describe the syndrome of adiposogenital dystrophy marked by genital hypoplasia, adiposity of the feminine type, changes in the secondary sex characteristics, etc. Recorded in 1900. Known as the *Babinski-Fröhlich disease* or *syndrome.*

Adiposogenital dystrophy

. . . See also under *Fröhlich's syndrome.*

Adrenal capsule, action of extracts of

. . . See under *Suprarenal capsule.*

Adrenal cortex is essential to life, recognition that

ARTUR BIEDL, Czechoslovakian physiologist, 1869 - 1933, demonstrated that the cortex of the adrenal gland is essential to life. Recorded in 1910.

Adrenal cortical extract in adrenal insufficiency

JULIUS MOSES ROGOFF, American physician, 1884-   , with George Neil Stewart, treated adrenal insufficiency with adrenal cortical extract, the first such application of the hormone on record. Published in 1929.

Adrenal cortical hormone, first extraction of

JULIUS MOSES ROGOFF, American physician, 1884-   , and GEORGE NEIL STEWART were the first to obtain adrenal cortical hormone. Published in 1927.

Adrenal cortical hormone, first practical method of preparing

JOSEPH JOHN PFIFFNER, American biochemist, 1903-   , with WILBUR W. SWINGLE, devised the first practical method for preparing extracts of the adrenal cortical hormone. Recorded in 1929.

Adrenal cortical hormone in Addison's disease

WILBUR WILLIS SWINGLE, American biologist, 1891-   , with JOSEPH JOHN PFIFFNER, prepared an adrenal cortical extract (eschatin) and found it effective in the treatment of Addison's disease. Published in 1930 and 1932.

Adrenal cortical hormone, isolation of—1934

EDWARD CALVIN KENDALL, American physiologist and chemist, 1886-   , isolated the adrenal cortical hormone in 1934. Recorded in 1934 and 1936.

Adrenal cortical hypofunction; Addison's disease

THOMAS ADDISON, English physician, 1793-1860, gave a classic description of the syndrome which later became known as Addison's disease. Recorded in 1849.

Adrenal cortical tumor, first recorded removal of

PERCY WILLIAM GEORGE SARGENT, English surgeon, 18??-   , was the first to excise an adrenal cortical tumor in a case of virilism. It was followed by recovery from the heterosexual condition. Recorded by Gordon Morgan Holmes, in 1925.

Adrenal gland sarcoma with skull metastases

ROBERT GRIEVE HUTCHISON, English physician, 1871 - 1943, described adrenal gland sarcoma in children, associated with metastases in the skull, exophthalmos, etc. Published in 1907. Known as *Hutchison's tumor.*

Adrenal glands and sex organs, relationship between

WILLIAM BULLOCH, English physician, 1868 - 1941, with JAMES HARRY SEQUEIRA, noted the relationship between the adrenal glands and the sexual organs and described the adrenogenital syndrome. Published in 1905.

Adrenal glands are essential to life, demonstration that

CHARLES EDOUARD BROWN-SÉQUARD, English physician in France, 1817-1894, experimented with the excision of the adrenals from animals and found that the glands are indispensable to life. Recorded in 1856.

Adrenal glands, first description of

. . . See under *Suprarenal glands.*

Adrenal glands, hemorrhage into

RUPERT WATERHOUSE, English physician, 1873-19??, described a condition of acute collapse due to hemorrhage into the adrenal glands in meningococcus meningitis. Recorded in 1911. Known as suprarenal apoplexy and *Waterhouse-Friderichsen syndrome.*

Adrenal pressor substance, discovery of

GEORGE OLIVER, English physician, 1841-1915, with E. A. SCHÄFER, studied the effects of injecting solutions of adrenal gland and noted a rise in blood pressure. Findings recorded in 1894.

Adrenaline in adrenal medulla, discovery of

EDME FÉLIX ALFRED VULPIAN, French physician, 1826-1887, discovered the presence of epinephrine in the adrenal medulla. Recorded in 1856.

Adrenaline, isolation of

. . . See under *Epinephrine.*

Adrenaline, naming of

JOKICHI TAKAMINE, Japanese chemist working in the United States, 1854-1922, named the pressor substance of the adrenal gland *adrenaline.* Reported in 1901.

Adrenocorticotropic hormone, isolation of pure

CHOH HAO LI, Chinese biochemist in the United States, 1913-   , with H. M. EVANS and M. E. SIMPSON, isolated the pure form of the adrenocorticotropic hormone from sheep pituitary glands. Recorded in 1943.

Adrenocorticotropic principle, isolation of

. . . See under *Pituitary, anterior,* etc.

Adrenogenital syndrome

. . . See under *Adrenal glands and sex organs, relationship between.*

Aegophony, **introduction of term**

RENÉ T. H. LAENNEC, French physician, 1781-1826, is credited with introducing the term *aegophony,* after his invention of the stethoscope. Published in 1819. It is based on the Greek *aix* (goat) and *phone* (sound).

Aerobic and anaerobic bacteria, differentiation between

LOUIS PASTEUR, French scientist and bacteriologist, 1822-1895, is credited with distinguishing between aerobic and anaerobic organisms, *circa* 1877.

Aerosporin, discovery of

G. C. AINSWORTH, English biochemist, 19??-   , with A. M. BROWN and G. BROWNLEE, discovered *aerosporin,* and antibiotic substance also known as polymyxin B sulfate. Recorded in 1947.

Affinity between chemical substances, concept of

HERMANN BOERHAAVE, Dutch physician, 1668-1738, introduced the concept of affinity between chemical substances. Reported in 1732.

African sleeping sickness

. . . See under *Sleeping sickness.*

Agglutination, specific, discovery of

HERBERT EDWARD DURHAM, Eng-lish bacteriologist, 1866-1945, with Max von Gruber (German bacteriologist, 1853-1927), discovered specific agglutination, in 1896. The phenomenon formed the basis of the Widal test for typhoid, reported in the same year. Known as *Gruber-Durham reaction.*

Agoraphobia, **introduction of term**

CARL FRIEDRICH OTTO WESTPHAL, German neurologist, 1833-1890, was the first to describe agoraphobia and to introduce the term. Recorded in 1871.

Agranulocytosis, first description of

WERNER SCHULTZ, German physician, 1878-1945, was the first to describe "agranulocytic angina," in 1922. He also introduced the term *agranulocytosis.* Known as *Schultz's disease.*

Agranulocytosis, first description of "complete"

WILHELM TÜRK, Austrian physician, 1871-1916, is said to have been the first to describe "complete" agranulocytosis. Recorded in 1907.

Agranulocytosis, **introduction of term**

. . . See under *Agranulocytosis, first description of.*

Agraphia, first adequate account of

JEAN ALBERT PITRES, French physician, 1848-1928, gave the first classic account of agraphia, in 1884.

Air composition, demonstration of

HENRY CAVENDISH, English scientist, 1731-1810, demonstrated the composition of the air. Published in 1784.

Albarran's glands

. . . See under *Bladder, subtrigonal glands of.*

Albumin and chloride shift between plasma and erythrocytes

HARTOG JAKOB HAMBURGER, Dutch physiologist, 1859-1924, described the phenomenon in which albumins and phosphates pass from the erythrocytes to the plasma when the blood is acid, and from the plasma to the erythrocytes when the blood is alkaline. The chlorides pass in the reverse direction. Reported *circa* 1902.

Albumin in urine, discovery of

FREDERIK DEKKERS, Dutch physician, 1648-1720, discovered the presence of albumin in urine by boiling the urine with acetic acid, in 1673.

Albumin in urine, early reagent for detecting

GEORGES HUBERT ESBACH, French physician, 1843-1890, invented a reagent for the detection of albumin in urine, in 1874.

Albumin standards, introduction of

CHARLES P. CLARK (American physician, 1879-1951) and FRANCIS B. KINGSBURY (American biochemist, 1886-   ) prepared permanent albumin standards used in connection with life-insurance tests for urinary proteins. Reported *circa* 1926. Known as the *Kingsbury-Clark albumin standards.*

Albuminuria in puerperal convulsions, first record of

JOHN CHARLES WEAVER LEVER, English physician, 1811-1858, was the first to record albuminuria in a patient with eclampsia. Published in 1843.

Albuminuria, recurrent physiologic

FREDERICK WILLIAM PAVY, English physician, 1829 - 1911, described a recurrent type of physiologic albuminuria, in 1885. Known as *Pavy's disease.*

Albumosuria, myelopathic, first description of

HENRY BENCE JONES, English physician, 1814-1873, was the first to describe the presence of a proteose in the urine of patients with multiple myeloma. Recorded in 1848. The proteose is known as *Bence Jones protein.*

Alcohol in breath, instrument for measuring

. . . See under *Drunkometer, invention of.*

Alcohol injection in neuralgia

CARL SCHLÖSSER, German ophthalmologist, 1857-1925, is credited with being the first to use deep alcohol injections in the treatment of neuralgia, in 1903.

Alcoholic neuritis, early description of

JAMES JACKSON, SR., American physician, 1777 - 1867, gave an early description of alcoholic neuritis, *arthrodynia a potu,* in 1822.

Alcoholic paraplegia, classic account of

SAMUEL WILKS, English physician, 1824-1911, gave a classic description of alcoholic paraplegia. Recorded in 1868.

Alcoholics, treatment of, with medicine said to contain strychnine and gold chloride

LESLIE E. KEELEY, American physician, 1832 - 1900, introduced a method for treating alcoholics by means of a preparation said to contain strychnine and gold chloride. Report published in 1881. Known as *Keeley cure* or *gold cure*. The method has also been used for other types of addiction, as with opium or morphine.

Alcoholism, early account of—1779

JOHN C. LETTSOM, Virgin Islands physician, 1744 - 1815, wrote an early original account of alcoholism. Recorded 1779-1787.

Alcometer, invention of

. . . See under *Drunkometer, invention of*.

Aleppo boil, early description of

ALEXANDER RUSSELL, English naturalist, 171?-1768, gave a good description of Aleppo boil, a form of cutaneous leishmaniasis. Published in 1756.

Aleppo boil, early medical description of

JEAN LOUIS MARC ALIBERT, French dermatologist, 1766 - 1837, described Aleppo boil, in 1829. Known also as *furunculosis orientalis* and *oriental sore*.

Alexin, introduction of term

HANS BUCHNER, German bacteriologist, 1850-1902, introduced the term *alexin* to describe "defensive proteids which attack bacteria." Reported in 1889.

Alimentary tract, submucous nerve plexus of

. . . See under *Nerve plexus, submucous, of alimentary tract*.

Alkaloids, agent used to identify

HUGO ERDMANN, German chemist, 1862-1910, invented a reagent composed of sulfuric and nitric acids and used in identifying alkaloids, in 1896. Called *Erdmann's reagent*.

Alkaptonuria, early report of

ALEXANDER J. G. MARCET, Scottish physician, 1772 - 1822, described a "singular variety of urine which turned black soon after being discharged," or alkaptonuria. Published in 1822-23.

Allergen-proof room, experiments with

WILLEM STORM VAN LEEUWEN, Dutch physician, 1882-1933, experimented with the construction of a room or chamber free from pollen. Recorded in 1925.

Allergy in tuberculosis, early understanding of

CLEMENS PETER PIRQUET VON CESENATICO, Austrian physician and pediatrician, 1874-1929, was first to point out the existence of allergy in tuberculosis. Published in 1908.

Allergy, introduction of term

CLEMENS PETER PIRQUET VON CESENATICO, Austrian pediatrician, 1874 - 1929, with BELA SCHICK (Austrian pediatrician, 1877-   ), introduced the term *allergy*, in 1907.

All-or-nothing law of heart muscle

HENRY PICKERING BOWDITCH, American physiologist, 1840-1911,

demonstrated the "all-or-nothing" principle of cardiac muscle contraction. Published in 1871.

All-or-nothing response of sensory nerve fibers

EDGAR DOUGLAS ADRIAN, English neurophysiologist, 1889-   , described the all-or-nothing response of sensory nerve fibers, in 1922.

Alphabet for blind, perfection and popularization of

LOUIS BRAILLE, French teacher of the blind, 1809-1852, perfected and popularized a system of dots, suggested in 1820 by Charles Barbier, which constitutes an alphabet for the blind. Introduced in 1830. Reported in 1837. Known as the *Braille system*.

Alphabet for blind

. . . See also under *Blind, alphabet for*.

Alternation of generation, introduction of doctrine of

JOHANNES JAPETUS SMITH STEENSTRUP, Swedish physician, 1813-1897, proposed the theory of alternation of generation, demonstrating that certain animals produce young which do not resemble them, the resemblance reappearing in the grandchildren. Recorded in 1842.

Alternation of generations, introduction of term

LUDWIG ADALBERT VON CHAMISSO, German poet and botanist, 1781-1838, is credited with being the first to use the expression *alternation of generations*, in 1819.

Aluminum, isolation of

FRIEDRICH WÖHLER, German chemist, 1800-1882, isolated metallic aluminum in the form of a gray powder, in 1827. Later, in 1845, he obtained the metal in massive form.

Amaurotic familial idiocy, cerebral changes in

BERNARD SACHS, American neurologist, 1858-1944, described the cerebral changes observed in amaurotic familial idiocy. Published in 1887. Amaurotic familial idiocy is known as *Tay-Sachs disease*.

Amaurotic familial idiocy, juvenile form of

FREDERICK EUSTACE BATTEN, English neurologist, 1865 - 1918, described "cerebral degeneration with symmetrical changes in the maculae in two members of a family." Published in 1903. The same condition was described by MARMADUKE STEPHEN MAYOU, English physician, 1876 - 1934, in 1904. Known as *Batten-Mayou disease*.

Amebiasis, incubation period of

ERNEST LINWOOD WALKER, Philippine bacteriologist, 1870-19??, with ANDREW WATSON SELLARDS, determined the incubation period of amebic infections. Recorded in 1913.

Amebiasis, stovarsol in treatment of

EMILE MARCHOUX, French physician, 1862-1943, introduced acetarsone or stovarsol in the treatment of amebiasis. Recorded in 1923.

Amebic dysentery, coinage of term

WILLIAM T. COUNCILMAN, American pathologist, 1854-1933, and HENRY A. LAFLEUR investigated amebic dysentery and originated the term, in 1890.

American Journal of Obstetrics, founding of

ABRAHAM JACOBI, American pediatrician, 1830-1919, with Emil Noeggerath (American gynecologist and obstetrician, 1827-1895), founded the *American Journal of Obstetrics,* in 1862.

Aminoacetic acid in myasthenia gravis

. . . See under *Myasthenia gravis.*

Aminopyrine, introduction of

WILHELM FILEHNE, German physician, 1844-1927, is credited with introducing aminopyrine (amidopyrine, pyramidon) into therapeutics. Published in 1896.

Ammonia, reagent for testing; Nessler's reagent

JULIUS NESSLER, German chemist, 1827-1905, devised a solution of potassium iodide, mercuric chloride, and potassium hydroxide, for testing the presence of ammonia in water, blood, urine, etc. Recorded in 1856. Known as *Nessler's reagent.*

Ammonia, synthesis of, from elements

FRITZ HABER, German chemist, 1868-1934, devised a method for producing ammonia by synthesis from the elements nitrogen and hydrogen, *circa* 1916. Received Nobel prize in 1919.

Ammonium acetate, discovery of

RAYMOND MINDERER, German military surgeon, 1572 - 1621, is credited with discovering ammonium acetate, *circa* 1610.

Amniography, introduction of

THOMAS ORVILLE MENEES, Grand Rapids, Mich., physician, 1890-1937, introduced amniography, roentgenography of the pregnant uterus after the injection of a radiopaque medium into the amniotic fluid. Recorded in 1930.

Amnioplastin, introduction of

KARL BURGER, German surgeon, 1893- , introduced the use of amnioplastin. Recorded in 1937. Its chief application is to the prevention of adhesions after craniotomy.

Amniotic bands of fetus

PIERRE JOSEPH CÉCILIEN SIMONART, Belgian obstetrician, 1817-1847, described amniotic bands formed by adhesions between the amnion and the fetus. Known as *Simonart's bands* or *threads.*

Amniotic fluid embolism of mother

PAUL EBY STEINER, American obstetrician, 1902- , with CLARENCE CHANCELUM LUSHBAUGH, described maternal pulmonary embolism by amniotic fluid as a cause of obstetric shock and death. Published in 1941.

Amniotic sac, puncture of, to check hemorrhage

JUSTINE DITRICHIN SIEGMUNDIN, German midwife, 1650-1705, introduced puncture of the amniotic sac to check hemorrhages in cases of placenta previa. Published in 1690.

Amphimixis, introduction of term

AUGUST FRIEDRICH LEOPOLD WEISMANN, German biologist, 1834-1914, introduced the term *amphimixis,* in 1891.

Ampules, hypodermic,
invention of
STANISLAUS LIMOUSIN, French pharmacist, 1842-1906, is credited with inventing hypodermic ampules, *circa* 1886.

Ampulla of common bile duct,
eponymic description of
ABRAHAM VATER, German anatomist, 1684-1751, described the dilatation of the common bile duct at the junction with the pancreatic duct. Published in 1720. Known as *ampulla of Vater*.

Ampulla of Vater
. . . See under *Ampulla of common bile duct*.

Amputation, first illustration
depicting an
HANS VON GERSSDORFF, German military surgeon, 1454-1517, wrote a field manual on the treatment of wounds which contains the first known illustration of an amputation. Published in 1517.

Amputation, hollow cone
method of
. . . See under *Hollow cone method of amputation*.

Amputations, use of ligature in
AMBROISE PARÉ, French surgeon, 1510-1590, described the use of ligatures in amputations. Published in 1564.

Amyl nitrite, discovery of
ANTOINE JEROME BALARD, French chemist, 1802-1876, is credited with the discovery of amyl nitrite, in 1844.

Amyl nitrite in treatment of angina
pectoris, introduction of
THOMAS LAUDER BRUNTON, Scot-

tish physician and pharmacologist, 1844-1916, introduced the use of amyl nitrite in the treatment of angina pectoris. Reported in 1867.

Amylene, early use of, as
anesthetic
JOHN SNOW, English physician, 1813-1858, was the first to use amylene as a general anesthetic on human beings. Recorded in 1858.

Amylocaine, introduction of
ERNEST F. A. FOURNEAU, French chemist and pharmacologist, 1872-1949, introduced amylocaine hydrochloride, a local anesthetic, in 1903. Also known as *stovaine*.

Amyloid degeneration with
deposit of lardacein
JOHN ABERCROMBIE, Scottish physician, 1780-1844, described a form of degeneration marked by the deposit of lardacein in the affected tissues. It is usually associated with impairment of nutrition, and is often observed in diseases marked by wasting. The condition is known as *Abercrombie's degeneration*. Date of first report not available.

Amyloidosis, primary, first
record of
CARL WILD, German physician, 184?-19??, provided the first description of primary amyloidosis. Published in 1886.

Amyotonia congenita; myatonia
congenita
HERMANN OPPENHEIM, Berlin neurologist, 1858-1919, described a congenital disease of children marked by subnormal tone of the muscles. Recorded in 1900. Known as *Oppenheim's disease*.

Anaesthesia and *anaesthetic*, introduction of terms

OLIVER WENDELL HOLMES, American physician and author, 1804-1894, suggested the use of the terms *anaesthesia* and *anaesthetic*, in 1846, in a letter to William T. G. Morton, American dentist.

Anal fistula, early operation for

JOHN OF ARDERNE, English physician, 1307-1380, is remembered for his operation for the treatment of anal fistula. Recorded in 1376.

Analyses of foods and fertilizers, first work in

JEAN B. J. D. BOUSSINGAULT, French physician and physiological chemist, 1802-1887, is believed to have been the first to analyze foods and fertilizer material. Reported in 1839.

Anaphase, introduction of term

. . . See under *Mitosis, three stages of*.

Anaphylactic reaction following subcutaneous injection of specific antigen

NICOLAS MAURICE ARTHUS, French physiologist, 1862 - 1945, described a local edema and necrosis following subcutaneous injection of the specific antigen in sensitized animals. Report published in 1903. Known as *Arthus' phenomenon*.

Anaphylactic shock, physiologic reactions in

JOHN AUER, American physician, 1875-1948, with PAUL A. LEWIS, described the physiologic reactions involved in fatal anaphylactic shock in the guinea pig. Published in 1910.

Anaphylaxis, early observations on—1798

EDWARD JENNER, English physician, 1749-1823, observed that a subsequent injection of variolous material at times produced violent reactions in subjects who tolerated the initial inoculation, in 1798.

Anaphylaxis, early observations on—1839

FRANÇOIS MAGENDIE, French physiologist, 1783-1855, demonstrated that repeated injections of egg albumin in rabbits who had tolerated the first injection sometimes resulted in death of the animals. Recorded in 1839.

Anaphylaxis, first full description of

PAUL JULES PORTIER, French physician, 1866-19??, with CHARLES ROBERT RICHET (French physiologist, 1850-1935), gave the first satisfactory description of anaphylaxis, in 1902.

Anaphylaxis, introduction of term

CHARLES ROBERT RICHET, French physiologist, 1850-1935, is credited with introducing the term *anaphylaxis, circa* 1902.

Anaphylaxis, passive, demonstration of

MAURICE NICOLLE, French physician, 1862-19??, demonstrated the phenomenon of passive anaphylaxis, in 1907.

Anaplasia, original description of

DAVID PAUL VON HANSEMANN, German pathologist, 1858 - 1920,

described anaplasia, the loss of normal differentiation, organization, and specific function in tumor cells. Published in 1902. Early report appeared in 1893.

Anastomosis of facial with hypoglossal nerve

CHARLES ALFRED BALLANCE, English surgeon, 1856-1936, devised an operation for the anastomosis of the facial with the hypoglossal nerve, in facial paralysis. Date not available.

Anastomosis of spinal accessory and facial nerves in facial paralysis

. . . See under *Facial paralysis.*

Anatomical tubercles

. . . See under *Dissecting - room warts.*

Anatomy, comparative, first comprehensive treatise on

GERARD BLAES, Dutch anatomist, 1625-1692, was the author of the first comprehensive treatise on comparative anatomy. Published in 1681.

Anatomy, comparative, founder of

ARISTOTLE, Greek scientist and philosopher, 384-322 B. C., is considered the founder of comparative anatomy; also one of the first embryologists.

Anatomy, Father of

HEROPHILUS, Greek physician and anatomist in Egypt, 335-280 B. C., is often credited with being the "Father of Anatomy."

Anatomy, Father of Modern

ANDREAS VESALIUS, Belgian anatomist, 1514-1564, is regarded as the "Father of Modern Anatomy." His main work, titled *De Corporis Humani,* was published in 1543.

Anatoxin, diphtheria, first preparation of

. . . See under *Diphtheria toxin, modification of, with formaldehyde.*

Ancylostomiasis as cause of pernicious anemia

JOSEPH LEIDY, American physician, 1823-1891, observed that the hookworm caused anemia in the cat and suggested that ancylostomiasis might be a cause of pernicious anemia in man. Published in 1886.

Ancylostomiasis, aspidium in treatment of

EDOARDO PERRONCITO, Italian physician, 1847-19??, introduced aspidium (*Dryopteris filix-mas*) as a vermifuge for the hookworm, *circa* 1910.

Ancylostomiasis, causative agent of

ANGELO DUBINI, Italian physician, 1813-1902, discovered the causative agent of hookworm disease to be a nematode worm (*Ancylostoma duodenale* or *Necator americanus*). Reported in 1843.

Ancylostomiasis, cause of American form of

CHARLES WARDELL STILES, American bacteriologist and parasitologist, 1867 - 1941, discovered the American species of hookworm, *Uncinaria americana* or *Necator americanus*. Recorded in 1902.

Ancylostomiasis, fecal examination for diagnosis of

GIOVANNI BATTISTA GRASSI, Italian pathologist, 1854-1925, introduced fecal examination in the diagnosis of hookworm disease; previously the diagnosis was made only *post mortem*. Recorded, with C. PARONA and E. PARONA, in 1878.

Ancylostomiasis in America, first recognition of

WALTER L. BLICKHAHN, American physician, 18??-19??, was the first to recognize ancylostomiasis under this name in America. Published in 1893.

Ancylostomiasis in Puerto Rico, recognition of

BAILEY KELLY ASHFORD, American physician, 1873-1934, was the first to recognize and publicize the prevalence of hookworm disease in Puerto Rico where one-third of the deaths were due to this disease. This led to a campaign for the eradication of ancylostomiasis. Published in 1900.

Ancylostomiasis, introduction of carbon tetrachloride in treatment of

MAURICE CROWTHER HALL, American physician, 1881 - 1938, is credited with introducing carbon tetrachloride in the treatment of hookworm infestation. Reported in 1921.

Ancylostomiasis, route of infection, through skin

ARTHUR LOOSS, German parasitologist, 1861-1923, demonstrated that the hookworm may enter by way of the skin, then travel through the lung to the intestine. Observed in 1898; reported in 1901.

Ancylostomiasis

. . . See also under *Hookworm*.

Androsterone, commercial synthesis of

LEOPOLD RUZICKA, Swiss biochemist, 1887-   , with M. W. GOLDBERG, J. MEYER, H. BRÜNGGER, and E. EICHENBERGER, devised a satisfactory method for the commercial synthesis of androsterone and testosterone. Recorded in 1934.

Androsterone, crystalline, isolation of

ADOLF FRIEDRICH JOHANN BUTENANDT, German biochemist, 1903-   , isolated the male sex hormone androsterone in crystalline form, *circa* 1931.

Anemia, achrestic, original description of

JOHN FREDERICK WILKINSON, English physician, 1897-   , with MARTIN CYRIL GORDON ISRAËLS, described achrestic anemia, a form resembling pernicious anemia but without the nervous system complications and without the absence of hydrochloric acid. Published in 1935.

Anemia, acute hemolytic, Lederer's

MAX LEDERER, American pathologist, 1885-1952, described a form of acute hemolytic anemia marked by presence of megaloblasts, high color index, etc. Published in 1925. Known as *Lederer's anemia*.

Anemia, aplastic, first description of

PAUL EHRLICH, German bacteriologist and pathologist, 1854-1915, was the first to differentiate aplastic anemia from other forms. Recorded in 1888.

Anemia, chronic infectious; eponymic description

ADOLF EDELMANN, Austrian physician, 1885-1939, was the first to describe chronic infectious anemia, in 1925. Known as *Edelmann's anemia* or *disease*.

Anemia, constitutional infantile, resembling pernicious anemia

GUIDO FANCONI, Swiss pediatrician, 1882-19??, described constitutional infantile anemia resembling pernicious anemia. Reported in Oct. 1927. Known as *Fanconi's disease*.

Anemia, Cooley's; thalassemia

. . . See under *Erythroblastic anemia, familial, in Mediterranean peoples*.

Anemia, iron deficiency type of

. . . See under *Iron deficiency anemia*, etc.

Anemia of hookworm disease, efficacy of iron in

WILLIAM BOSWORTH CASTLE, American physician, 1897-   , proved the effectiveness of iron in the treatment of anemia associated with hookworm disease, even in the presence of the parasites. Reported in 1931.

Anemia of pregnancy, first accurate description of

HERMANN NASSE, German physician, 1807-1892, was the first to give an adequate description of anemia of pregnancy, in 1836.

Anemia, introduction of term

GABRIEL ANDRAL, French physician, 1797-1876, is believed to have introduced the term *anemia* (or *anaemia*), *circa* 1829.

Anemia, pernicious, early account of

JAMES SCARFE COMBE, Scottish physician, 1796 - 1883, described a case of anemia which is now believed to have been pernicious anemia. Recorded in 1824, some 25 years before Addison presented his classic account.

Anemia, pernicious, first description of

THOMAS ADDISON, English physician, 1793-1860, first described the condition in 1849. ANTON BIERMER, German physician, 1827-1892, followed with a more complete description in 1868 and still another in 1872. The disease is known by several eponyms, such as *Addison's anemia, Addison-Biermer anemia, Biermer's disease*, etc., and refers to a macrocytic form of anemia marked by increased blood destruction, gastric achylia, nervous disorders, and, often, glossitis.

Anemia, refractile bodies seen in erythrocytes in certain types of

. . . See under *Erythrocytes, refractile bodies in*, etc.

Anemia, ringlike bodies in erythrocytes in some forms of

. . . See under *Ringlike bodies in erythrocytes*.

Anemia, sickle-cell, first clear description of

JAMES BRYAN HERRICK, American

physician, 1861-1954, is credited with presenting the first accurate description of sickle-cell anemia, in 1910. Known as *Herrick's anemia, drepanocytic anemia, sicklemia,* and *Dresbach's anemia.*

Anemias, classification of, on basis of hemoglobin content, etc.

MAXWELL MYER WINTROBE, American hematologist, 1901-   , devised a classification of anemias based on the hemoglobin content of the erythrocytes and the differences in the size of the cells. Published in 1930.

Anesthesia by intratracheal insufflation, first description of

SAMUEL JAMES MELTZER, American physiologist, 1851-1920, with JOHN AUER, devised a method of anesthesia by intratracheal insufflation of air containing an anesthetic vapor, for use in thoracic surgery. Reported in 1909. Known as *Meltzer's method.* Earlier, in 1905, intratracheal insufflation was attempted by FRANZ KUHN, German physician, 1866-1929.

Anesthesia, general, by rectal injection of ether and oil

JAMES T. GWATHMEY, American surgeon, 1863-1944, developed a method for producing general anesthesia without inhalation, by the injection into the rectum of ether and oil. First report dated 1913. Known as *Gwathmey's method.*

Anesthesia, hypnotic, early induction of

JAMES ESDAILE, English surgeon, 1808-1859, was successful with his attempts to induce hypnotic anesthesia in Hindus, but not so successful with Europeans. Recorded in 1846.

Anesthesia, infiltration, pioneer work in

WILLIAM S. HALSTED, American surgeon, 1852 - 1922, did original work in the field of infiltration anesthesia, with cocaine. Reported in 1885.

Anesthesia, intravenous, first use of, in man

PIERRE CYPRIEN ORÉ, French physician, 1833-18??, was the first to use intravenous anesthesia in man, by means of chloral. Recorded in 1874. In 1872 Oré used the same method in animals.

Anesthesia, local, by use of ice and salt

NEILS ARNOTT, Scottish physician, 1788-1874, devised a method for local anesthesia by the use of a freezing mixture composed of ice and salt. Probable date of report, 1851. Called *Arnott's anesthesia.*

Anesthesia, peridural, introduction of

FIDEL PAGES MIRAVE, Spanish surgeon, 18?? - 1924, introduced the method of peridural anesthesia. Recorded in 1921.

Anesthesia, regional block, introduction of

WILLIAM S. HALSTED, American surgeon, 1852 - 1922, is credited with introducing regional nerve block anesthesia by the use of cocaine. Reported in 1885.

Anesthesia, spinal, first clinical trial of

RUDOLPH MATAS, American surgeon, 1860-19??, is credited with being the first to try spinal anesthesia clinically, in 1899.

Anesthesia, spinal, in animals
JAMES LEONARD CORNING, American neurologist, 1855-1923, experimented with spinal anesthesia in dogs, using cocaine. Recorded in 1885.

Anesthesia
. . . See also under particular kind of anesthesia, as *Ether anesthesia*, etc.

Anesthetics, inhalation device
  for administration of,
  by drop method
. . . See under *Inhalation device*.

Aneurysm, distal ligation in
JAMES WARDROP, English surgeon, 1782-1869, was the first to use distal ligation in treating aneurysm of the carotid artery. Recorded in 1827. Known as *Wardrop's operation*.

Aneurysm, first operative
  treatment of
ALFRED ARMAND LOUIS MARIE VELPEAU, French surgeon, 1795-1867, is said to have been the first to attempt treating aneurysm by operation. Recorded in 1831.

Aneurysm in which arterial sac
  communicates with two veins
HENRY PARK, English surgeon, 1744-1831, described a type of arteriovenous aneurysm in which the artery communicates with two veins, *circa* 1783. Known as *Park's aneurysm*.

Aneurysm, ligation of iliac and
  femoral arteries in a case of
GURDON BUCK, American surgeon,

1807 - 1877, ligated the iliac and femoral arteries in a case involving aneurysm. Reported in 1858.

Aneurysm needle with
  eye near point
ALBERT REVERDIN, Swiss surgeon, 1881-1929, devised an aneurysm needle having an eye near the point. Date not available. Known as *Reverdin's needle*.

Aneurysm of abdominal and
  thoracic aorta in living subject
ANDREAS VESALIUS, Belgian anatomist, 1514-1564, was probably the first to diagnose aneurysm of the abdominal and thoracic aorta in a living subject, in 1555.

Aneurysm of terminal
  pulmonary arteries
FRITZ VALDEMAR RASMUSSEN, Danish physician, 1834-1877, described aneurysm or dilatation of the terminal pulmonary arteries in tuberculosis, often leading to massive hemorrhage. Published in 1868. Known as *Rasmussen's aneurysm*.

Aneurysm, traumatic, treatment
  of, by ligation
DOMINIQUE ANEL, French surgeon, *circa* 1678-1730, treated a case of traumatic aneurysm by litigation, in 1710.

Aneurysm, treatment of,
  by galvanopuncture
LUIGI CINISELLI, Italian surgeon, 1803-1878, devised a method for treating aneurysm by means of galvanopuncture, to stimulate clot formation. Reported in 1869.

Aneurysm, treatment of, by
  insertion of a watch spring
GUIDO BACCELLI, Italian physician,

1832-1916, devised a method for treating aneurysm by inserting a watch spring or a wire thread into the sac, to stimulate coagulation. Reported in 1877.

Aneurysm, treatment of, by introducing fine wire in sac

CHARLES HEWITT MOORE, English surgeon, 1821-1870, introduced a method for treating aneurysm by inserting fine wire in the sac. Reported in 1864.

Aneurysmorrhaphy, first recorded

RUDOLPH MATAS, American surgeon, 1860-19??, is credited with performing the first recorded aneurysmorrhaphy on April 6, 1888.

Aneurysms, distinction between true and false

ANTONIO SCARPA, Italian anatomist and surgeon, 175?-1832, is credited with differentiating between true and false aneurysms. Published in 1804.

Aneurysms, idiopathic and traumatic, recognition of

ANTYLLUS, Greek physician and surgeon, *circa* 220-280 A. D., recognized two forms of aneurysm, the idiopathic or congenital and the traumatic. Exact date not available.

Angina pectoris, amyl nitrite in treatment of

THOMAS LAUDER BRUNTON, Scottish physician and pharmacologist, 1844-1916, introduced the use of amyl nitrite in the treatment of angina pectoris. Recorded in 1867.

Angina pectoris, cervical sympathectomy for relief of

THOMAS JONNESCO, (Toma Iones-cu), Rumanian surgeon, 1860-1926, introduced cervical sympathectomy for the relief of angina pectoris, in 1916. Reported in 1920.

Angina pectoris, early description of—1759

EWDARD HYDE, 1st Earl of Clarendon, 1609-1674, described angina pectoris suffered by his father, Henry Hyde. Published in 1759. This is probably the first recorded case.

Angina pectoris, early description of—1768

NICOLAS FRANÇOIS ROUGNON DE MAGNY, French physician, 1727-1799, described a case of what is now believed to have been angina pectoris. Recorded in 1768.

Angina pectoris, first accurate description of—1768

WILLIAM HEBERDEN, *père*, English physician, 1710-1801, gave the first clear description of angina pectoris, *circa* 1768. Report published after his death, in 1802. Heberden is also credited with introducing the term *angina pectoris*.

Angina pectoris, introduction of term

WILLIAM HEBERDEN, *père*, English physician, 1710-1801, is credited with introducing the term *angina pectoris, circa* 1768. Known also as *Heberden's asthma* and *Rougnon-Heberden disease*.

Angina pectoris is associated with coronary occlusion, early suggestion that

ALLAN SCOTT, Scottish physician and anatomist, 1781-1813, suggested that angina pectoris is associated with or caused by coronary occlusion. Reported in 1809.

Angina pectoris, retrosternal pain in

. . . See under *Retrosternal pain in angina pectoris.*

Angina pectoris, theobromine sodium salicylate in treatment of

SIEGFRIED ASKANAZY, German physician, 1838 - 1916, suggested the use of diuretin, theobromine sodium salicylate, for the relief of angina pectoris. Recorded in 1895.

Angina pectoris, treatment of, by paravertebral injection of alcohol

FRITZ BRUNN, Austrian surgeon, 1888 - 19??, with FELIX MANDL, Austrian surgeon, 1892-   , introduced a method for treating angina pectoris by paravertebral injection of alcohol. Recorded in 1924.

Angina pectoris, treatment of, by paravertebral injection of novocain

GEORGE ARTHUR LÄWEN, German surgeon, 1876-19??, introduced the use of paravertebral injection of novocain in the treatment of angina pectoris. Recorded in 1922.

Angiocardiography, introduction of

GEORGE PORTER ROBB, American physician, 1898-   , with ISRAEL STEINBERG, devised a method of visualizing the chambers of the heart and the great vessels, after injection of a contrast medium. Published in 1938.

Angiokeratoma, eponymic description of

VITTORIO MIBELLI, Italian dermatologist, 1860 - 1910, described a skin disease marked by telangiectases and warty growths which are arranged in groups, thickening of the epidermis, etc. Published in 1889. Known as *Mibelli's disease No. 1,* and as *telangiectatic warts.*

Angiokeratoma, original description of

E. WYNDHAM COTTLE, English physician, 185?-1919, was the first to describe angiokeratoma, later known as Mibelli's disease. Recorded in 1877.

Angiomatosis retinae

. . . See under *Retina, angiomatosis of,* etc.

Angioneurotic edema, earliest description of

JOHN LAWS MILTON, Scottish physician, 1820-1898, gave the first description of angioneurotic edema, which he called "giant urticaria," in 1876.

Angioneurotic edema, eponymic description of

HEINRICH IRENAEUS QUINCKE, German physician, 1842 - 1922, gave a classic description of angioneurotic edema, published in 1882. Known as *Quincke's edema* or *disease.*

Angioneurotic hematuria

. . . See under *Renal epistaxis, early description of.*

Angstrom unit of wavelength, introduction of

ANDERS JÖNS ÅNGSTRÖM, Swedish physicist, 1814-1879, proposed a standard unit of wavelength before the Stockholm Academy, in 1853. An Angstrom unit is one-tenth of a millimicron long, or 1/100 millionth of a centimeter. It is used for designating wavelengths of x-rays, radium radiation, visible light, etc.

Animal calorimetry, early experiments on

ADAIR CRAWFORD, English physician, 1748 - 1795, performed the first recorded experiments on animal calorimetry. Published in 1779.

Animal egg, germinal spot of, discovery of

JEAN J. M. C. V. COSTE, French embryologist, 1807 - 1873, discovered and described the germinal spot of the animal egg. Reported in 1837.

Animal magnetism, popularization of concept of

FRANZ ANTON MESMER, German physician, 1734-1815, was an ardent advocate of the doctrine of animal magnetism, a concept said to have been introduced by one VALENTINE GREATARICK, in 1666. In 1766 Mesmer published a paper on the magnetism of heavenly bodies; his paper on animal magnetism appeared in 1779. The doctrine is known as *Mesmerism*.

Animals and plants, binomial classification of

. . . See under *Binomial nomenclature,* etc.

Anion, introduction of term

MICHAEL FARADAY, English chemist and physicist, 1791-1867, introduced the term *anion,* to describe those ions which move in the electrolyte toward the anode. Reported in 1833.

Ankle joint, Syme's amputation at

JAMES SYME, Scottish surgeon, 1799-1870, performed the first successful operation at the ankle joint on Sept. 8, 1842. Recorded in 1843. Known as *Syme's amputation.*

Ankylosis of hip, subtrochanteric osteotomy for correction in case of

WILLIAM ADAMS, English surgeon, 1820-1900, devised an operation for the correction of deformity due to bony ankylosis of the hip, by subtrochanteric osteotomy. Reported in 1871. It is a modification of the Barton operation, reported in 1826.

Ankylosis of knee, operation involving removal of V-shaped piece of bone for relief of

JOHN RHEA BARTON, American surgeon, 1794-1871, devised an operation for ankylosis of the knee joint in which a V-shaped segment of bone is removed. Recorded in 1826.

Ankylosis, operative, for relief of disability due to flaccid paralysis

. . . See under *Arthrodesis of joints.*

Annulus ovalis; limbus fossae ovalis

RAYMOND VIEUSSENS, French anatomist, 1641-1715, described the rounded margin of the fossa ovalis, the annulus ovalis. Published in 1705. Known as *Vieussens' annulus.*

**Anociassociation, introduction
of concept and method of**
GEORGE WASHINGTON CRILE,
American surgeon, 1864-1943, introduced a procedure in which local
and general anesthesia are combined with other methods to elim-
inate preoperative fear and postoperative shock by minimizing painful stimuli. Recorded in 1913.

Anode, **introduction of term**
MICHAEL FARADAY, English chemist and physicist, 1791-1867, introduced the term *anode,* on the basis
of the Greek *ana* (up) and *hodos*
(way), in allusion to the carbon
electrode where the current came
up or "rose." Reported in 1833.

**Anorexia nervosa, introduction of
term, and description of**
WILLIAM W. GULL, English physician, 1816-1890, is credited with
being first to describe the condition
anorexia nervosa and to introduce
the term. Reported in 1873. Known
also as *apepsia hysterica* and *apepsia nervosa.*

**Ansa subclavia, eponymic
description of**
RAYMOND VIEUSSENS, French anatomist, 1641-1715, described
nerve fibers extending around the
subclavian artery in the region of
the middle and inferior cervical
ganglia. Recorded in 1705. Known
as *ansa of Vieussens.*

Antabuse, introduction of
. . . See under *Tetraethylthiuram
disulfide.*

**Anterior horn cells, degeneration
of, in progressive muscular
atrophy**
. . . See under *Progressive muscular
atrophy,* etc.

**Anterior pituitary-like factor,
discovery of, in placenta**
JAMES BERTRAM COLLIP, Canadian
physician and biochemist, 1892-
, discovered an ovary-stimulating hormone in the placenta,
which he called anterior pituitary-
like factor. Preliminary report in
1930.

**Anthrax bacillus, cultivation
of—1863**
CASIMIR J. DAVAINE, French physician, 1812-1882, cultivated the anthrax bacillus and transmitted the
disease from one animal to another,
in 1863.

Anthrax bacillus, discovery of
FRANZ ALOYS ANTOINE POLLEND-
ER, German physician, 1800-1879,
discovered the anthrax bacillus in
the blood of sheep that died of anthrax, in 1849. Recorded in 1855.

**Anthrax bacillus, growth of,
in pure cultures**
ROBERT KOCH, German bacteriologist, 1843-1910, demonstrated the
growth of the anthrax bacillus in
pure cultures, in 1876.

**Anthrax bacillus, spore
formation of**
ROBERT KOCH, German bacteriologist, 1843-1910, demonstrated that
the anthrax bacillus is capable of
forming spores which later trans-
form into bacilli, in 1876.

**Anthrax, first adequate
description of**
PHILIBERT CHABERT, French veterinarian, 1737-1814, gave the first
clear account of anthrax, in 1780.
So good was the description, that
the condition became known as
Chabert's disease, a term now re-

served for the disease in sheep, cattle, and goats.

Anthrax pustule, areola around, description of

FRANÇOIS CHAUSSIER, French physician, 1746-1828, gave a clear description of the inflammatory areola which surrounds the anthrax pustule. Reported *circa* 1807.

Anthrax, salvarsan in treatment of

GEORG BECKER, German physician, 1874-19??, is credited with introducing the use of salvarsan in the treatment of anthrax. Published in 1911.

Anthrax serum, early preparation of

ACHILLE SCLAVO, Italian bacteriologist, 1861-1930, prepared a specific anti-anthrax serum, in 1895.

Anthrax, thermoprecipitin reaction for diagnosis of

ALBERTO ASCOLI, Italian veterinarian, 1877-19??, devised a thermoprecipitin reaction test for the diagnosis of anthrax. Recorded in 1910.

Anthropologists, Society of, in Paris

PIERRE PAUL BROCA, French surgeon and anthropologist, 1824-1880, founded the Society of Anthropologists in Paris, in 1859.

Anthropology, founder of modern

JOHANN FRIEDRICH BLUMENBACH, German anthropologist, 1752-1840, is considered the founder of modern anthropology. He is noted for the classification of the subdivisions of the human race and for his studies in craniology. Blumen-

bach's division of the races was based mainly on the habitat and the color of the skin. Published in 1775.

Anthropometry, application of, to aesthetics

ALBRECHT DÜRER, German engraver and illustrator, 1471-1528, produced a great work on the proper proportions of the human body, titled *"Vier Bücher von menschlicher Proportion."* In it Dürer makes the first application of anthropometry to aesthetics. Published in 1528.

Antihistamine, description of first

G. UNGAR, French scientist, 19??-, with J. L. PARROT and D. BOVET, described the first antihistamine, "933 F," in 1937.

Antipneumococcal serum, preparation of new

FRED NEUFELD, German bacteriologist, 1861-1945, with LUDWIG HAENDEL, developed the new antipneumococcal serum. Published in 1910.

Antipneumococcal serum, preparation of old

GEORG KLEMPERER, German physician, 1865-19??, with FELIX KLEMPERER (German physician, 1866-1932), used immune rabbit serum in the treatment of pneumonia. Published in 1891.

Antipyrine, introduction of

WILHELM FILEHNE, German physician, 1844-1927, is credited with introducing antipyrine into therapeutics, as an analgesic, antirheumatic, etc. Recorded in 1884.

Antireticular cytotoxic serum, introduction of

ALEXANDER A. BOGOMOLETS, Russian physician and biochemist, 1881-1946, introduced antireticular cytotoxic serum, made by inoculating horses with an extract of spleen and bone marrow. Date not available.

Antisepsis, introduction of, in France

JUST M. M. LUCAS-CHAMPIONNIÈRE, French surgeon, 1843-1913, is credited with introducing antiseptic techniques in France. His *Chirurgie Antiseptique* was published in 1876.

Antivenin, early production of

. . . See under *Cobra antivenin*.

Antivenom serum, early development of

LÉON CHARLES ALBERT CALMETTE, French bacteriologist, 1863-1933, developed the first effective antivenom serum. First report published in 1894.

Antivirus, introduction of term

ALEXANDRE BESREDKA, French physician, 1870-1940, is believed to have introduced the term *antivirus, circa* 1903.

Antrum of Highmore

. . . See under *Sinus, maxillary, eponymic description of*.

Anus, artificial, early operation for

PHILIP SYNG PHYSICK, American surgeon, 1768-1837, devised an operation for the construction of an artificial anus. Recorded in 1826.

Anus, artificial, first successful construction of

C. DURET, French surgeon, 1762-1804, was the first to construct successfully an artificial anus in an infant with congenital atresia. Published in 1798.

Aorta, abdominal, ligation of

ASTLEY PASTON COOPER, English surgeon, 1768-1841, performed a ligation of the abdominal aorta in 1817. Recorded in 1818.

Aorta, dilatation of proximal part of

JOSEPH HODGSON, English physician, 1788-1869, described an aneurysmal dilatation of the proximal part of the aorta, often accompanied by hypertrophy of the heart. Reported in 1815. Known as *Hodgson's disease*.

Aorta, semilunar valves of, tubercles in

. . . See under *Corpora arantii*.

Aortic aneurysm, first description of

ANTOINE SAPORTA, French physician, 15??-1573, is credited with being the first to describe aneurysm of the aorta, in 1554.

Aortic aneurysm, tracheal tug in

WILLIAM HENRY PORTER, Irish physician, 1790 - 1861, described tracheal tug as a sign of aortic aneurysm. Published in 1826.

Aortic insufficiency, alternate blanching of nails in

. . . See under *Fingernails, alternate flushing and blanching of*.

Aortic insufficiency, early description of—1706

WILLIAM COWPER, English surgeon, 1666-1709, described aortic insufficiency, "of ossifications or petrifactions in the coats of the arteries, particularly in the valves of the great artery," in 1706.

Aortic insufficiency, early description of—1829

THOMAS HODGKIN, English physician, 1798-1866, described aortic insufficiency in 1829.

Aortic insufficiency, early description of—1832

DOMINIC JOHN CORRIGAN, Irish physician, 1802 - 1880, described aortic insufficiency in a classic account published in 1832.

Aortic medionecrosis

. . . See under *Medionecrosis of aorta.*

Aortic paraganglia; Zuckerkandl's bodies

EMIL ZUCKERKANDL, Austrian anatomist, 1849-1910, described chromaffin bodies situated along the course of the aorta and associated with the sympathetic ganglia, *circa* 1880.

Aortic sinus, eponymic description of

ANTONIO MARIA VALSALVA, Italian anatomist, 1666-1723, described the dilatation of the aorta opposite the segments of the semilunar valve. Recorded in 1740. Known as *sinus of Valsalva.*

Aortic stenosis, early description of

LAZARE RIVIÈRE, French physician, 1589-1655, is said to have been the first to describe aortic stenosis. Published in 1674.

Aortitis, syphilitic, early description of

. . . See under *Syphilitic aortitis.*

Apepsia hysterica; apepsia nervosa

. . . See under *Anorexia nervosa.*

Aphakia, definition of

FRANS C. DONDERS, Dutch physician, 1818-1889, described the condition of aphakia, congenital absence of the crystalline lens, in 1864.

Aphasia, early description of—1745

CARL VON LINNÉ (Linnaeus), Swedish physician and naturalist, 1707-1778, was probably first to describe aphasia, in 1745.

Aphasia related to lesion in anterior cerebral lobes

JEAN BAPTISTE BOUILLAUD, French physician, 1796-1881, pointed out the relation of aphasia with a lesion in the anterior cerebral lobes, thus identifying the anterior cerebral lobes as the speech center. Reported in 1825.

Aphasia, subcortical, in which patient is able to indicate the number of syllables in a word

LUDWIG LICHTHEIM, German physician, 1845-1928, described a form of subcortical aphasia in which the patient is able to determine mentally and to indicate by signs the number of syllables in a given word, although he is unable to pronounce it. Published in 1885. Known as *Lichtheim's disease.*

Aphemia, **introduction of term**

PIERRE PAUL BROCA, French surgeon and anthropologist, 1824-1880, suggested the word *aphemia* (now *aphasia*) in connection with his discovery of the speech center in the third left frontal convolution. Reported in 1861.

Aphthae of palate of newborn, original description of

ALOIS BEDNAR, Austrian pediatrician, 1816-1888, described aphthae of the hard palate of infants, known as *Bednar's aphthae.* Recorded in 1850-53.

Aplanatic foci, law of

JOSEPH JACKSON LISTER, English optician, 1786-1869, discovered the law of aplanatic foci of lenses, *circa* 1825.

Aplasia axialis extracorticalis congenita

. . . See under *Familial centrolobar sclerosis.*

Apoplexy, recognition of nature of

JOHANN JACOB WEPFER, German physician, 1620-1695, demonstrated that apoplexy is caused by hemorrhage into the brain. Recorded in 1658.

Apparatus for extracting fatty material

FRANZ RITTER VON SOXHLET, German chemist, 1848-1926, devised a glass apparatus consisting of flask, condenser, and intermediate tube, used to extract fatty matter, as from vegetable drugs, in 1882. Known as *Soxhlet apparatus.*

Apparatus for keeping organs alive outside of body

. . . See under *Perfusion apparatus,* etc.

Apparatus for stretching shortened muscles

ROBERT JONES, English orthopedist, 1858-1933, devised an apparatus for stretching shortened muscles, as in Volkmann's ischemic paralysis. Recorded in 1908.

Appendectomy, first recorded successful

CLAUDIUS AMYAND, English surgeon, 168?-1740, is credited with performing the first recorded successful appendectomy. Published in 1736.

Appendectomy, incision for, in which muscles are separated by blunt dissection

CHARLES MCBURNEY, American surgeon, 1845-1913, devised an incision, for appendectomy, in which the muscle fibers are separated by blunt dissection rather than by cutting. Published in 1894. Known as *McBurney's incision.*

Appendicitis, chronic, first recognition of

FRANÇOIS MÉLIER, French physician, 1798-1866, was the first to recognize chronic appendicitis as a clinical entity. He suggested operative treatment. Recorded in 1827.

Appendicitis, early description of—1554

JEAN FRANÇOIS FERNEL, French physician, 1497-1558, gave an early description of appendicitis, which he called coarctation of intestine, in 1554.

Appendicitis, first complete understanding of—1886

REGINALD H. FITZ, American physician, 1843-1913, was the first to give an adequate description of appendicitis, demonstrating the symptoms and the pathology involved. Reported in 1886.

Appendicitis, first elective operation for

THOMAS GEORGE MORTON, American surgeon, 1835-1903, is credited with performing the first elective and successful operation for appendicitis, in April 1887. Recorded by Frank Woodbury in 1887.

Appendicitis, first recorded postmortem on a case of

LORENZ (LAURENTIUS) HEISTER, German surgeon and anatomist, 1683-1758, is credited with performing the first postmortem in a case of fatal appendicitis, in 1711.

Appendicitis, first reported case of, in English

JOHN PARKINSON, English surgeon, 1774-1842, is credited with being the first to record a case of appendicitis in English, in 1812.

Appendicitis, first successful operation for, in America

WILLARD PARKER, American surgeon, 1800-1884, is credited with being the first to operate for appendicitis in the United States, in 1864. Published in 1867.

Appendicitis, first successful operation for, in England

HENRY HANCOCK, London surgeon, 1809-1880, is credited with performing the first successful operation for peritonitis resulting from appendicitis, in England, in 1848.

***Appendicitis,* introduction of term**

REGINALD H. FITZ, American physician, 1843-1913, is credited with the introduction of the term *appendicitis,* about 1886.

Appendicitis, point of special tenderness in

CHARLES MCBURNEY, American surgeon, 1845-1913, described the point of special tenderness in appendicitis as follows: "The seat of greatest pain, determined by the pressure of one finger, has been very exactly between an inch and a half and two inches from the anterior spinous process of the ilium on a straight line drawn from that process to the umbilicus." Published in 1889. Known as *McBurney's point* or *sign.*

Appendicitis with perforation and peritonitis

JEAN BAPTISTE LOUYER - VILLERMAY, French surgeon, 1776-1837, reported cases of appendicitis with perforation and fatal peritonitis. This is said to have resulted in the recognition of appendicitis as a clinical entity. Recorded in 1824.

Appendicitis with perforation, first successful operation for

RICHARD JOHN HALL, American surgeon, 1854-19??, is credited with performing the first successful operation for the removal of a perforated appendix. Published in 1886.

Appendicostomy, introduction of

ROBERT FULTON WEIR, American surgeon, 1838-1927, introduced the method of appendicostomy, the opening of the appendix for the purpose of irrigating the large intestine. Published in 1902. Known as *Weir's operation*.

Appendix, first description of
. . . See under *Vermiform appendix*.

Appendix, valve at opening of
JOSEPH GERLACH, German surgeon, 1820-1896, described a fold of mucous membrane at the opening of the appendix into the cecum. Published in 1847. Known as *Gerlach's valve*.

**Apraxia, clinical tests for,
    as aid in diagnosis of
    brain disease**
ISADOR HENRY CORIAT, Boston neurologist, 1875 - 19??, studied apraxia and developed clinical tests for the disorder, of value also in the diagnosis of allied brain diseases. Recorded in 1911.

**Apraxia due to involvement
    of corpus callosum**
HUGO CARL LIEPMANN, German neurologist, 1863 - 1925, demonstrated that a case of apraxia involving the left side of the body was based on involvement of the corpus callosum. Recorded in 1900.

Apraxia, first clear description of
HUGO CARL LIEPMANN, German neurologist, 1863-1925, is credited with giving the first clear description of apraxia and differentiating the various forms of the disease. Monograph published in 1900.

**Apraxia, frontal, early
    description of**
FRITZ HARTMANN, German neu-

rologist, 1871 - 1937, described a frontal type of apraxia, in 1907.

**Aqueduct of cerebrum, eponymic
    description of**
FRANCISCUS SYLVIUS (Franciscus de le Boë), Dutch physician, 1614-1672, described the cerebral aqueduct, *circa* 1650. Known as *aqueduct of Sylvius*.

Aqueduct of Sylvius
. . . See under *Aqueduct of cerebrum*.

Aqueduct of vestibule, discovery of
DOMENICO COTUGNO, Italian anatomist, 1736-1822, discovered the aqueduct of the inner ear. Recorded in 1761. Known as *aqueduct of Cotunnius*, Cotunnius being the Latinized form of Cotugno.

**Arachnodactyly with ectopia
    of crystalline lens**
ANTONIN BERNARD JEAN MARFAN, French pediatrician, 1858 - 1942, described a syndrome marked by arachnodactyly, ectopia of the crystalline lens, and abnormal flexibility of the joints. Recorded in 1896. Known as *Marfan's syndrome*.

**Arachnoid, granulations
    or elevations of**
ANTONIO PACCHIONI, Italian anatomist, 1665-1726, described small arachnoid elevations which form clusters on the surface of the dura mater and produce depressions on the inner surface of the cranium. Pacchioni thought they were glands concerned with the production of lymph. Published in 1705. Known as *Pacchionian bodies*.

Arachnoid, **introduction of term**
HEROPHILUS, Greek physician and

atamonist in Egypt, 335-280 B. C., is credited with the introduction of the term *arachnoid*, in allusion to the resemblance of the structure to a spider's web, on the basis of the Greek *arachnes* (spider) and *eidos* (form).

Archiv für Klinische Chirurgie, founding of

BERNHARD R. K. VON LANGENBECK, German surgeon, 1810 - 1887, founded the *Archiv für Klinische Chirurgie*, the Archives of Clinical Surgery, in 1861. Known as *Langenbeck's Archiv*.

Archives of Neurology, founding of

JEAN MARTIN CHARCOT, French neurologist, 1825 - 1893, founded the *Archives of Neurology*, in 1880. He was the editor until his death.

Arcuate ligament of diaphragm, early description of

. . . See under *Ligament, arcuate, of diaphragm.*

Areola, application of term, to pigmented area around nipple

GASPARD BAUHIN, Swiss anatomist, 1560-1624, introduced the term *areola* to designate the pigmented area around the nipple, *circa* 1592.

Areola, enlargement of sebaceous glands of

WILLIAM FETHERSTON MONTGOMERY, Irish obstetrician, 1797-1859, described the enlarged sebaceous glands of the areola of the breast, seen in late pregnancy and during lactation. Published in 1837. Known as *Montgomery's glands* or *tubercles.*

Areola surrounding anthrax pustule

. . . See under *Anthrax pustule, areola around,* etc.

Argon, discovery of

JOHN WILLIAM STRUTT RAYLEIGH, English physicist, 1842-1919, with WILLIAM RAMSAY, discovered argon, in 1894. The word *argon* means, in substance, "inert," and is an allusion to the property of the element.

Argyll Robertson pupil, original description of

DOUGLAS MORAY COOPER LAMB ARGYLL ROBERTSON, Scottish physician, 1837 - 1909, described the pupil which reacts to accommodation but not to light, in 1869. The title of the original paper was *Four Cases of Spinal Myosis; with remarks on the action of light on the pupil.*

Ariboflavinosis, early description of

. . . See under *Riboflavin deficiency.*

Army Medical Museum, founder of

WILLIAM ALEXANDER HAMMOND, American neurologist, 1828-1900, was the founder of the Army Medical Museum.

Arnold Pick disease

. . . See under *Cerebral atrophy with aphasia.*

Arrhenoblastoma, record of, with relation to sex characteristics

ROBERT MEYER, German gynecologist, 1864-1947, studied ovarian tumors, especially those having defeminizing or masculinizing power, i.e., arrhenoblastomas. Published in 1930.

Arsenic cancer, first description of
JOHN AYRTON PARIS, English physician, 1785-1856, is credited with giving the first description of arsenic cancer. Recorded in 1820.

Arsphenamine, discovery of
PAUL EHRLICH, German bacteriologist and pathologist, 1854-1915, and SAHACHIRO HATA (Japanese physician and bacteriologist, 1873-1938) discovered arsphenamine, in 1909. Called also *salvarsan*.

Arsphenamine erythema, eponymic description of
GASTON MILIAN, French dermatologist, 1871-1945, described an erythematous eruption appearing usually on the ninth day after an injection of an arsphenamine preparation. Published in 1932. Known as *Milian's erythema*.

Arsphenamine, use of, in rat-bite fever
SAHACHIRO HATA, Japanese physician and bacteriologist, 1873-1938, was the first to use arsphenamine in the treatment of rat-bite fever, in 1912.

Artane in treatment of parkinsonism
. . . See under *Parkinsonism*.

Arteria thyreoidea ima
. . . See under *Artery, deep thyroid*.

Arterial circle of Robinson
FRED BYRON ROBINSON, American surgeon and anatomist, 1857-1910, described an arterial circle formed by branches of the abdominal aorta, uterine and ovarian arteries, and the hypogastric and common iliac arteries. Recorded in 1903. Known as *Robinson's circle*.

Arteriectomy in arterial thrombosis
RENÉ LERICHE, French surgeon, 1879-19??, with R. FONTAINE and S. M. DUPERTIUS, described excision of a portion of an artery in arterial thrombosis. Published in 1937.

Arteries and veins, first clear differentiation between
HEROPHILUS, Greek physician and anatomist in Egypt, 335-280 B. C., was the first to make a clear distinction between veins and arteries, saying that arteries are "six times as thick" as veins.

Arteries can be transplanted after being stored
ALEXIS CARREL, French surgeon, 1873-1944, demonstrated that arteries which have been stored for some time can still be transplanted. Reported *circa* 1908.

Arteries, expansion of, during systole, early observation on
JEAN FRANÇOIS FERNEL, French physician, 1497-1558, noted that during systole of the heart the arteries increase in size. Reported in his book published in 1542.

Arteries, ossification of
JOHANN GEORG C. F. M. LOBSTEIN, Alsatian pathologist, 1777 - 1835, wrote an early report on the ossification of arteries, in 1833. In this account he introduced the word *arteriosclerosis* (*arteriosclerose*).

Arteriocapillary fibrosis, early description of—1872

WILLIAM W. GULL, English physician, 1816-1890, with HENRY G. SUTTON (English physician, 1837-1891), described arteriocapillary fibrosis or generalized arteriosclerosis, in 1872. Known as *Gull-Sutton's disease*.

Arteriogram, first recording of

... See under *Cerebral encephalography and arteriography*.

Arterioles, smooth muscle in, discovery of

FRIEDRICH G. J. HENLE, German anatomist, 1809-1885, was first to establish the presence of smooth muscle fibers in coat of smaller arteries, a finding which led to the concept of a vasomotor function. Reported in 1841.

Arteriosclerosis affecting medium and small arteries

JOHANN GEORG MÖNCKEBERG, German pathologist, 1877-1925, described a type of arteriosclerosis affecting the middle coat of the small and medium arteries. Recorded in 1903. Known as *Mönckeberg's arteriosclerosis*.

Arteriosclerosis, experimental production of

OTTO JOSUÉ, French physician, 1869-1923, produced experimental arteriosclerosis, by repeated injections of adrenaline. Recorded in 1903.

Arteriosclerosis, generalized

... See under *Arteriocapillary fibrosis*.

Arteriosclerosis, introduction of term

JOHANN GEORG C. F. M. LOBSTEIN, Alsatian pathologist, 1777-1835, introduced the term *arteriosclerosis* (in the original, *arteriosclerose*) in a treatise published in 1833.

Arteriosclerosis produced experimentally by high cholesterol diet

... See under *Cholesterol-rich diet*.

Arteriovenous aneurysm, early description of—1753

WILLIAM HUNTER, Scottish surgeon and obstetrician, 1718-1783, is believed to have been first to describe arteriovenous aneurysm, in 1753.

Arteritis obliterans, early description of

... See under *Thromboangiitis obliterans*.

Artery, deep thyroid; arteria thyreoidea ima

JOHANN ERNST NEUBAUER, German anatomist, 1742-1777, described the deep or inferior thyroid artery, in 1772. Known as *Neubauer's artery*.

Artery, external iliac, operation for ligation of

... See under *External iliac artery*, etc.

Artery, fenestrated membrane of

FRIEDRICH G. J. HENLE, German anatomist, 1809-1885, described a "fenestrated" membrane (layer of elastic tissue) in the coats of certain arteries. *Circa* 1840. Known as *Henle's fenestrated membrane*.

Artery, internal maxillary

. . . See under *Internal maxillary artery*.

Artery, middle cerebral;
  eponymic description of

FRANCISCUS SYLVIUS (Franciscus de le Boë), Dutch physician, 1614-1672, described the middle cerebral artery, about 1645. Known as *Sylvian artery*.

Artery, spaces in external coat of

CHARLES PHILIPPE ROBIN, French physician and histologist, 1821-1885, described small spaces in the external coat of arteries communicating with the lymphatic system. Recorded in 1868. Similar spaces in the vessels of the brain were described by RUDOLPH LUDWIG KARL VIRCHOW about 1872. Known as *Robin's spaces* and *Virchow-Robin spaces*.

Artery, vein, and nerve,
  association of

ERASISTRATUS, Greek anatomist and physician, *circa* 300-250 B. C., was the first to note and describe the anatomical association of artery, vein, and nerve.

Arthritic general pseudoparalysis,
  eponymic description of

MAURICE KLIPPEL, French neurologist, 1858-1942, was first to describe arthritic general pseudoparalysis. Published in 1892. Known as *Klippel's disease*.

Arthritis, chronic, in children

ANDRÉ VICTOR CORNIL, French physician, 1837-1898, was the first to describe chronic arthritis in children. Recorded in 1864.

Arthritis deformans, joint
  swellings in

JOHN HAYGARTH, English physician, 1740-1827, described peculiar joint swellings in the fingers and elsewhere observed in arthritis deformans, in 1805.

Arthrodesis for relief of disability
  in flaccid paralysis

EDUARD ALBERT, Austrian surgeon, 1841-1900, did original work on arthrodesis for the relief of disability resulting from flaccid paralysis. Recorded in 1882.

Arthus' phenomenon of
  anaphylaxis

. . . See under *Anaphylactic reaction following subcutaneous injection of specific antigen*.

Artificial circulation to keep
  organs and other excised
  parts alive

. . . See under *Perfusion to keep excised organs alive*.

Artificial culture of cells,
  first recorded

. . . See under *Cells, first artificial culture of*.

Artificial insemination, early
  record of

JOHN HUNTER, Scottish surgeon in England, 1728-1793, suggested the method of artificial insemination to a patient, in 1790. The patient effected the insemination with a syringe. Recorded by EVERARD HOME in 1799.

Artificial respiration, arm-lift
  method of

HOLGER NIELSEN, Copenhagen physician, 1866 - 19??, devised a method for administering artificial respiration in which the patient lies prone and the operator extends or lifts the patient's arms for inspiration and exerts pressure on the scapulae for expiration. Recorded in 1932. Known as the *Holger Nielsen resuscitation technique*.

Artificial respiration, early method of—1856

MARSHALL HALL, English physician, 1790-1857, described a prone method of artificial respiration, in 1856.

Artificial respiration, early method of—1858

HENRY ROBERT SILVESTER, English physician, 1828 - 1908, devised a method for artificial respiration in which the subject is placed on his back and his arms are raised and lowered against the chest. Recorded in 1858. Known as *Silvester's method*.

Artificial respiration in asphyxia of newborn

HARVEY L. BYRD, American physician, 1820-1884, with JAMES H. DEW (American physician, 1843-1914), devised a method for administering artificial respiration to newborn in cases of asphyxia. Known as *Byrd-Dew method*. Date not available.

Artificial respiration, Schafer's prone pressure method of

EDWARD ALBERT SHARPEY-SCHAFER, English physician, 1850-1935, devised a prone pressure method of artificial respiration. Recorded in 1904. Known as *Schafer's method*.

Arytenoid cartilages, early description of

BERENGARIUS OF CAPRI, Italian anatomist, 1480-1550, gave an early description of the arytenoid cartilages, in 1521.

Aryvocalis muscle, eponymic description of

WILHELM FRIEDRICH VON LUDWIG, German surgeon, 1790-1865, described the aryvocalis muscle, a slip of the vocalis muscle inserted into the vocal fold. Date not available. Known as *muscle of Ludwig*.

Asbestosis, fatal case of uncomplicated, in U. S.

KENNETH MERRILL LYNCH, American pathologist, 1887-   , reported what is believed to be the first fatal case of asbestosis in the United States, in 1931.

Ascending neuritis, first description of

SILAS WEIR MITCHELL, American physician and physiologist, 1829-1914, gave the first description of ascending neuritis, in 1872.

Aschner's phenomenon or reflex

. . . See under *Oculocardiac reflex*.

Aschoff nodules or bodies

. . . See under *Myocarditis, rheumatic, characteristic lesions of*.

Ascites, relief of, by omentopexy

. . . See under *Omentopexy for relief of cirrhosis of liver*.

Aselli's glands or pancreas, eponymic description of

. . . See under *Lymph nodes near pancreas*.

Aspetic meningitis, introduction
of term

JAMES BOURNE AYER, American
neurologist, 1882-   , introduced
the term *aseptic meningitis,* to describe the meningeal reaction to
aseptic irritation. Published in
1920.

Aspidium in treatment of
ancylostomiasis

. . . See under *Ancylostomiasis.*

Assezat's triangle

. . . See under *Triangle formed by
lines uniting alveolar point with
basion and nasion.*

Association neurones, first
description of

THEODOR HERMANN MEYNERT,
German neurologist and psychiatrist in Austria, 1833-1892, is credited with giving the earliest
description of "association neurones," in 1868.

Astasia-abasia, description of

PAUL OSCAR BLOCQ, French physician, 1860-1896, described the condition astasia-abasia, in which the
subject is unable to stand or walk
although the legs are otherwise not
disabled, in 1888.

Asthenic body type,
eponymic description of

BERTHOLD STILLER, German physician in Hungary, 1837-1922, described an asthenic body type
associated with enteroptosis. Published in 1907. Known as *Stiller's
disease.*

Asthenopia in relation to headache

. . . See under *Eye strain as cause
of headache,* etc.

Asthenopia, introduction
of term

WILLIAM MACKENZIE, Scottish
opthalmologist, 1791-1868, is credited with introducing the concept
and term of *asthenopia.* Recorded
in 1830.

Asthma and catarrh
caused by pollen

. . . See under *Pollen as cause of
catarrh and asthma.*

Asthma, animal emanations
as cause of

HENRY HYDE SALTER, English physician, 1823-1871, called attention
to emanations from rabbits, cats,
dogs, etc. as cause of asthma. Recorded in 1860.

Asthma, high altitudes in

WILLIAM STORM VAN LEEUWEN,
Dutch physician, 1882-1933, demonstrated the benefit of high altitudes in cases of asthma. Recorded
in 1925.

Astigmatism as cause of headache,
early observation on

SILAS WEIR MITCHELL, American
neurologist, 1829-1914, noted the
relation of astigmatism to headache. Published in 1874.

Astigmatism chart consisting of
triple parallel lines

HEINRICH OTTO BECKER, German
opthalmologist, 1828-1890, invented a test chart for astigmatism consisting of triple parallel lines placed
at various meridians. Recorded in
1883.

Astigmatism, early description of

GEORGE BIDDELL AIRY, English
physician, 1801 - 1892, described

astigmatism and corrected it with cylindrical lenses. Recorded in 1827.

Astigmatism, first description of

THOMAS YOUNG, English physician, 1773-1829, is said to have been the first to describe astigmatism, in 1801.

Astigmatometer, invention of—1867

LOUIS EMILE JAVAL, French ophthalmologist, 1839-1907, is credited with the invention of the astigmatometer, in 1867.

Astral hyalitis, first description of

ARTHUR H. BENSON, English ophthalmologist, 1855-19??, described an inflammation of the vitreous humor, characterized by the presence of star-shaped bodies. Recorded *circa* 1890.

Astrocytes; Golgi's cells

CAMILLO GOLGI, Italian histologist, 1844-1926, described two types of nerve cells situated in the posterior horns of the spinal cord and characterized by their short processes. In *type I* the axons of the cells emerge from the gray matter; in *type II* the axons do not pass out of the gray matter. Published in 1880 and 1885.

Astrocytes of neuroglia, early description of

OTTO F. K. DEITERS, German anatomist, 1834 - 1863, described the star-shaped cells of the neuroglia, *circa* 1865.

Astrocytes of neuroglia, early description of

SANTIAGO RAMÓN Y CAJAL, Span-

ish neurologist, 1852 - 1934, described the astrocytes of the neuroglia, in 1881. Known as *Cajal's cells.*

A.T.10 in treatment of tetany

. . . See under *Tetany, dihydrotachysterol in treatment of.*

Atabrine in treatment of malaria

. . . See under *Malaria.*

Ataxia analgica hysterica, eponymic description of

PAUL BRIQUET, French physician, 1796-1881, gave the first description of ataxia analgica hysterica, a condition marked by anesthesia of the skin and muscles of the leg. Published in 1859. Known as *Briquet's ataxia.*

Ataxia, hysterical, eponymic description of

. . . See under *Ataxia analgica hysterica.*

Atelectasis in dead infants

EDUARD JOERG, German-American physician, 1808 - 1878, described pulmonary atelectasis in infants and interpreted its significance in determining whether or not air has entered the lungs of a dead newborn. Reported in 1832.

Athetosis, eponymic description of

WILLIAM ALEXANDER HAMMOND, American neurologist, 1828-1900, described athetosis, a disorder marked by vermicular movements of the hands and feet, occurring mostly in children. First report in 1871. Known as *Hammond's disease.*

Athetosis relieved by excision of precentral cortex

VICTOR ALEXANDER HADEN HORSLEY, English surgeon, 1857-1916, proved that removal of the precentral cortex in man relieves or abolishes athetosis. Published in 1909.

Atlas of diseases of eye, early edition of, before era of ophthalmoscopy

FRIEDRICH AUGUST VON AMMON, Dresden ophthalmologist, 1799-1861, produced an atlas of diseases of the eye which is considered the most comprehensive work for the era preceding ophthalmoscopy. Published in 1838.

Atlas of pathological anatomy, first complete

ROBERT CARSWELL, English physician, 1793-1857, prepared an atlas of pathological anatomy containing about 2000 hand-colored illustrations of excellent quality. Published in 1838.

Atom, first use of term

LEUCIPPUS OF MILETUS, Greek philosopher, 5th century B. C., was probably the first to use the term *atom.*

Atomic theory, development of

JOHN DALTON, English chemist and physicist, 1766 - 1844, developed and promulgated the atomic theory of matter. Proposed in 1803-1807.

Atomic theory, earliest reference to

ANAXAGORAS, Greek philosopher, *circa* 500-428 B. C., was probably the first to teach a crude form of the atomic theory.

Atomic theory, early reference to

DEMOCRITUS OF ABDERA, Greek philosopher, *circa* 460-370 B. C., suggested that all matter is composed of atoms, an atom being a small indivisible particle.

Atomic weight, introduction of concept of

JOHN DALTON, English chemist and physicist, 1766 - 1844, introduced the idea of atomic weight, *circa* 1803.

Atoms, representation of, by arbitrary symbols

JOHN DALTON, English chemist and physicist, 1766 - 1844, introduced the use of arbitrary symbols to represent atoms or elements, *circa* 1802.

Atoms, representation of, by letters

JONS JAKOB BERZELIUS, Swedish chemist, 1779-1848, introduced the use of letters to represent atoms or elements, in 1819.

Atom-smashing, pioneer work in

JOHN D. COCKCROFT, English physicist, 1897- , and ERNEST T. S. WALTON, Irish physicist, 1903- , did notable research in nuclear physics. They received the Nobel prize in physics for their work in atom-smashing, in 1951.

Atoxyl in treatment of trypanosomiasis

. . . See under *Trypanosomiasis.*

Atrioventricular bundle, classic description of

WILHELM HIS, *fils,* German physiologist, 1863 - 1934, described a muscular band containing some nerve fibers which links the auricles with the ventricles of the heart. Published in 1893. Known as *bundle of His*. The structure was also described by ALBERT F. S. KENT, English physiologist, in the same year.

Atrioventricular bundle, early description of

WALTER HOLBROOK GASKELL, English physiologist and anatomist, 1847-1914, gave an early but incomplete description of the atrioventricular bundle *circa* 1882. Known as *Gaskell's bridge*.

Atrioventricular node, first description of

SUNAO TAWARA, Japanese pathologist, 1873-19??, is credited with the first description of the atrioventricular node, in 1906. Known as *Tawara's node*.

Atrioventricular valves, nodules on free edges of, in infants

. . . See under *Nodules on free edges*.

Atrium of heart, fibers extending across right

. . . See under *Fibers extending across right atrium*.

Atrium, right, intervenous tubercle of

. . . See under *Tubercle, intervenous, of heart*.

Atrophoderma pigmentosum

. . . See under *Xeroderma pigmentosum, eponymic description of*.

Atrophy, hereditary familial spinal muscular

. . . See under *Progressive muscular atrophy*.

Atrophy of anterior horns of spinal cord in poliomyelitis

JEAN MARTIN CHARCOT, French neurologist, 1825 - 1893, with ALEXIS JOFFROY, French physician, 1844-1908, discovered the atrophy of the anterior horns of the spinal cord in poliomyelitis. Recorded in 1869.

Atrophy of bone associated with inflamatory conditions of the extremities

ROBERT KIENBOCK, Austrian radiologist, 1871-1953, described acute atrophy of bone occurring in certain inflammatory conditions of the extremities. Published in 1901. Known as *Kienbock's atrophy*.

Atrophy of muscles of face and scapulohumeral region

LOUIS T. J. LANDOUZY, French physician, 1845-1917, described a type of atrophy affecting the muscles of the face and the scapulohumeral region, in 1885. Another report, with J. J. Dejerine, was published in 1886. Known as *Landouzy-Dejerine atrophy*.

Atrophy of newborn, Parrot's

. . . See under *Parrot's atrophy of the newborn*.

Atrophy of optic nerve, peripheral

. . . See under *Optic nerve, peripheral atrophy of*.

Atropine and hyoscyamine in eye examination

FRANZ REISINGER, German ophthalmologist, 1787-1855, was first to use hyoscyamine and atropine in examination of the eye. Recorded in 1825.

Atropine, isolation of
PHILIPP L. GEIGER, German pharmacologist, 1785-1836, and HERMANN HESSE (German pharmacologist of nineteenth century) isolated atropine in 1833.

Aubert's phenomenon, first report of
. . . See under *Optical illusion in which a vertical line seems to incline.*

Audiometer, introduction of first
ARTHUR HARTMANN, German physician, 1849-1931, is credited with devising the first audiometer. Recorded in 1878.

Auditory organs, early description of
GIULIO CASSERIO, Italian anatomist, 1561-1616, gave one of the earliest descriptions of the ear, *circa* 1600.

Auditory tube, classic description of
BARTOLOMMEO EUSTACHIUS, Italian anatomist, 1524-1574, gave a classic description of the auditory tube, in 1563. The eponymic designation *Eustachian tube* was originated by ANTONIO M. VALSALVA, in 1704.

Auditory tube, diverticulum of; eponymic description
WILHELM KIRCHNER, German otologist, 1849-1935, described a diverticulum of the auditory tube. Known as *Kirchner's diverticulum.* Recorded *circa* 1890.

Auditory tube, early references to
ALCMAEON, Greek writer, 550-500

B. C., is believed to have discovered the auditory tube, later described by ARISTOTLE and EUSTACHIUS.

Auditory tube
. . . See also under *Eustachian tube.*

Auerbach's ganglion, discovery of
. . . See under *Ganglion of Auerbach's plexus.*

Auerbach's plexus, discovery of
LEOPOLD AUERBACH, German anatomist, 1828 - 1897, described the myenteric plexus or plexus of autonomic nerve fibers situated between the circular and longitudinal muscular coats of the intestine. Reported in 1862.

Aura in epilepsy, first mention of
ARETAEUS THE CAPPADOCIAN, Greek physician in Rome, *circa* 81-138, was the first to record the aura in epilepsy. Exact date not available.

Aural speculum with illumination and mirror reflectors
. . . See under *Speculum for mouth.*

Aural vertigo; Ménière's syndrome
. . . See under *Ménière's syndrome.*

Aureomycin, introduction of
BENJAMIN MINGE DUGGAR, American scientist, 19??- , with his associates, discovered and introduced aureomycin. Recorded in 1948.

Auricular fibrillation, action of digitalis in
JAMES MACKENZIE, Scottish cardiologist in England, 1853 - 1925, demonstrated the action of digitalis

in auricular fibrillation. Published in 1905.

Auricular fibrillation as cause of permanent arrhythmia

THOMAS LEWIS, English cardiologist, 1881-1945, was the first to describe auricular fibrillation as a cause of permanent clinical arrhythmia. Recorded in 1909.

Auricular fibrillation, early description of—1909

THOMAS LEWIS, English cardiologist, 1881-1945, gave the first clear description of auricular fibrillation. Recorded in 1909.

Auricular fibrillation, effectiveness of quinidine in

WALTER FREY, German physician, 1884- , demonstrated that quinidine is the most effective of the cinchona alkaloids in controlling auricular fibrillation. Published in 1918.

Auricular fibrillation in man, first recognition of

ARTHUR R. CUSHNY, Scottish physician and pharmacologist, 1866-1926, with CHARLES W. EDMUNDS (American physician, 1873-1941), was the first to recognize and describe auricular fibrillation in man, in 1901. Reported in 1906.

Auricular fibrillation, introduction of term

THOMAS LEWIS, English cardiologist, 1881-1945, is credited with introducing the term *auricular fibrillation,* in 1909.

Auricular flutter, experimental production of

JOHN ALEXANDER MACWILLIAM, Aberdeen physician, 1857 - 1937, demonstrated that auricular flutter can be produced experimentally by the injection of poisons into the blood stream. Recorded in 1887.

Auricular flutter in man, early recognition of—1905

WILLIAM THOMAS RITCHIE, Scottish physician, 1873-1945, was first to recognize auricular flutter in man, in 1905.

Auricular flutter, introduction of term

WILLIAM ADAM JOLLY, English physician, 1878-1939, with WILLIAM THOMAS RITCHIE, Scottish physician, 1873-1945, introduced the term *flutter.* Published in 1910.

Auricular paroxysmal tachycardia, description of

LEON BOUVERET, French physician, 1850-1929, described paroxysmal auricular tachycardia, in 1889. Known as *Bouveret's syndrome.*

Auriculopalpebral reflex

. . . See under *Intracranial pressure, increased, pain reflex in.*

Autohemotherapy, early use of

FRIEDRICH LUITHLEN, German physician, 1869-1927, introduced autohemotherapy in the treatment of skin diseases, in 1913.

Autonomic nerve fibers situated between the muscular coats of the intestine

. . . See under *Auerbach's plexus.*

Autonomic nervous system, control of, by hypothalamus

WALTER RUDOLF HESS, Swiss physiologist, 1881-195?, pioneered in the study of the control of the autonomic nervous system by the hypothalamus. For this and for his work on the reaction of animals to electric shock, he was the co-winner of the Nobel prize in 1949.

Autonomic nervous system, introduction of term

JOHN NEWPORT LANGLEY, English physiologist, 1852 - 1925, introduced the title *autonomic nervous system, circa* 1898. Published in 1903.

Autonomic nervous system pathways, mapping of—1889

JOHN NEWPORT LANGLEY, English physiologist, 1852 - 1925, studied the autonomic nervous system and mapped many of its pathways. Research began *circa* 1889; early report published in 1894.

Autosuggestion, introduction of term

EMILE COUÉ, French pharmacist, 1857-1926, is believed to have originated the basis of the term *autosuggestion,* in 1922.

Autotechnicon, invention of

HARRY GOLDBLATT, American-pathologist, 1891-   , with LOUIS GROSS, invented the Autotechnicon, a device for the automatic fixation, dehydration, and impregnation of tissue specimens. Reported in 1929.

Avellis's syndrome

. . . See under *Soft palate, recurrent paralysis of.*

Avertin, clinical introduction of

OTTO BUTZENGEIGER, German physician, 1885-   , introduced the use of avertin and reported his clinical experience in 1927.

Avertin

. . . See also under *Tribromethanol.*

Axilemma, eponymic description of

LUDWIG MAUTHNER, Bohemian ophthalmologist in Austria, 1840-1894, described the axilemma, the sheath of an axon, in 1882. Known as *axolemma* or *axilemma* of *Mauthner* and *Mauthner's sheath.*

Axis cylinder, eponymic description of

ROBERT REMAK, German physiologist and neurologist, 1815-1865, described the axis cylinder or axon, in 1838. Known as *Remak's band.*

Axis cylinder, transverse lines in

CARL FROMMANN, German anatomist, 1831-1892, discovered transverse lines or striae in the axis cylinder of myelinated nerve fibers, made visible by staining with silver nitrate. Known as *Frommann's lines.* Date not available.

Axis of birth canal, curve describing

CARL GUSTAV CARUS, German obstetrician, 1789-1869, described the longitudinal axis of the pelvic canal as a curved line having the symphysis pubis as its center. Reported in 1820. Known as *curve of Carus.*

Axis-traction forceps; Tarnier's forceps

ÉTIENNE STÉPHANE TARNIER, French obstetrician, 1828-1897, invented an axis-traction forceps, in 1877.

Axon, eponymic description of

. . . See under *Axis-cylinder.*

Axon, lumen of, dissertation on

JOHANNES EVANGELISTA VON PUR-
KINJE, Bohemian physiologist,
1787-1869, described the existence
of a lumen in the axis-cylinders of
nerves. Recorded in 1838.

**Axon of medullated fibers,
transverse lines in**

. . . See under *Axis cylinder.*

**Axon, sheath of; eponymic
description**

. . . See under *Axilemma, eponymic
description of.*

**Ayerza's disease, eponymic
description of**

ABEL AYERZA, Argentinian physician, 1861-1918, described, in a lecture, a syndrome marked by chronic
cyanosis, dyspnea, erythremia, and
sclerosis of the pulmonary artery,
in 1901. Published in 1925 by LUIS
AYERZA.

***Ayerza's disease,* introduction
of name**

FRANCISCO C. ARRILAGA, Argentinian physician, 1870-19??, is credited with introducing the eponymic
name *Ayerza's disease,* about 1912.

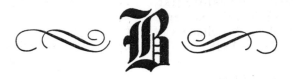

Babes-Ernst bodies or corpuscles, description of

VICTOR BABES, Rumanian microbiologist, 1854-1926, with PAUL ERNST, German pathologist, described the metachromatic granules seen in the protoplasm of bacteria. These granules are more refractive than the surrounding protoplasm and stain deeply with anilin dyes. Reported in 1888. Known as *Babes-Ernst bodies.*

Babinski toe reflex or sign

JOSEPH F. F. BABINSKI, Polish neurologist in France, 1857-1932, noted that in organic disease of the pyramidal tract stimulation of the sole causes the great toe to extend (dorsiflexion) while the other toes fan out or flex. This sign distinguishes organic from hysterical hemiplegia. Report published in 1896.

Babinski-Fröhlich disease or syndrome

. . . See under *Adiposogenital dystrophy, first description of.*

Bacillary dysentery, bacteriology of—1898

KIYOSHI SHIGA, Japanese bacteriologist, 1870-19??, discovered the organism, *Shigella dysenteriae,* causing the most virulent form of dysentery, in 1898. The *Shiga bacillus* elaborates a neurotropic exotoxin in addition to the endotoxin elaborated by all members of the *Shigella* group of organisms.

Bacillary dysentery, bacteriology of—1900

WALTHER KRUSE, German bacteriologist, 1864-1943, investigated the bacteriological picture of bacillary dysentery, especially with reference to *Shigella dysenteriae,* which is also known as *Shiga-Kruse bacillus.* Recorded in 1900. In the same year, SIMON FLEXNER, American pathologist and bacteriologist, 1863-1946, isolated *Shigella paradysenteriae* in cases of tropical dysentery. This organism was at first believed to be identical with *Shigella dysenteriae.* Known as *Flexner's bacillus.*

Bacillary dysentery in children, sulfaguanidine in treating

. . . See under *Sulfaguanidine.*

Bacillus abortus, discovery of

. . . See under *Brucella abortus.*

Bacillus acidophilus, discovery of

. . . See under *Lactobacillus acidophilus.*

Bacillus aerogenes capsulatus, discovery of

WILLIAM HENRY WELCH, American pathologist, 1850-1934, with GEORGE H. F. NUTTALL, discovered *Bacillus aerogenes capsulatus,* the causative agent of gas gangrene. Reported in 1892. Also known as *Bacillus perfringens, Clostridium welchii, Welch bacillus,* and *Bacillus achalme.*

Bacillus anthracis, discovery of

... See under *Anthrax bacillus.*

Bacillus botulinus, discovery of

EMILE P. M. VAN ERMENGEM, Belgian physician and bacteriologist, 1851 - 1932, discovered *Bacillus botulinus,* in cases of food poisoning, in 1897.

Bacillus bulgaricus, discovery of

... See under *Lactobacillus bulgaricus.*

Bacillus granulosis, isolation of, from case of trachoma

HIDEYO NOGUCHI, Japanese bacteriologist in America, 1876-1928, isolated the *Bacillus granulosis* from American Indian trachoma. Recorded in 1927. Noguchi believed the organism to be the cause of trachoma and he experimented with the production of trachoma in monkeys.

Bacillus icteroides, isolation of

GIUSEPPE SANARELLI, Italian bacteriologist, 1864 - 1940, isolated *Bacillus (Salmonella) icteroides.* Reported in 1894. Known as *Sanarelli's bacillus.*

Bacillus, introduction of term

OTTO FRIEDRICH MÜLLER, Danish bacteriologist, 1730-1784, is generally credited with the introduction of the term *bacillus,* about 1773.

Bacillus leprae, cultivation of

ERNEST REINHOLD ROST, English physician in India, 1872-19??, succeeded in cultivating the *bacillus leprae,* in 1904.

Bacillus odontolyticus, isolation of

JAMES McINTOSH, English physician, 1881 - 19??, with W. W. JAMES and P. LAZARUS-BARLOW, isolated the *Bacillus odontolyticus* from scrapings of carious teeth. Recorded in 1922.

Bacillus paratyphosus B, isolation of

EMILE CHARLES ACHARD, French physician, 1860-1944, with RAOUL BENSAUDE (French physician, 1866 - 1938) studied paratyphoid fever and isolated *Bacillus paratyphosus B,* now called *Salmonella paratyphi B.* Report published in 1896.

Bacillus psittacosis, discovery of

EDMOND ISIDORE ETIENNE NOCARD, French veterinarian, 1850 - 1903, discovered *Bacillus psittacosis,* which he thought was the cause of psittacosis. The organism was later proved to be identical with *Bacillus aertrycke,* and shown not to be the cause of the disease. Reported in 1892.

Bacillus subtilis, first description of

CHRISTIAN GOTTFRIED EHRENBERG, German bacteriologist, 1795-1876, was the first to describe *Bacillus subtilis*. Published in 1838.

Bacillus

. . . See also under *Bacterium, Brucella, Escherichia, Lactobacillus,* etc., and under the name of the particular disease.

Bacitracin, discovery of

BALBINA A. JOHNSON, H. ANKER, and F. L. MELENEY, American scientists, isolated bacitracin, a product of a particular strain of *Bacillus subtilis,* in 1943. Published in 1945. The term is based on the name of a patient, Margaret Tracy, from whom the bacillus was obtained.

Bacteria, early classification of—1773

OTTO FRIEDRICH MÜLLER, Danish scientist, 1730 - 1784, is credited with being first to attempt a classification of bacteria. Early report published in 1773-74.

Bacteria, filtration of, first attempts with

THEODOR ALBRECHT EDWIN KLEBS, German bacteriologist, 1834-1913, is credited with being the first to filter bacterial growths and to test the effects of the filtrate. Recorded in 1872.

Bacteria, first observation of—1675

ANTONJ VAN LEEUWENHOEK, Dutch naturalist, 1632 - 1723, is credited with being first to observe bacteria, with the aid of his crude microscope, in 1675.

Bacteria, method of making smears of

ROBERT KOCH, German bacteriologist, 1843 - 1910, introduced the method of making bacterial smears and fixing them with heat. Recorded in 1877.

Bacteria, staining of

. . . See under *Staining of bacteria, first experiments in.*

Bacterial chains and clumps, early observation of

ANTONJ VAN LEEUWENHOEK, Dutch naturalist, 1632 - 1723, observed the arrangement of bacteria in chains and clumps, using his crude microscope, *circa* 1677.

Bacterial culture, attenuated, first use of

LOUIS PASTEUR, French scientist and bacteriologist, 1822 - 1895, is credited with being first to use an attenuated bacterial culture for therapeutic purposes, *circa* 1880.

Bacterial endocarditis, Bracht-Wächter bodies in

ERICH BRACHT, German physician, 1882- , with ?. ?. WÄCHTER, described areas of necrosis in the myocardium containing a serous exudate and polymorphonuclear leukocytes, in bacterial endocarditis. Recorded in 1909.

Bacterial endocarditis, isolation of causative agent of

HUGO SCHOTTMÜLLER, German physician and bacteriologist, 1867-1936, isolated *Streptococcus viridans* from cases of bacterial endocarditis and demonstrated it to be the cause of the disease. Published in 1910. The organism is also known as *Schottmüller's bacillus.*

Bacterial endocarditis, subcutaneous nodes in

WILLIAM OSLER, Canadian - English physician, 1849 - 1919, described small painful swellings on the hands and feet, especially on the fingertips and the tips of the toes, associated with bacterial endocarditis. Osler first observed the nodes in 1888; reported in 1909.

Bacterial hemolysis, discovery of

JULES J. B. V. BORDET, Belgian bacteriologist and pathologist, 1870-19??, was the first to describe bacterial hemolysis, in 1898.

Bactericidal power of immune serum is destroyed by heat

HANS BUCHNER, German bacteriologist, 1850-1902, demonstrated that the bactericidal power of immune serum is destroyed by heat. Reported in 1889.

Bacteriophage, introduction of term

FREDERICK WILLIAM TWORT, English bacteriologist, 1877 - 1950, is credited with introducing the term *bacteriophage, circa* 1917.

Bacteriophagia, discovery of—1915

FREDERICK WILLIAM TWORT, English bacteriologist, 1877 - 1950, discovered the phenomenon of transmissible bacterial lysis, bacteriophagia, *circa* 1915. Known as the *Twort-d'Herelle phenomenon.*

Bacteriophagia, discovery of—1917

FELIX H. D'HERELLE, Canadian physician in the U. S. S. R., 1873-1949, described the phenomenon of bacteriophagia (transmissible bacterial lysis) in 1917. Known as the *Twort-d'Herelle phenomenon.*

Bacteriotropins, early description of

FRED NEUFELD, German bacteriologist, 1861-1945, described bacteriotropins and also introduced the term. Recorded in 1904.

Bacterium coli, first description of

. . . See under *Escherichia coli.*

Bacterium, first pure culture of a

JOSEPH LISTER, English surgeon, 1827-1912, is credited with being the first to grow a bacterium in a pure culture. He accomplished this with *B. lactis,* in 1874. Recorded in 1877.

Bacterium paratyphosum A, isolation of

NORMAN BEECHEY GWYN, American physician, 1875-19??, isolated the *Bacterium paratyphosum A,* in 1898.

Bacterium paratyphosum B, isolation of

EMILE CHARLES ACHARD, French physician, 1860-1944, with RAOUL BENSAUDE, isolated the *Bacterium paratyphosum B.* Recorded in 1896.

Bacterium paratyphosum C, isolation of

LUDWIK HIRSCHFELD, Swiss physician, 1884-1954, isolated and described the *Bacterium paratyphosum C.* Published in 1919.

Baelz's disease, classic description of

... See under *Myxadenitis labialis.*

Bag for capturing expired air in studies of respiratory exchange

CLAUDE G. DOUGLAS, English physiologist, 1882 - 19??, invented a rubber bag used to capture expired air in experiments to determine the total respiratory exchange in man. Reported in 1911.

Bag, obstetric, for dilating cervix uteri

... See under *Obstetric bag,* etc.

Bag, rubber, for controlling bleeding in suprapubic prostatectomy

JAMES EMMONS BRIGGS, American surgeon, 1869 - 1942, invented a dilatable rubber bag used to control bleeding after suprapubic prostatectomy. Reported in 1906. Known as *Briggs's bag.*

Baker's cyst

... See under *Cyst formed by herniation of synovial membrane of a joint.*

Balantidium coli, discovery of

PEHR HENRIK MALMSTEN, Swedish physician, 1811-1883, discovered the *Balantidium coli* in 1857. This organism is believed to have been the first parasitic protozoon to be discovered and identified as such.

Ballistocardiograph, introduction of

ISAAC STARR, American physician, 1895-   , with A. J. RAWSON, H. A. SCHROEDER, and N. R. Jos-

EPH, introduced the ballistocardiograph, a device for recording the stroke volume of the heart. Published in 1939.

Balloon, use of, in recording stomach movements, in animals

ANTON JULIUS CARLSON, American physiologist, 1875 - 19??, studied and recorded the movements of the stomach in animals by means of a balloon inserted through a fistula. Reported in 1912.

Baló's disease

... See under *Encephalitis, periaxial concentric.*

Balsam, use of, in glass slide preparations

JOHANNES EVANGELISTA VON PURKINJE, Bohemian physiologist, 1787-1869, is credited with being the first to use Canada balsam in making glass slide preparations, *circa* 1830.

Band, metal, in treating fracture of long bones

... See under *Fracture, treatment of, with metal band.*

Bandage for support of arm in fracture of clavicle

ALFRED ARMAND L. M. VELPEAU, French surgeon, 1795 - 1867, devised a bandage to support the arm in case of fracture of the clavicle. Published in 1839. Known as *Velpeau's bandage.*

Bandage impregnated with starch and bismuth, for burns

ADOLF VON BARDELEBEN, German physician, 1861 - 1914, invented a bandage dressing impregnated with a mixture of bismuth and starch, for use in burns. Date not available.

Bandage-tourniquet to secure bloodless operative field

JOHANN FRIEDRICH A. VON ESMARCH, German military surgeon, 1823-1908, devised a rubber bandage used as a tourniquet to secure a bloodless field in operations upon limbs. Published in 1873.

Bandl's ring

. . . See under *Uterus, contraction ring of.*

Bárány's caloric test

. . . See under *Caloric differential test for labyrinthine function.*

Barbital, introduction of

EMIL FISCHER, German chemist, 1852-1919, with JOSEPH VON MERING, German physician, 1849-1908, introduced barbital or veronal, *circa* 1902.

Bärensprung's disease

. . . See under *Tinea cruris.*

Barium, discovery of

KARL WILHELM SCHEELE, Swedish chemist, 1742-1786, is credited with discovering barium, in 1774, by treating pyrolusite with sulfuric acid.

Barium, introduction of term

HUMPHRY DAVY, English chemist and physicist, 1778 - 1829, introduced the term *barium*, on the basis of the Greek *barys* (heavy), because of the presence of the element in barytes or heavy spar.

Barnes's bags for dilating cervix of uterus

. . . See under *Rubber bag for dilating cervix.*

Barraquer's disease; Barraquer-Simons disease

. . . See under *Lipodystrophia progressiva.*

Barraquer's operation for cataract

. . . See under *Cataract extraction by suction.*

Bartholin's glands; major vestibular glands

. . . See under *Vestibular glands, major.*

Barth's hernia

. . . See under *Hernia of intestine between persistent vitelline duct and abdominal wall.*

Bartonella bacilliformis

. . . See under *Verruga peruana.*

Basal cell carcinoma, eponymic description of

. . . See under *Rodent ulcer, eponymic description of.*

Basal metabolism standards, establishment of

EUGENE F. DU BOIS, American physiologist, 1882-19??, established basal metabolism standards expressed in tabular form, on the basis of calories per square meter per hour. *Circa* 1924.

Basement membrane, discovery and naming of

WILLIAM BOWMAN, English ophthalmologist and anatomist, 1816-1892, described the delicate noncellular layer which lies under the epithelium of secreting glands and mucous membranes, and named it *basement membrane,* in 1842.

Basement membrane of mucosa of intestinal tract, bronchi, bronchia, and trachea

MAURICE GEORGES DEBOVE, French physician, 1845-1920, described the basement membrane, the noncellular layer underlying the epithelium of the bronchial and tracheal mucosa, the alimentary tract, etc. Published *circa* 1882.

Basle Nomina Anatomica; Basle anatomical nomenclature; BNA

WILHELM HIS, SR., German anatomist, 1831-1904, is credited with being instrumental in the formulation of a list of anatomical terms, in Latin, adopted in 1895 by the German Anatomical Society in Basle. Known as the *Basle Nomina Anatomica* or BNA.

Basophilism, pituitary, original description of

HARVEY W. CUSHING, Boston surgeon, 1869-1939, described a condition due to overgrowth of the basophil cells of the anterior lobe of the pituitary, in 1932. The condition is marked by adiposity, kyphosis, amenorrhea or impotence, hypertension, etc. Known as *Cushing's disease* or *syndrome.*

Bassini's operation for inguinal hernia

. . . See under *Inguinal hernia, Bassini's operation for.*

Bastian-Bruns law

. . . See under *Spinal cord, transverse lesion of.*

Batten-Mayou disease

. . . See under *Amaurotic familial idiocy, juvenile form of.*

Battey's operation of ovariotomy

. . . See under *Ovariotomy for treatment of non-ovarian diseases.*

Battle's incision for abdominal section

WILLIAM HENRY BATTLE, English surgeon, 1855-1936, introduced a vertical incision of the rectus sheaths with retraction of the rectus muscle inward. Recorded in 1895. Known as Battle-Jalaguier-Kammerer incision. ADOLPHE JALAGUIER modified the incision in 1897. In the same year FREDERIC KAMMERER added his modification.

BCG vaccine

. . . See under *Tuberculosis, development of preventive vaccine for.*

Bead test for digestive function

MAX EINHORN, American physician, 1862-1953, devised a method for studying digestive function by having the patient smallow a capsule containing a sample of food wrapped in gauze to which a colored glass bead is attached for identification. Reported in 1906.

Beard's disease; neurasthenia

. . . See under *Neurasthenia, first description of.*

Beau's lines on fingernails

. . . See under *Lines, transverse, on fingernails.*

Bechterev-Mendel reflex

. . . See under *Toes, dorsal flexion of, when dorsum of foot is tapped.*

Bechterev's fibers

. . . See under *Cerebral cortex, layer of fibers parallel to tangential fibers of.*

Bed, seesawing, for cardiovascular and peripheral vascular disease

CLARENCE ELMER SANDERS, American physician, 1885-1949, devised an automatically seesawing bed for use in cardiovascular and peripheral vascular disease. Published in 1936. Known as *Sanders' bed, oscillating bed,* and *vaso-oscillator bed.*

Bed, surgical, for supporting patient in semisitting posture

WILLIS D. GATCH, American surgeon, 1878-19??, devised a surgical bed with an adjustable frame for supporting the patient in a sitting or semisitting posture, as in postoperative care. Reported in 1909.

Bed, use of, for delivering parturient women

. . . See under *Deilvery of parturient women in bed,* etc.

Behçet's syndrome, eponymic description of

HULUSI BEHÇET, Turkish dermatologist, 1889 - 1948, described a condition marked by recurrent ulceration of the genitalia, lesions of the mouth, uveitis, etc. Published in 1937.

Bellini's ducts

. . . See under *Kidney, papillary ducts of.*

Bellini's tubules

. . . See under *Uriniferous tubules, discovery of.*

Bell-Magendie law of spinal nerve roots

. . . See under *Motor function of anterior roots of spinal nerves.*

Bell's palsy

. . . See under *Facial paralysis.*

Bence Jones protein

. . . See under *Albumosuria, myelopathic,* etc.

Benzene ring, theory of closed

FRIEDRICH AUGUST KEKULÉ, German chemist, 1829-1896, promulgated his theory of the closed benzene ring in 1865.

Benzhexol in treatment of parkinsonism

. . . See under *Parkinsonism.*

Benzoic acid compounds, discovery of

JUSTUS VON LIEBIG, German chemist, 1803 - 1873, with FRIEDRICH WÖHLER (German chemist, 1800-1882), discovered benzoic compounds and studied their properties, in 1832.

Benzoic acid, early description of

BLAISE DE VIGENÈRE, French chemist and cryptologist, 1546-1619, is credited with the first description of benzoic acid, in 1608.

Benzyl alcohol, introduction of, as local anesthetic

DAVID ISRAEL MACHT, Baltimore pharmacologist, 1882- , studied the properties of benzyl alcohol and introduced it as a local anesthetic. Recorded in 1918.

Berger's paresthesia

. . . See under *Paresthesia of lower limbs in young persons.*

Beriberi, discovery of cause of

CHRISTIAAN EIJKMAN, Dutch bacteriologist and physiologist, 1858-1930, produced polyneuritis in chickens by feeding them polished rice, and thus paved the way to the discovery that beriberi is caused by lack of vitamin B in the diet. Reported in 1890.

Beriberi, early modern description of

JACOBUS BONTIUS, Dutch physician, 1592-1631, is credited with writing the first modern scientific account of beriberi, as he saw it in the East Indies. Published posthumously in 1642.

Beriberi, experimental production of

CHRISTIAAN EIJKMAN, Dutch bacteriologist and physiologist, 1858-1930, produced experimental beriberi in fowls by feeding them a diet consisting of over-milled rice. Published in 1890.

Beriberi, Japanese, dietary origin of

KANEHIRO TAKAKI, Japanese physician, 1849 - 1915, demonstrated the dietary origin of kakke or Japanese beriberi. Recorded in 1885.

Beriberi, outbreak of, in Tokyo, in 1881

ERWIN VON BAELZ, German physician, 1849-1913, described the outbreak of beriberi in Tokyo, in 1881. The report was an important contribution to the understanding of the disease.

Berkefeld filter, introduction of

ALBERT NORDTMEYER, German inventor, 1858 - 19??, observed that even ground water in the vicinity of the Kieselguhr mine in Hannover, Germany, was perfectly clear, and concluded that the earth must have special filtering properties. This led to his introduction of the Berkefeld filter in 1891. The name is derived from WILHELM BERKEFIELD (also Berkefeld), German manufacturer, 1836-1897, the owner of the Kieselguhr mine.

Bernhardt's disease, description of

. . . See under *Meralgia paraesthetica*.

Beta-oxybutyric acid, isolation of

RUDOLPH EDUARD KÜLZ, German biochemist, 1845 - 1895, isolated beta-oxybutyric acid from urine. Recorded in 1884.

Beurmann-Gougerot disease

. . . See under *Sporotrichosis, first complete description of*.

Bibliography, Father of

CONRAD GESNER, Swiss physician and bibliographer, 1516-1565, compiled numerous bibliographies in many fields. He is regarded as the Father of Bibliography.

Biett's disease, first complete description of

. . . See under *Lupus erythematosus*.

Bifocal lenses, invention of

BENJAMIN FRANKLIN, American statesman and scientist, 1706-1790, invented bifocal lenses for spectacles. Introduced *circa* 1756.

Bigelow's method for reducing dislocation of hip

. . . See under *Dislocation of hip, method of reducing, using iliofemoral ligament*.

Bile, importance of, in digestion

THEODOR SCHWANN, German anatomist, 1810-1882, working with an artificial biliary fistula in a dog, demonstrated that bile is essential to digestion. Recorded in 1844.

Bile pigments can be formed by tissues other than liver tissue

JOHN WILLIAM McNEE, Scottish physician, 1887-   , demonstrated that bile pigments can be formed by tissues other than liver tissue, thus disproving the theory held previously. Recorded in 1914.

Bile pigments, van den Bergh test for

ALBERT ABRAHAM HIJMANS VAN DEN BERGH, Dutch physician, 1869-1943, devised a test for the presence of bile pigments in the blood. Published in 1913.

Bile salts, first test for

MAX JOSEF VON PETTENKOFER, German chemist and hygienist, 1818-1901, was first to introduce a test for bile or bile salts. Recorded in 1844.

Bilharzia haematobia, naming of

THOMAS SPENCER COBBOLD, English parasitologist, 1828-1886, introduced the name *Bilharzia haematobia,* circa 1864.

Bilharziasis, discovery of fluke of

THEODOR MAXIMILLIAN BILHARZ, German physician and zoologist, 1825-1862, discovered the parasite causing bilharziasis or schistosomiasis in tropical countries, especially Egypt, in 1851. Recorded in 1852. The organism was at first named *Distoma haematobium* and *Bilharzia haematobia.* It is known now as *Schistosoma haematobium.*

Biliary cirrhosis; hypertrophic biliary cirrhosis; obstructive biliary cirrhosis

VICTOR CHARLES HANOT, French physician, 1844 - 1896, described hypertrophic cirrhosis of the liver due to either chronic cholangitis (hypertrophic biliary cirrhosis) or obstruction of the bile ducts (obstructive biliary cirrhosis). Reported in 1875. Known as *Hanot's disease.*

Billroth I and Billroth II operations

. . . See under *Pylorus, resection of.*

Binocular vision, early understanding of

ALHAZEN, Arabian mathematician, physicist, and optician, *circa* 965-1039, was one of the earliest to appreciate the phenomena of binocular vision. Date not available.

Binomial nomenclature for plants and animals, early suggestion of—1640

JOACHIM JUNG, German scientist, 1587-1657, was probably the first to suggest a binomial nomenclature for plants and animals, about 1640. Such a classification was not adopted, however, until LINNAEUS proposed his system.

Binomial nomenclature for plants and animals, early suggestion of—1690

AUGUSTUS QUIRINUS RIVINUS, German anatomist and botanist, 1652-1723, is credited with suggesting a binomial nomenclature for classifying plants and animals, in 1690. The method was, however, not adopted until LINNAEUS proposed his system.

Binomial nomenclature for plants and animals, successful development of

CARL VON LINNÉ (Linnaeus), Swedish physician and naturalist, 1707 - 1778, developed the first workable modern classification for animals and plants in which the binomial system of genus and species is used, comparable to a system of family name and given name. Linné reported his suggestions and observations in a work titled *Systema Naturae*, first published in 1735. The tenth edition, considered the most important, was published in 1758.

Biotin, isolation of—alpha form

FRITZ KÖGL, German biochemist, 1897-   , with E. J. HAM, isolated α-biotin. Recorded in 1943.

Biotin, isolation of—beta form

VINCENT DU VIGNEAUD, American biochemist, 1901-   , with D. B. MELVILLE, P. GYÖRGY, and C. S. ROSE, isolated β-biotin and demonstrated its identity with vitamin H. Published in 1940.

Biotin, synthesis of

STANTON AVERY HARRIS, American biochemist, 1902-   , with D. E. WOLF, R. MOZINGO, and K. FOLKERS, synthesized biotin. Published in 1943.

Biparietal obliquity of fetal head

. . . See under *Naegele's obliquity*.

Bipp, introduction of

. . . See under *Bismuth iodoform paraffin paste*.

Birth canal, curved line forming longitudinal axis of

CARL GUSTAV CARUS, German obstetrician, 1789-1869, described the longitudinal axis of the pelvic canal as a curved line having the symphysis pubis as its center. Reported in 1820. Known as *curve of Carus*.

Bismuth in treatment of syphilis

. . . See under *Syphilis*.

Bismuth iodoform paraffin paste, introduction of

JAMES RUTHERFORD MORISON, English surgeon, 1853-1939, introduced the use of *bipp*, bismuthiodoform - paraffin paste, in the treatment of wounds. Recorded in 1916.

Bismuth meal, introduction of

WALTER BRADFORD CANNON, American physiologist, 1871-1945, introduced the bismuth meal in roentgenographic procedures. Published in 1898.

Bismuth paste in diagnosis and treatment of tuberculous sinuses

EMIL G. BECK, Chicago surgeon, 1866-1932, devised a bismuth subnitrate paste for the diagnosis and treatment of tuberculous sinuses and cavities and fistulous tracts. Reported in 1908. Known as *Beck's paste*.

Bite-wing radiography, introduction of

HOWARD RILEY RAPER, American dentist, 18??-19??, introduced the method of bite-wing radiography by which the crowns of the upper and lower teeth are photographed simultaneously. Published in 1925.

Bizzozero's blood platelet
. . . See under *Achromacyte, early description of*.

Bladder, aeroscopic examination of
HOWARD ATWOOD KELLY, Baltimore gynecologist, 1858-1943, introduced the method of aeroscopic examination of the bladder. Recorded in 1893.

Bladder and symphysis pubis, space between
. . . See under *Prevesical space of Retzius*.

Bladder diverticula, first operation for
JULES ÉMILE PÉAN, French surgeon, 1830-1898, is credited with being the first to operate for diverticula of the bladder. Recorded in 1895.

Bladder, extrophy of, early successful operation for
JOSEPH PANCOAST, American surgeon, 1805-1882, performed a successful operation for extrophy of the urinary bladder, in 1859.

Bladder, extrophy of, implantation of ureters into rectum for relief of
. . . See under *Ureters, implantation of*.

Bladder, extrophy of, in female; first operation
DANIEL AYRES, American surgeon, 1822-1892, is credited with performing the first successful plastic operation for the correction of congenital extrophy of the female urinary bladder. Published in 1859.

Bladder, non-prostatic obstruction at the neck of
GEORGE JAMES GUTHRIE, English surgeon, 1785 - 1856, is credited with being the first to describe non-prostatic obstruction at the neck of the bladder. Published in 1834.

Bladder, subtrigonal glands of
JOAQUIN ALBARRAN Y DOMINGUEZ, Cuban surgeon and urologist in France, 1860-1912, described the subtrigonal glands of the urinary bladder. Published in 1892. Known as *Albarran's glands*.

Bladder, trigone of urinary
. . . See under *Trigone of urinary bladder*.

Blastoderm, external layer of
AUGUST ANTINOUS RAUBER, German anatomist, 1845 - 1917, described the outermost of the three layers of cells which form the blastoderm of the embryo, in 1888. Known as *Rauber's layer*.

Blastomycosis, North American, eponymic description of
THOMAS CASPAR GILCHRIST, American dermatologist, 1862-1927, described a generalized blastomycosis (caused by *Blastomyces dermatitidis*), in 1896. Known as *Gilchrist's disease*.

Blastomycosis of skin, European
ABRAHAM BUSCHKE, German physician, 1868 - 1943, and OTTO BUSSE, German physician, 1847-

1922, reported cryptococcosis or European blastomycosis of the skin, independently, in 1895. Known as *Busse-Buschke disease.*

Blind, alphabet for, based on Roman letters

WILLIAM MOON, English physician, 1818-1894, devised a raised alphabet for the blind in which the letters retained a partial resemblance to Roman type. Introduced in 1845. Published in 1847.

Blind, alphabet for, consisting of dots

CHARLES BARBIER, French officer, 1789-1859, devised an alphabet for the blind which consisted of dots instead of embossed lines, *circa* 1820. This system of elevated dots was later modified by Braille.

Blind, alphabet for, early form of

VALENTIN HAUY, French physician and teacher of the blind, 1745-1822, originated the use of embossed paper or raised letters in teaching the blind to read. Reported in 1786.

Blind, alphabet for, improved—by Braille

LOUIS BRAILLE, French teacher of the blind, 1809-1852, perfected and popularized a system of dots, suggested in 1820 by CHARLES BARBIER, which constitutes an alphabet for the blind. Introduced in 1830. Reported in 1837. Known as the *Braille system.*

Blind spot of retina, discovery of

EDME MARIOTTE, French scientist, 1620 - 1684, discovered the blind spot of the retina. Recorded in 1668.

Blind, systematic education of, introduction of method for

VALENTIN HAUY, French physician and teacher of the blind, 1745-1822, is credited with being the first to introduce a system for the education of the blind, in 1784.

Blindness, sudden, caused by embolism of retinal artery, recognition of

FRIEDRICH W. E. A. VON GRAEFE, German ophthalmologist, 1828-1870, was first to recognize embolism of the retinal artery as a cause of sudden blindness. Reported in 1859.

Blocking of nerve trunk with local anesthesia

GEORGE W. CRILE, American surgeon, 1864 - 1943, developed a method for blocking nerve trunks with local anesthesia. Reported in 1901. Known as *block anesthesia.*

Blood, arterial and venous, both contain oxygen and carbon dioxide

GUSTAV MAGNUS, German physician, 1802-1870, demonstrated that both arterial blood and venous blood contain oxygen and carbon dioxide. Published in 1837.

Blood bank, early mention of

OSWALD HOPE ROBERTSON, American physician, 1886-195?, suggested the use of preserved blood and the establishment of blood banks, in 1918.

Blood bank, establishment of first

BERNARD FANTUS, Chicago physician, 1874 - 1940, described the establishment of the first blood bank at the Cook County Hospital, in 1937.

Blood circulation, discovery
of mechanism of
WILLIAM HARVEY, English physician, 1578 - 1657, discovered the mechanism of the circulation of the blood and described it in his *Exercitatio Anatomica de Motu Cordis et Sanguinis in Animalibus,* in 1628. This work has been called the most important book in the history of medicine.

Blood, classification of, in
four groups—1907
JAN JANSKY, Czechoslovakian physician, 18??-1921, classified human blood in four groups, numbered from I to IV, in 1907. Known as *Jansky's grouping.*

Blood, classification of, in
four groups—1910
WILLIAM LORENZO MOSS, American hematologist, 1876-19??, classified human blood in four groups, independently of Jansky, in 1910.

Blood, classification of
. . . See also under *Blood grouping.*

Blood clotting, essential
part of fibrinogen in
. . . See under *Fibrinogen, part of, in blood clotting.*

Blood coagulation, essential
part of calcium in
. . . See under *Calcium in blood coagulation,* etc.

Blood count, differential,
basis of
PAUL EHRLICH, German bacteri-

ologist and pathologist, 1854-1915, is credited with formulating the basis of the differential blood count technique. Recorded in 1879.

Blood, defibrinated, for
animal transfusions
JEAN LOUIS PRÉVOST, French physician, 1790-1850, with JEAN B. A. DUMAS, successfully used defibrinated blood in animal transfusions. This is said to have been the first attempt to prevent coagulation in the process of transfusion and the first successful result. Recorded in 1821.

Blood, examination of, in disease,
first proponent of
GABRIEL ANDRAL, French physician, 1797-1876, was first to urge the examination of the blood in disease, possibly in 1843.

Blood exposed to air changes
color, observation that
JOHN MAYOW, English physiologist, 1643 - 1679, observed the changing color of blood which is exposed to air and concluded that respiration involves the exchange of gases between the blood and the air. Published in 1674.

Blood flow, instrument for
measuring velocity of
KARL FRIEDRICH W. LUDWIG, German physiologist, 1816 - 1895, invented a "stromuhr," an instrument for measuring the speed of the blood stream. Recorded in 1867. In the same year, but independently of Ludwig, a similar device was invented by JAN DOGIEL, Russian physiologist, 1830-1905.

**Blood gases, analysis of;
earliest record**

HEINRICH GUSTAV MAGNUS, German physician, 1802 - 1870, made the first quantitative analysis of the blood gases, demonstrating that arterial blood has a higher concentration of oxygen than the venous blood while the venous blood contains more carbon dioxide. Reported in 1837.

**Blood gases, early
investigation of**

LOTHAR MEYER, German physician, 1830-1895, studied the gases of the blood, especially the concentration of carbon dioxide. Recorded in 1857 and 1858.

**Blood grouping, development
of basis for—1900**

KARL LANDSTEINER, American pathologist, 1868-1943, discovered three of the four main blood groups and thus laid the foundation for blood grouping. Reported in 1900.

**Blood grouping in jurisprudence
of paternity, early report
on—1921**

REUBEN OTTENBERG, New York physician, 1882 - 19??, developed methods for typing blood and wrote on the medicolegal applications of blood grouping to paternity. Published in 1921.

**Blood groups are inherited,
demonstration that**

EMIL VON DUNGERN, German physician, 1876 - 19??, with LUDWIK HIRSZFELD, demonstrated that blood groups are inherited in accordance with the Mendelian laws. Recorded in 1910.

Blood, iron in, discovery of

V. MENGHINI, German physiologist, 17?? - 178?, discovered the presence of iron in the blood. Reported in 1746.

**Blood oxygen not in simple
solution**

LOTHAR MEYER, German physician, 1830-1895, demonstrated that the oxygen in the blood is held in something other than simple solution, since reduction of the air pressure was not followed by a commensurate liberation of the gas. Published in 1857.

***Blood platelet*, introduction
of term**

GIULIO BIZZOZERO, Italian physician, 1846-1901, is credited with coining the term blood *platelet*, about 1882.

**Blood platelets, first accurate
count of**

GEORGES HAYEM, French physician, 1841-1933, devised a method for the first accurate count of the blood platelets. Recorded in 1878.

**Blood platelets, first
description of**

ALFRED DONNE, French physician, 1801-1878, is believed to have been the first to describe the blood platelets as a third element of the blood, in 1842.

**Blood platelets, megakaryocytes
in formation of**

JAMES HOMER WRIGHT, American pathologist, 1869-1928, is credited with discovering the role played by the megakaryocytes in the formation of blood platelets. Published in 1906.

**Blood pressure determination,
application of stethoscope
to brachial artery in**

NIKOLAI SERGEEVICH KOROTKOV,
Russian physician, 1874-19??, introduced the modern method of
placing the stethoscope on the
brachial artery in the bend of the
elbow, below the blood-pressure
cuff, while measuring the blood
pressure. Published in 1905.

**Blood pressure, earliest
measurement of**

STEPHEN HALES, English physiologist and clergyman, 1677 - 1761,
performed the earliest known experiments to determine blood pressure in animals. He observed the
height to which the blood rose in a
tube inserted directly into the artery. The experiments were performed about 1705, and reported
in the preface to a book on plants,
published in 1727.

**Blood pressure in man, direct
measurement of**

J. FAIVRE, French physician, 1824-
1879, is said to have made the first
accurate measurements of the blood
pressure in man by connecting a
mercury manometer with an artery.
Recorded in 1856.

**Blood pressure, pioneer
in recording of**

. . . See under *Sphygmomanometer,
invention of.*

**Blood pressure, use of stetho-
scope in measuring**

. . . See under *Stethoscope, use of,
in measuring systolic and diastolic
blood pressure.*

**Blood serum, specific gravity of,
early determination of—1719**

JAMES JURIN, English scientist,
1684-1750, determined the specific
gravity of the blood serum to be
1.030. Recorded in 1719.

**Blood, specific gravity of, early
determination of—1719**

JAMES JURIN, English scientist,
1684-1750, determined the specific
gravity of blood to be 1.053. Recorded in 1719.

**Blood transfusion by
slow-drip method**

HUGH LESLIE MARRIOT, London
physician, 1900-   , with ALAN
KEKWICK (English physician,
1909-   ), introduced the continuous, slow-drip method of blood
transfusion. Published in 1935.

**Blood transfusion, early
accomplishment of**

FRANCESCO FOLLI, Italian physician, 1624-1685, is credited with
being one of the early advocates of
transfusion of blood. He is said to
have accomplished transfusion by
the use of a combination silver tube,
bone cannula, and animal blood
vessel, in 1654.

**Blood transfusion, first
description of**

GIOVANNI FRANCISCO COLLE, Italian physician, 1558-1631, gave the
first definite description of a blood
transfusion, in 1628.

**Blood transfusion in treatment
of shock due to burns**

GUSTAV RIEHL, German physician,
1855-1943, is credited with introducing the method of blood trans-

fusion in treating shock due to burns. Published in 1925.

Blood transfusion

. . . See also under *Transfusion of blood.*

Blood vessels, end-to-end anastomosis of

ALEXIS CARREL, French surgeon, 1873-1944, developed a technique for end - to - end anastomosis of blood vessels. Recorded in 1907.

Blood volume, first determination of

HERMANN WELCKER, German physiologist, 1822-1897, is believed to have been the first to determine the total blood volume and the volume of the red blood cells. Recorded in 1858.

Blood volume, measurement of, with carbon monoxide

CHARLES EUGÈNE QUINQUAUD, French physician, 1841-1894, with NESTOR GRÉHANT (French physician, 1838-1910), devised a method for determining the volume of the blood by the use of carbon monoxide. Reported in 1882.

Blood volume, method for determining, by use of dye

JOHN T. GERAGHTY, American urologist, 1876-1924, with LEONARD G. ROWNTREE (American physician, 1883-19??) and NORMAN M. KEITH (American physician, 1885-19??), devised a method for determining the blood and plasma volume by the use of an intravenous injection of a dye. Reported in 1915.

Bloodless fold of Treves

. . . See under *Ileocecal fold, bloodless.*

Blue line in gums in chronic lead poisoning, first observation of

HENRY BURTON, English physician, 1799-1849, was the first to take note of the blue line in the gums of subjects suffering from chronic lead poisoning. Reported in 1840.

Blumenbach's process

. . . See under *Uncinate process.*

Blush-and-blanch phenomena

. . . See under *Menstruation, study of, by intraocular endometrial transplants.*

Boarding out of children from tuberculous households

. . . See under *Children from tuberculous households,* etc.

Boas' breakfast test meal

ISMAR ISIDOR BOAS, German physician, 1858-1938, devised a breakfast test meal consisting of a tablespoonful of oats boiled down in a quart of water to form a pint of meal, in 1885. Recorded in 1890.

Bockhart's impetigo

. . . See under *Impetigo circumpilaris infantilis.*

Bodies of Arantius, discovery of

. . . See under *Corpora arantii.*

Body build, description of types of

ERNST KRETSCHMER, German psychiatrist, 1888-   , described several types of body build, including the leptosome, pyknic, etc. Published in 1927.

Body build in relation to character and mentality

ERNST KRETSCHMER, German psychiatrist, 1888-   , attempted to establish the relationship of body build and constitution to character and mentality. Published in 1921.

Body of Highmore

... See under *Mediastinum testis, eponymic description of.*

Body temperature, brain center of

ISAAC OTT, American physiologist, 1847-1916, described a heat regulating center in the brain. Published in 1887.

Body temperature, nervous regulation of

ISAAC OTT, American physiologist, 1847-1916, studied and reported the nervous mechanism by which body temperature is regulated. Published in 1884.

Bombyx mori, life history of

... See under *Silk worm, metamorphosis of,* etc.

Bone atrophy following injury

PAUL HERMANN MARTIN SUDECK, German surgeon, 1866-1938, described acute bone atrophy sometimes following injury. Published in 1900. Known as *traumatic osteoporosis* and as *Sudeck's atrophy.*

Bone, canals in, for blood vessels

ALFRED WILHELM VOLKMANN, German physiologist, 1800 - 1877, described canals in compact bone which transmit blood vessels from the periosteum. Published in 1863. Known as *Volkmann's canals.*

Bone, canals of, containing blood and lymph vessels

CLOPTON HAVERS, English anatomist, 1653-1702, described the anastomosing canals of bone tissue which contain blood and lymph vessels, nerves, and marrow. Reported in 1691. Known as *Haversian canals.*

Bone graft, first record of—1668

JOB JANSZOON VAN MEEKEREN, Dutch surgeon, 1611-1666, is credited with reporting the first successful bone graft operation in which a piece of bone from the skull of a dog was transplanted into a cranial defect of a Russian soldier. Meekeren did not perform the operation but merely quoted the report of a missionary in Russia. Published in 1668.

Bone grafts as internal splints, first use of

FRED HOUDLETT ALBEE, American surgeon, 1876 - 1945, is credited with being the first to utilize living bone grafts as internal splints, as in treating Pott's disease. Published in 1911 and 1915.

Bone grafts, preservation of

ALBERTO FRANCIS INCLAN, English surgeon, 1916-   , studied methods for the preservation of bone. His work laid the foundation for the modern use of refrigerated bone. Published in 1942.

Bone marrow, biopsy of, by sternal puncture

CARLY PAUL SEYFARTH, German surgeon, 1890 -   , introduced

sternal puncture as a method of obtaining bone marrow for diagnostic purposes. Published in 1923.

Bone marrow, biopsy of, first suggestion for

ALFRED WOLFF, German physician, 1881-   , experimented with trephining the long bones of experimental animals for the purpose of obtaining marrow, and suggested that biopsy of bone marrow in human beings be made a part of diagnostic procedure. Published in 1903.

Bone marrow, biopsy of; introduction into practice

G. GHEDINI, Italian physician, 18?? - 19??, introduced biopsy of bone marrow as a clinical procedure. He obtained the marrow by puncturing the shaft of the tibia. Recorded in 1908.

Bone saw for cutting bone grafts

FRED HOUDLETT ALBEE, American surgeon, 1876-1945, devised a saw for cutting bone grafts. It consists of electrically operated, double rotary, adjustable blades. First reported in 1919. Known as *Albee's saw*.

Bone wax, iodoform, invention of

ALBERT VON MOSETIG-MOORHOF, Austrian surgeon, 1838-1907, devised a bone wax, consisting of iodoform, spermaceti, and sesame oil, for use in filling bone defects. Recorded in 1903. Known as *Mosetig-Moorhof bone wax*.

Boöphilus bovis

. . . See under *Texas cattle fever*, etc.

Boot for producing vacuum around a limb, early invention of—1834

VICTOR THEODORE JUNOD, French physician, 1809-1881, invented a boot which could be fitted hermetically about a leg or arm and from which the air could be removed by an air pump. Reported in a study on the effect of compression and rarefaction of the air about a limb, in 1834. Known as *Junod's boot*.

Bordet-Gengou bacillus, discovery of

. . . See under *Hemophilus pertussis*.

Bornholm disease, first description of

. . . See under *Epidemic pleurodynia*.

Boron, isolation of, from boric acid

HUMPHRY DAVY, English chemist and physicist, 1778-1829, isolated boron from boric acid, in 1808.

Boron, isolation of, from boron trioxide

JOSEPH L. GAY - LUSSAC, French chemist and physicist, 1778-1850, and LOUIS J. THENARD (French chemist, 1777-1857) isolated boron by heating boron trioxide with potassium, in 1808.

Borrelia recurrentis (Spirochaeta obermeieri), discovery of

OTTO HUGO FRANZ OBERMEIER, German physician, 1843-1873, discovered the causative agent of the European louse-borne form of relapsing fever, the *Spirillum recurrentis*, now known as *Borrelia recurrentis*, during the German epidemic of 1872. Recorded in 1873.

Botryomycosis, causative agent of

JOSEPH EMILE MAGROU, French physician, 1883- , demonstrated that botryomycosis is caused by a staphylococcus, now known as *Micrococcus ascoformans*. Reported in 1914.

Botryomycosis in horses, first description of

OTTO VON BOLLINGER, German physician, 1843-1909, was the first to describe botryomycosis, a granulomatous disease of horses, camels, and, sometimes, cattle. Bollinger described the disease in horses. Recorded in 1870.

Bottle operation for hydrocele

... See under *Hydrocele, operation for, by complete eversion of tunica vaginalis.*

Botulism, early description of

CHRISTIAN ANDREAS JUSTINUS KERNER, German physician, 1786-1862, was probably the first to describe the condition now known as botulism. Recorded in 1820.

Bougie for auditory tube, invention of

JEAN ANTOINE SAISSY, French physician, 1756-1822, invented a bougie for the Eustachian tube and was the first to use such an instrument. Recorded in 1829.

Bougies, wax-tipped, introduction of; for locating stones in urinary tract

HOWARD ATWOOD KELLY, Baltimore gynecologist, 1858-1943, introduced the use of wax-tipped bougies for locating stones in the urinary tract. Reported in 1900.

Bourneville's disease

... See under *Brain, tuberous sclerosis of.*

Bovine tubercle bacilli in man

MAZŸCK PORCHER RÁVENEL, American physician, 1861-1946, is credited with isolating bovine tubercle bacilli from tuberculous children, in 1902.

Brachial artery, utilization of, in hemopiezometry

... See under *Blood pressure determination, etc.*

Brachial plexus, naming of nerves of

JOSEPH G. DUVERNEY, French anatomist, 1648-1730, named the nerves which form the brachial plexus, in 1697. Before this the nerves were designated by numbers.

Brachial plexus, partial paralysis of, due to birth injury

WILHELM H. ERB, German neurologist, 1840-1921, described a partial paralysis of the brachial plexus due to birth injury. Reported in 1874. Called *Erb's palsy* or *paralysis,* also *Erb-Duchenne paralysis.*

Brachialgia statica paresthetica

ROBERT WARTENBERG, American neurologist, 1887- , described nocturnal arm paresthesia or brachialgia statica paresthetica, *circa* 1920.

Brachycephalic skulls

... See under *Dolichocephalic and brachycephalic skulls.*

Braille system for the blind

... See under *Alphabet for blind, perfection and popularization of.*

Brain abscess, first accurate account of

HERMANN LEBERT, French physician, 1813-1878, gave the first accurate account of brain abscess, in 1856.

Brain abscess, first successful operation for

SAUVEUR FRANÇOIS MORAND, French surgeon, 1697-1773, is credited with performing the first successful operation for temporosphenoidal abscess, following an ear infection, in 1752. Recorded in 1768.

Brain, action currents of

. . . See under *Electroencephalogram, early findings leading to.*

Brain, areas of human, delineation of

. . . See under *Map of human cortex.*

Brain concussion, first description of

LANFRANCHI of Milan, Italian phycian, 12??-1315, was the first to describe cerebral concussion, in 1296. Published in 1565.

Brain currents, early investigation of

FRANCIS GOTCH, English physiologist, 1853-1913, with VICTOR ALEXANDER HADEN HORSLEY, English surgeon, 1857-1916, demonstrated that the mammalian brain in action produces electrical currents. They recorded these currents with sensitive string galvanometers. Recorded in 1891.

Brain, cytoarchitectonic map of

OTFRID FOERSTER, German neurologist, 1873-1941, studied the human brain and developed a well-known cytoarchitectonic map of the human cerebral cortex. Published in 1936.

Brain, electric stimulation of, early work on

. . . See under *Cerebral cortex, electric stimulation of.*

Brain infection, trephining and draining in

HARRIS PEYTON MOSHER, American surgeon, 1867-19??, is credited with introducing the modern method of trephining the skull and draining in inflammatory conditions of the brain. Published in 1916.

Brain, posterior occipital convolution of

. . . See under *Occipital convolution, posterior,* etc.

Brain, tuberous sclerosis of; eponymic description

DÉSIRÉ MAGLOIRE BOURNEVILLE, French neurologist, 1840-1909, described tuberous sclerosis of the brain, a condition marked by the formation of tumors on the surfaces of the lateral ventricles and sclerotic areas of the surface of the brain. Published in 1880. Known as *Bourneville's disease.*

Brain tumor, first accurate localization and removal of

ALEXANDER HUGHES BENNETT, English surgeon, 1848-1901, with RICKMAN JOHN GODLEE, made the first recorded accurate clinical localization of a brain tumor which was removed on November 25, 1884. The patient survived the operation for one month. Recorded in 1884.

Brain tumors, electroencephalo-graphic localization of

WILLIAM GREY WALTER, English physiologist, 1911-   , developed a method for the localization of brain tumors by means of electroencephalography. Published in 1936.

Brain ventricles, early notice of

HEROPHILUS, Greek physician and anatomist in Egypt, 335-280 B.C., noted and described the ventricles of the brain. Exact date not available.

Brass-founders' ague, early investigation of

CHARLES TURNER THACKRAH, English physician, 1795-1833, is credited with being first to investigate brass-founders' ague, a disease which is said to have a picture simulating malarial fever. Published in 1831.

Brazilian yaws, discovery and description of

ACHILLE BREDA, Italian dermatologist, 1850-1933, discovered and described Brazilian yaws, in 1895. Known as *Breda's disease.*

Breast, cancer and hypertrophy of

LANFRANCHI of Milan, Italian physician, 12??-1315, was the first to differentiate between hypertrophy and cancer of the breast. Work written in 1296; published in 1565.

Breast, hyperplastic cystic disease of

ASTLEY PASTON COOPER, English surgeon and anatomist, 1768-1841, gave an early description of hyperplastic cystic disease of the female breast. Recorded in 1829. Cooper called it "hydatid" disease.

Breast, neuralgia of; early description

ASTLEY PASTON COOPER, English surgeon and anatomist, 1768-1841, described neuralgia of the breast and its relation to the condition of the pelvic organs. Published in 1829.

Breast, plastic surgery of

HIPPOLYTE MORESTIN, French surgeon, 1869-1919, devised an operation for the reconstruction of the female breast. Recorded in 1902.

Breast, suspensory ligaments of; early description

ASTLEY PASTON COOPER, English surgeon and anatomist, 1768-1841, described the fibrous processes in the breast which attach the glandular structure to the skin. Published in 1845. Known as the suspensory ligaments of the breast.

Breasts, enlarged, plastic operation for

HANS KRASKE, German surgeon, 1878-19??, devised a plastic operation for the reduction in size of enlarged or pendulous breasts. Published in 1923.

Breasts, painless cystic enlargement of

PAUL RECLUS, French surgeon, 1847-1914, described a bilateral involvement of the female breast marked by cystic enlargement due to multiple dilatations of the ducts and acini. Recorded in 1883. Known as *Reclus' disease* of the breast.

Bregma, introduction of, as craniometric point

PIERRE PAUL BROCA, French surgeon and anthropologist, 1824-

1880, defined *bregma* as a craniometric point. Exact date not available.

Brenner's tumor

. . . See under *Oophoroma folliculare.*

Brill's disease

. . . See under *Typhus, recrudescence of epidemic.*

Broad ligament of uterus, cyst of

CASPAR FRIEDRICH WOLFF, German anatomist, 1733-1794, described the mesonephros, the excretory organ of the embryo. The vestige of this organ occasionally forms a cyst in the broad ligament of the uterus and is, therefore, called *wolffian cyst.* Date not available.

Broadbent's sign

. . . See under *Pericardium, adherent, retraction of intercostal tissue in.*

Brodie's abscess

. . . See under *Tuberculous inflammation of head of a bone.*

Brodie's ligament

. . . See under *Transverse humeral ligament.*

Brodmann's areas

. . . See under *Occipital and preoccipital areas of cerebral cortex.*

Bromine, discovery and naming of

ANTOINE JEROME BALARD, French chemist, 1802-1876, discovered the element bromine in sea water, in 1826. He called the substance *muride,* in allusion to the Latin *muria,* brine, but later changed the name to *brome,* on the basis of the Greek *bromos,* stench, because of the unpleasant odor of bromine fumes. The form *bromine* was introduced by J. T. TURNER, in 1827.

Bromsulphalein liver function test

SANFORD MORRIS ROSENTHAL, American physician, 1897-   , with EDWIN CLAY WHITE, introduced bromsulphalein as an agent for testing liver function. Published in 1924.

Bronchi, introduction of medicaments into

HORACE GREEN, American laryngologist, 1802-1866, is credited with being the first to attempt the introduction of medicinal substances into the bronchi. The degree of success attained is questioned by some. Recorded in 1846.

Bronchial blood vessels, first description of

FREDERIK RUYSCH, Dutch anatomist, 1638-1731, is credited with being the first to describe the bronchial blood vessels. Recorded in his *Thesaurus Anatomicus,* published 1701-1716.

Bronchial tubes, muscular fibers of

FRANZ DANIEL REISSEISEN, German anatomist, 1773-1828, was first to give a clear account of the muscular elements of the bronchi, in 1804. Known as *Reisseisen's muscles.*

Bronchiectasis, first accurate description of

RENÉ T. H. LAENNEC, French physician, 1781-1826, was first to give a clear description of bronchiectasis, in 1819. It is said that the condition was first observed by one of his pupils in 1808.

Bronchiectatic lobe, first successful removal of

WERNER KÖRTE, German surgeon, 1853-1937, is said to have been the first to successfully excise a bronchiectatic lobe. Published in 1908.

Bronchitis, introduction of term

CHARLES BADHAM, English physician, 1780-1845, is credited with introducing the term *bronchitis*, circa 1808.

Bronchoscopy, direct, introduction of

GUSTAV KILLIAN, German laryngologist, 1860-1921, is credited with introducing the method of direct bronchoscopy, in 1898.

Bronchoscopy, first textbook on

CHEVALIER JACKSON, American bronchoesophagolaryngologist, 1865-19??, wrote the first textbook on bronchoscopy. Published in 1907.

Bronchoscopy, therapeutic, introduction of

FRANZ NOWOTNY, German physician, 1872-1925, is credited with introducing bronchoscopy in the treatment of asthma. Recorded in 1907.

Bronchoscopy

. . . See also under *Tracheo-bronchoscopy*.

Bronchospirochetosis, discovery and description of

ALDO CASTELLANI, Italian pathologist, 1878-19??, was the first to describe an infectious disease caused by *Spirochaeta bronchialis*. It is characterized by chronic bronchitis and hemoptysis. Reported in 1920. Known as *bronchospirochetosis, hemorrhagic bronchitis,* and *Castellani's bronchitis* or *disease.*

Bronchovesicular respiration, introduction of term

AUSTIN FLINT, American physician, 1812-1886, is credited with having introduced the term *bronchovesicular respiration, circa* 1856.

Brow presentation, early description of

FRANÇOIS MAURICEAU, French obstetrician, 1637-1709, described fetal brow presentation, *circa* 1668.

Brownian movement of minute particles, description of

ROBERT BROWN, Scottish botanist, 1773-1858, was the first to give an adequate description of the oscillating movement exhibited by minute particles suspended in a liquid. Observed in 1827; reported in 1828. Known as *Brownian movement.*

Brown-Sequard paralysis or syndrome

CHARLES EDOUARD BROWN-SEQUARD, British physiologist in France, 1817-1894, described a syndrome marked by a motor paralysis of one side of the body and loss of sensation on the other side. It is caused by a lesion involving one side of the spinal cord. Reported in 1850.

Brucella abortus, discovery of

BERNHARD LAURITS FREDERIK BANG, Danish physician, 1848-1932, discovered *Brucella abortus,* the organism causing infectious abortion in cattle and brucellosis in man. Reported in 1897.

Bruce's septicemia, causative agent of
. . . See under *Malta fever.*

Bruch's membrane
. . . See under *Choroid, basilar membrane of.*

Bubonic plague, flea as vector of
MASAKI OGATA, Tokyo physician, 1864-1919, was first to demonstrate that the flea, especially *Xenopsylla cheopis,* is the only or at least principal vector of the bubonic plague. Published in 1897.

Buccal cavity, diverticulum of, in embryo
MARTIN HEINRICH RATHKE, German anatomist, 1783-1860, discovered a diverticulum arising from the embryonic buccal cavity; from it arises the anterior lobe of the pituitary. Recorded in 1839. Known as *Rathke's pouch, craniobuccal pouch, neurobuccal pouch.*

Bucky diaphragm
. . . See under *Diaphragm used in roentgenography to prevent secondary rays from reaching the plate.*

Budinger-Ludloff-Läwen disease
. . . See under *Patella, pathologic fracture of cartilage of.*

Buerger's disease
. . . See under *Thromboangiitis obliterans, eponymic description of.*

Bufagin, isolation of
JOHN JACOB ABEL, Baltimore phar-

macologist and physiologist, 1857-1938, isolated bufagin, the digitalis-like substance found in the parotid glands of the toad *Bufo agua.* He reported the observations in 1911, in cooperation with DAVID I. MACHT, Baltimore pharmacologist, 1882-19??.

Bulbar paralysis, chronic progressive
GUILLAUME B. A. DUCHENNE, French neurologist, 1806-1875, gave the first accurate description of chronic progressive bulbar paralysis, marked by progressive atrophy and paralysis of the muscles of the mouth, lips, tongue, pharynx, and larynx, due to degeneration of the nerve nuclei in the floor of the fourth ventricle. Published in 1860.

Bulbourethral glands, description of—1684
JEAN MÉRY, French surgeon, 1645-1722, described two glands near the bulb of the corpus spongiosum. They communicate with the cavernous part of the urethra. Reported in 1684. Known as *Méry's glands* and *Cowper's glands.*

Bulbourethral glands, description of—1700
WILLIAM COWPER, English surgeon, 1666-1709, described the bulbourethral glands in an account "of two new glands and their excretory ducts lately discovered in human bodies," in 1700. Known as *Cowper's glands* and as *Méry's glands.*

Bullets in tissues, instrument for detecting
JOHN HARVEY GIRDNER, American physician, 1856-1933, devised an electric probe for the detection of

bullets or other metallic masses embedded in the tissues. Reported in 1887.

Bundle of His

. . . See under *Atrioventricular bundle, classic description of.*

Bundle of Lenhossek

. . . See under *Vagus and glossopharyngeal nerves, ascending roots of.*

Bundle-branch block as expressed in electrocardiogram

HANS EPPINGER, Austrian physician, 1879-1946, with OSCAR STOERK (German physician, 1870-1926), gave the first description of the electrocardiogramic changes associated with bundle-branch block. Published in 1910.

Bunsen burner, invention of

ROBERT W. BUNSEN, German chemist, 1811-1899, invented a gas burner provided with an adjustable opening near the base of the tube which allows an influx of air for complete oxidation of the burning gas. *Circa* 1855.

Bunyan bag in treatment of burns

JOHN BUNYAN, English naval surgeon, 1907-   , with WILLIAM STANNARD, developed a bag of water-proof material for use over wet dressings and in treatment of burns. Recorded in 1940.

Burdach's column

. . . See under *Cuneate fasciculus of spinal cord.*

Burnett's disinfecting solution

. . . See under *Zinc chloride disinfectant solution.*

Burns as cause of duodenal ulceration

. . . See under *Duodenal ulceration due to burns of skin.*

Burns, earliest classification of—1607

WILHELM FABRY (Fabricius Hildanus), German surgeon, 1560-1634, made the earliest known classification of burns, in 1607.

Burns, early classification of

GUILLAUME DUPUYTREN, French surgeon, 1777-1835, formulated an early classification of burns, in 1832.

Burns, treatment of, with Bunyan bag

. . . See under *Bunyan bag.*

Burns, treatment of, with gentian violet

ROBERT HENRY ALDRICH, Boston surgeon, 1902-   , is credited with introducing gentian violet in the treatment of burns. Recorded in 1933.

Burns, treatment of, with tannic acid and silver nitrate

. . . See under *Tannic acid-silver nitrate method.*

Burns's space

. . . See under *Triangular space above manubrium, between layers of cervical fascia.*

Burow's solution

. . . See under *Solution of aluminum acetate.*

Bursa, pharyngeal, in infants

HUBERT VON LUSCHKA, German anatomist, 1820-1875, described the pharyngeal bursa, a recess in the pharynx of a fetus or a young infant resulting from the ingrowth of epithelium along the course of the degenerating notochord. Published in 1873. Known as *Luschka's bursa.*

Butterfat in milk, determination of percentage of

STEPHEN MOULTON BABCOCK, American agricultural chemist, 1843-1931, invented a method for determining the butterfat content of milk by centrifuging a mixture of equal quantities of sulfuric acid and the milk to be tested. Reported in 1890.

***B*-wave, original description of**

. . . See under *Pulse, mid-diastolic wave in.*

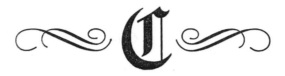

**C-4-dicarboxylic acid,
   catalytic role of**

ALBERT SZENT-GYÖRGYI, Hungarian biochemist, 1893-   , discovered the catalytic action of C-4-dicarboxylic acid in tissue respiration, *circa* 1930. Received the Nobel prize in 1937.

**Cachexia strumipriva,
   introduction of term**

EMIL THEODOR KOCHER, Swiss surgeon, 1841-1917, is credited with introducing the term *cachexia strumipriva,* to describe myxedema following total excision of the thyroid. Published in 1883.

Cadaver blood in transfusion

SERGEI SERGEIEVICH YUDIN, Moscow physician, 1892-1954, experimented with the use of cadaver blood in transfusion. Reported in 1933 and 1936. In 1937 he reported the conclusions derived from a thousand cases. The first attempt to use cadaver blood is said to have been made by DR. SAMOV, of Kharkov, in 1927.

**Cadaveric position of vocal
   cords in total paralysis**

CARL ADOLPH CHRISTIAN JACOB GERHARDT, German physician, 1833-1902, introduced the term *ca-daveric position,* to describe the position of the vocal cords in total paralysis. Published in 1872.

**Caesarean section, early
   successful**

HENDRIK VAN ROONHUYZE, Dutch surgeon, 1622-1672, performed several successful caesarean sections. Recorded in 1663.

**Caesarean section, lower-
   segment type of**

FRIEDRICH BENJAMIN OSIANDER, German surgeon, 1759-1822, introduced the lower-segment method of caesarean section, *circa* 1812.

**Caesarean section, Portes'
   classic method of**

LOUIS PORTES, French gynecologist, 1891-   , is credited with introducing the classic caesarean section in which the uterus is temporarily delivered from the abdominal cavity, emptied, and reintegrated. Recorded in 1924. Known as *Portes' operation.*

**Caesarean section, Saenger's
   operation of**

MAX SAENGER, German gynecologist, 1853-1903, devised the once classic operation in which the uterus was delivered through a long abdominal incision, emptied of its content, and then returned to the abdominal cavity. Recorded in 1882. Known as *Saenger's operation.*

Caesarean section, suprasymphyseal transperitoneal

FRITZ FRANK, German gynecologist, 1856-1923, introduced the suprasymphyseal transperitoneal caesarean section. Recorded in 1907.

Caesarean section, vaginal method of

ALFRED DÜHRSSEN, German gynecologist, 1862-1933, was the first to perform vaginal caesarean section, in April 1895. Recorded in 1898.

Caesarean section with hysterectomy and adnexectomy

EDOARDO PORRO, Italian surgeon, 1842-1902, introduced an operation combining caesarean section with excision of the uterus and adnexa. Recorded in 1876. Known as *Porro's operation.*

Caesarean section

... See also under *Cesarean section.*

Caisson disease due to liberation of nitrogen

PAUL BERT, French physician, 1833-1886, proposed the theory that the symptoms of caisson disease are due to the injury caused by the rapid liberation of nitrogen bubbles from the blood. Published in 1871.

Caisson disease, first description of

BRIAN POL, French surgeon, 182?-1888, with T. J. J. WATELLE, studied the effects of increased atmospheric pressure and described the condition now known as *caisson sickness* or *disease.* Published in 1854.

Calamus scriptorius, description and naming of

HEROPHILUS, Greek physician and anatomist in Egypt, 335-280 B.C., described and named the *calamus scriptorius,* the Latin for "writer's pen," a space at the lower part of the fourth ventricle. Exact date not available.

Calcaneus, epiphysitis of; eponymic description

JAMES WARREN SEVER, Boston orthopedic surgeon, 1878- , described epiphysitis of the *os calcis* or calcaneus, in 1908. Known as *Sever's disease.*

Calciferol, isolation of crystalline

ROBERT BENEDICT BOURDILLON, English biochemist, 1889- , with H. M. BRUCE, C. FISCHMANN, R. G. C. JENKINS, and T. A. WEBSTER, isolated crystalline calciferol (vitamin D-2) from irradiated ergosterol. Recorded in 1931.

Calcium in blood coagulation, first mention of essential part of

NICOLAS MAURICE ARTHUS, French physiologist, 1862-1945, established the importance of calcium in the process of blood coagulation. His report, published in 1890, is believed to be the earliest on this subject.

Calcium metabolism is controlled by parathyroid glands

WILLIAM GEORGE MACCALLUM, Baltimore pathologist, 1874-1944, with CARL VOEGTLIN (American pharmacologist, 1879-19??), demonstrated that the calcium metabolism is controlled by the parathyroid glands. Recorded (in Johns Hopkins Hospital Bulletin) in 1908.

Calomel ointment as prophylactic against syphilis

... See under *Syphilis.*

Caloric differential test for labyrinthine function

ROBERT BÁRÁNY, Austrian physician, 1876-1936, devised an irrigation test for the ear in which hot water produces one type of nystagmus while cold water causes an opposite type. If the labyrinth is diseased there is no nystagmus. Reported in 1907.

Caloric feeding of infants, introduction of

... See under *Infants, caloric requirements of.*

Campbell's area of cortex

... See under *Precentral area of cerebral cortex.*

Camptocormia in soldiers, early description of

ACHILLE ALEXANDER SOUQUES, French neurologist, 1860-1944, described camptocormia as seen in soldiers. Recorded in 1915.

Campus Foreli

... See under *Subthalamic region,* etc.

Canada balsam, early use of

... See under *Balsam, use of, in glass slide preparations.*

Canada balsam, use of, in histologic technique

JACOB A. L. CLARKE, English phy-

sician, 1817-1880, introduced the use of Canada balsam in mounting histologic specimens, a step which was an important advance in histologic technique. Recorded in 1851.

Canal for passage of auricular branch of vagus

FRIEDRICH ARNOLD, German anatomist, 1803-1890, described the passage in the petrous portion of the temporal bone for the auricular branch of the vagus. Reported in 1828. Known as *Arnold's canal.*

Canal of Hunter; subsartorial canal

JOHN HUNTER, Scottish surgeon, 1728-1793, described a space or canal on the medial aspect of the middle third of the thigh, under the sartorius muscle. It contains the femoral vessels and the saphenous vein. Reported in 1786. Known also as *canalis adductorius.*

Canal of Nuck

... See under *Round ligament, peritoneal diverticulum of.*

Canal of Schlemm, eponymic description of

FRIEDRICH S. SCHLEMM, German anatomist, 1795-1858, described the venous sinus of the sclera, a circular canal near the junction of the sclera with the cornea, which gives rise to the anterior ciliary veins. Published in 1830. Known as *Schlemm's canal* and *Lauth's canal.*

Canals of diploe, early description of

GILBERT BRESCHET, French anatomist, 1784-1845, gave the first accurate description of the canals of the diploe, in 1819. Known as *Breschet's canals.*

Canals of Petit; zonular spaces

FRANÇOIS POURFOUR DU PETIT, French physician and physiologist, 1664-1741, described spaces which surround the capsule or periphery of the crystalline lens, *circa* 1715.

Cancer, experiment in transmission of

BERNARD PEYRILHE, French physician, 1735-1804, attempted to transmit cancer by injecting material from a human breast cancer into a dog. Recorded in 1774.

Cancer, first successful use of radium in

S. W. GOLDBERG, Russian physician, 1872-19??, with EFIM SEMENOVICH LONDON (Russian physician, 1869-1939), used radium successfully in the treatment of cancer. Published in 1902.

Cancer, first successful use of x-rays in

. . . See under *Roentgen rays in treatment of cancer,* etc.

Cancer incidence in mice reduced by oophorectomy

. . . See under *Mammary cancer incidence in mice,* etc.

Cancer resulting from irritation by tar and paraffin

RICHARD VON VOLKMANN, German surgeon, 1830-1889, was the first to describe cancer resulting from irritation of the skin by coal tar and paraffin. Recorded in 1873.

Cancer, transmission of, by cell-free filtrate

FRANCIS PEYTON ROUS, American physician, 1879-19??, demonstrated the transmission of chicken sarcoma by injection of cell-free filtrates. Published in 1910. This form of chicken sarcoma is also known as *Rous sarcoma.*

Cancer, transmission of, by inoculation

CARL OLUF JENSEN, Copenhagen veterinary surgeon and pathologist, 1864-1934, demonstrated that carcinoma and sarcoma can be transplanted, and even retransplanted, in mice and rats. Report published in 1902.

Cancer, transplantation of, in mammals

ARTHUR NATHAN HANAU, German pathologist, 1858-1900, is credited with being first to transplant carcinoma in mammals, in the rat. Reported in 1889.

Candida albicans, discovery of—1839

BERNHARD RUDOLPH CONRAD VON LANGENBECK, German surgeon, 1810-1887, is said to have discovered *Candida albicans,* in 1839. F. T. BERG later proved the organism to be the causative agent of thrush.

Candida albicans, discovery of—1841

FREDRIK THEODOR BERG, Swedish physician, 1806-1887, discovered *Candida albicans* in a case of thrush, demonstrating that the organism is the causative agent of the disease. Recorded in 1841.

Candida albicans in thrush

. . . See also under *Thrush.*

Canthoplasty for correction of divergent strabismus

CORNELIUS REA AGNEW, American

ophthalmologist, 1830-1888, devised several operative procedures, including cantholplasty, for the correction of divergent squint, for chalazion, etc. The operation for divergent strabismus was reported in 1866.

Capillaries, distribution of, in muscles

AUGUST KROGH, Danish physiologist, 1874-1949, studied the distribution of the capillaries in the muscles and the oxygen pressure necessary for supplying the tissues. Reported in 1919.

Capillaries in muscle fibers of heart

. . . See under *Heart, capillaries in muscle fibers of*.

Capillary circulation, demonstration of, in the lungs

MARCELLO MALPIGHI, Italian anatomist, 1628-1694, is credited with discovering the capillary circulation in the lungs. Reported in 1661. This discovery filled the gap in Harvey's concept of the blood circuit.

Capillary pulse observed under fingernails

HEINRICH IRENAEUS QUINCKE, German physician, 1842-1922, described capillary pulsation visible under the fingernails. Recorded in 1868. Known as *Quincke's pulse*.

Capillary tubes, Poiseuille's law regarding flow in

. . . See under *Poiseuille's law*, etc.

Capon-comb test, introduction of

ANTOINE PEZARD, French physician, 18??-19??, is credited with in-

troducing the capon-comb test for the evaluation of androgens. Recorded in 1911.

Capsule surrounding renal glomerulus, description of

WILLIAM BOWMAN, English ophthalmologist and anatomist, 1816-1892, described the double-walled dilatation which surrounds the renal glomerulus and forms the beginning of a uriniferous tubule, in 1842. Known as *Bowman's capsule*.

Caramiphen in parkinsonism

. . . See under *Parkinsonism*.

Carbasone in treatment of amebiasis

ALFRED CUMMINGS REED, American physician, 1884-   , with H. H. ANDERSON, N. A. DAVID, and C. D. LEAKE, introduced the use of carbasone in the treatment of amebiasis. Recorded in 1932.

Carbohydrate breakdown, theory of, through stages involving citric acid

HANS ADOLF KREBS, English biochemist, 1900-   , proposed a theory of carbohydrate breakdown through stages involving citric acid. Known as *citric acid cycle. Circa* 1937.

Carbohydrate oxidation, aerobic, theory of

HANS ADOLF KREBS, English biochemist, 1900-   , promulgated a theory of aerobic carbohydrate oxidation. *Circa* 1937.

Carbolic acid, antispetic property of

FRANÇOIS JULES LEMAIRE, French scientist, 1814-1886, is credited with discovering the antiseptic quality of carbolic acid. Published in 1860.

Carbolic acid, diluted, impregnation of surgical dressings with

JOSEPH LISTER, English surgeon, 1827-1912, introduced the method of impregnating surgical dressings with diluted carbolic acid, in 1865. Reported in 1867.

Carbolic acid from coal tar

FRIEDLIEB FERDINAND RUNGE, German chemist, 1795-1867, was the first to prepare phenol by the destructive distillation of coal. Published in 1834.

Carbolic acid spray in operating room

JOSEPH LISTER, English surgeon, 1827-1912, introduced the use of a carbolic acid spray in the operating room as a sterilizing measure, in 1865. Reported in 1867.

Carbolic acid, use of, in obstetrics

ÉTIENNE STÉPHANE TARNIER, French obstetrician, 1828-1897, was first to use a solution of carbolic acid in obstetrics. Recorded in 1894.

Carbolic acid, use of, in treating tetanus

. . . See under *Tetanus*.

Carbon chain, theory of open

FRIEDRICH AUGUST KEKULÉ, German chemist, 1829-1896, announced his theory of the open carbon chain, in 1865.

Carbon dioxide, distribution of, between plasma and corpuscles

EDWARD PALMER POULTON, Eng-

glish physiologist, 1883-1939, with JACK JOFFA, investigated the partition or distribution of carbon dioxide between plasma and corpuscles in both reduced and oxygenated blood. Recorded in 1920.

Carbon dioxide gas as anesthetic

HENRY HILL HICKMAN, English surgeon, 1800-1830, rendered animals unconscious by the exclusion of air and the substitution of carbon dioxide, and demonstrated that operations could be performed without pain and with good results. Recorded in 1824.

Carbon dioxide is given off by skin, demonstration that

WILLIAM C. CRUIKSHANK, English surgeon, 1745-1800, demonstrated that the skin gives off carbon dioxide. Reported under the title "Experiments upon the insensible perspiration of the human body," in 1795.

Carbon dioxide, isolation of

JOSEPH BLACK, Scottish chemist, 1728-1799, is credited with isolating carbon dioxide, in 1754.

Carbon dioxide, liquefaction of

. . . See under *Liquefaction of gases,* etc.

Carbon monoxide in medicinal gases, apparatus for detecting

JAKOB EDWARD SCHMIDT, American physician and lexicographer, 1905-   , devised an apparatus and "shunt" method for the detection of carbon monoxide in gases, by the use of iodine pentoxide. Reported in the U.S.P. XI, in 1935.

Carbonic anhydrase, isolation of

NORMAN URQUHART MELDRUM,

English chemist, 1907-1933, with FRANCIS J. W. WORSLEY, isolated and studied carbonic anhydrase, the enzyme which catalyzes the decomposition of carbonic acid into carbon dioxide and water and thus assists the transfer of carbon dioxide from the tissues to the blood and the alveolar air. Recorded in 1933.

Carbon-zinc electric cell, invention of

ROBERT W. BUNSEN, German chemist, 1811-1899, devised an electric or galvanic cell in which the carbon element was placed in dilute nitric acid and the zinc electrode in dilute sulfuric acid, in 1841.

Carcinoma, first successful transplantation in mammals

. . . See under *Cancer.*

Carcinoma mucocellulare

. . . See under *Carcinoma of ovary, marked by signet-ring-like cells.*

Carcinoma of breast, spread of, by lymphatics

WILLIAM SAMPSON HANDLEY, English surgeon, 1872-19??, was probably the first to stress the importance of the lymphatics in the spread of mammary carcinoma, in 1906.

Carcinoma of bronchus, first successful removal of entire lung for

. . . See under *Lung, removal of,* etc.

Carcinoma of ovary, marked by signet-ring-like cells

FRIEDRICH ERNST KRUKENBERG, German pathologist, 1871-1946, described a type of carcinoma of the ovary, often metastatic, marked by

areas of degeneration and signet-ring-like cells. Published in 1896. Known as *Krukenberg's tumor, carcinoma mucocellulare,* and *fibrosarcoma ovarii mucocellulare.*

Carcinoma of uterine cervix, Schiller test for

WALTER SCHILLER, American pathologist, 1887-   , introduced an iodine test for the detection of carcinoma of the uterine cervix. The suspected area is painted with Lugol's solution and the appearance of white spots is considered a positive reaction. Published in 1933.

Cardiac asthma, eponymic description of

LÉON ROSTAN, French physician, 1790-1866, described cardiac asthma, in 1817. Known as *Rostan's asthma.*

Cardiac catheterization

. . . See under *Heart, catheterization of.*

Cardiac ganglion, eponymic description of

HEINRICH AUGUST WRISBERG, German anatomist, 1739-1808, described a ganglion of the superficial cardiac plexus situated under the aortic arch. Recorded in 1764. Known as *Wrisberg's ganglion.*

Cardiac muscle, scroll-like structure of

RICHARD LOWER, English physician, 1631-1691, is credited with discovering the scroll-like structure of the heart muscle. Recorded in 1669.

Cardiac output, determination of, by acetylene method

ARTHUR GROLLMAN, American

physiologist, 1901-   , studied the cardiac output of man by the use of the acetylene method. Reported in 1929.

Cardiac output, determination of, by gasometry

ADOLF FICK, German physiologist, 1829-1901, devised a method for determining cardiac output by gasometry. Reported in 1870. Known as *Fick's principle*.

Cardinal ligament

. . . See under *Mackenrodt's ligament*.

Cardiolysis, introduction of

LUDOLPH BRAUER, German physician, 1865-1951, was the first to suggest the method of cardiolysis for relief of adhesive pericarditis. The operation is said to have been performed by DR. PETERSEN. Recorded in 1902.

Cardio-omentopexy, introduction of

CLAUDE SCHAEFFER BECK, American surgeon, 1894-   , with VLADIMIR LESLIE TICHY, introduced an operation in which a portion of the omentum is drawn through the diaphragm and sutured to the heart, to provide collateral circulation to the cardiac muscle. Published in 1935.

Cardioptosis; Rummo's disease

. . . See under *Heart, downward displacement of*.

Carotid artery, ligation of

ASTLEY PASTON COOPER, English surgeon, 1768-1841, ligated the common carotid artery for aneurysm on Nov. 1, 1805. In this case the patient died, but another operation, performed June 22, 1808, proved successful and the patient lived until 1821.

Carotid body tumors, early account of pathology of

FELIX JACOB MARCHAND, German pathologist, 1846-1928, gave what is probably the first description of the pathology of carotid body tumors, in 1891.

Carotid sinus depressor reflex

TORALD HERMANN SOLLMANN, American pharmacologist, 1874-19??, described the carotid sinus depressor reflex, the slowing of the heart rate when pressure is applied on the carotid artery at the level of the cricoid cartilage, in 1912.

Carotid sinus depressor reflex

HEINRICH E. HERING, German physiologist, 1866-1948, described the carotid sinus reflex, a slowing of the heart caused by pressure on the carotid artery at the level of the cricoid cartilage. Recorded in 1923.

Carotid sinus, discovery of function of

CORNEILLE HEYMANS, Belgian pharmacologist, 1892-   , discovered the function of the carotid sinus in the regulation of respiration and blood pressure. Reported in 1929, 1933, etc. Received the Nobel prize in 1938.

Carotid sinus syndrome; original description as such

SOMA WEISS, Boston physician, 1898-1942, with JAMES PORTER BAKER, described the carotid sinus in health and disease, especially its role in the causation of fainting and convulsions. Recorded in 1933.

Carotid sinus syndrome

. . . See also under *Vasovagal syncope.*

Carotid tubercle of sixth cervical vertebra

EDOUARD P. M. CHASSAIGNAC, French surgeon, 1804-1879, noted and described a well-developed anterior tubercle on the transverse process of the sixth cervical vertebra. Known as *Chassaignac's tubercle.* Recorded *circa* 1845.

Carrel-Dakin solution for irrigation of wounds

. . . See under *Solution of chlorinated soda and sodium bicarbonate.*

Carrel-Dakin treatment of wounds

ALEXIS CARREL, French surgeon, 1873-1944, with HENRY DRYSDALE DAKIN and associates, introduced the Carrel-Dakin method for treating wounds by means of Dakin's solution. Recorded in 1915.

***Carrión's disease,* introduction of term**

ERNESTO ODRIOZOLA, Peruvian physician, 1862-1921, introduced the name *Carrión's disease* in honor of DANIEL A. CARRIÓN (a student in Peru, 1850-1885) who died of the disease while studying it. Published in 1895. Known also as *Oroya fever.*

Cartilage of first branchial arch, eponymic description of

JOHANN FRIEDRICH MECKEL (the younger), German anatomist, 1781-1833, described the cartilage of the mandibular or first branchial arch, in 1805. Known as *Meckel's cartilage.*

Cartilage of hyoid arch of embryo

KARL BOGISLAUS REICHERT, German anatomist, 1811-1883, described the cartilage of the hyoid arch of the embryo which gives rise to the styloid process, the lesser cornu of the hyoid bone, and other structures. Recorded in 1836. Known as *Reichert's cartilage.*

Cartilage of Luschka

. . . See under *Vocal cord, cartilaginous nodule in.*

Casein coat surrounding milk globules, discovery of

FERDINAND MORITZ ASCHERSON, German physician, 1798-1879, discovered the casein membrane or coat which surrounds milk globules. Reported in 1831.

Catalytic metabolism of glycogen

. . . See under *Glycogen, catalytic metabolism of.*

Cataract extraction by suction with a special instrument

IGNACIO BARRAQUER, Spanish ophthalmologist, 1884-   , devised a method for extracting a cataract by means of suction with a special instrument. Reported in 1917. Known as *Barraquer's operation.*

Cataract, extraction of lens in, modern method of

JACQUES DAVIEL, French ophthalmologist, 1693-1762, is believed to have originated the modern method of extracting the lens in cataract, in 1748.

Cataract, opacity of lens in

ANTOINE MAITRE-JAN, French ophthalmologist, 1650-1730, demonstrated that cataract consists of an opacity in the lens. Previously, cataract was explained by the assumed presence of a pellicle inside of the capsule of the lens. Noted in 1692; published in 1707.

Catatonia as disease entity, recognition of

KARL LUDWIG KAHLBAUM, German psychiatrist, 1828-1899, described catatonia as a separate disease entity, in 1869.

Catgut ring in intestinal anastomosis

ROBERT ABBE, American surgeon, 1851-1928, developed the catgut rings used for supporting the ends of the intestine in the operation for intestinal anastomosis. Reports published in 1889 and 1892.

Catheterization of heart

. . . See under *Heart, catheterization of.*

Catheterization of individual ureters in male

HOWARD ATWOOD KELLY, Baltimore gynecologist, 1858-1943, developed a method for the catheterization of the individual ureters in the male. Recorded in 1898.

Catheterization of ureters, systematization of

JOAQUIN ALBARRAN Y DOMINGUEZ, Cuban urologist in France, 1860-1912, is associated with inventions of cystoscopes and the systematization of catheterization of ureters. Reports published in 1889 and 1909.

Catheters, French scale for

. . . See under *Scale for measuring size of urethral sounds and catheters.*

Cathode, introduction of term

MICHAEL FARADAY, English chemist and physicist, 1791-1867, introduced the term *cathode,* to designate the electrode in which, in his concept, the electric current went down or "set." The word is derived from the Greek *kata* (down) and *hodos* (way). Recorded in 1833.

Cation, introduction of term

MICHAEL FARADAY, English chemist and physicist, 1791-1867, introduced the term *cation,* to describe those ions which move in the electrolyte toward the cathode. Reported in 1833.

Caudal anesthesia, introduction of

FERNARD CATHELIN, French surgeon, 1873-1945, is credited with introducing caudal anesthesia in which the anesthetic was injected into the epidural space through the sacrococcygeal ligament. Published in 1901.

Causalgia, first description of

SILAS WEIR MITCHELL, American neurologist, 1829-1914, was first to describe causalgia resulting from injury to peripheral nerves, as observed in the United States General Hospital, in Philadelphia. Recorded in 1864.

Cautery punch in urologic procedures

JOHN ROBERTS CAULK, American urologist, 1881-1938, introduced the so-called cautery punch in urologic practice. Recorded in 1920.

Caval valve

. . . See under *Valvula venae cavae.*

Cavernous respiration, introduction of term

AUSTIN FLINT, American physician, 1812-1886, is credited with having introduced the term *cavernous respiration, circa* 1856.

Cavum septi pellucidi, early description of

JULIUS CAESAR ARANTIUS, Italian physician, 1530-1589, gave an early, and possibly the first, description of the median cleft between the two laminae of the septum pellucidum, in 1571. Also called *ventricle of Arantius, fifth ventricle,* and *pseudocele.*

Cecostomy, first recorded case of

P. PILLORE, French surgeon, 1748-1809, is credited with performing cecostomy in 1776. Recorded by J. Z. AMUSSAT, in 1839.

Celiac disease, early description of—1888

SAMUEL JONES GEE, English pediatrician, 1839-1911, was the first to describe a diarrheal disease of children, similar to or identical with sprue, in 1888. The condition was described later, in 1908, by CHRISTIAN A. HERTER (American physician, 1865-1910). Known as *Gee-Herter disease.*

Cell division, changes involved in

WALTHER FLEMMING, German anatomist, 1843-1905, described the changes involved in cell division. Published in 1879.

Cell structure of plants, discovery of

MATTHIAS JAKOB SCHLEIDEN, Hamburg botanist, 1804-1881, demonstrated that plants are made of tissues which are composed of cells. He also held that growth is accomplished by increase in the number of cells. Published in 1838.

Cell theory, founder of

THEODOR SCHWANN, German anatomist, 1810-1882, is regarded as the founder of the cell theory as applied to animals. Schwann was aided by SCHLEIDEN's recognition that the cell is the unit of plant structure. Published in 1839.

Cells, first artificial culture of

LEO LOEB, American pathologist, 1869-19??, is credited with being first to culture cells artificially, in 1898.

Cells in cerebral cortex with ascending axons

GIOVANNI MARTINOTTI, Italian pathologist, 1857-1928, described fusiform cells in the cerebral cortex with ascending axis-cylinder processes running toward the surface and ramifying horizontally, in 1898. Known as *Martinotti's cells.*

Cells in crypts of Lieberkühn in small intestine

JOSEF PANETH, German physician, 1857-1890, described cells in the fundus of the crypts of Lieberkühn containing eosinophil granules. Published in 1888. Known as *cells of Paneth.*

Cells of Hensen

. . . See under *Organ of Corti, outermost cells covering.*

Cells of Paneth

. . . See under *Cells in crypts of Lieberkühn in small intestine.*

Cementum fibrils; Ebner's fibrils
. . . See under *Fibrils in dentin and cementum of tooth.*

Centigrade thermometer or scale
ANDERS CELSIUS, Swedish astronomer, 1701-1744, devised a thermometer scale in which the interval between the boiling point and the freezing point is divided into one hundred parts or degrees. Reported in 1742.

Central canal of vitreous
. . . See under *Hyaloid canal of eye.*

Centrifugation in separating red from white corpuscles
MAGNUS GUSTAV BLIX, Swedish physician, 1849-1904, is credited with suggesting the use of centrifugal force in separating red from white corpuscles. Recorded in 1884.

Centrosome, discovery of
EDOUARD VAN BENEDEN, Belgian embryologist, 1846-1910, and WALTHER FLEMMING, German anatomist, 1843-1905, working independently, discovered the centrosome, in 1876.

Centrosome, first application of term
THEODOR BOVERI, German zoologist, 1862-1915, was the first to apply the word *centrosome* to the body now bearing this name, which was discovered by FLEMMING and VAN BENEDEN. Reported in 1888.

Centrum ovale, first correct description of
RAYMOND VIEUSSENS, French anatomist, 1641-1715, is credited with giving the first correct description of the centrum ovale. Published in 1685.

Cephalic version, combined, introduction of
MARMADUKE BURR WRIGHT, American obstetrician, 1803-1879, introduced the method of combined cephalic version. Published in 1854.

Cephalotribe, invention of
LOUIS AUGUSTE BAUDELOCQUE, French obstetrician, 1800-1864, invented the cephalotribe in 1833.

Cerebellar sclerosis, hereditary
. . . See under *Hereditary cerebellar sclerosis.*

Cerebellum as center of static and tonic functions
LUIGI LUCIANI, Italian physiologist, 1840-1919, investigated the cerebellum, working with decerebellated dogs, and showed it to be the organ concerned with tonic and static functions. Published in 1891.

Cerebellum, branching neurons in cortex of
JOHANNES EVANGELISTA VON PURKINJE, Bohemian physiologist, 1787-1869, described large branching neurons in the middle layer of the cerebellar cortex Recorded in 1837. Known as *Purkinje's cells* or *corpuscles.*

Cerebellum is organ of coordination, demonstration that
MARIE J. P. FLOURENS, French physiologist, 1794-1867, experimented with pigeons and demonstrated that removal of the cerebellum resulted in loss of coordination and equilibrium. Reported in 1823.

Cerebellum, naming of
ERASISTRATUS, Greek anatomist and physician, *circa* 300-250 B.C.,

described and named the cerebellum.

Cerebral atrophy with aphasia

ARNOLD PICK, Prague neurologist, 1851-1924, described a form of circumscribed cerebral atrophy marked by progressive dementia and aphasia. Published in 1892. Known as *Arnold Pick disease*.

Cerebral cortex, cells in, with ascending axons

... See under *Cells in cerebral cortex with ascending axons*.

Cerebral cortex, electric stimulation of

GUSTAV T. FRITSCH, German neurologist, 1838-1927, with EDUARD HITZIG (German neurologist and psychiatrist, 1838-1907), experimented with electric stimulation of the frontal lobe of the cerebral cortex, demonstrating the existence of a motor area. Reported in 1870.

Cerebral cortex, layer of fibers parallel to tangential fibers of

VLADIMIR MICHAILOVICH BECHTEREV, Russian neurologist, 1857-1927, described a layer of fibers in the cerebral cortex situated parallel to the tangential fibers. Reported in 1891. Known as *Bechterev's fibers*.

Cerebral cortex, line running parallel to surface of

FRANCESCO GENNARI, Italian anatomist, *circa* 1750-1795, described one of two bands of white fibers running parallel to the surface of the cerebral cortex and seen on section. Reported in 1782. Known as the *line* or *stripe* of *Gennari*.

Cerebral cortex, motor and sensory areas, early mapping of—1876

PAUL EMIL FLECHSIG, German neurologist, 1847-1929, charted the motor and sensory areas of the cerebral cortex, in 1876.

Cerebral cortex reflex; Haab's reflex

... See under *Pupillary contraction without accommodation or convergence*.

Cerebral encephalography and arteriography, introduction of

ANTONIO C. A. F. EGAS MONIZ, Portuguese neurologist, 1874-19??, introduced arterial encephalography and obtained the first arteriogram. Reported in 1927.

Cerebral function, early attempt at localization of

FRANZ JOSEPH GALL, German anatomist, 1758-1828, with JOHANN CASPAR SPURZHEIM, made an attempt to localize cerebral function. Although the results were inaccurate, the work stimulated further research in the field, and, among other things, laid the foundation of phrenology. Published between 1810 and 1819.

Cerebral function localization, fundamental work on

DAVID FERRIER, Scottish neurologist in England, 1843-1928, laid the foundation of the knowledge concerning localization of cerebral functions. Work published in 1876.

Cerebral hernia, artificial, as means of decompression in brain tumor

HARVEY W. CUSHING, Boston surgeon, 1869-1939, established a

method for decompressing in cases of inaccessible brain tumors by forming an artificial cerebral hernia. Reported in 1905.

Cerebral inhibition of spinal reflexes

. . . See under *Spinal reflexes,* etc.

Cerebral spastic paralysis, congenital; eponymic description

WILLIAM JOHN LITTLE, English surgeon, 1810-1894, described a form of congenital spastic paralysis in infants, due to insufficient development of the pyramidal tracts. Reported in a series of lectures, in 1843. Known as *Little's disease.*

Cerebroside lipoidosis; Gaucher's disease

. . . See under *Familial splenic anemia.*

Cerebrospinal fever, description of—1805

GASPARD VIEUSSEUX, Geneva physician, 1746-1814, gave the earliest description of cerebrospinal fever, in 1805.

Cerebrospinal fever, first report of epidemic

THOMAS WILLIS, English physician and anatomist, 1621-1675, is believed to have been the first to record an epidemic of cerebrospinal fever, in 1661. Published in 1684.

Cerebrospinal fever in America, use of serum for

SIMON FLEXNER, American pathologist and bacteriologist, 1863-1946, developed a serum for cerebrospinal fever, in 1907. Known as *Flexner's serum.*

Cerebrospinal fever in Germany, use of serum for

GEORG JOCHMANN, German physician, 1874-1915, developed a serum for use against meningococcic infections, in 1906.

Cerebrospinal fever

. . . See also under *Cerebrospinal meningitis.*

Cerebrospinal fluid, chemical constituents of

WILLIAM MESTREZAT, French neurologist, 1883-1928, gave the first accurate description of the chemical constituents of the cerebrospinal fluid. Published in 1911.

Cerebrospinal fluid, demonstration of origin of

WALTER E. DANDY, Baltimore neurosurgeon, 1886-1946, demonstrated the origin of the cerebrospinal fluid, in 1913.

Cerebrospinal fluid, excess of globulin in

. . . See under *Globulin in cerebrospinal fluid.*

Cerebrospinal fluid, first description of

DOMENICO COTUGNO, Italian anatomist, 1736-1822, was the first to describe the cerebrospinal fluid, in 1764.

Cerebrospinal fluid, pathways of escape of

LEWIS HILL WEED, American anatomist, 1886-1952, studied the pathways of escape of the cerebrospinal fluid from the subarachnoid space. Recorded in 1914.

Cerebrospinal meningitis, epidemic, first description of

ELISHA NORTH, American physician, 1771-1843, is credited with being first to describe epidemic cerebrospinal meningitis, in 1811.

Cerebrospinal meningitis, Kernig's sign of

VLADIMIR MICHAILOVICH KERNIG, Russian physician, 1840-1917, discovered a method for testing meningeal irritation by extending the leg at the knee with the thigh flexed at right angle to the body. In meningitis, this maneuver meets with resistance or elicits pain. Published in 1882. Known as *Kernig's sign* or *maneuver.*

Cerebrospinal meningitis

. . . See also under *Cerebrospinal fever.*

Cerebrospinal syphilis, treatment of, with blood serum of patient

HOMER F. SWIFT, American physician, 1881-1953, with ARTHUR W. M. ELLIS (English physician, 1883-), devised a method for treating general paresis or cerebrospinal syphilis by intradural injection of the patient's blood serum taken after the injection of arsphenamine. Reported in 1912. Known as the *Swift-Ellis treatment.*

Cerebrum is organ of cerebration or thought, demonstration that

MARIE J. P. FLOURENS, French physiologist, 1794-1867, experimented with pigeons and demonstrated that the removal of the cerebrum leaves the reflexes intact but causes loss of cerebration. Reported in 1823.

Cerebrum, naming of

ERASISTRATUS, Greek anatomist and physician, *circa* 300-250 B.C.,

described and named the cerebrum. Exact date not available.

Cerium, discovery of

JÖNS JAKOB BERZELIUS, Swedish chemist, 1779-1848, discovered the element cerium in 1803. The name is based on the asteroid *Ceres,* prominent at that time.

Ceruminous glands, first mention of

NIELS STENSEN, Danish anatomist, 1638-1686, is credited with being first to describe the cerumen-producing glands of the body. Published in 1662.

Cervical carcinoma, smear diagnosis of

GEORGE NICHOLAS PAPANICOLAOU, Greek anatomist and physician in the United States, 1883- , with HERBERT FREDERICK TRAUT, developed the method of diagnosing carcinoma of the cervix by the use of vaginal smears. Recorded in 1941.

Cervical dilator made of steel, by Bossi

LUIGI MARIA BOSSI, Italian obstetrician, 1859-1919, devised a steel instrument which he used to dilate the cervical canal. Reported in 1892.

Cervical dilators, by Hegar

ALFRED HEGAR, German gynecologist, 1830-1914, invented a series of metal bougies or sounds of varying sizes for dilating the cervix of the uterus. Recorded in 1872.

Cervical rib, scalenotomy for relief of symptoms due to

. . . See under *Scalenotomy for relief,* etc.

Cervical sympathetic, paralysis of, syndrome resulting from

JOHANN FRIEDRICH HORNER, Swiss ophthalmologist, 1831-1886, described a syndrome resulting from paralysis of the cervical sympathetic nerves, in 1869. It is marked by ptosis of the upper lid, enophthalmos, miosis, anhidrosis, etc. Known as *Horner's syndrome*.

Cervical vertebrae, congenital fusion of

MAURICE KLIPPEL, French neurologist, 1858-1942, with ANDRÉ FEIL (French physician, 1884-   ), described congenital fusion of the cervical vertebrae, marked by shortness of the neck, limitation of movement, etc. Published in 1892. Known as *Klippel-Feil* syndrome.

Cervical zone of uterus, definition of

ROBERT BARNES, English obstetrician, 1817-1907, gave a definitive description of the cervical zone of the uterus, limiting it to the lowest fourth of the internal surface of the uterus. *Circa* 1880.

Cervix, first successful excision of, in America

JOHN B. STRACHAN, American surgeon, 1788-1861, is credited with being the first to perform a successful cervicectomy in America. Reported by T. F. Gillian in 1829.

Cervix, laceration of; early account of repair

THOMAS ADDIS EMMET, American gynecologist, 1828-1919, performed surgical repair of cervical laceration. Recorded in 1869.

Cesarean section, first, in United States

JOHN LAMBERT RICHMOND, Newton, Ohio, surgeon, 1785-1855, is said to have performed the first successful cesarean section in the United States, on April 22, 1827.

Cesarean section for women dying in late pregnancy

NUMA POMPILIUS, second king of Rome, 715-673 B.C., ordered abdominal section for women dying in late pregnancy or in childbirth, in order to deliver the child. Known as *lex regia;* under the Caesars it was called *lex Caesaria.* Exact date not available.

Cesarean section

. . . See also under *Caesarean section*.

Cesium, discovery of

ROBERT W. BUNSEN, German chemist, 1811-1899, discovered the element cesium in 1860, in collaboration with G. R. KIRCHHOFF, German physicist. The name is derived from the Latin *caesius,* bluish-gray, in allusion to the two blue lines of its spectrum.

Cesium, effect of, on rate of oxidation of sewage

JAKOB EDWARD SCHMIDT, American physician and lexicographer, 1905-   , investigated the problem of catalysis in sewage disposal and found that the addition of small quantities of cesium, rubidium, and certain other metals greatly accelerated the rate of oxidation of the sewage. Recorded in 1934.

Chabert's disease

. . . See under *Anthrax, first adequate clinical description of*.

Chair for surgical and obstetrical operations, invention of

CHRISTOPHER JOHNSTON, American surgeon, 1822-1891, devised an operating chair for surgical and obstetrical operations and vaginal examinations. Recorded in 1860.

Chalazion, operation for treatment of

CORNELIUS REA AGNEW, American ophthalmologist, 1830-1888, devised several operative procedures for the treatment of eye defects, including one for chalazion. Reported *circa* 1866.

Chalazion

. . . See also under *Meibomian cyst.*

Chancre, hard, eponymic description of

JOHN HUNTER, Scottish surgeon in England, 1728-1793, described the primary lesion of syphilis, after inoculating himself experimentally with the discharge of a patient who had both gonorrhea and syphilis, in 1767. Recorded in 1786. Known as *Hunterian chancre.*

Chancre, lymphatic; Nisbet's chancre

WILLIAM NISBET, English physician, 1759-1822, described ulcerative nodules in the penis, following lymphangitis resulting from chancroid. Published in 1787.

Chancre, mixed form of

JOSEPH PIERRE ROLLETT, French physician, 1824-1894, demonstrated the existence of mixed lesions which are the result of syphilis and some other infection. Published in 1866. Known as *mixed chancre* and *Rollett's disease.*

Chancres, soft and hard, demonstration of

PHILIPPE RICORD, French urologist and dermatologist, 1800-1889, described the chancre and differentiated between a soft chancre (*ulcus molle*) and a hard chancre (*ulcus durum*), in 1838.

Chancroid, causative organism of

AUGUSTO DUCREY, Italian physician, 1860-1940, discovered *Hemophilus ducreyi,* the causative agent of chancroid. Published in 1889.

Chancroid, first clear description of

LEON BASSEREAU, French physician, 1811-1888, gave the first clear description of chancroid, in 1852.

Chapman bag, invention of

. . . See under *Ice bag for application to the spine.*

Characteristics, acquired, may be transmitted to next generation

. . . See under *Theory of inheritance of acquired characteristics.*

Charcot-Leyden crystals

. . . See under *Crystals occurring in sputum in bronchial asthma and bronchitis.*

Charcot-Marie-Tooth disease

. . . See under *Neuropathic muscular atrophy, progressive,* etc .

Charcot's joint

. . . See under *Neurogenic arthropathy.*

Chaulmoogra oil, introduction of, to Western medicine

FREDERIC JOHN MOUAT, English physician in Indian Service, 1816-

1897, is credited with introducing the use of chaulmoogra oil in the treatment of leprosy to Western medicine, in 1854. The oil was, however, used by Chinese physicians and others many centuries earlier.

Chaulmoogra oil, use of, in leprosy

HARRY T. HOLLMANN, Hawaiian physician, 1878-19??, with A. L. DEAN, described the use of chaulmoogra oil in the treatment of leprosy, in 1919.

Check ligaments
. . . See under *Odontoid ligaments, lateral.*

Cheek, fat pad in, description of
. . . See under *Fat pad in cheek.*

Cheilitis glandularis apostematosa
. . . See under *Myxadenitis labialis.*

Cheiropompholyx, original description of

JONATHAN HUTCHINSON, English surgeon, 1828-1913, wrote a classic description of cheiropompholyx, a condition marked by the formation of vesicles on the palms and soles. Recorded in 1875.

Chemical equilibrium, introduction of concept of

CLAUDE LOUIS BERTHOLLET, French chemist, 1748-1822, introduced the concept of chemical equilibrium, in 1801.

Chemical formulae, structural, introduction of

FRIEDRICH A. KEKULÉ VON STRADONITZ, German chemist, 1829-1896, devised a structural formula for benzene in 1865, and thus started the trend for using such formulae to designate other chemical compounds.

Chemical structure in relation to physiologic action

ALEXANDER CRUM BROWN, Scottish physiologist, 1838-1922, and THOMAS RICHARD FRASER, Scottish pharmacologist, 1841-1919, were the first to study the relationship between chemical structure of drugs and physiologic action. Published in 1868-9.

Chemical symbols and formulas, modern system of

JÖNS JAKOB BERZELIUS, Swedish chemist, 1779-1848, introduced the modern system of expressing chemical symbols and formulas by using the Latin names of the elements followed by a numerical notation. *Circa* 1820.

Chemistry, first substantial textbook of

ANDREAS LIBAVIUS (Libau), German chemist, 1546-1616, compiled the contemporary knowledge of chemistry and published a book titled *Alchymia*, in 1595. This book is regarded by some as the first real textbook on chemistry.

Chemistry, founder of modern

ANTOINE LAURENT LAVOISIER, French chemist, 1743-1794, is regarded as the founder of modern chemistry.

Chick, development of, as seen through microscope

MARCELLO MALPIGHI, Italian anatomist, 1628-1694, wrote several dissertations on the development of the chick, as seen through the microscope. Recorded in 1673 and 1675.

Chickenpox and scarlet fever, distinction between

GIOVAN FILIPPO INGRASSIA, Italian physician and anatomist, 1510-1580, is credited with distinguishing between scarlet fever and chickenpox, in 1553.

Chickenpox and smallpox, distinction between

WILLIAM HEBERDEN, *père,* English physician, 1710-1801, gave one of the earliest clear descriptions of chickenpox and differentiated it from smallpox, *circa* 1764. Reported in 1768.

Chickenpox, inclusion bodies in

ERNEST EDWARD TYZZER, American pathologist, 1875-19??, was the first to describe inclusion bodies in varicella. Recorded in 1905-6.

Chigoe or jigger, first description of

DON GONÇALO FERNANDEZ DE OVIDEO Y VALDÉS, Spanish naturalist, 1478-1557, was the first to describe the chigoe (jigger), a sand flea of tropical America. Published in 1525.

Child with congenital syphilis will not infect its mother if mother has no signs of the disease

ABRAHAM COLLES, Irish surgeon, 1773-1843, promulgated the axiom that a child with congenital syphilis will not infect its mother if the mother shows no signs of the disease. Reported in 1837. The same maxim was announced by PIERRE P. F. BAUMES, French physician, 1791-1871, in 1840. Known as *Colles' law, Baumes' law,* and *Colles-Baumes law.*

Childbirth, nitrous oxide-oxygen anesthesia in

. . . See under *Nitrous oxide-oxygen anesthesia.*

Children, dosage of medicine for

THOMAS YOUNG, English physician, 1773-1829, devised a formula for the determination of dosage for children over two years of age; it is expressed by adding 12 to the age and dividing the sum by the age. Published in 1813. Known as *Young's rule.*

Children from tuberculous households, boarding out of

JACQUES JOSEPH GRANCHER, French physician, 1843-1907, introduced the system of boarding out children from tuberculous households, in France. Known as *Grancher's system.* Established in 1903.

Children of tuberculous parents are not born with the disease but are prone to be affected later

GEORGES KUSS, French physician, 1867-1936, established that the children of tuberculous parents are not born with tuberculosis but are prone to be affected later. Reported in 1898.

Children's dispensary, first, in Europe

GEORGE ARMSTRONG, English pediatrician, 1719-1789, is credited with being the founder of the first children's dispensary in Europe, in 1769.

Chimney sweep's cancer of scrotum

PERCIVALL POTT, English surgeon, 1714-1788, described cancer of the scrotum, an occupational disease of chimney sweeps. Published in 1775. This is said to be the first record of cancer due to industrial or occupational injury.

Chiralgia paresthetica; neuritis of branch of radial nerve

ROBERT WARTENBERG, American neurologist, 1887- , described an isolated neuritis of the superficial branch of the radial nerve, known as chiralgia paresthetica, *circa* 1917.

Chloral, appreciation of, as a hypnotic

MATHIAS E. O. LIEBREICH, German physician, 1839-1908, recognized the pharmacologic action of chloral and introduced it as a hypnotic. Reported in 1869.

Chloral, discovery of

JUSTUS VON LIEBIG, German chemist, 1803 - 1873, discovered that chloral is formed by the interaction of chlorine and alcohol. He derived the name chloral from *chlor*ine and *al*cohol. Discovery made in 1831; report published in 1832.

Chloramphenicol, production of

JOHN EHRLICH, American scientist, 1907- , with Q. R. BARTZ, R. M. SMITH, D. A. JOSLYN, and P. R. BURKHOLDER, discovered chloramphenicol. It was first isolated from *Streptomyces venezuelae* contained in a sample of soil taken near Caracas, Venezuela. Published in 1947.

Chloride shift

. . . See under *Albumin and chloride shift between plasma and erythrocytes.*

Chlorine, discovery of

KARL WILHELM SCHEELE, Swedish chemist, 1742-1786, is credited with discovering chlorine, which he thought was a form of hydrochloric acid, in 1774.

Chlorine, naming of

HUMPHRY DAVY, English chemist and physicist, 1778 - 1829, introduced the name *chlorine*, based on the Greek *chloros* (green), in allusion to the greenish color of the gas. Published in 1811.

Chloroform administered through tracheal tube

WILLIAM MACEWEN, Scottish surgeon, 1848-1924, was the first to administer chloroform by means of a tracheal tube inserted through the mouth. Recorded in 1880.

Chloroform, discovery of—1831

EUGENE SOUBEIRAN, French chemist, 1793-1858, discovered chloroform in 1831. Published in 1831.

Chloroform, discovery of—1832

SAMUEL GUTHRIE, American physician, 1782-1848, discovered chloroform, probably in 1831. Published in 1832.

Chloroform, discovery of—1832

JUSTUS VON LIEBIG, German chemist, 1803-1873, is credited with discovering chloroform in 1831, but the report was published in 1832.

Chloroform, discovery of anesthetic properties of—1847

MARIE J. P. FLOURENS, French

physiologist, 1794 - 1867, discovered the anesthetic properties of chloroform, *circa* 1847.

Chloroform, introduction of, in obstetrics

JAMES YOUNG SIMPSON, Scottish obstetrician, 1811-1870, is credited with being the first to use chloroform anesthesia in obstetrics, in England. Recorded in 1847.

Chloroma, first case of

ALLAN BURNS, Scottish physician and anatomist, 1781-1813, is believed to have been the first to describe a case of chloroma, in 1811. Also called *chlorosarcoma* and *green cancer*.

Chloromycetin, discovery of

. . . See under *Chloramphenicol*.

Chloromycetin in typhus

. . . See under *Typhus*, etc.

Chlorophyll, early recognition of—1779

JAN INGENHOUSZ, Dutch physician and naturalist, 1730-1799, discovered that only the green parts of plants are able to absorb carbon dioxide in the presence of light. Recorded in 1779.

Chlorophyll, early recognition of—1837

RENÉ JOACHIM HENRI DUTROCHET, French physiologist, 1776 - 1847, demonstrated that only those plant cells which contain green pigment are capable of absorbing carbon dioxide in the presence of light. Published in 1837.

Chlorosis, blood in, deficient in iron

FERDINAND FOEDISCH, German physician, 178?-18??, demonstrated that the blood of chlorotic patients is deficient in iron. Published in 1832.

Chlorosis, description of, as a clinical entity

FRIEDRICH HOFFMANN, German physician, 1660 - 1742, is credited with giving an accurate description of chlorosis and recognizing it as a clinical entity. Reported in 1730.

Chlorosis, Egyptian, is due to ancylostomiasis

WILHELM GRIESINGER, German neurologist, 1817-1868, recognized the relationship between ancylostomiasis and Egyptian chlorosis. Recorded in 1854. The condition was once known as *Griesinger's disease*.

Chlorosis, first definite description of

JOHANN LANGE, German physician, 1485-1565, is credited with giving the first definite description of chlorosis, in 1554.

Chlorosis marked by reduction in hemoglobin content

JOHN DUNCAN, Scottish physician, 1839-1899, is credited with demonstrating that in chlorosis the hemoglobin content is diminished but the number of red blood cells is almost unchanged. Reported in 1867.

Chlorosis, pills of iron sulfate and potassium carbonate in treatment of

PIERRE BLAUD, French physician, 1774-1858, introduced the use of "Blaud's pills," now known as pills of ferrous carbonate, in the treatment of chlorosis. Published in 1832.

Chocolate cysts of ovary

JOHN ALBERTSON SAMPSON, American surgeon, 1873-1946, described chocolate cysts of the ovary resulting from endometriosis. Published in 1921.

Cholangiography, first use of

ADOLPH REICH, American gynecologist, 1864-19??, is said to have been the first to obtain cholangiograms, after "accidental injection of bile ducts with petrolatum and bismuth paste." Recorded in 1918.

Cholecystectomy, first recorded successful

CARL JOHANN AUGUST LANGENBUCH, German surgeon, 1846-1901, performed the first successful excision of the gallbladder, on July 15, 1882.

Cholecystography, introduction of successful

EVART AMBROSE GRAHAM (American surgeon, 1883-   ) and WARREN HENRY COLE, (American surgeon, 1898-   ) introduced successful cholecystography in 1924. Known as *Graham - Cole test*.

Cholecystokinin, description of

ANDREW CONWAY IVY, American physiologist, 1893-   , described cholecystokinin, a hormone secreted by the intestinal mucosa which stimulates the motility of the gallbladder. Recorded in 1928.

Cholecystotomy for removal of stones from gallbladder, first operation of

JOHN STOUGH BOBBS, American surgeon, 1809-1870, was the first to perform cholecystotomy for the removal of stones from the gallbladder, in 1868.

Cholelithectomy in a living patient

. . . See under *Gallstone, first removal of*, etc.

Cholera, discovery of causative organism of

ROBERT KOCH, German bacteriologist, 1843-1910, discovered *Vibrio cholerae* (*Vibrio comma*), the causative organism of Asiatic cholera in man, in 1883.

Cholera, early account of, in modern times

GARCIA DEL HUERTO, Spanish physician in Italy and India, 1490-1570, was the first European to give an account of Asiatic cholera in modern times. Recorded in 1563.

Cholera, inoculation against, using two vaccines

WALDEMAR M. W. HAFFKINE, Russian bacteriologist, 1860-1930, developed a method of inoculation against cholera using two kinds of vaccine, first an attenuated culture of *Vibrio comma*, then, sometime later, a virulent culture. Reported *circa* 1892.

Cholera, spread of, by water supplies, first mention of

JOHN PARKIN, English physician, 1801-1886, was first to suggest the posibility that cholera is spread by water supplies. Published in 1832.

Cholera, spread of, by water supplies, proof of

JOHN SNOW, English physician, 1813-1858, studied a number of outbreaks of cholera and demonstrated that they are related to water supplies. Published in 1849.

Cholera vaccine made of killed organisms

WILHELM KOLLE, German bacteriologist, 1868 - 1935, introduced a vaccine prepared from killed cholera bacilli for use in immunizing against Asiatic cholera. Recorded in 1896.

Cholesterol-rich diet in production of arteriosclerosis

NIKOLAI NIKOLAIEVICH ANICHKOV, Russian physician, 1885-19??, with S. S. CHALATOW, produced arteriosclerosis in animals experimentally by feeding them a high cholesterol diet. Recorded in 1913.

Chondrin and glutin, discovery of

JOHANNES MÜLLER, German anatomist and physiologist, 1801-1858, discovered chondrin and glutin in cartilage and bone. Recorded in 1837.

Chondrodystrophy can be inherited

ERNST TRIER MØRCH, Danish physician, 1908-   , demonstrated that chondrodystrophy can be inherited. Published in 1941.

Chondro-osteodystrophy; eccentro-osteochondrodysplasia

LUIS MORQUIO, Uruguayan physician, 1867-1935, described a type of abnormal ossification marked by the presence of multiple discrete centers, instead of one ossification center, resulting in moderate dwarfishness, bodily deformities, etc. Published in 1929. Known as *Morquio-Brailsford disease* and *Morquio's disease*.

Chorda dorsalis, discovery of

. . . See under *Notochord*.

Chorda tympani, early description of—1561

GABRIEL FALLOPIUS, Italian anatomist, 1523 - 1562, described the chorda tympani in a work published in 1561.

Chorda tympani, identification of, as a nerve

BARTOLOMMEO EUSTACHIUS, Italian anatomist, 1524-1574, described the chorda tympani and identified it as a nerve. Recorded in 1563.

Chordoma, introduction of term

MORITZ WILHELM HUGO RIBBERT, Swiss pathologist, 1855-1920, introduced the term *chordoma*. He also demonstrated that the tumor originates from the embryonic remains of the notochord. Published in 1894.

Chorea, chronic hereditary, earliest description of

ROBLEY DUNGLISON, American physiologist, 1798-1869, gave the earliest known description of chronic hereditary chorea, in 1842. The disease was described later by GEORGE HUNTINGTON, whose name it bears.

Chorea, chronic hereditary, eponymic description of

GEORGE HUNTINGTON, American physician, 1851-1916, gave a classic description of chronic progressive hereditary chorea, marked by irregular movements, speech disturbances, and a progressive dementia, in 1872. Known as *Huntington's chorea*.

Chorea, chronic hereditary, in adults; early account

CHARLES OSCAR WATERS, American physician, 1816-1892, described a case of chronic hereditary chorea in an adult, later to be known as Huntington's chorea. Recorded by ROBLEY DUNGLISON (American physician, 1798-1869), in 1842.

Chorea, electric, description of

ANGELO DUBINI, Italian physician, 1813-1902, described electric chorea, a variety with sudden and violent movements, in 1846. Known as *Dubini's disease.*

Chorea minor; Sydenham's chorea

THOMAS SYDENHAM, English physician, 1624-1689, gave a classic description of chorea minor, the ordinary chorea marked by moderate involuntary movements. Published in 1686.

Chorea, post-paralytic, first description of

SILAS WEIR MITCHELL, American neurologist, 1829-1914, is credited with being first to describe post-paralytic chorea, in 1874. Known also as *posthemiplegic chorea.*

Choroid, basilar membrane of; eponymic description

KARL WILHELM LUDWIG BRUCH, German anatomist, 1819-1884, described the *lamina basalis chorioideae,* in 1844. Known as *Bruch's membrane.*

Choroid neoplasms, treatment of, with radon seeds

ROBERT FOSTER MOORE, English ophthalmologist, 1878-19??, introduced the method of treating neoplasms of the choroid by the use of intraocular radon seeds. Reported in 1930. Called *Foster Moore's technique.*

Choroid, whorls of capillary vessels of

JACOBUS BENIGNUS WINSLOW, Danish anatomist in France, 1669-1760, described whorls of capillaries which give rise to the vorticose veins of the choroid, in 1720. Published in 1732. Known as *Winslow's stars.*

Choroiditis guttata senilis, early description of

JONATHAN HUTCHINSON, English surgeon, 1828-1913, described *choroiditis guttata senilis,* a condition of the choroid marked by degeneration and the formation of yellow spots around the macula, seen in elderly persons. Published in 1875.

Choroiditis guttata senilis, eponymic description of

WARREN TAY, English physician, 1843-1927, described *choroiditis guttata senilis,* a degenerative condition of the choroid (observed in amaurotic familial idiocy) characterized by the development of yellow spots around the macula. Reported in 1881. Known as *Tay's choroiditis.*

Chromatolysis, introduction of term

GEORGES MARINESCO, Rumanian pathologist, 1864-1938, is credited with introducing the term *chromatolysis,* in 1909.

Chromhidrosis, early description of—1858

ALFRED LEROY DE MERICOURT,

French physician, 1825-1901, described blue and black chromhidrosis, in 1858.

Chromosome, introduction of term

HEINRICH WILHELM GOTTFRIED WALDEYER, German anatomist, 1836-1921, is credited with introducing the term *chromosome,* in 1888. It is based on the Greek *chromos* or *chroma* (color) and *soma* (body).

Chromosomes, accessory, as determinants of sex

CLARENCE ERWIN MCCLUNG, Philadelphia zoologist, 1870-19??, declared the accessory chromosomes to be sex determinants. Reported in 1902. Known as *sex chromosomes, X and Y chromosomes, McClung's chromosomes.*

Chromosomes as agents of heredity, discovery of

THOMAS HUNT MORGAN, American geneticist, 1866-1945, is credited with discovering and demonstrating the function of chromosomes in heredity. Published between 1913 and 1916. Received the Nobel prize in 1933.

Chromosomes, discovery of 48, in man

HERBERT M. EVANS, American biologist, 1882-19??, is credited with the discovery of the 48 chromosomes in man, *circa* 1920.

Chromosomes, splitting of, in reproduction

... See under *Splitting of chromosomes in act of reproduction.*

Chromosomes, X and Y

... See under *Chromosomes, accessory, as determinants of sex.*

Chronaxy, introduction of term and concept of

LOUIS LAPIQUE (also LAPICQUE), French physiologist 1866-19??, introduced the term *chronaxie* (now usually *chronaxy*), in 1909. It designates the duration of time that a current twice as strong as the galvanic threshold must flow in order to excite the test tissue. The word is based on the Greek *chronos* (time) and *axia* (value).

Chronic cystic mastitis, classic description of

PAUL RECLUS, French surgeon, 1847-1914, gave a classic description of chronic cystic mastitis. Recorded in 1883.

Chronic cystic mastitis, first description of

ASTLEY PASTON COOPER, English physician and anatomist, 1768-1841, is credited with giving the first description of chronic cystic mastitis, in 1831.

Chronic, cystic mastitis, introduction of term

P. KÖNIG, German physician, *floruit* not available, is credited with introducing the term *chronic cystic mastitis,* in 1893.

Chronic hypertrophic myocarditis, early description of

JEAN N. CORVISART DES MARETS, French physician, 1755-1821, described chronic hypertrophic myocarditis in 1806.

Chronic idiopathic xanthomatosis

. . . See under *Hand-Schüller-Christian disease.*

Chronic mastitis, ovarian hormone in

. . . See under *Ovarian hormone.*

Chronic nephritis, classic description of

RICHARD BRIGHT, English physician, 1789-1858, gave a classic description of chronic nephritis, in 1827. Known as *Bright's disease.*

Chvostek's sign

. . . see under *Tetany, Chvostek's sign of.*

Cicatricial hypertrophy resembling keloid

CAESAR HENRY HAWKINS, English surgeon, 1798-1884, described scar hypertrophy resembling keloid tissue, in 1833.

Cilia, epithelial, motion of

JOHANNES EVANGELISTA VON PURKINJE, Bohemian physiologist, 1787-1869, gave a classic description of the motion of epithelial cilia, in 1835.

Cilia on inner surface of ciliary body, early description of

FRIEDRICH AUGUST VON AMMON, Dresden ophthalmologist, 1799-1861, described the fine hairs on the inner surface of the ciliary body, the pyriform scleral fissure of early fetal life, and the posterior scleral protuberance, in 1838-1847.

Ciliary body, early description of

HEROPHILUS, Greek physician and anatomist in Egypt, 335-280 B.C., was probably the first to describe the ciliary body, *circa* 290 B.C.

Ciliary body, introduction of term

GABRIEL FALLOPIUS, Italian anatomist, 1523-1562, is credited with the introduction of the term *ciliary body,* about 1551. He applied the term to the entire anterior border of the choroid.

Ciliary body, limitation of term

FRIEDRICH GUSTAV JAKOB HENLE, German anatomist, 1809-1885, limited the term ciliary body to the ciliary muscle and the corona ciliaris or pars plicata. Exact date not available.

Ciliary ganglion, early description of

ANDERS ADOLF RETZIUS, Swedish anatomist, 1796 - 1860, described the ciliary ganglion, a ganglion in the posterior part of the orbit supplying fibers to the muscles of the ciliary process and the iris, *circa* 1840.

Ciliary glands, eponymic description of

JACOB ANTONIUS MOLL, Dutch ophthalmologist, 1832 - 1914, gave the first satisfactory description of the modified sweat glands situated on the margins of the eyelids and opening, in some instances, into the hair follicles of the eyelashes; *circa* 1865. Known as *Moll's glands.*

Ciliary muscle, inner circular part of

HEINRICH MÜLLER, German anatomist, 1820-1864, described the innermost fibers of the circular portion of the ciliary muscle. Recorded in 1858. Known as *muscle of Müller.*

Ciliary muscle, radial fibers of

WILLIAM BOWMAN, English ophthalmologist and anatomist, 1816-1892, described the ciliary muscle, especially the radial fibers, in 1847.

Ciliated epithelium, first accurate description of

FRIEDRICH G. J. HENLE, German anatomist, 1809-1885, gave the first clear description of ciliated epithelium, in 1837.

Cinchona, early appreciation of

SEBASTIANO BADO, Italian physician, *circa* 1640-1676, wrote a work expounding the beneficial properties of cinchona bark. Published in 1663.

Cinchona, first publication on

PEDRO BARBA, Spanish physician, 1608-1671, is credited with being the first to write a treatise on cinchona and its use in the treatment of malaria. Published in 1642.

Cinchona in treatment of malaria, in Italy

FRANCESCO TORTI, Italian physician and pharmacologist, 1658-1741, is credited with introducing the use of cinchona in the treatment of malaria in Italy, in 1712.

Cinchona, introduction of, in England

THOMAS SYDENHAM, English physician, 1624-1689, is credited with popularizing the use of cinchona in England, where the drug was introduced in 1653. At this time the drug was known as *Peruvian bark, Jesuit's powder, powder of the Fathers,* etc.

Cinchona, introduction of, in Spain

SEBASTIANO BADO, Italian physician, *circa* 1640-1676, described the introduction of cinchona into Spain in 1632. Recorded in 1663.

Cinchona, introduction of term

CARL VON LINNÉ, Swedish physician and naturalist, 1707-1778, introduced the term *cinchona,* to describe the tree, in 1740. The name was coined in honor of the Countess Cinchon (also Chinchon), whose cure by the powdered bark served to popularize the drug.

Cinchona, isolation of active principle of

BERNARDINO ANTONIO GOMES, Spanish scientist, 1769-1823, was the first to isolate an active principle from cinchona bark, in 1810. He named it *cinchonino.* The effectiveness was proved later by PELLETIER and CAVENTOU.

Cinchona

. . . See also under *Malaria, Quinine,* etc.

Cinchophen, introduction of, as diuretic

ARTHUR NICOLAIER, German physician, 1862-19??, introduced cinchophen as a diuretic in gout and rheumatism. Recorded in 1908.

Circle of Haller

. . . See under *Nerve, optic, vascular circle surrounding.*

Circle of Willis, original description of

THOMAS WILLIS, English physician and anatomist, 1621-1675, described a vascular circle formed by the internal carotid artery, the anterior and posterior cerebral arteries, and the posterior communicating arteries. Published in 1664.

Circulation time, use of decholin sodium in measuring

LEONARD TARR, American physician, 1901-   , with B. S. OPPENHEIMER and R. V. SAGAR, measured the circulation time by the use of sodium dehydrocholate (sodium decholin). Published in 1933.

Circulus arteriosus halleri

. . . See under *Nerve, optic, vascular circle surrounding.*

Circulus venosus halleri

. . . See under *Nipple, circle of veins beneath areola of.*

Cirrhosis of liver, production of experimental—1901

LUDVIG HEKTOEN, American pathologist, 1863-1951, produced experimental bacillary cirrhosis of the liver. Reported in 1901.

Cirrhosis of

. . . See also under name of particular organ or structure.

Cisternal puncture, introduction of

JAMES BOURNE AYER, American neurologist, 1882-19??, introduced cisternal puncture for the purpose of withdrawing cerebrospinal fluid. Recorded in 1920.

Citrated blood, first use of

LUIS AGOTE, Argentinian physician, 1869-19??, is said to have been the first to transfuse citrated blood. Recorded in 1914-15. The anticoagulant effect of sodium citrate was discovered by ALBERT HUSTIN, in 1914. See under *Sodium citrate.*

Citric acid cycle

. . . See under *Carbohydrate breakdown, theory of, through stages invloving citric acid.*

Clarke's column; dorsal nucleus of Clarke

. . . See under *Intermediolateral cell column of spinal cord.*

Classification of animals and plants, binomial

. . . See under *Binomial nomenclature for plants and animals,* etc.

Clavicle, first successful excision of

CHARLES MCCREARY, Kentucky surgeon, 1785-1826, excised the clavicle in a case of osteosarcoma, in 1811 or 1813. Recorded in 1852.

Cleft palate, early operation for

CARL FERDINAND VON GRAEFE, German surgeon, 1787-1840, devised an operation for the treatment of congenital cleft palate. Published in 1820.

Cleidocranial dysostosis, first description of

SAUVEUR FRANÇOIS MORAND, French surgeon, 1697-1773, gave the first recorded description of cleidocranial dysostosis, in 1766.

Cleidocranial dysostosis, introduction of term

PIERRE MARIE, French neurologist, 1853-1940, with PAUL SAINTON, introduced the term of *cleidocranial dysostosis,* in 1898.

Clinic for children, first free, establishment of

ABRAHAM JACOBI, American pediatrician, 1830-1919, is credited with establishing the first free clinic for children in the United States. Founded in New York, in 1862.

Clinical lectures in Great Britain, first, given in English

WILLIAM CULLEN, Scottish physician, 1710-1790, was the first to give clinical lectures in Great Britain in English, instead of in Latin, in 1757.

Clinical records, collections of; the *Consilia*

TADDEO ALDEROTTI, Italian physician and teacher, *circa* 1223-1303, introduced a new form of medical literature by presenting collections of clinical records, known as the *Consilia* (or *Concilia*). Exact date not available.

Cloquet's ganglion, discovery of

. . . See under *Nasopalatine nerve, ganglion of*.

Clostridium histolyticum, isolation of

MICHEL WEINBERG, French bacteriologist, 1868-1940, with P. SEGUIN, isolated *Clostridium histolyticum*. Published in 1916.

Clostridium oedematiens, isolation of

MICHEL WEINBERG, French bacteriologist, 1868-1940, with P. SEGUIN, isolated *Clostridium oedematiens (Cl. novyi)*. Recorded in 1915.

Clostridium septique, discovery of

. . . See under *Vibrion septique*.

Clostridium tetani, pure culture of

. . . See under *Tetanus bacillus, pure culture of*.

Clostridium welchii

. . . See under *Bacillus aerogenes capsulatus*.

Clubfoot, pathologic anatomy of

ANTONIO SCARPA, Italian anatomist and surgeon, 175?-1832, is credited with giving the first full description of the morbid anatomy of clubfoot. Published in 1803.

Clubfoot, subcutaneous section of Achilles tendon in

. . . See under *Achilles tendon*.

Coal miner's safety lamp, invention of

HUMPHRY DAVY, English chemist and physicist, 1778-1829, made many contributions to industrial hygiene and devised the well-known coal miner's safety lamp, in 1815.

Cobra antivenin, early production of

THOMAS RICHARD FRASER, English pharmacologist, 1841-1919, did original work in the field of immunization against cobra venom, and produced antivenin in 1895.

Cocaine as local anesthetic; early suggestion

SIGMUND FREUD, Austrian psychiatrist, 1856-1939, was one of the first to suggest the use of cocaine as a surface anesthetic. Reported in 1884.

Cocaine as local anesthetic; first suggestion

THOMAS MORÉNO Y MAIZ, French pharmacologist, 182?-18??, is credited with being the first to suggest that cocaine be used as a local anesthetic. Recorded in 1868.

Cocaine as local anesthetic, first use of

CARL KOLLER, Austrian-American ophthalmologist, 1857-1944, is credited with being the first to use cocaine as a local anesthetic, on Sept. 16, 1884. Koller used the drug upon the eye.

Cocaine, isolation of, from coca leaves

ALBERT NIEMANN, German pharmacologist, *circa* 1825-1890, isolated cocaine from Peruvian coca leaves. Reported in 1860.

Coccidioidomycosis, eponymic description of

ROBERT JOHANN WERNICKE, Argentinian pathologist, 1873-19??, described coccidioidomycosis, in 1892. The condition was also described by ARTUS POSADA, Argentinian physician, in the same year. Known as *Posada-Wernicke disease, Posada's disease, valley fever,* etc.

Coccobacillus foetidus ozaenae, isolation and naming of

FERNAND PEREZ, Argentinian bacteriologist, 1863-1935, is credited with isolating and naming the *Coccobacillus foetidus ozaenae,* the organism assumed to be the cause of ozena. Recorded in 1899. Known as *Perez's bacillus* and *Salmonella foetida.*

Coccygeal ganglion; ganglion impar

AUGUSTIN FRIEDRICH WALTHER, German anatomist, 1688-1746, described a ganglion located on the anterior surface of the coccyx, near the tip, *circa* 1722. Known as *Walther's ganglion.*

Cochlea, cells of, on basilar membrane

ARTHUR BÖTTCHER, German anatomist, 1831-1889, discovered and described dark polyhedral cells occurring in a single layer on the basilar membrane, between the basilar membrane and the cells of Claudius. Recorded in 1868. Known as *Böttcher's cells.*

Cochlea, early description of—450 B.C.

EMPEDOCLES OF AGRIGENTUM, Greek philospher and medical writer, *circa* 490-430 B.C., observed the cohlea of the ear and referred to it in his writing, *circa* 450 B.C. This is probably the earliest description of the structure.

Cochlea, early description of—1552

BARTOLOMMEO EUSTACHIUS, Italian anatomist, 1524-1574, described and illustrated the cochlea in 1552.

Cochlea, introduction of term

GABRIEL FALLOPIUS, Italian anatomist, 1523-1562, is believed to have been the first to use the term *cochlea,* in 1561.

Cochlea, membranous canal of

ERNST REISSNER, Riga anatomist, 1824-1878, described the membranous canal of the cochlea, in 1851. Called *canal of Reissner.*

Cochlea, spiral canal of

ISIDOR ROSENTHAL, German physiologist, 1836-1915, described the spiral tube which turns around the modiolus of the cochlea, about 1890. Known as *Rosenthal's canal.*

Cock's testes, transplantation of

. . . See under *Internal secretion, first demonstration of.*

Cod liver oil in rickets, early appreciation of

DIETRICH SCHÜTTE, German physician, 1790-1854, presented what is probably the first report on the beneficial effect of cod liver oil in the treatment of rickets. Recorded in 1824.

Cod liver oil, introduction of, in England

THOMAS PERCIVAL, English physician, 1740-1804, is credited with introducing cod liver oil in English therapeutics, in 1782.

Cod liver oil, popularization of, in continental Europe

JOHANN HEINRICH SCHENK, German physician, 1782-1855, advocated the use of cod liver oil in the treatment of rickets, an effort which resulted in the general use of the oil on the continent of Europe. Recorded in 1822.

Codeine, isolation of

PIERRE JEAN ROBIQUET, French physician, 1780-1840, is credited with isolating codeine, in 1832.

Coefficient for estimating renal function based on urea index

LÉON AMBARD, French physiologist and pharmacologist, 1876-19??, worked out a coefficient for estimating renal function, based on a formula showing the relation between the amount of urea in the blood and the amount excreted by the kidneys. Reported in 1910.

Coenzyme A, discovery of

FRITZ A. LIPMANN, German bi-ochemist in the United States, 1899- , discovered and isolated coenzyme A, *circa* 1950. Received the Nobel prize, with HANS A. KREBS, in 1953.

Cold pack in treating fevers, in England

JAMES CURRIE, English physician, 1756-1805, is said to have been the first to use cold packs in the treatment of fevers, in England. Recorded in 1797.

Cold pack in treating fevers, in Germany

JOHANN SIGMUND HAHN, German physician, 1696-1773, is credited with introducing the use of cold packs in the treatment of fevers, in Germany. Published report appeared in 1737.

Cold water cure, introduction of

VINCENZ PRIESSNITZ, German farmer, 1799-1851, was an ardent advocate of hydrotherapy and became known for his treatise on the so-called cold water cure, which he introduced in the 1830s. His cold-water compress is known as *Priessnitz's bandage.*

Colles' fascia, introduction of term

JOHN STRUTHERS, English physician, 1812-1884, introduced the term *Colles' fascia,* in 1854, to designate the fascia which ABRAHAM COLLES described in 1811.

Colles' fracture

. . . See under *Radius, fracture of, with "silver-fork" deformity.*

Colloid and crystalloid substances, distinction between

THOMAS GRAHAM, Scottish chemist, 1805-1869, is credited with differentiating between the two classes of substances, the colloids and the crystalloids, *circa* 1850.

Colloid, introduction of term

THOMAS GRAHAM, Scottish chemist, 1805-1869, introduced the term *colloid* to describe a form of dispersed matter, *circa* 1850.

Colloid milium, first description of

ERNST LEBERECHT WAGNER, German pathologist, 1829-1888, was the first to describe colloid milium, a yellowish papule in the chorium of the skin undergoing colloid degeneration. Published in 1866. Known as *Wagner's disease.*

Collodion in microscopic technique, introduction of

MATHIAS MARIE DUVAL, French anatomist, 1844-1907, is credited with introducing collodion for the embedding of histologic preparations. Published in 1879.

Colon, diverticula of, early description—1849

JEAN CRUVEILHIER, French pathologist, 1791-1874, gave an early description of diverticula of the colon, in 1849.

Colon, idiopathic congenital dilatation of

CALEB HILLIER PARRY, English physician, 1755-1822, is regarded as being the first to record a case of congenital idiopathic dilatation of the colon. Recorded in his *Collected Works,* in 1825.

Colon, kinking of, resulting in stasis

ERWIN PAYR, German surgeon, 1871-1947, described a condition of colonic stasis resulting from a kinking of the colon at the splenic or the hepatic flexure, or a kinking of an adhesion between the transverse and descending portions of the colon. Published in 1910. Known as *Payr's disease.*

Color blindness, early description of—1798

JOHN DALTON, English chemist and physicist, 1766-1844, described color blindness in a paper titled "Extraordinary facts relating to the vision of colors." First read in 1794; published in 1798.

Color blindness, first definite record of

JOSEPH HUDDARD, English physician, 1741-1816, gave the first definite and reliable description of color blindess in a letter written to JOSEPH PRIESTLEY. Published in 1777.

Color perception, test for, by use of colored skeins

HERMANN L. COHN, German ophthalmologist, 1838-1906, developed a test for color perception by means of color skeins and colored embroidery patterns. Reported in 1879.

Color vision, chemical theory of

KARL E. K. HERING, German physiologist, 1834-1918, proposed a theory to explain color vision on the basis of chemical changes taking place in the retina under the influence of light having different wavelengths. Reported in 1872.

Color vision, Helmholtz theory of

HERMANN LUDWIG FERDINAND VON HELMHOLTZ, German physiologist

and physicist, 1821-1894, developed YOUNG's theory of color vision, stating that it depends on three sets of retinal fibers corresponding to red, green, and violet. Published in 1852.

Color vision test based on discernment of figures formed of colored dots

SHINOBU ISHIHARA, Japanese ophthalmologist, 1879-19??, developed a test for color vision based on the discernment of figures or patterned lines formed from colored dots placed in a field of dots of another color. First published in 1917. Known as *Ishihara test.*

Color vision, test of, with wool skeins

. . . See under *Wool skein test.*

Color vision, theory of, based on evolution

CHRISTINE LADD-FRANKLIN, Baltimore physician and psychologist, 1847-1930, promulgated a theory of color vision developed on a basis of evolution. Reported in 1892.

Colorimeter, photoelectric, introduction of

CHARLES SHEARD, American biophysicist, 1883-   , with ARTHUR HAWLEY SANFORD, developed a photoelectric colorimeter, for the determination of hemoglobin. Published in 1930. Known as *Sheard-Sanford photelometer.*

Colorimeter with colored glass standards

HARRY SIDNEY NEWCOMER, American physician, 1887-19??, devised a small colorimeter with colored glass standards, for the determination of hemoglobin. Recorded in 1923. Known as *Newcomer's hemoglobinometer.*

Colostomy, first recorded, for obstruction

PIERRE FINE, French surgeon, 1760-1814, performed the first recorded colostomy for the relief of intestinal obstruction, in 1797. The patient is said to have lived for about 3½ months after the operation. Recorded in 1805.

Colostomy, first successful

KAREL MAYDL, Bohemian surgeon, 1853-1903, is credited with performing the first successful colostomy. Recorded in 1888.

Colostomy, first suggestion of, in intestinal obstruction

ALEXIS LITTRE, French surgeon and anatomist, 1658-1726, is credited with being the first to suggest the operation of colostomy for the relief of intestinal obstruction, in 1710. Known as *Littre's operation.*

Colostomy just above inguinal ligament

. . . See under *Inguinal colostomy.*

Colostomy, lumbar, for relief of intestinal obstruction

. . . See under *Lumbar colostomy,* etc.

Columbus, syphilitic sailors of

. . . See under *Syphilitic sailors of Columbus,* etc.

Columnar epithelium, accurate description of

FRIEDRICH G. J. HENLE, German anatomist, 1809-1885, gave the first clear description of columnar epithelium, in 1837.

Columns of Morgagni
. . . See under *Rectal columns.*

Common bile duct, ampulla of
. . . See under *Ampulla of common bile duct,* etc.

Common cardinal veins, description of
GEORGES L. C. F. CUVIER, French naturalist, 1769 - 1832, described the common cardinal veins, *circa* 1800. Known as *ducts of Cuvier.*

Common iliac artery, first ligation of
WILLIAM GIBSON, American surgeon, 1788-1868, is credited with being the first to ligate the common iliac artery, on July 27, 1812. Recorded in 1820.

Commotio retinae, description of
. . . See under *Retina, traumatic edema of.*

Complement deviation phenomenon—1901
MAX NEISSER, German bacteriologist, 1869-1938, described the phenomenon of complement deviation, with R. LUBOWSKI, in 1901. The phenomenon was noted independently by FRIEDRICH WECHSBERG in the same year. Known as *Neisser-Wechsberg phenomenon.*

Complement-fixation reaction, discovery of
JULES J. B. V. BORDET, Belgian bacteriologist and pathologist, 1870-19??, working with OCTAVE GENGOU, discovered the complement-fixation reaction. Reported in 1900.

Compound A, preparation of
EDWARD CALVIN KENDALL, Ameri-can physiologist and chemist, 1886-, prepared Compound A (11-dehydro-corticosterone) by partial synthesis, in 1944.

Compound ointment of sulfur, introduction of
FERDINAND VON HEBRA, Austrian dermatologist, 1816-1880, originated compound ointment of sulfur, for treatment of parasitic skin diseases, *circa* 1856. Known as *Hebra's itch ointment.*

Compound Spirit of Ether
FRIEDRICH HOFFMANN, German physician, 1660 - 1742, originated *Compound Spirit of Ether* by combining *Spirit of Ether* with ethereal oil. Reported 1729-1739. Known as *Hoffmann's Anodyne.*

Compression diaphragm for intensifying action of roentgen rays
HEINRICH ERNST ALBERS-SCHÖNBERG, German surgeon, 1865-1921, invented a compression diaphragm which intensifies the action of roentgen rays, by cutting out secondary rays. Report published in 1903.

Compression fracture of vertebra; Kümmell's disease
. . . See under *Vertebra, compression fracture of.*

Condenser of microscope, invention of
. . . See under *Microscope condenser.*

Conditioned reflex, introduction of concept and name of
IVAN PETROVICH PAVLOV, Russian physiologist, 1849-1936, using his

stomach pouch method, discovered the conditioned reflex, a reflex initiated by a stimulus not normal to the reaction but associated with it by repeated procedures. Reported *circa* 1898.

Conduction anesthesia, introduction of

MAX OBERST, German surgeon, 1849-1925, is credited with introducing conduction anesthesia (also known as block or regional anesthesia), *circa* 1890. Recorded by Oberst's pupil LUDWIG PERNICE, in 1890.

Condylomata, syphilitic and non-syphilitic, distinction between

GABRIEL FALLOPIUS, Italian anatomist, 1523-1562, distinguished between syphilitic and non-syphilitic condylomata, in a work published in 1563.

Congenital ectodermal dysplasia, eponymic description of

HERMANN WERNER SIEMENS, German dermatologist, 1891-   , described congenital ectodermal dysplasia, a condition marked by glossiness of the skin, absence of sweat glands, defective teeth, etc. Known as *Siemens' syndrome*. Date not available.

Congenital hemolytic anemia, fragility of erythrocytes in

ANATOLE MARIE EMILE CHAUFFARD, French physician, 1855-1932, was the first to note the fragility of the red blood cells in congenital hemolytic anemia. Published in 1907.

Congress of Anthropologists, first meeting of

The first Congress of Anthropolo-

gists was called in 1861. One of those actively concerned with it was KARL ERNST VON BAER, German embryologist born in Estonia, 1792-1876.

Conjunctivitis, diplobacillary form of

KARL THEODOR PAUL POLYKARPOS AXENFELD, German ophthalmologist, 1867-1930, described a diplobacillary form of chronic conjunctivitis, in 1896.

Conjunctivitis, filtration of virus of

ALBERT BOTTERI, German ophthalmologist, 1879-19??, recorded the filtration of the virus of inclusion conjunctivitis, in 1912.

Conjunctivitis, infectious, caused by a leptothrix

HENRI PERINAUD, French ophthalmologist, 1844 - 1905, described a form of infectious conjunctivitis, transferred to man from animals, believed to be caused by a leptothrix. Published in 1889. Known as *Perinaud's conjunctivitis*.

Conjunctivitis, infectious tuberculous

HENRI PARINAUD, French ophthalmologist, 1844-1905, with XAVIER GALEZOWSKI, described a form of tuberculous conjunctivitis observed in both animals and man. Published in 1889. Known as *Parinaud's oculo-glandular syndrome*.

Conjunctivitis, isolation of diplobacillus in

KARL THEODOR PAUL POLYKARPOS AXENFELD, German ophthalmologist, 1867-1930, and VICTOR MORAX, French physician, 1866-

1935, independently isolated a diplobacillus which causes a form of chronic conjunctivitis, in 1896. Known as *Morax - Axenfeld haemophilus*.

Conjunctivitis

. . . See also under name of particular conjunctivitis, as *Vernal conjunctivitis*.

**Conservation of energy,
acceptance of principle of**

HERMANN LUDWIG FERDINAND VON HELMHOLTZ, German physiologist and physicist, 1821-1894, performed basic experiments which led to the universal acceptance of the doctrine of the conservation of energy. Published in 1847.

**Conservation of energy in
physiological processes**

JULIUS ROBERT VON MAYER, German scientist, 1814-1878, demonstrated that the principle of conservation of energy holds true with regard to physiological processes. Published in 1842.

***Consilia*, introduction of, in
medical literature**

. . . See under *Clinical records, collections of*.

**Contact lenses, development of
modern methods for**

LEOPOLD HEINE, German ophthalmologist, 1870-19??, is credited with introducing the modern methods used in fitting contact lenses. Recorded in 1930.

**Contact lenses, practical,
introduction of**

JOSEF DALLOS, German ophthalmologist, 18??-19??, is credited

with introducing practical contact lenses. Published in 1933.

Contraction currents of heart

. . . See under *Heart, contraction current of*.

**Contracture of muscles due to
injury or pressure**

RICHARD VON VOLKMANN, German surgeon, 1830-1889, described ischemic contracture of muscles resulting from injury or pressure. Published in 1881. Known as *Volkmann's contracture*.

Contracture of

. . . See also under name of organ or structure involved.

**Convex lenses, early
experiments with**

ALHAZEN, Arabian mathematician, physicist, and optician, *circa* 965-1039, is known to have experimented with convex lenses with regard to refraction and application in opticianry.

Cooling of traumatized and potentially infected limbs

. . . See under *Surgical refrigeration*.

**Coprolalia and echolalia,
condition marked by**

. . . See under *Echolalia and coprolalia*.

**Coprostanol, discovery of,
in normal feces**

WILLIAM MARCET, English physician, 1829-1900, described the presence of coprosterin or coprostanol in the feces of normal subjects. Published in 1858.

Coracobrachialis muscle, first good description of

GIULIO CASSERIO, Italian anatomist, 1561-1616, was the first to give a complete description of the coracobrachialis muscle, previously recognized by Arantius, in 1594.

Coracobrachialis muscle, recognition of, as a separate muscle

JULIUS CAESAR ARANTIUS, Italian physician, 1530-1589, was first to describe the coracobrachialis muscle as a separate structure. Exact date unknown; probably in 1571.

Cordotomy for relief of pain in lower part of body

WILLIAM GIBSON SPILLER, American neurologist, 1863-1940, with EDWARD MARTIN, introduced the treatment of persistent pain of organic origin in the lower part of the body by division of the anterolateral column of the spinal cord. Recorded in 1912.

Cornea, brown line of degeneration in

JEAN STÄHLI, Swiss ophthalmologist, 1890-   , described a horizontal brown line in the lower part of the cornea resulting from senile degeneration. Recorded in 1918. Known as *Stahli's pigment line*.

Cornea, outgrowth of cells at periphery of, in elderly persons

FRIEDRICH G. J. HENLE, German anatomist, 1809-1885, described hyaline excrescences on the back part of the periphery of the cornea, in elderly persons. *Circa* 1839. Known as *Henle's warts*.

Cornea, ring around, formed by thickened Descemet's membrane

. . . See under *Descemet's membrane*.

Cornea, serpiginous ulcer of

EDWIN THEODOR SAEMISCH, German ophthalmologist, 1833-1909, described a serpiginous ulcer of the cornea, in 1870. Known as *Saemisch's ulcer*.

Corneal corpuscles, eponymic description of

JOSEPH TOYNBEE, English otologist, 1815-1866, described the corneal corpuscles, stellate cells within the corneal spaces. Published in 1841. Known as *Toynbee's corpuscles*.

Corneal curvature, early work on

HERMANN JAKOB KNAPP, German-American ophthalmologist, 1831-1911, did important research in the field of corneal curvature. Published in 1859.

Corneal grafting, development of

ANTON ELSCHNIG, Czechoslovakian ophthalmologist, 1863-1939, improved the method of corneal grafting introduced by Arthur von Hippel, and obtained good results in many operations on the human eye. Published in 1930.

Corneal grafting, introduction of

. . . See under *Keratoplasty*.

Corneal opacity, first description of

PHILIPP FRANZ VON WALTHER, German physician, 1782-1849, is credited with being first to describe a corneal opacity. Recorded in 1845.

Corneal transplantation
. . . See under *Corneal grafting* and *Keratoplasty*.

Corniculate cartilages
. . . See under *Larynx, corniculate cartilages of*.

Cornu cutaneum, first description of
EVERARD HOME, English surgeon, 1756-1832, was the first to describe cornu cutaneum, also known as cornu humanum, in 1791.

Coronary arteries, entrance of blood into
JOSEPH HYRTL, Hungarian anatomist, 1810-1894, demonstrated that the entrance to the coronary arteries is not covered by the semilunar valves during systole, as had been believed, and that the blood does not enter these arteries during diastole. Recorded in 1854.

Coronary occlusion, association of, with angina pectoris
. . . See under *Angina pectoris*.

Coronary occlusion, classic description of
. . . See under *Coronary thrombosis, classic description of*.

Coronary thrombosis, classic description of
JAMES BRYAN HERRICK, American physician, 1861-1954, gave a classic description of the clinical features observed in cases involving sudden obstruction of the coronary arteries. Recorded in 1912.

Coronary thrombosis, first diagnosis of, before death
ADAM HAMMER, Austrian physician, 1818-1878, is credited with being the first to make a diagnosis of coronary thrombosis in a living patient. Recorded in 1878.

Coronary valves, eponymic description of
ADAM CHRISTIAN THEBESIUS, German physician, 1686-1732, was the first to describe the valves of the coronary sinus. Published in 1708. Known as *Thebesian valves*.

Coronary vein, valve in large
RAYMOND VIEUSSENS, French anatomist, 1641-1715, was the first to describe the valve of the large coronary vein. Published in 1705.

Coronary vessels, first accurate description of
RAYMOND VIEUSSENS, French anatomist, 1641-1715, is credited with giving the first accurate description of the course of the coronary vessels. Published in 1705.

Corpora arantii, discovery of
JULIUS CAESAR ARANTIUS, Italian physician, 1530-1589, discovered and described the small tubercles at the tips of the cusps of the aortic and pulmonary valves of the heart. One tubercle is found in each of the semilunar valves of the aorta and pulmonary arteries. They are also known as the *bodies of Arantius*. The description appeared in the text *De Humano Foetu*, published in 1571.

Corpora cavernosa, fibrosis of; Peyronie's disease
. . . See under *Penis, fibrosis of corpora cavernosa of*.

Corpus callosum, degeneration of, in alcoholism

ETTORE MARCHIAFAVA, Italian pathologist, 1847-1935, noted primary degeneration of the corpus callosum in alcoholic patients. Date not available.

Corpus callosum, median raphe of

. . . See under *Raphe of corpus callosum.*

Corpus striatum syndrome; status marmoratus

CECIL VOGT, German neurologist, 1875-19??, with OSKAR VOGT (German neurologist, 1870-19??), described a condition marked by athetosis, hyperkinesis, etc, due to disease of the corpus striatum. Published in 1920. Known as *Vogt's syndrome* or *disease.*

Corpuscles, tactile, in fingertips, etc.

. . . See under *Tactile nerve endings in tips of fingers and toes.*

Corrigan pulse in aortic insufficiency

. . . See under *Water-hammer pulse,* etc.

Corsets, bad effects of tight

SAMUEL THOMAS SOEMMERRING, German physician, 1755-1830, published a paper, in 1793, listing the bad effects of wearing tight corsets upon the internal organs. The result was a falling off in popularity of tight corsets and hoop skirts.

Cortex, human, areas of

. . . See under *Map of human cortex.*

Cortex, sensory, functional subdivisions of, in rhesus monkey

JOHANNES G. DUSSER DE BARENNE, Dutch physiologist, 1885-1940, was the first to describe and outline the major functional subdivisions of the sensory cortex of the rhesus monkey. Reported in 1924.

Cortical motor centers in man

JEAN MARTIN CHARCOT, French neurologist and clinician, 1825-1893, with JEAN ALBERT PITRES, French neurologist, 1848-1928, demonstrated the existence of cortical motor centers in man. Published in 1877, 1878, and 1883.

Cortical visual center, discovery of

SALOMON EBERHARD HENSCHEN, Swedish pathologist, 1847-1930, discovered the cortical visual center, in 1888.

Corticosterone, isolation of—1936

HAROLD LAWRENCE MASON, American chemist, 1901-   , with C. S. MYERS and E. C. KENDALL, isolated corticosterone (Kendall compound B), in 1936.

Corticosterone, isolation of—1937

P. DE FREMERY, French biochemist, 1894-   , with E. LAQUEUR, T. REICHSTEIN, R. W. SPANHOFF, and I. E. UYLDERT, isolated corticosterone. Recorded in 1937.

Cortin, crystalline, isolation of

EDWARD CALVIN KENDALL, American physiologist and chemist, 1886-   , with H. L. MASON, B. F. MCKENZIE, C. S. MYERS, and G. A. KOELSCHE, succeeded in isolating cortin in crystalline form. Reported in 1934.

Cortisone, discovery of
. . . See under *Cortisone, isolation of.*

Cortisone, effect of, on rheumatic fever, rheumatoid arthritis, etc.
EDWARD CALVIN KENDALL, American physiologist and chemist, 1886- , with his colleagues HENCH, POLLEY, and SLOCUMB, demonstrated the effect of cortisone on rheumatoid arthritis, rheumatic fever, etc., in 1948.

Cortisone in treatment of rheumatic fever
. . . See under *Rheumatic fever.*

Cortisone in treatment of rheumatoid arthritis
. . . See under *Rheumatoid arthritis.*

Cortisone, isolation of
EDWARD CALVIN KENDALL, American physiologist and chemist, 1886- , with H. L. MASON, C. S. MYERS, and W. D. ALLERS, isolated nine related steroid hormones from adrenal cortical extracts, one of which was Compound E, later, in 1939, named cortisone. The isolation of the nine hormones was recorded in 1936.

Cortisone, isolation of
TADEUS REICHSTEIN, Polish-Swiss biochemist, 1897- , isolated Compound F-a, which is identical with Compound F and Compound E. Recorded in 1936.

Cortisone, isolation of
OSKAR PAUL WINTERSTEINER, American biochemist, 1898- , with JOSEPH JOHN PFIFFNER, American biochemist, 1903- , isolated Compound F, which is identical with Kendall's Compound E or cortisone, in 1935-36.

***Corynebacterium diphtheriae,* discovery of**
THEODOR A. E. KLEBS, German bacteriologist, 1834-1913, discovered the *Corynebacterium diphtheriae* in 1833. Known also as *Klebs-Loeffler bacillus.*

***Corynebacterium diphtheriae,* isolation and identification of**
FRIEDRICH A. J. LOEFFLER, German bacteriologist, 1852-1915, isolated and gave the first full description of *Corynebacterium diphtheriae* in 1884. The organism is also known as the *Klebs-Loeffler bacillus.*

***Corynebacterium diphtheriae,* three types of**
JAMES STIRLING ANDERSON, English bacteriologist, 18??- , with F. C. HAPPOLD, J. W. McLEOD, and J. G. THOMSON, distinguished three types of *Corynebacterium diphtheriae,* the *gravis, mitis,* and *intermedius.* Published in 1931.

Corynebacterium pseudo-tuberculosis
. . . See under *Pseudotuberculosis in cattle, sheep, etc., causative agent of.*

Countertraction utilizing well leg
. . . See under *Well-leg countertraction.*

Coventry treatment
. . . See under *Sponge, burnt, in treatment of goiter.*

Cowper's glands

. . . See under *Bulbourethral glands.*

Cowpox vaccination, earliest record of

BENJAMIN JESTY, Dorsetshire farmer, 1737-1816, is credited with being first to perform successfully cowpox vaccination on cows and on his wife and sons, in 1774.

Coxsackie virus in poliomyelitis, isolation of

EDWARD CHARLES CURNEN, American microbiologist, 1909- , with associates, isolated the Coxsackie virus from poliomyelitis patients. Published in 1949.

Coxsackie virus, isolation of

GILBERT JULIUS DALLDORF, American microbiologist, 1900- , with GRACE MARY SICKLES, isolated the Coxsackie virus from the stools of children. Published in 1948.

Coxalgic pelvis, early description of

CARL C. T. LITZMANN, German gynecologist and obstetrician, 1815-1890, described the coxalgic female pelvis (deformity caused by hip joint disease), in 1853.

Cracked-pot note on percussion in case of fracture of skull

WILLIAM MACEWEN, Scottish surgeon, 1848-1924, described a cracked-pot note obtained on percussing the skull in case of fracture. Published in 1893.

Craigia, discovery of

. . . See under *Paramoeba, discovery and naming of.*

Cranial bones, study of sound transmission through

. . . See under *Sound transmission through cranial bones,* etc.

Cranial nerves, classification of—1778

SAMUEL THOMAS SOEMMERRING, German anatomist, 1755 - 1830, classified the cranial nerves in 1778. This classification superseded that of THOMAS WILLIS, published in 1664.

Cranial nerves, first pair, function of

ALESSANDRO ACHILLINI, Italian anatomist, 1463-1512, studied the olfactory nerves and is believed to have been the first investigator to recognize their function. Exact date not available.

Cranial nerves

. . . See also under name of particular nerve.

Craniobuccal pouch

. . . See under *Buccal cavity, diverticulum of, in embryo.*

Craniofacial dysostosis; hypertelorism

. . . See under *Hypertelorism.*

Craniohypophysial xanthomatosis, first description of

THOMAS SMITH, English pathologist, 1833-1909, is credited with being the first to describe the condition now known as *Hand-Schüller-Christian disease,* or craniohypophysial xanthomatosis. Recorded in 1865 and 1876. It was described by HAND in 1893, by SCHÜLLER in 1915, and by CHRISTIAN in 1919.

Craniometric plane passing through nasion and basion

CHRISTOPHER THEODORE AEBY, Swiss anatomist, 1835-1885, described a craniometric plane passing through the nasion and basion, perpendicular to the median plane of the cranium. Published in 1867. Known as *Aeby's plane*.

Craniometry, founder of modern

PIERRE PAUL BROCA, French surgeon and anthropologist, 1824-1880, is regarded as the founder of modern craniometry. His *"Mémoires d'anthropologie"* appeared in 1871-77.

Creatine, isolation of, from muscle

MICHEL E. CHEVREUL, French chemist, 1786-1889, isolated creatine from muscle. Reported in 1832.

Crepitation, introduction of term

RENE T. H. LAENNEC, French physician, 1781-1826, is credited with introducing the term *crepitation*, after his invention of the stethoscope and his study of auscultation. Published in 1819.

Crescent-shaped cells beneath neurilemma of medullated nerve fibers

ALBERT ADAMKIEWICZ, Polish pathologist, 1850-1921, described the demilunes or crescent-shaped cells found beneath the neurilemma of medullated nerve fibers. Reported in 1885. These cells are also known as the *demilunes of Adamkiewicz*.

Cretinism and endemic goiter, association of

BOMBASTUS AB HOHENHEIM (PARACELSUS), Swiss physician, chemist, and reformer, 1493-1541, was the first to record the coincidence of cretinism and endemic goiter. Published account appeared in 1603.

Cretinism and myxedema are due to lack of thyroid function

FELIX SEMON, English laryngologist, 1849-1921, recognized that myxedema, cretinism, and cachexia strumipriva are related and are caused by loss of thyroid function. Recorded in 1883.

Cretinism, first accurate clinical aspect of

THOMAS B. CURLING, English surgeon, 1811-1888, is believed to have been the first to give an accurate clinical picture of cretinism, in 1850. He pointed to thyroid deficiency as the probable cause.

Cretinism, prevention of, by iodine

GASPARD ADOLPH CHATIN, French physician, 1813-1901, demonstrated that iodine can prevent the development of cretinism and endemic goiter. Published in 1850.

Cretinism, sporadic and endemic, differentiation of

FRIEDRICH PINELESS, German physician, 1868-1936, distinguished between sporadic cretinism and endemic cretinism associated with goiter. Published in 1902.

Criminal type, introduction of concept of a

CESARE LOMBROSO, Italian physician and criminologist, 1836-1909, propounded the theory of a "criminal type" of personality, holding that criminals have a definite physical and mental constitution. His studies showed that the incidence of physical, mental, and nervous anomalies and disorders was higher among criminals. Report published in 1876.

Cross-hatching as a means of depicting shades

ALBRECHT DÜRER, German engraver and illustrator, 1471-1528, was the first to employ the method of cross-hatching to represent shadows and degrees of shading in wood engraving. This is illustrated in his *"Vier Bücher von Menschlicher Proportion,"* published in 1528.

Crush syndrome, first description of

SEIGO MINAMI, Japanese physician, 1890- , is credited with giving the first description of the crush syndrome, marked by manifestations of renal failure and caused by the crushing of a part. Published in 1923.

Cryoscopy of urine, introduction of

SÁNDOR KORÁNYI, Hungarian physician, 1866-1944, introduced cryoscopy of the urine as a criterion of kidney function. Published in 1894.

Cryptococcosis; European blastomycosis

. . . See under *Blastomycosis of skin, European.*

Cryptococcus neoformans infection in man

. . . See under *Torula histolytica infection in man.*

Crypts of Lieberkühn, cells in

. . . See under *Cells in crypts of Lieberkühn,* etc.

Crystalline insulin, production of

. . . See under *Insulin, crystalline,* etc.

Crystals, double refraction of

CHRITIAAN HUYGENS, Dutch physicist and mathematician, 1629-1695, discovered the phenomenon of double refraction in crystals. *Circa* 1678.

Crystals in prostatic fluid, discovery of

ARTHUR BÖTTCHER, German anatomist, 1831-1889, discovered the so-called spermin crystals in prostatic fluid. The crystals are seen when a solution of ammonium phosphate is added to prostatic fluid. Known as *Böttcher crystals.* Exact date not available.

Crystals occurring in sputum in bronchial asthma and in bronchitis

FRIEDRICH ALBERT ZENKER, German pathologist, 1825-1898, described colorless, needle-like crystals of phosphate found in the sputum of patients with bronchial asthma and other conditions. Recorded in 1851. The crystals were also noted and described by JEAN MARTIN CHARCOT, French neurologist, 1824-1893, in 1853, and by ERNST VIKTOR VON LEYDEN, German neurologist, 1832-1910, in 1869. Known as *Charcot-Leyden-Zenker* or *Charcot- Leyden* crystals.

Crystals, right-handed and left-handed forms of

LOUIS PASTEUR, French scientist and bacteriologist, 1822-1895, is credited with discovering the existence of right- and left-handed forms of crystals, *circa* 1846.

Cuboidodigital reflex

. . . See under *Toes, dorsal flexion of, when dorsum of foot is tapped.*

Cullen's sign of ruptured ectopic pregnancy

. . . See under *Ectopic pregnancy, ruptured, sign of.*

Cultivation of tissue in vitro, introduction of

ALEXIS CARREL, French surgeon, 1873-1944, in collaboration with M. T. BURROWS, devised a method for cultivating tissue in vitro. Recorded in 1910.

Cuneate fasciculus of spinal cord, early adequate description of

KARL FRIEDRICH BURDACH, German anatomist and physiologist, 1776-1847, gave the first complete account of the cuneate fasciculus of the spinal cord (fasciculus cuneatus), in 1806. Known as *Burdach's column.*

Cuneate nucleus, lateral part of

LEONID V. BLUMENAU, Russian neurologist, 1862-1931, described the lateral part of the cuneate nucleus. Published in 1907.

Cuneiform cartilages of larynx

HEINRICH AUGUST WRISBERG, German anatomist, 1739-1808, gave a clear description of the cuneiform cartilages of the larynx. Published in 1764. Known as *Wrisberg's corpuscles.*

Cupping device or artificial leech

CHARLES L. S. HEURTELOUP, French surgeon, 1793-1864, designed an artificial leech or cupping device, *circa* 1822, which is termed a *heurteloup.*

Curare in anesthesia, introduction of

HAROLD RANDALL GRIFFITH, American anesthesiologist, 1894- , with G. Enid Johnson, introduced curare in anesthesia. Published in 1942.

Curling's ulcer

. . . See under *Duodenal ulceration due to burns of skin.*

Curschmann's spirals, original description of

. . . See under *Spirals of mucin threads in sputum of asthmatics.*

Curve having its center at the sacral promontory

ROBERT BARNES, English obstetrician, 1817-1907, described an imaginary curve having its center at the sacral promontory, in relation to the mechanism of labor, especially with reference to Naegele's obliquity. Reported in 1884.

Curved line forming axis of birth canal

. . . See under *Axis of birth canal.*

Cushing's disease and syndrome

. . . See under *Basophilism, pituitary,* etc.

Cusp, fifth, on lingual surface of molar teeth

GEORG CARABELLI, Hungarian dentist, 1787-1842, described a tubercle or fifth cusp on the lingual surface of upper molar teeth. Said to be hereditary. Reported in 1844. Known as *Carabelli's cusp* or *tubercle.*

Cyanogen, isolation of

JOSEPH L. GAY-LUSSAC, French chemist and physicist, 1778-1850, isolated cyanogen by heating silver cyanide, in 1815. It was the first "compound radical" isolated.

Cyclodialysis, introduction of, in treating glaucoma

LEOPOLD HEINE, German ophthalmologist, 1870-1940, is credited with introducing cyclodialysis in the treatment of glaucoma, an operation in which a communication is formed between the suprachoroidal space and the anterior chamber of the eye. Published in 1905.

Cyclopropane, experimental use of, as anesthetic

GEORGE HERBERT WILLIAM LUCAS, Canadian pharmacologist, 1894- , with VELYIEN EWART HENDERSON, studied the properties of cyclopropane as an anesthetic in animals. Recorded in 1929.

Cyclopropane, first clinical use of, as an anesthetic

JOHN ALDEN STILES, American physician, 1905- , with W. B. NEFF, E. A. ROVENSTINE, and R. M. WATERS, reported the first clinical use of cyclopropane as an anesthetic, in 1934.

Cyclopropane, first preparation of

AUGUST VON FREUND, German chemist, 1851-1918, is credited with being first to prepare cyclopropane, used as an inhalant general anesthetic. Published in 1882.

Cylindrical lenses in astigmatism

GEORGE BIDDELL AIRY, English physician, 1801-1892, fitted cylindrical lenses for the correction of astigmatism. Recorded in 1827.

Cyon's nerve

. . . See under *Depressor nerve of the heart*, etc.

Cyst formed by herniation of synovial membrane of a joint through opening in capsule

WILLIAM MORRANT BAKER, London surgeon, 1839-1896, described cysts formed in the popliteal space by the herniation of synovial membrane through openings in the capsule. Others describe the condition as inflammation of the popliteal bursa. Recorded in 1877. Known as *popliteal bursitis* and as *Baker's cyst*.

Cyst of broad ligament of uterus

. . . See under *Broad ligament of uterus*.

Cyst, retention, of a sweat gland

. . . See under *Hidrocystoma, eponymic description of*.

Cystic duct, spiral valve of, early description—1720

LORENZ (LAURENTIUS) HEISTER, German surgeon and anatomist, 1683-1758, described spiral folds of mucous membrane in the cystic duct and in the neck of the gallbladder. Published in 1720. Known as *Heister's valve*.

Cystography, introduction of

FRIEDRICH VOELCKER, German surgeon, 1872-19??, was the first to produce cystograms. Published, with ALEXANDER VON LICHTENBERG, in 1905.

Cystoscope, electrically lighted, invention of

MAX NITZE, German urologist, 1848-1906, invented an electrically lighted cystoscope, *circa* 1879.

Cystoscope, invention of

MAX NITZE, German urologist,

1848-1906, constructed the first cystoscope, with the assistance of an instrument maker named LEITER, in 1877.

Cystoscope, operative, invention of

MAX NITZE, German urologist, 1848-1906, modified his original cystoscope to adapt it for operative procedures, as for the excision of bladder tumors. Recorded in 1897.

Cystoscope, prismatic type, invention of

MAX NITZE, German urologist, 1848-1906, improved his original cystoscope by introducing a system of prisms. Recorded in 1894.

Cystoscopic cutting instrument operating under water

. . . See under *Resectoscope*.

Cystoscopy, systematization of

JOAQUIN ALBARRAN Y DOMINGUEZ, Cuban urologist in France, 1860-1912, is associated with the invention and modification of special cystoscopes, and with systematizing the methods of cystoscopy. Reports published in 1889 and 1909.

Cystotomy, early performance of—1851

WILLARD PARKER, American surgeon, 1800-1884, performed an operation for cystotomy in a case involving cystitis, tuberculosis of the kidney, and other complications, in 1851.

Cytoarchitectonic map of human cerebral cortex

. . . See under *Brain, cytoarchitectonic map of*.

Cytotrophoblast, eponymic description of

THEODOR LANGHANS, German anatomist and pathologist in Switzerland, 1839-1915, described the cytotrophoblast, the inner cellular layer of the trophoblast, in 1870. Known as *Langhans' layer*. The cells which form the layer are known as *Langhans' cells*.

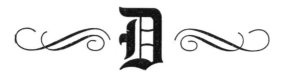

Dacryocystorhinostomy, introduction of

ADDEO TOTI, Italian ophthalmologist, 1861-19??, devised the operation of dacryocystorhinostomy, in 1904. The communication between the lacrimal sac and the middle meatus is made through the lacrimal bone.

Dacryolith consisting of *Nocardia foersteri*

LOUIS A. DESMARRES, French ophthalmologist, 1810-1882, described a type of dacryolith consisting of masses of *Nocardia foersteri,* in 1847. Known as *Desmarres' dacryolith.*

Dacryon, introduction of, as craniometric point

PIERRE PAUL BROCA, French surgeon and anthropologist, 1824-1880, defined *dacryon* as a craniometric point. Exact date not available.

Danielssen-Boeck disease

. . . See under *Leprosy, early modern account of.*

Darier's disease

. . . See under *Keratosis follicularis, early description of.*

Dark adaptation, early description of

HERMANN AUBERT, German physiologist, 1826-1892, described dark adaptation in a work published in 1865.

Darling's histoplasmosis

. . . See under *Histoplasmosis, original description of.*

Darwin's tubercle; tuberculum auriculae

. . . See under *Tuberculum auriculae.*

Davidsohn's sign

. . . See under *Pupil, illumination of, by light placed in mouth.*

DDT, early compounding of

OTHMAR ZEIDLER, German chemist, 182?-1892, is credited with having compounded DDT from chloral and brombenzal, in 1874.

DDT, synthesis and evaluation of

PAUL MÜLLER, Swiss chemist, 1900-   , synthesized dichloro-diphenyl-trichloro-ethane (DDT) and discovered its insecticidal properties. Recorded in 1939.

Deaf and dumb, first school for, in Great Britain

THOMAS BRAIDWOOD, Scottish

teacher, 1715-1806, founded the first school for the deaf and dumb in Great Britain, in 1760.

Deaf and dumb, teaching of, by combined system

JUAN PABLO BONET, Spanish physician, 1575-1630, devised a method of teaching the deaf to speak. He also taught the dumb to communicate by finger-spelling and other expressions. Recorded in 1620.

Deaf-mutes, alphabet for, introduction of

GEORGE DALGARNO, Scottish educator, 162?-1687, devised a special alphabet to be used by deaf-mutes. Published in 1680.

Deaf-mutes, method of instructing

JAN COENRAAD AMMAN, Dutch educator, 1669-1730, did considerable work on methods of instruction for deaf-mutes. Report published in 1700.

Deaf-mutes, sign language for

. . . See under *Sign language.*

Deafness due to obstruction of auditory tube

ASTLEY PASTON COOPER, English surgeon and anatomist, 1768-1841, described a form of deafness due to obstruction of the auditory tube. Published in 1801.

Decapitation instrument for use in difficult labor

GUSTAV AUGUST VON BRAUN, Austrian obstetrician, 1829-1911, invented a hook for use in decapitation of the fetus in cases of difficult labor. Reported in 1861.

Decerebrate rigidity, description of

CHARLES SCOTT SHERRINGTON, English neurophysiologist, 1857-1952, demonstrated decerebrate rigidity, the rigid extension of an animal's legs resulting from section of the brain stem, in 1897. Published in 1898.

Decholin sodium in circulation time

. . . See under *Circulation time.*

Decidua, introduction of term

WILLIAM HUNTER, Scottish surgeon and obstetrician, 1718-1783, introduced the term *decidua* in his *The Anatomy of the Human Gravid Uterus,* published in 1774.

Decidual tissue formed as result of mechanical stimulation

LEO LOEB, American pathologist, 1869-19??, produced decidual tissue (deciduomata) in the uterus of mice by mechanical stimulation, in 1907.

Decompression in brain tumor by means of artificial cerebral hernia

. . . See under *Cerebral hernia, artificial,* etc.

Decompression sickness

. . . See under *Caisson disease.*

Decussation in form of letter X, early mention of

ARETAEUS THE CAPPADOCIAN, Greek physician in Rome, *circa* 81-138, was the first to formulate the pattern of the motor pathway as a decussation in the shape of the letter X. Exact date not available.

Deep layer of superficial perineal fascia, description of

ABRAHAM COLLES, Irish surgeon, 1773-1843, gave a complete description of the deep layer of the superficial perineal fascia, in 1811. Known as *Colles' fascia*.

Deep x-ray therapy, first use of

LEOPOLD FREUND, Vienna physician, 1868-1944, is credited with being the first to use deep x-ray therapy. Recorded in 1897.

Defibrinated blood, bactericidal action of

GEORGE H. F. NUTTALL, American biologist, 1862-1937, discovered the bactericidal action of the defibrinated blood of certain animals. Recorded in 1888.

Degeneration, amyloid, with deposits of lardacein

. . . See under *Amyloid degeneration*.

Deglutition, classic description of—1813

FRANÇOIS MAGENDIE, French physiologist, 1783-1855, gave a classic description of the mechanism of deglutition, in 1813.

Deglutition, reflex nature of

ANGELO MOSSO, Italian physiologist, 1846-1910, studied the mechanism of deglutition and demonstrated that it is reflex in character. Recorded in 1876.

Dejerine-Sottas disease or neuropathy

. . . See under *Progressive hypertrophic interstitial neuropathy*.

Dejerine's neurotabes

. . . See under *Neuritis, peripheral, first description of*.

Déléage's disease

. . . See under *Dystrophia myotonica*.

Delhi sore, *Leishmania tropica* in

JAMES HOMER WRIGHT, American pathologist, 1869-1928, discovered *Leishmania tropica* in oriental or Delhi sore. Published in 1903.

Delirium tremens, early description of

THOMAS SUTTON, English physician, 1767-1835, described delirium tremens and differentiated it from other forms of delirium or frenzy. Recorded in 1813.

Delirium tremens, first complete description of

JOHN WARE, American physician, 1795-1864, was the first to give a full account of delirium tremens, in 1831.

Delirium tremens, introduction of term

THOMAS SUTTON, English physician, 1767-1835, is credited with introducing the term *delirium tremens*, in 1813.

Delivery of parturient women in bed, introduction of

FRANÇOIS MAURICEAU, French obstetrician, 1637-1709, is credited with introducing the practice of delivering parturient women in a bed instead of an obstetric chair. His book on obstetrics, which is said to have elevated obstetrics to the status of a science, was published in 1668.

Dementia paralytica and congenital syphilis

THOMAS SMITH CLOUSTON, English physician, 1840-1915, was the first to demonstrate the relationship between congenital syphilis and dementia paralytica. Recorded in 1877. Clouston reported a case of general paralysis in a patient sixteen years old.

Dementia paralytica, first classic description of

ANTOINE L. J. BAYLE, French physician, 1799-1858, presented the first classic description of dementia paralytica or general paralysis of the insane, in 1822. Known as *Bayle's disease.*

Dementia paralytica, histopathology of

FRANZ NISSL, German neurologist, 1860-1919, gave the first accurate account of the histopathology of general paralysis. Published in 1904.

Dementia paralytica marked by aphasia, convulsions, monoplegia, etc.

HEINRICH LISSAUER, German neurologist, 1861-1891, described an atypical general paralysis characterized by aphasia, monoplegia, convulsions, etc. Published posthumously in 1901. Known as *Lissauer's paralysis.*

Dementia paralytica, syphilis as cause of

JEAN ALFRED FOURNIER, French syphilologist, 1832-1914, demonstrated statistically the etiologic relationship of syphilis to dementia paralytica and to tabes dorsalis. Recorded in 1894.

Dementia paralytica

. . . See also under *Paralysis, general.*

Dementia praecox, introduction of concept of

EMIL KRAEPELIN, German psychi-

atrist, 1856-1926, is credited with introducing the psychiatric concept of dementia praecox, *circa* 1879.

Demilunes found beneath neurilemma of medullated nerve fibers

. . . See under *Crescent-shaped cells beneath neurilemma.*

Dengue, causative agent of, is a filtrable virus

PERCY MOREAU ASHBURN, American army surgeon, 1872-1940, with CHARLES FRANKLIN CRAIG (American physician, 1872-1950), demonstrated that the organism responsible for dengue is a filtrable virus. Recorded in 1907.

Dengue, demonstration of vector of

JAMES STEVENS SIMMONS, American physician and bacteriologist, 1890-1954, proved that *Aëdes albopictus* is a vector of dengue. Published in 1931.

Dengue, first definite account of

DAVID BYLON, physician in Dutch East Indies, 1748-1802, gave the first definite account of dengue in his description of the Dutch East Indies epidemic of 1779. Published in 1780.

Dengue, mosquito vector of

THOMAS LANE BANCROFT, Australian physician, 1860-1933, is credited with being the first to demonstrate that *Aëdes aegypti* is a vector of dengue. Published in 1906.

Dengue, Philadelphia outbreak of

BENJAMIN RUSH, American physician, 1745-1813, described the Philadelphia outbreak of dengue in 1780. Published in 1789.

Dental capsule, persistent; Nasmyth's membrane

ALEXANDER NASMYTH, Scottish anatomist and dentist, 180?-1848, described the structure and pathology of the persistent capsular investments of teeth. Recorded in 1839.

Dental caries, chemical and parasitic origin of

WILLOUGHBY DAYTON MILLER, American physician and dentist, 1853-1907, is credited with introducing the chemo-parasitic theory to explain the origin of dental caries. Published in 1889.

Dental index, introduction of

WILLIAM HENRY FLOWER, English anatomist, 1831-1899, introduced the concept of dental index, a figure obtained by multiplying the dental length by 100 and dividing by the length of the basinasal line. Known as *Flower's index*. Date not available.

Dental radiography in America, introduction of

WILLIAM JAMES MORTON, New York physician, 1846-1920, is credited with introducing dental radiography in America. Recorded in 1896.

Dental radiography in England, introduction of

CHARLES ALEXANDER CLARK, English dentist, 1860-1939, is credited with introducing the practice of dental radiography in England, *circa* 1896. Published in 1901.

Dentin fibrils; Ebner's fibrils

. . . See under *Fibrils in dentin and cementum of tooth.*

Dentin, lamination lines of

SAMUEL JAMES AUGUSTUS SALTER, English dentist, 1825-1897, described lines in dentin which are regarded as incremental, separating the growth layers or laminae. Published in 1874. Known as *Salter's lines*.

Dentistry, Father of French

PIERRE FAUCHARD, French dentist, 1678-1761, is regarded as the Father of Dentistry in France.

Dentition, first accurate description of

BARTOLOMMEO EUSTACCHIO, Italian anatomist, 1520-1574, gave the first clear and accurate description of the processes of first and second dentitions. Recorded in 1563.

Depressor nerve of heart, discovery of; Cyon's nerve

ELIE DE CYON, Russian physiologist, 1843-1912, with KARL FRIEDRICH W. LUDWIG (German physiologist, 1816-1895), discovered a branch of the vagus nerve (in the rabbit) the stimulation of which causes a lowering of the blood pressure. Published in 1866.

Depressor urethrae muscle, eponymic description of

JEAN FRANÇOIS JARJAVAY, French physician, 1815-1869, described the depressor urethrae muscle, a slender branch of the *sphincter urethrae membranaceae*. Reported in 1856. Known as *Jarjavay's muscle*.

Dermacentroxenus rickettsi

. . . See under *Rocky Mountain spotted fever, naming of causative agent of.*

Dermatitis exfoliativa, eponymic description of

WILLIAM JAMES ERASMUS WILSON, English dermatologist, 1809-1884, gave the first clear description of dermatitis exfoliativa, in 1870. Known as *Wilson's disease.*

Dermatitis exfoliativa of newborn

GOTTFRIED RITTER VON RITTERSHAIN, Austrian dermatologist, 1820-1883, was the first to describe dermatitis exfoliativa of infants or the newborn. Recorded in 1878. Known as *Ritter's disease.*

Dermatitis gangrenosa infantum

. . . See under *Ecthyma gangrenosum.*

Dermatitis herpetiformis, early description of

LOUIS ADOLPHUS DUHRING, American dermatologist, 1845-1913, described a form of dermatitis characterized by erythematous papular, vesicular, pustular, or bullous lesions occurring in groups and in combinations, and accompanied by itching or burning. Reported in 1884. Known as *Duhring's disease* and as *dermatitis multiformis* or *herpetiformis.*

Dermatitis herpetiformis, original description of

WILLIAM TILBURY FOX, English dermatologist, 1836-1879, gave the first description of dermatitis herpetiformis or hydroa, in 1880.

Dermatitis infectiosa eczematoides

MARTIN FEENEY ENGMAN, American dermatologist, 1869-19??, described infectious eczematoid dermatitis, a condition accompanying or following, in many cases, some other infection. Reported in 1902. Called *Engman's disease.*

Dermatofibrosarcoma, description of

JEAN F. DARIER, French dermatologist, 1856-1938, described a type of multiple sarcoid with a wide variation in malignancy, known as dermatofibrosarcoma, in 1904. Called also *Darier-Roussy sarcoid,* in allusion to GUSTAVE ROUSSY, French pathologist, 1874-1948, who described the same condition.

Dermatology, founder of modern

FERDINAND VON HEBRA, Austrian dermatologist, 1816-1880, is considered to be the founder of modern dermatology.

Dermatolysis, **coinage of term**

JEAN LOUIS ALIBERT, French dermatologist, 1766-1837, invented the word *dermatolysis,* which he reported in 1832.

Dermatomyositis, first description of

ERNST LEBERECHT WAGNER, German pathologist, 1829-1888, was the first to describe dermatomyositis, an inflammation of muscle and overlying tissue. Published in 1863.

Dermatoses, **coinage of term**

JEAN LOUIS ALIBERT, French dermatologist, 1766-1837, is believed to have coined the term *dermatoses,* which he reported in 1832.

Dermoid cysts of ovary, early description of

... See under *Ovary, dermoid cysts of.*

Descemet's membrane, eponymic description of

JEAN DESCEMET, French anatomist, 1732-1810, gave a complete description of the posterior elastic lamina, now known as *Descemet's membrane,* in 1759. The part was described earlier, in 1729, by BENEDICT DUDDELL, English ophthalmologist, 1690-1752.

Descemet's membrane, pre-eponymic description of

BENEDICT DUDDELL, English ophthalmologist, 1690-1752, described the posterior elastic lamina, in 1729. The structure was described later, in 1759, by JEAN DESCEMET, French anatomist, 1732-1810.

Descemet's membrane, thickening of, forming ring

JOHANN IGNAZ J. DOELLINGER, German physician, 1770-1841, described a form of thickening of Descemet's membrane which forms a ring around the cornea. Reported in 1817. Known as *Doellinger's ring.*

Descending paralysis, progressive unilateral

CHARLES KARSNER MILLS, American neurologist, 1845-1931, described a case of unilateral progressive descending paralysis, in 1906.

Desoxycorticosterone acetate, isolation of

MARGUERITE STEIGER, Swiss biochemist, 19??-   , with TADEUS

REICHSTEIN (Swiss biochemist, 1897-   ), synthesized and isolated desoxycorticosterone acetate, in 1937.

Deuterium; heavy hydrogen; isolation of

HAROLD CLAYTON UREY, American physical chemist, 1893-   , isolated heavy hydrogen or deuterium. Date not available.

Developmental mechanics, introduction of concept of

WILHELM HIS, SR., German anatomist, 1831 - 1904, introduced the concept of *developmental mechanics,* which explains the formation of the various organs and structures on the basis of local inequalities in growth and the differences in the consistencies of the tissues. Published in 1874.

Devergie's disease, early description of

... See under *Pityriasis rubra pilaris.*

Device for alternating pressure around a limb

... See under *Boot for producing vacuum around a limb.*

Devic's disease, original account of

... See under *Neuromyelitis optica.*

Devonshire colic due to lead poisoning

GEORGE BAKER, Devonshire physician, 1722 - 1809, found that the cause of the endemic colic in Devonshire was due to lead poisoning, caused by lead-contaminated cider. Reported in 1767.

**Devonshire colic, early
  explanation of**

... See under *Lead colic of Devonshire.*

**Dew point, recognition of
  importance of**

WILLIAM CHARLES WELLS, American physician, 1757 - 1817, described the concept and importance
of the dew point. Recorded in 1814.

**Dextran, introduction of,
  as plasma substitute**

ANDERS JOHAN TROED GRÖNWALL,
Swedish scientist, 1912-   , with
BJÖRN INGELMAN, introduced dextran, a gummy substance derived
from milk and other sources, as a
plasma substitute. Published in
1944.

**Dextrocardia with situs inversus
  viscerum, early account of**

MATTHEW BAILLIE, English physician, 1761-1823, described a case
of congenital dextrocardia associated with situs inversus viscerum,
in 1788.

**Dextrose and levulose,
  synthesis of**

EMIL FISCHER, German chemist,
1852 - 1919, synthesized dextrose
and levulose, *circa* 1887.

**Diabetes insipidus and diabetes
  mellitus, differentiation
  between**

JOHANN PETER FRANK, German
physician, 1745 - 1821, is credited
with being first to differentiate between diabetes mellitus and diabetes insipidus. *Circa* 1794. The
distinction was pointed out earlier,
in 1674, by THOMAS WILLIS, Eng-

lish physician and anatomist, 1621-
1675.

**Diabetes insipidus, production of,
  by hypothalamic injury**

JOHN HENRY BIGGART, Scottish
physician, 19??-   , with GEORGE
LIONEL ALEXANDER, produced diabetes insipidus in dogs by experimentally injuring the hypothalamus. Published in 1939.

**Diabetes insipidus, relation of,
  to posterior lobe of pituitary**

ALFRED E. FRANK, German physician, 1884-   , showed the relationship of the posterior lobe of the
hypophysis to diabetes insipidus, in
1912. He demonstrated that the
posterior lobe produces an "anti-
diuretic" hormone.

**Diabetes mellitus, acetone
  in urine in**

RUDOLF VON JAKSCH, German physician, 1855 - 1947, described acetone in the urine of diabetics.
Recorded in 1885.

**Diabetes mellitus and diabetes
  insipidus, distinction between**

THOMAS WILLIS, English physician and anatomist, 1621 - 1675,
differentiated between diabetes
mellitus and diabetes insipidus. Recorded in 1674. The credit for the
differentiation is, however, generally given to JOHANN PETER
FRANK, German physician, 1745-
1821, who recorded his findings
circa 1794.

**Diabetes mellitus and pancreas,
  relation between**

THOMAS CAWLEY, English physician, 174? - 18??, is credited with
being the first to suggest that injury

to or disease of the pancreas is the cause of diabetes. Published in 1788.

Diabetes mellitus associated with hirsutism in female

. . . See under *Hirsutism and diabetes in female*.

Diabetes mellitus, beta-oxybutyric acid in

ERNST STADELMANN, German biochemist, 1853-19??, discovered the presence of beta-oxybutyric acid in the urine of diabetics. Published in 1883.

Diabetes mellitus, early description of—2nd century

ARETAEUS THE CAPPADOCIAN, Greek physician in Rome, *circa* 81-138 A.D., described diabetes, in his book on the causes and symptoms of acute and chronic diseases. Exact date not available.

Diabetes mellitus, exclusive meat diet in

. . . See under *Meat diet*.

Diabetes mellitus, experimental production of

JOSEPH VON MERING, German physician, 1849 - 1908, produced experimental diabetes by the use of phloridzin. Published in 1886.

Diabetes mellitus, improvement in, after hypophysectomy, in animals

BERNARDO ALBERTO HOUSSAY, Argentinian physiologist, 1887-19??, is credited with being the first to observe an improvement in the diabetic symptoms of depancreatized animals after hypophysectomy. Reported in 1930.

Diabetes mellitus in dogs induced by puncture of floor of fourth ventricle

. . . See under *Fourth ventricle, puncture of*.

Diabetes mellitus, islands of Langerhans in

WILLIAM GEORGE MACCALLUM, Baltimore pathologist, 1874-1944, pointed out the relationship between the islands of Langerhans and the glycosuria of diabetes mellitus. Recorded in 1909.

Diabetes mellitus, retinitis in

HENRY DEWEY NOYES, American ophthalmologist, 1832 - 1900, was the first to study and record retinitis associated with diabetes mellitus. Published in 1867-68.

Diabetes mellitus, starvation treatment for

. . . See under *Starvation treatment for diabetes*.

Diabetic coma, labored breathing of; Kussmaul's respiration

ADOLF KUSSMAUL, German physician, 1822-1902, gave a classic description of the labored breathing or air hunger observed in diabetic coma. Published in 1874. Known as *Kussmaul's respiration* or *sign*.

Diabetic coma, softness of eyeball in

DAVID RIESMAN, American physician, 1867-1940, described the soft eyeball in diabetic coma as a diagnostic sign. Recorded in 1916. Known as *Riesman's eyeball sign* in diabetic coma.

Diabetic sugar is glucose, proof that

MICHEL E. CHEVREUL, French

chemist, 1786 - 1889, investigated the sugar in diabetic urine and proved it to be glucose. Reported in 1815.

Diabetic urine contains sugar, proof that

MATTHEW DOBSON, English physician, *circa* 1745-1784, evaporated diabetic urine and demonstrated that it contained sugar. Recorded in 1776.

Diabetic urine, sweetness of

THOMAS WILLIS, English physician and anatomist, 1621-1675, is credited with being the first to record the fact that the urine of diabetics is sweet. Published in 1674.

Diabetogenic action of extract of anterior pituitary

... See under *Pituitary extract, diabetogenic effect of*.

Diapedesis, demonstration of

JULIUS FRIEDRICH COHNHEIM, German pathologist, 1839-1884, studied inflammation and showed that the leukocytes are derived by diapedesis. Reported in 1867 and 1873.

Diapedesis, first recognition of

WILLIAM ADDISON, English physician, 1802-1881, is believed to have been the first to recognize diapedesis, *circa* 1843.

Diaphragm, congenital defects in

GIOVANNI BATTISTA MORGAGNI, Italian anatomist and pathologist, 1682-1771, described openings in the diaphragm, due to congenital defects, close behind the sternum, often the sites of hernia. Recorded

circa 1717. Known as *foramen* (or *foramina*) of *Morgagni*.

Diaphragm, hysterical paralysis of

PAUL BRIQUET, French physician, 1796-1881, described a syndrome involving hysterical paralysis of the diaphragm, shortness of breath, and aphonia. Published in 1859. Known as *Briquet's syndrome*.

Diaphragm used in roentgenography to prevent secondary rays from reaching the plate

GUSTAV BUCKY, German roentgenologist in America, 1880-19??, invented a type of diaphragm used in roentgenography to prevent secondary rays from reaching the plate, thus preventing distortion of contrast and definition. Reported in 1913.

Diascopy, introduction of, in dermatology

PAUL GERSON UNNA, German dermatologist, 1850-1929, is credited with introducing the method of diascopy in examination of the skin. Reported in 1894.

Diastase, isolation of, and notes on industrial applications

ANSELME PAYEN, French physiologist, 1795-1871, is credited with isolating diastase and studying its industrial applications. Recorded in 1833.

Diathermy, introduction of, and coinage of term

KARL FRANZ NAGELSCHMIDT, German physician, 1875-1952, is credited with introducing the method of diathermy treatment and with coining the term *diathermy*. Recorded in 1909.

Dichlorodiethyl sulfide (mustard gas), discovery of

. . . See under *Mustard gas, discovery of*.

Dictionary, medical, first to be published in the British Isles

. . . See under *Medical dictionary*.

Dicumarol, isolation of

MARK ARNOLD STAHMANN, American biochemist, 1914- , with C. F. HUEBNER and K. P. LINK, identified and synthesized the "hemorrhagic agent" dicumarol. Published in 1941.

Dienestrol, introduction of

EDWARD CHARLES DODDS, English chemist, 1899- , with L. GOLDBERG, W. LAWSON, and R. ROBINSON, introduced dienestrol, in 1938.

Diethylstilbestrol, discovery of

. . . See under *Stilbestrol*.

Dietl's crisis, original description of

JÓZEF DIETL, Polish physician, 1804 - 1878, described attacks marked by nephralgia, chills, nausea, etc., resulting from a partial twisting of the kidney pedicle. Published in 1864.

Diffuse infantile familial cerebral sclerosis

KNUD H. KRABBE, Danish neurologist, 1885-19??, described a condition known as diffuse infantile familial cerebral sclerosis or familial infantile diffuse sclerosis. Published in 1934. Known as *Krabbe's disease*.

Digalen, discovery and isolation of

MAX CLOETTA, Swiss pharmacologist, 1868-1940, isolated digalen, a digitalis preparation suitable for injection. Published in 1904.

Digestion, normal, possible without bacteria in alimentary tract

GEORGE H. F. NUTTALL, American biologist, 1862 - 1937, with HANS THIERFELDER, demonstrated that normal digestion and good health may be had without the presence of bacteria in the alimentary tract. Published in 1895.

Digestion, process of, in living subject

WILLIAM BEAUMONT, United States Army surgeon, 1785-1853, was the first to study digestion in the living subject by observing the process in the gastric fistula of ALEXIS SAN MARTIN, who acquired the fistula as a result of a stomach wound. Recorded in 1825.

Digitalin, amorphous, isolation of

AUGUSTINE EUGÈNE HOMOLLE, French physician, 1808-1875, isolated amorphous digitalin, in 1845.

Digitalis, introduction of, in medical practice

WILLIAM WITHERING, English physician, 1741 - 1799, is credited with introducing digitalis in medical practice, about 1778. He was not, however, the first to use it, the drug having been mentioned in the literature long before. Withering was influenced to try digitalis when he observed the beneficial results obtained by housewives who used it in treating dropsy. Digitalis was accepted by the Edinburgh pharmacopoeia in 1783. Withering published his report in 1785.

Digitalization, rapid, early advocate of

CARY EGGLESTON, American physician, 1884- , was an early advocate of rapid digitalization by large doses of the drug given at frequent intervals. Published in 1915.

Digoxin, isolation of, from *Digitalis lanata*

SYDNEY SMITH, English chemist, 1902- , isolated the cardiotonic glycoside digoxin, from *Digitalis lanata,* in 1930.

Dihydrotachysterol in treatment of tetany

... See under *Tetany,* etc.

Dilaudid, introduction of

RUDOLF GOTTLIEB, Heidelberg pharmacologist, 1864-1924, introduced dilaudid into therapeutics. Published in 1926.

Dimorphism, discovery of phenomenon of

ERNST EILHARD MITSCHERLICH, German chemist, 1794-1863, is credited with discovering and describing the phenomenon of dimorphism. Recorded in 1826.

…ics of eye

… e under *Refraction of eye.*

… in parkinsonism

… under *Parkinsonism.*

… alum-precipitated …r

… THOMAS GLENNY, …sician, 1882-19??, pre…m-precipitated toxoid

for active immunization against diphtheria. Recorded in 1930.

Diphtheria antitoxin, first production of

EMIL ADOLF VON BEHRING, German bacteriologist, 1854-1917, with SHIBASABURO KITASATO (Japanese bacteriologist, 1852-1931) developed effective diphtheria antitoxin. Reported in 1890.

Diphtheria, causative organism of, isolation and identification of—1884

FRIEDRICH A. J. LOEFFLER, German bacteriologist, 1852-1915, isolated and gave the first full description of the diphtheria bacillus (*Corynebacterium diphtheriae*) in 1884. The organism is known also as the *Klebs-Loeffler bacillus.*

Diphtheria, causative organism of, recognition of—1883

THEODOR A. E. KLEBS, German bacteriologist, 1834-1913, discovered the diphtheria bacillus (*Corynebacterium diphtheriae*) and reported the finding in 1883. The organism is known eponymically as the *Klebs-Loeffler bacillus.*

Diphtheria, classic work on

SAMUEL BARD, American physician, 1742-1821, wrote a classic monograph on the subject of diphtheria, in 1771. It was titled *An enquiry into the nature, cause, and cure of the angina suffocativa or sore throat distemper.*

Diphtheria, early description of—2nd century

ARETAEUS THE CAPPADOCIAN, Greek physician in Rome, *circa* 81-138, recognized and described diphtheria. Exact date not available.

Diphtheria, first complete description of

FRANCIS HOME, Scottish physician, 1719-1813, is credited with writing the first complete account of diphtheria. Published in 1765.

Diphtheria, introduction of term

PIERRE F. BRETONNEAU, French pathologist, 1778-1862, is credited with introducing the term *diphtheria,* in 1821.

Diphtheria, recognition as distinct disease

PIERRE F. BRETONNEAU, French pathologist, 1778 - 1862, was the first to differentiate diphtheria from similar affections and to recognize it as a distinct disease entity, in 1826.

Diphtheria susceptibility, skin test for

BELA SCHICK, Austrian pediatrician, 1877- , devised a skin test for the determination of susceptibility to diphtheria. Published in 1908 and 1913. Known as the *Schick test.*

Diphtheria toxin and antitoxin, determination of potency of

GASTON RAMON, French bacteriologist, 1885- , developed a vitro test for estimating the potency of diphtheria toxins and antitoxins, in flocculation units. Recorded in 1924. Known as *Ramon's flocculation test.*

Diphtheria toxin, isolation of

PIERRE P. E. ROUX, French bacteriologist, 1853-1933, with ALEXANDRE E. J. YERSIN (French bacteriologist, 1863-1943), demonstrated the existence of a soluble diphtheria toxin (exotoxin) by passing a culture of the diphtheria bacilli through a porcelain filter. Reported in 1888.

Diphtheria toxin, modification of, with formaldehyde

GASTON RAMON, French bacteriologist, 1885- , treated diphtheria toxin with formaldehyde, to destroy the toxic properties while retaining the antigenic power, in 1923. Recorded in 1928. The modified toxin was called *toxoid* or *anatoxin.*

Diphtheria toxin-antitoxin, development of

EMIL ADOLF VON BEHRING, German bacteriologist, 1854 - 1917, developed a toxin-antitoxin preparation for immunization against diphtheria, in 1912. Recorded in 1914.

Diphtheria toxin-antitoxin, use of, in children, for active immunization

EMIL ADOLF VON BEHRING, German bacteriologist, 1854-1917, was the first to use toxin-antitoxin mixtures in children to produce active immunization against diphtheria, in 1913.

Diplococcus intracellularis meningitidis, discovery of

. . . See under *Meningococcus.*

Diploe, canals of; early description

. . . See under *Canals of diploe.*

Disease, early classification of—1763

CARL VON LINNÉ (LINNAEUS), Swedish physician and naturalist,

1707-1778, devised a classification of disease, *Genera morborum in auditorium usum,* in 1763.

Diseases of children, first book on

THOMAS PHAER, English physician, 1510-1560, wrote a treatise on the diseases of children, considered the first work on the subject. Published in 1545.

Diseases mentioned in the Bible, book on

THOMAS BARTHOLIN, Danish anatomist, 1616-1680, wrote an important work on the diseases mentioned in the Bible. Published in 1672.

Dislocation of hip, method of reducing, using iliofemoral ligament

HENRY JACOB BIGELOW, American surgeon, 1818 - 1890, devised a method for reducing dislocation of the hip by using the iliofemoral ligament as a fulcrum. Reported in 1869. Known as *Bigelow's method.*

Dispersion of light, early explanation of

THOMAS YOUNG, English physician, 1773 - 1829, gave an early explanation of the phenomenon involving dispersion of light. Published in 1802.

Dissecting-room warts; verrucae necrogenicae

SAMUEL WILKS, English physician, 1824 - 1911, described warty growths on the hands occurring in persons who do postmortem work or dissections. Recorded in 1862. Known also as *anatomical tubercles, postmorterm warts,* etc.

Disseminated sclerosis, early description of

. . . See under *Multiple sclerosis.*

Distal myopathy, original description of

WILLIAM RICHARD GOWERS, English neurologist, 1845 - 1915, described "distal myopathy," a form of progressive muscular atrophy, in 1902.

Distichia, operation for correction of

CARL FERDINAND VON ARLT, Vienna ophthalmologist, 1812 - 1887, devised an operation for distichia in which the ciliary bulbs are excised and transplanted away from the edge of the lid. Reported *circa* 1854. Known as *Arlt's operation* and *Arlt-Jaesche technic.*

Diuretin in treatment of angina pectoris

. . . See under *Angina pectoris, theobromine sodium salicylate in.*

Divergent strabismus, canthoplasty for correction of

. . . See under *Canthoplasty.*

Diverticular hernia

. . . See under *Hernia of diverticulum.*

Diverticulum, false, of sigmoid colon

ERNST GRASER, German surgeon, 1860-1929, described the condition of false diverticulum of the sigmoid colon, in 1899. Known as *Graser's diverticulum.*

Diverticulum of embryonic buccal cavity

. . . See under *Buccal cavity, diverticulum of, in embryo.*

Diverticulum of ileum derived from persistent yolk stalk

JOHANN FRIEDRICH MECKEL (the younger), German anatomist, 1781-1833, described an inconstant appendage or sacculation of the ileum resulting from an unobliterated yolk stalk. Recorded in 1809. Known as *Meckel's diverticulum*.

Divinyl ether, introduction of—1930

CHAUNCEY D. LEAKE, American physiologist, 1896-   , is credited with introducing divinyl ether, an inhalation anesthetic, in 1930.

Divinyl ether, introduction of—1933

SAMUEL GELFAN, Canadian pharmacologist, 1903-   , with I. R. BELL, studied the clinical applications of divinyl ether. Published in 1933.

Döderlein's bacillus, isolation of

ALBERT SIEGMUND GUSTAV DÖDERLEIN, German obstetrician, 1860-1941, discovered a large grampositive bacillus in the normal secretion of the vagina. Recorded in 1892.

Dolichocephalic and brachycephalic skulls

ANDERS ADOLF RETZIUS, Swedish anatomist, 1796-1860, divided human skulls into two classes, the dolichocephalic and the brachycephalic, on the basis of the cephalic or cranial index. Recorded in 1842.

Donder's law of rotation of the eyeball

. . . See under *Eye, rotation of, around line of sight.*

Dorsal nucleus; Clarke's column

. . . See under *Intermediolateral cell column of spinal cord.*

Dorsocuboidal reflex

. . . See under *Toes, dorsal flexion of, when dorsum of foot is tapped.*

Dorsolateral tract; marginal tract

HEINRICH LISSAUER, German neurologist, 1861 - 1891, described a tract of the spinal cord composed of fibers from the dorsal roots and also from the fasciculus proprius. Published in 1885. Known as *Lissauer's tract, marginal bundle, fasciculus dorsolateralis,* etc.

Dover's powder, introduction of

. . . See under *Powder of opium and ipecac.*

Drainage tube, intestinal, with double channel

. . . See under *Intestinal drainage tube with double channel.*

Drepanocytic anemia

. . . See under *Anemia, sickle-cell, first clear description of.*

Dresbach's anemia

. . . See under *Anemia, sickle-cell, first clear description of.*

Dropsy, albuminuria and hemoglobinuria in

WILLIAM CHARLES WELLS, American physician, 1757-1817, was the first to describe hematuria and albuminuria in dropsy. Published in 1812.

Dropsy, congenital generalized, first description of

HERMANN SCHRIDDE, German

pathologist, 1875 - 19??, described congenital generalized dropsy, in 1910. Known as *Schridde's disease.*

Dropsy, differentiation of cardiac from renal

RICHARD BRIGHT, English physician, 1789 - 1858, distinguished between renal and cardiac dropsy in a report published in 1827.

Dropsy, renal, detection of albuminuria in

JOHN BLACKALL, English physician, 1771-1860, detected the presence of albumin in the urine of patients with renal dropsy. Reported in 1813.

Drunkometer, invention of

ROLLA NEIL HARGER, Indianapolis chemist, 1890-   , invented an instrument (called *drunkometer, intoximeter,* or *alcometer*) which allows rapid measurement of alcohol in the expired air of a person suspected of drunkenness. Reported in 1938.

D-tubocurarine chloride, isolation of

HAROLD KING, English pharmacologist, 1887-   , is credited with isolating *d*-tubocurarine chloride from curare. Published in 1935.

Du Bois' abscess of thymus, in syphilitic infants

. . . See under *Thymus, abscess of, in congenital syphilis.*

Ducts, embryonic, which in female develop into reproductive organs

. . . See under *Embryonic ducts which in female,* etc.

Ducts, smaller, of sublingual glands

. . . See under *Glands, sublingual, smaller ducts of.*

Ductus arteriosus, early description of, in 1571

JULIUS CAESAR ARANTIUS, Italian physician, 1530-1589, described the ductus arteriosus in his comprehensive text on embryology, published in 1571.

Ductus arteriosus, eponymic description of

LEONARDO BOTALLUS, Italian physician, 1530-15??, gave one of the earliest descriptions of the ductus arteriosus. Exact date not available. Known as *ductus botalli.*

Ductus arteriosus, formation of artificial

. . . See under *Pulmonary artery stenosis or atresia.*

Ductus epoophori longitudinalis

. . . See under *Gartner's duct, eponymic description of.*

Ductus venosus, early description of, in 1571

JULIUS CAESAR ARANTIUS, Italian physician, 1530-1589, gave a classic description of the ductus venosus (*ductus venosus arantii*) in his text *De Humano Foetu,* published in 1571.

Duhring's disease, original description of

. . . See under *Dermatitis herpetiformis.*

Dumping syndrome, original description of

ARTHUR FREDERICK HERTZ (also HURST), English physician, 1879-

1944, was the first to describe the so-called "dumping syndrome," sometimes occurring after gastrectomy and marked by hot flushes, cold perspiration, palpitation, etc. Published in 1913. The name "dumping syndrome" was suggested by C. L. MIX, in 1922.

Duncan's folds

. . . See under *Uterus, peritoneal folds of, seen after delivery.*

Duodenal cap deformity in duodenal ulcer, as seen in roentgenograms

ÅKE OLOF ÅKERLUND, Swedish roentgenologist, 1887-   , described a deformity of the duodenal cap as seen in roentgenograms of duodenal ulcer. It consists of an indentation in addition to the niche. The disfigurement is called *Åkerlund's deformity*. Exact date not available.

Duodenal fossa, inferior, eponymic description of

WENZEL TREITZ, Austrian physician and anatomist, 1819-1872, described the inferior duodenal fossa, a recess at the lower and external part of the ascending portion of the duodenum. Published in 1857. Known as *Treitz's fossa*.

Duodenal fossae considered as one

HEINRICH WILHELM GOTTFRIED WALDEYER-HARTZ, German anatomist, 1836-1921, described the two duodenal fossae with reference to hernia. Recorded in 1868. Known as *Waldeyer's fossa*.

Duodenal glands, description of

. . . See under *Duodenum, racemose mucous glands in submucous layer of.*

Duodenal ulcer, first recorded case of

GEORG ERHARD HAMBERGER, German surgeon, 1697-1755, gave the first description of duodenal ulcer which terminated in perforation. Recorded in 1746.

Duodenal ulcer, perforating, early description of

JACOPO PENADA, Italian physician, 1748-1828, described a perforating duodenal ulcer in 1793.

Duodenal ulcer, smooth diet for

WALTER CLEMENT ALVAREZ, American physician, 1884-   , introduced a smooth diet in the treatment of duodenal ulcer. Published in 1922.

Duodenal ulceration due to burns of skin

THOMAS B. CURLING, English surgeon, 1811-1888, gave a description of acute ulceration of the duodenum resulting from burns of the skin and superficial tissues. First report published in 1842. A case of an acute perforating ulcer of the duodenum due to burns was reported in 1866. The condition is known as *Curling's ulcer*.

Duodenopancreatectomy in treating carcinoma, introduction of

ALEXANDER BRUNSCHWIG, American surgeon, 1901-   , introduced an operation for the resection of the duodenum and the head of the pancreas, for carcinoma. Described in 1937.

Duodenum, aspiration of, in 1889

ISMAR ISIDOR BOAS, German physician, 1858-1938, performed an aspiration of the duodenum in 1889.

Duodenum, introduction
of term

HEROPHILUS, Greek surgeon and anatomist in Egypt, 335-280 B.C., is credited with introducing the term *duodenum*, so called because the length of the part is about twelve fingers' breadth. Based on the Latin *duodeni*, twelve each.

Duodenum, racemose mucous
glands in submucous layer of

JOHANN CONRAD BRUNNER, Swiss anatomist, 1653 - 1727, discovered and described the racemose mucous glands in the submucous layer of the duodenum. Reported in 1687. Known as *Brunner's glands*.

Dupuytren's abscess

. . . See under *Abscess in right iliac fossa*.

Dupuytren's fracture

. . . See under *Fibula, fracture of lower end of*.

Duroziez's disease

. . . See under *Mitral stenosis, congenital, first description of*.

Duval's nucleus in
medulla oblongata

MATHIAS MARIE DUVAL, French anatomist, 1844-1907, described a mass of multipolar ganglion cells situated in the medulla oblongata, ventrolaterad from the hypoglossal nucleus. Published in 1883.

Dynamite, invention of

ALFRED BERNARD NOBEL, Swedish munitions manufacturer, 1833-1896, invented dynamite, consisting of nitro-glycerine absorbed by a porous material, in 1866.

Dyschondroplasia, eponymic
description of

LÉOPOLD LOUIS X. E. OLLIER, French surgeon, 1830 - 1900, described dyschondroplasia, an abnormal growth of cartilage in long bones with the formation of bony and cartilaginous tumors on the shafts. Published in 1889. Known as *Ollier's disease, multiple cartilaginous exostoses, hereditary deforming chondrodysplasia*, etc.

Dysentery, amebic, early
mention of ipecac for

SAMUEL PURCHAS, English compiler of travelogues, 1575-1626, was the first to record the use of ipecac in the treatment of amebic dysentery, in his *Pilgrimes*, in 1625.

Dysentery, bacillary, first
important work on

JOHANN GEORG ZIMMERMANN, German physician, 1728 - 1795, is credited with writing the first important work on bacillary dysentery, in 1767.

Dysentery, bacillary, sulfaguanidine in treatment of

ELI KENNERLY MARSHALL, JR., American pharmacologist, 1889- , with A. C. BRATTON, L. B. EDWARDS, and E. L. WALKER, introduced sulfaguanidine in the treatment of bacillary dysentery. Recorded in 1941.

Dysentery, bacillary

. . . See also under the names of the causative agents.

Dyshidrosis, pompholyx, original
description of

. . . See under *Pompholyx*.

Dyslexia, application of,
to word blindness

RUDOLF BERLIN, German ophthalmologist, 1833-1897, suggested the term *dyslexia* in a paper on "an unusual kind of word blindness," published in 1887.

Dysphagia with glossitis
and anemia

HENRY STANLEY PLUMMER, American physician, 1874 - 1936, described a syndrome of dysphagia, glossitis, and anemia, often accompanied by splenomegaly and atrophy of oral and pharyngeal tissue. Recorded in 1912. The condition was also described by D. R. PATERSON, in 1919, and by PORTER PAISLEY VINSON (American physician, 1890-   ), in 1922. Known as *Plummer-Vinson syndrome.* An earlier report by Vinson is dated 1919.

Dyspituitarism marked by
tachycardia, hypotension,
oliguria, etc.

LOUIS RENON, French physician, 1863-1922, with ARTHUR DELILLE (French physician, 1876 - 1950), described a dyspituitarism syndrome marked by tachycardia, hypotension, oliguria, insomnia, hyperhidrosis, etc. Reported in 1908. Known as *Renon-Delille syndrome.*

Dyspnea of effort, early
description of

JEAN NICOLAS CORVISART DES MARETS, French physician, 1755-1821, was the first to describe dyspnea of effort. Recorded in 1806.

Dystocia, bilateral pelviotomy
for relief of

JOHN A. AITKEN, Scottish surgeon, 172?-1790, devised a bilateral pelviotomy for relief of dystocia in case of narrow pelvis. Published in 1784.

Dystonia musculorum
deformans—1907

MARCUS WALTER SCHWALBE, German neurologist, 1883 - 19??, described torsion spasm or dystonia musculorum deformans, a disease marked by involuntary, irregular, clonic contractions of the muscles of the body and extremities. Recorded in 1907. Known eponimically as *Ziehen-Oppenheim disease,* after the two investigators who described it in 1911.

Dystonia musculorum deformans—
January 16, 1911

GEORG THEODOR ZIEHEN, German psychiatrist, 1862-1924, described torsion spasm or dystonia musculorum deformans. Published January 16, 1911. Known as *Ziehen-Oppenheim disease.*

Dystonia musculorum deformans—
October 1, 1911

HERMANN OPPENHEIM, German neurologist, 1858-1919, described dystonia musculorum deformans, or torsion spasm, October 1, 1911. Known as *Ziehen-Oppenheim disease.*

Dystrophia myotonica, first
description of

FRANCISQUE DÉLÉAGE, French physician, 1862-19??, gave the first recorded description of dystrophia myotonica. Published in 1890. Known as *Déléage's disease.*

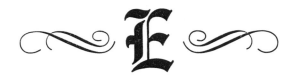

Ear, division of, into internal, middle, and external

ANTONIO MARIA VALSALVA, Italian anatomist, 1666 - 1723, is credited with dividing the ear into three parts, the internal ear, the middle ear, and the external ear. Recorded in 1704.

Ear, early description of

GIULIO CASSERIO, Italian anatomist, 1561-1616, gave one of the earliest descriptions of the ear, *circa* 1600.

Ear, first book on anatomy, physiology, and diseases of

JOSEPH G. DUVERNEY, French anatomist, 1648-1730, wrote the first book dealing with the anatomy, physiology, and pathology of the ear. Published in 1683.

Ear, helical apex of

THOMAS WOOLNER, English sculptor and poet, 1825-1892, described the apex of the helix of the ear, *circa* 1860. Known as *Woolner's tip*.

Ear, inner, aqueduct of; first description

. . . See under *Aqueduct of vestibule*.

Ear, internal, acute imflammation of

FRIEDRICH EDUARD RUDOLPH VOL- TOLINI, German otolaryngologist, 1819-1889, described an acute inflammation of the internal ear, associated with cerebral and constitutional symptoms. Recorded in 1867. Known as *Voltolini's disease*.

Ear, projection from each, is bilateral

WALTER FREDERICK MOTT, English neurologist, 1853-1926, studied the propagation of auditory impulses and demonstrated that the projection from each ear is bilateral. Recorded in 1886.

Ear with obliterated folds, as stigma of degeneracy

BENOIT AUGUSTIN MOREL, French alienist, 1809-1873, described a deformed ear, a stigma of degeneracy, marked by partial obliteration of the folds, a thin edge, and general prominence. Published in 1857. Known as *Morel ear*.

Ears, congenital asymmetry of

HENRI M. D. DE BLAINVILLE, French anthropologist, 1777-1850, was the first to describe congenital asymmetry of the two ears. Known as *Blainville's ears*. Published in 1814.

Ears

. . . See also under the name of the particular part or structure sought.

Ebers papyrus, discovery of

. . . See under *Medical document, oldest.*

Ecchymoses under pleura in suffocation

AUGUSTE AMBROISE TARDIEU, French physician, 1818-1879, described ecchymotic spots found under the pleura in subjects dying from suffocation or strangulation. Published in 1859. Known as *Tardieu's ecchymoses.*

Ecchymosis of perineum involving scrotum or labia, as sign of fracture of pelvis

GEORGE P. COOPERNAIL, American surgeon, 1876-19??, described ecchymosis of the perineum and adjacent parts, as the scrotum or labia, as a sign in fracture of the pelvis. Reported in 1916.

Echinococcus, introduction of term

KARL ASMUND RUDOLPHI, Dutch physician, 1771-1832, is said to have introduced the term *echinococcus, circa* 1808.

Echolalia and coprolalia, condition marked by

GEORGES GILLES DE LA TOURETTE, French neurologist, 1857-1904, described a condition marked by tics, motor incoordination, echolalia, and coprolalia, in 1884.

Eck's fistula

. . . See under *Portal vein and vena cava, communication between.*

Eclampsia, albuminuria in

. . . See under *Albuminuria in puerperal convulsions.*

Ecthyma gangrenosum, first description of

WHITLEY STOKES, Irish physician, 1763-1845, was first to describe dermatitis gangrenosa infantum or ecthyma gangrenosum. Recorded in 1807. Also called *ecthyma terebrans.*

Ectoderm, mesoderm, and endoderm, early definition of

ROBERT REMAK, German physiologist and neurologist, 1815-1865, is said to have been first to define the three primary layers, the ectoderm, the mesoderm, and the entoderm, in 1851.

Ectodermal dysplasia, hereditary, first description of

FERDINAND GEORG DANZ, German physician, 1761-1793, was the first to describe hereditary ectodermal dysplasia, marked by absence of hair, teeth, etc. Published in 1792.

Ectodermosis erosiva pluriorificialis

. . . See under *Stevens-Johnson syndrome in children.*

Ectopic pregnancy, ruptured, first successful operation for

ROBERT LAWSON TAIT, English gynecologist, 1845-1899, performed the first successful operation for ruptured ectopic pregnancy on March 1, 1883.

Ectopic pregnancy, first successful operation for, in America

JOHN BARD, American physician, 1716-1799, performed the first recorded successful operation for ectopic pregnancy in America, in 1759. Recorded in 1764.

Ectopic pregnancy, ruptured, sign of

THOMAS S. CULLEN, Baltimore gnyecologist, 1868-1953, described a bluish discoloration of the skin around the umbilicus as a sign of a ruptured ectopic pregnancy. Published in 1919. Known as *Cullen's sign*.

Ectopic pregnancy

. . . See also under *Pregnancy,* and under particular type of ectopic pregnancy.

Eczema, acute and chronic, differentiation between

PIERRE FRANÇOIS OLIVE RAYER, French dermatologist, 1793-1867, was the first to draw a distinction between acute and chronic eczema, *circa* 1826.

Eczema marginatum, first description of

. . . See under *Tinea cruris.*

Eczema marginatum, fungous origin of

. . . See under *Tinea cruris, fungous origin of.*

Eddowes' syndrome, eponymic description of

ALFRED EDDOWES, English physician, 1850-1946, described a syndrome marked by osteosclerosis, blueness of the scleras, fragility of the bones, etc., occurring on a familial pattern. Published in 1900.

Edelmann's anemia

. . . See under *Anemia, chronic infectious; eponymic description.*

Edinger's nucleus

. . . See under *Nucleus beneath aqueduct of Sylvius.*

Effort syndrome, early description of

. . . See under *Irritable heart.*

Effort syndrome, introduction of term

THOMAS LEWIS, English cardiologist, 1881-1945, was the first to use the term *effort syndrome,* in 1917, in a report by the Medical Research Committee on soldiers returned as cases involving "disordered action of the heart" or "valvular disease of the heart."

Egophony, introduction of term

. . . See under *Aegophony.*

Ehlers-Danlos syndrome, original description of

. . . See under *Skin, hyperelasticity of,* etc.

Elbow, first excision of

PHILIPP BRIAN MOREAU, French surgeon, 1758-1817, is credited with the first recorded excision of the elbow, in 1786. Published in 1803.

Elbow, first excision of, in the United States

JAMES MANN, United States Army surgeon, 1759-1832, is credited with being the first in the United States to excise the elbow joint. Recorded in 1822.

Electric cell composed of metallic zinc and copper

JOHN FREDERIC DANIELL, English physicist and chemist, 1790-1845, invented a form of two-fluid cell having as its electrodes metallic copper and zinc, *circa* 1843.

Electric convulsion therapy, introduction of

UGO CERLETTI, Italian physician,

19?? -   , with Lucio Bini, introduced electric convulsion therapy.
Reported in 1938.

Electric current, magnetic action of

Hans Christian Oersted, Danish
physicist, 1777-1851, discovered, in
1819, that a magnetic needle placed
near a wire through which current
is flowing will assume a position
perpendicular to the path of the
current. Reported in 1820. The
observation gave the start to the
science of electromagnetism.

Electric cystoscopic instrument operating under water

. . . See under *Resectoscope.*

Electric lamp having a filament of oxides of rare-earth metals

Walter Hermann Nernst, German physicist, 1864-1941, invented
an electric lamp whose filament is
composed of magnesia and the oxides of rare-earth metals. Such a
filament once brought to incandes-
cence remains so with low current
and without a vacuum. Produced
in 1897. Known as *Nernst lamp.*
Nernst received the Nobel prize in
1920.

Electric potential difference between injured nerve and its muscle

. . . See under *Potential difference
between,* etc.

Electric properties of living tissue, discovery of

Luigi Galvani, Italian physician,
1737-1798, laid the foundation for
modern electrophysiology when he
discovered, in experiments with
frog legs, the electric properties of
animal tissue, in 1791.

Electrical phenomena involved in the excitatory process of the heart

John Scott Burdon-Sanderson,
English physiologist, 1828-1905,
with F. J. M. Page, studied the electrical phenomena involved in the
excitatory process of the heart in
the frog and tortoise. Reported in
1883.

Electricity, animal, discovery of

The fact that certain animals are
able to give a shock was known to
the ancients. But in 1773, John
Walsh and Jan Ingenhousz
proved, by ingenious experiments,
that the shock of the torpedo fish
was electrical in nature.

Electricity, conduction and non-conduction of

Stephen Gray, English naturalist
and physicist, 1695-1736, discovered the fact that some substances
conduct electricity while others do
not. Recorded in 1729.

Electricity, earliest form of condenser for

. . . See under *Leyden jar, invention of.*

Electricity, introduction of term

William Gilbert, English physician and naturalist, 1540-1603, is
credited with introducing the word
electricity, on the basis of the Greek
elektron, amber. His work on the
subject was published in 1600.

Electricity, positive and negative, concept of

C. F. de C. du Fay, French chemist, 1699-1739, is credited with the
discovery that there are two kinds
of electricity, positive and negative,

circa 1725. The concept was further developed by BENJAMIN FRANKLIN.

Electricity produced by rubbing amber, early references to

The fact that static electricity may be produced by rubbing amber was known to the ancients. THALES OF MILETUS, Greek sage and philosopher, *circa* 640-546 B.C., was one of the early observers of this phenomenon. THEOPHRASTUS (Greek botanist, 370-285 B.C.) and PLINY the elder (Roman author, 23-79 A.D.) recorded the observation in their writings.

Electrocardiogram, changes in, in bundle-branch block

HANS EPPINGER, German physiologist, 1879-19??, with CARL JULIUS ROTHBERGER, performed the first experiments to determine the electrocardiogramic changes in bundle-branch block. Published in 1910.

Electrocardiogram changes in coronary disease

HAROLD E. B. PARDEE, American cardiologist, 1886-   , described constant changes in the electrocardiogram associated with coronary arteries disease. Recorded in 1920.

Electrocardiograph, invention of

WILLEM EINTHOVEN, Dutch physiologist, 1860-1927, invented the electrocardiograph in 1903, when he demonstrated that his sensitive string galvanometer was capable of registering the electrical changes occurring in the human heart during its activity.

Electrocardiography, introduction of chest leads in

CHARLES CHRISTIAN WOLFERTH, American physician, 1887-   , with FRANCIS CLARK WOOD, introduced the use of chest leads in electrocardiography. Published in 1932.

Electrocardiography, pioneer work in

THOMAS LEWIS, English cardiologist, 1881-1945, did fundamental research in the field electrocardiography, associating the clinical picture and the pathological findings with the graphic results obtained by the use of the electrocardiograph. Early reports published in 1910.

Electrocardiography, unipolar leads in

. . . See under *Unipolar leads*, etc.

Electrode, introduction of term

MICHAEL FARADAY, English chemist and physicist, 1791-1867, introduced the term *electrode*, on the basis of *electricity* and the Greek *hodos*, a way or path; i.e., a path for the electricity. Reported in 1833.

Electrodes, application of, to human cortex

. . . See under *Faradization of human cortex*.

Electrodes, first use of, in study of heart currents

AUGUSTUS DÉSIRÉ WALLER, English physiologist, 1856-1922, was the first to use electrodes in studying the electric currents of the beating heart. Recorded in 1887.

Electroencephalogram, early findings leading to

RICHARD CATON, English surgeon, 1842-1926, was the first to succeed in leading off and recording the action currents of the brains of animals. This achievement led to the development of the electroencephalograph. Published in 1875.

Electroencephalogram in man, first description of

JOHANNES (HANS) BERGER, German neurologist, 1873-1941, demonstrated that the electric activity of the human brain could be recorded through the intact scalp, and described the first electroencephalogram in man. Published in 1929.

Electrolysis, discovery of

The phenomenon of electrolysis was discovered by W. NICHOLSON and A. CARLISLE shortly after the invention of the electric cell by ALESSANDRO VOLTA in 1800. The discovery was made accidentally when the observers noticed bubbles of gas being liberated at the surface of electrodes submerged in water. Exact date not available.

Electrolysis, introduction of term

MICHAEL FARADAY, English chemist and physicist, 1791-1867, introduced the term *electrolysis*, based on *electricity* and the Greek *lyein*, to loose. Reported in 1833.

Electrolysis, quantitative studies of

MICHAEL FARADAY, English chemist and physicist, 1791-1867, investigated the phenomenon of electrolysis in detail and formulated the law that the weight of a substance deposited or liberated electrolytically is proportional to the strength of the current passing through the solution. Reported in 1833.

Electrolytic dissociation

. . . See under *Theory of electrolytic dissociation*.

Electromagnet, use of, in ophthalmology

JULIUS HIRSCHBERG, German ophthalmologist, 1843-1925, is credited with introducing the use of the electromagnet in ophthalmology, in 1885.

Electromagnetic induction, discovery of

MICHAEL FARADAY, English chemist and physicist, 1791-1867, discovered electromagentic induction, *circa* 1831.

Electromagnetism, discovery of

. . . See under *Electric current, magnetic action of*.

Electrophysiology, founder of modern

EMIL H. DU BOIS-REYMOND, German physiologist, 1818-1896, is considered the founder of modern electrophysiology.

Electrotherapy, founder of

GUILLAUME B. A. DUCHENNE, French neurologist, 1806-1875, is considered to be the founder of modern electrotherapy.

Electrotherapy, high-frequency currents in

. . . See under *High-frequency currents*.

Electrotonus, description of

EMIL H. DU BOIS-REYMOND, German physiologist, 1818-1896, described electrotonus, the condition of a muscle or nerve when a galvanic current is applied to a portion of its length. Published in 1843.

Elements, use of letters to represent

. . . See under *Atoms, representation of, by letters.*

Elephantiasis congenita, eponymic description of

MAX NONNE, German neurologist, 1861-19??, described elephantiasis congenita hereditaria (hereditary lymphedema), in 1891. Known as *Nonne-Milroy-Meige disease.*

Elephantiasis, ligation of carotids in

JOHN MURRAY CARNOCHAN, American surgeon, 1817-1887, introduced ligation of the carotids as a means of treating elephantiasis. Recorded in 1867.

Elephantiasis, mosquito serving as host to parasite of

PATRICK MANSON, Scottish parasitologist, 1844-1922, established that the mosquito *Culex fatigans* is the intermediate host to the parasite, *Wuchereria bancrofti* or *Filaria sanguinis-hominis,* which causes elephantiasis. Recorded in 1879.

Elliptocytes, description of

MELVIN DRESBACH, American physician, 1874-1946, described elliptical human red blood cells. Published March 18, 1904.

Embolectomy, first successful

ERNEST MOSNY, French physician, 1861-1918, and J. DUMONT, recorded the first successful embolectomy performed by DR. G. LABEY, on November 16, 1911.

Embolectomy, first successful, in England

GEOFFREY JEFFERSON, English surgeon, 1886-   , is credited with being the first in Britain to perform embolectomy successfully. Recorded in 1925.

Embolism as cause of sudden death

CHARLES DELUCENA MEIGS, American physician, 1792-1869, called attention to embolism as sudden death in "childbed." Previous to Meigs's discovery, such deaths were regarded as due to "syncope." Recorded in 1849.

Embolism due to intracardiac clots, classic description of

WILLIAM SENHOUSE KIRKES, English physician, 1823-1864, described "some of the principal effects resulting from the detachment of fibrinous deposits from the interior of the heart and their mixture with the circulating blood." Published in 1852.

Embolism of mother by amniotic fluid

. . . See under *Amniotic fluid embolism of mother.*

Embryo, first point of cell differentiation in

WARREN HARMON LEWIS, Baltimore anatomist and embryologist, 1870-19??, is credited with being first to note that the dorsal lip of the blastopore is the point where cell differentiation begins. Recorded in 1907.

Embryo, germinal vesicle of

JOHANNES EVANGELISTA VON PURKINJE, Bohemian physiologist, 1787-1869, gave the first description of the germinal vesicle of the embryo. Recorded in 1825. Known as *Purkinje's vesicle.*

**Embryo, human, formula for
estimating age of**

FRANKLIN PAINE MALL, American
embryologist, 1862-1917, developed a formula for estimating the
age of a human embryo. Reported
in 1893. Known as *Mall's formula.*

**Embryo, need of air for
development of**

THEODOR SCHWANN, German anatomist, 1810-1882, demonstrated
that the embryo requires air for its
development. He experimented
with an embryonic chick. Published
in 1834.

**Embryology, comparative, first
book on**

RUDOLPH ALBERT VON KÖLLIKER,
Swiss anatomist and histologist,
1817-1905, is credited with writing
the first book on comparative embryology. Published in 1861.

Embryology, early text on, in 1571

JULIUS CAESAR ARANTIUS, Italian
physician, 1530-1589, published a
comprehensive text on embryology
in 1571. It was titled *De Humano
Foetu* and described many parts
previously not recognized, as the
foramen ovale, ductus arteriosus,
etc.

**Embryology, founder of
modern human**

WILHELM HIS, *père*, Swiss anatomist and embryologist, 1831-1904,
is considered the founder of modern human embryology.

**Embryology, laboratory of, of the
Carnegia Institute, founder of**

FRANKLIN PAINE MALL, American
embryologist, 1862-1917, was the
founder of the laboratory of embryology of the Carnegie Institu-
tion.

Embryology, modern, father of

KARL ERNST VON BAER, German
embryologist born in Estonia, 1792-
1876, is considered the father of
modern embryology. He discovered the mammalian ovum, promulgated the germ layer theory, and
made many other significant contributions to embryology.

**Embryology, wax-plate method
of reconstruction in**

. . . See under *Wax-plate method
of reconstruction.*

**Embryonal carcinosarcoma
of kidney**

MAX WILMS, German surgeon,
1867-1918, described embryonal
carcinosarcoma of the kidney, in
1899. Known as *Wilms's tumor.*

**Embryonic ducts which in female
develop into reproductive
organs**

JOHANNES MÜLLER, German anatomist and physiologist, 1801-1858,
described two embryonic ducts
which empty into the cloaca and
which in the female become the vagina, uterus, and oviducts. Recorded in 1825 and 1830. Known
as *Müller's ducts* or *Müllerian
ducts.*

**Embryos, dissection of;
first record**

HIERONYMUS FABRICIUS AB AQUA-
PENDENTE, Italian anatomist and
surgeon, 1537-1619, was the first to
record the dissection of embryos.
Published in 1600.

Emetine, amebicidal action of

EDWARD BRIGHT VEDDER, American physician, 1878-1952, demonstrated the effectiveness of emetine against the ameba in the intestinal tract. Published in 1911. Vedder's work led to the use of emetine in the treatment of amebic dystentery.

Emetine, first recorded use of, for amebiasis

JAMES LOMAX BARDSLEY, English physician, 1801-1876, was the first to record the use of emetine in the treatment of amebiasis in 1829. Published in 1830.

Emetine, isolation of

PIERRE J. PELLETIER, French chemist, 1788-1842, isolated the alkaloid emetine, in 1817.

Emetine, isolation of, in pure form

BENJAMIN H. PAUL, English chemist, 1828-1902, with A. J. COWNLEY, isolated the alkaloid emetine in pure form. Recorded in 1894.

Emetine, subcutaneous use of

LEONARD ROGERS, English physician, 1868-19??, demonstrated that the soluble salts of emetine can be used subcutaneously in treating amebiasis. Recorded in 1912.

Emotion and facial expression, relation between

GUILLAUME BENJAMIN AMAND DUCHENNE DE BOULOGNE, French neurologist, 1806-1875, produced an atlas of photographs depicting the mechanism of facial expression in states of emotion. Published in 1862.

Emphysema, early account of—1726

JOHN FLOYER, English physician, 1649-1734, gave possibly the first account of the changes in the lungs occurring in emphysema. Published in 1726.

Emphysema, early account of — 1857

WILLIAM JENNER, English physician, 1815-1898, gave a clear account of emphysema of the lungs, in 1857.

Enamel cuticle, primary; eponymic description of

ALEXANDER NASMYTH, Scottish anatomist and dentist, 180?-1848, described the primary enamel cuticle, in 1839. Known as *Nasmyth's membrane*.

Enamel, mottled; dental fluorosis; early report on

GREENE V. BLACK, American dentist, 1836-1915, described the pathologic histology of mottled enamel due to fluorosis. Published in 1916.

Encephalitis, eastern equine, virus of, in man

LEROY DRYDEN FOTHERGILL, American physician, 1901- , with J. H. DINGLE, S. FARBER, and M. L. CONNERLEY, isolated the virus of eastern equine encephalitis from man. Recorded in 1933.

Encephalitis, epidemic

. . . See under *Encephalitis, lethargic,* etc.

Encephalitis, epidemic, first satisfactory description of

. . . See under *Lethargic encephalitis.*

Encephalitis, Japanese, experimental transmission of

MICHITOMO HAYASHI, Japanese physician, 1889- , was the first

to transmit the Japanese type of encephalitis experimentally. Recorded
in 1934.

Encephalitis, Japanese, isolation of virus of

TENJI TANIGUCHI, Japanese bacteriologist, 1900-   , with M.
HOSOKAWA and S. KUGA, isolated
the virus of Japanese encephalitis,
in the epidemic of the summer of
1935. Published in 1936.

Encephalitis, lethargic and Japanese forms of

RENJIRO KANEKO, Japanese physician, 1886-   , with Y. AOKI,
differentiated between lethargic
encephalitis and Japanese encephalitis. Recorded in 1928.

Encephalitis, lethargic, experimental transmission of

LEO LOEWE, American physician,
1896-   , with ISRAEL STRAUSS,
transmitted lethargic encephalitis
experimentally. Recorded in 1919.

Encephalitis, lethargic, first description of

JEAN RENÉ CRUCHET, French physician, 1875-19??, was the first to
describe epidemic or lethargic encephalitis. Recorded April 27,
1917. ECONOMO's more adequate
description appeared on May 10,
1917.

Encephalitis lethargica as cause of parkinsonism

ACHILLE ALEXANDER SOUQUES,
French neurologist, 1860-1944,
demonstrated the importance of
encephalitis lethargica as a cause
of parkinsonism. Recorded in
1921.

Encephalitis, lethargic

. . . See also under *Lethargic encephalitis*.

Encephalitis, myoclonic epidemic, description of

ANGELO DUBINI, Italian physician,
1813 - 1902, described the myo-
clonic form of epidemic encephalitis, in 1846.

Encephalitis, periaxial concentric, eponymic description of

JÓZSEF BALÓ, Hungarian neurologist, 1896-   , described encephalitis periaxialis concentrica, in
1927. Known as *Balo's disease*.

Encephalitis periaxialis diffusa, eponymic description of

PAUL FERDINAND SCHILDER, German physician, 1886 - 1940, described encephalitis periaxialis diffusa, an inflammation of the white
matter of the cerebrum, occurring
mostly in children. Published in
1912. Known as *Schilder's disease*.

Encephalitis, St. Louis type, isolation of virus of

RALPH S. MACKENFUSS, St. Louis
physician, 1898-   , with
CHARLES ARMSTRONG and HOW-
ARD A. MCCORDOCK, is credited
with isolating the virus of St. Louis
encephalitis. Reported in 1933.

Encephalitis, western equine, virus of, in man

BEATRICE FAY HOWITT, American
bacteriologist, 1891-   , isolated
the virus of western equine encephalitis from man. Recorded in
1938.

End organ or corpuscle of Ruffini

. . . See under *Ruffini's corpuscle
or end organ*.

Endocarditis, atypical verrucous

EMANUEL LIBMAN, American cardiologist, 1872 - 1946, with B. SACKS, described a form of valvular and mural endocarditis. Published in 1923. Known as *Libman-Sacks disease.*

Endocarditis due to gonococcus

. . . See under *Gonococcus as cause of ulcerative endocarditis.*

Endocarditis, early clear description of—1554

JEAN FRANÇOIS FERNEL, French physician, 1497 - 1558, gave the earliest clear description of endocarditis, in 1554.

Endocarditis, early clear description of—1809

ALLAN BURNS, Scottish physician and anatomist, 1781-1813, is remembered for his description of endocarditis. Published in 1809.

Endocarditis is due to bacterial infection

EMANUEL FREDRIK HAGBARTH WINGE, Norwegian physician, 1827-1894, is said to have been the first to explain endocarditis on the basis of bacterial infection. Recorded in 1869.

Endocrine glands are affected by emotions

WALTER BRADFORD CANNON, American physiologist, 1871-1945, demonstrated that the endocrine glands are influenced by emotion. He showed that cats worried by dogs respond by an elevation of the level of blood sugar, increase in blood pressure, and an increased output of epinephrine. Published in 1915.

Endocrinology, introduction of term

NICOLO PENDE, Italian physician, 1880-19??, is credited with introducing the term *endocrinology*, in 1909.

Endometrium, cyclic changes in

FRITZ HITSCHMANN, German gynecologist, 1870-1926, with LUDWIG ADLER, described the cyclic changes in the endometrium and established their normal nature. Reported in 1908.

Endometrium, hyperplasia of; early study

THOMAS STEPHEN CULLEN, Baltimore gynecologist, 1868-1953, gave the first complete description of hyperplasia of the endometrium. Published in 1900.

End-organ of hearing

. . . See under *Acoustic apparatus, end-organ of.*

Endosmosis, introduction of term

RENÉ J. H. DUTROCHET, French physiologist, 1776-1847, is credited with the introduction of the term *endosmosis*, in 1827.

Endothelial myeloma; Ewing's tumor or sarcoma

JAMES EWING, American pathologist, 1866-1943, described a form of bone sarcoma which usually affects the shaft of long bones. Reported in 1921.

Energy transformation in living tissue with relation to chemical reactions

OTTO FRITZ MEYERHOF, German biochemist, 1884-1951, did basic research on the relation between chemical reactions taking place in living tissues, especially muscles, and the energy transformation involved. Recorded in 1918. Meyerhof shared the Nobel prize with A. V. HILL, in 1922.

Entamoeba histolytica and *Entamoeba coli,* differentiation between

HEINRICH IRENAEUS QUINCKE, German physician, 1842 - 1922, with ERNST ROOS, differentiated between *Entamoeba coli* and *Entamoeba histolytica.* Published in 1893.

Entamoeba histolytica, discovery of

FRIEDRICH LÖSCH, German physician, 184?-19??, discovered *Entamoeba histolytica,* the causative agent of amebic dysentery, thus differentiating the amebic type from the other forms of dysentery. Reported in 1875.

Entamoeba histolytica in liver abscess

STEPHANOS KARTULIS, Greek physician, 1852-1920, was the first to isolate *Entamoeba histolytica* from a tropical abscess of the liver. Recorded in 1886. The discovery led to the recognition of the amebae as the cause of dysentery in man.

Entamoeba histolytica, pure culture of

D. WARD CUTLER, English bacteriologist, 1888- , is credited with being the first to obtain *Entamoeba histolytica* in pure culture. Recorded in 1918.

Entamoeba histolytica, special medium for cultivation of

WILLIAM CHARLES BOECK, American scientist, 1894- , with JAROSLAV DRBOHLAV, developed a culture medium which enabled them to cultivate *Entamoeba histolytica* for long periods of time. Published in 1925.

Enteric coated pills, invention of

PAUL GERSON UNNA, German dermatologist, 1850-1929, is credited with introducing the use of enteric coated pills. Reported in 1884.

Enteric fever, introduction of term

CHARLES RITCHIE, English physician, 1799 - 1878, introduced the term *enteric fever,* in an essay distinguishing between typhoid and typhus, in 1846.

Enterocele, partial

. . . See under *Hernia in which only part of intestinal lumen is involved.*

Enterogastrone, description of

ANDREW CONWAY IVY, American physiologist, 1893- , described enterogastrone, a duodenal hormone which inhibits gastric secretion. *Circa* 1925.

Enterogastrone, description of

T. KOSAKA, Chinese physiologist, 189?- , with ROBERT KHO-SENG LIM, described enterogastrone, in 1930.

Enterogenous cyanosis, introduction of term

BAREND JOSEPH E. STOKVIS, Dutch physician, 1834-1902, introduced the term *enterogenous cyanosis* to describe a condition marked by cyanosis, enteritis, etc. Published in 1902.

Enterokinase, introduction of term
IVAN PETROVICH PAVLOV, Russian physiologist, 1849-1936, is credited with introducing the term *enterokinase,* to describe the enzyme of the intestinal juice which activates the proteolytic enzyme of the pancreatic juice, in 1899. It is said that the discovery of enterokinase was made by one of Pavlov's students.

Enteroptosis, early description of
FRANTZ GLENARD, French physician, 1848-1920, described enteroptosis and gastroptosis. Recorded in 1885.

Enterotome for construction of artificial anus
GUILLAUME DUPUYTREN, French surgeon, 1777-1835, invented an enterotome or cutting forceps which he used in his operation for the construction of an artificial anus. Published in 1828.

Entropion, operation for, by resection of orbicularis
ANDREAS ANAGNOSTAKIS, Cretan surgeon, 1826 - 1897, devised an operation for treating entropion. It involves the resection of a strip of orbicularis muscle through an incision running the length of the tarsal plate. Date not available.

Enucleation of uterine fibroids by vaginal route
. . . See under *Uterine fibroids, enucleation of, etc.*

Envelope method for treating burns by irrigation
. . . See under *Irrigation method with sodium hypochlorite.*

Enzymes, crystallization of
JOHN HOWARD NORTHROP, American scientist, 1891-   , crystallized pepsin and other enzymes. Recorded in 1930. Received Nobel prize in 1946.

Enzymes of autoxidation in plants
A. BACH, German biologist, 1865-19??, is credited with discovering oxygenase and peroxidase, the enzymes of autoxidation in plants. Recorded in 1903.

Enzymes
. . . See also under name of particular enzyme.

Eosin-methylene blue stain, introduction of
DMITRI LEONIDOVICH ROMANOVSKY, Russian physician, 1861-1921, devised the original eosin-methylene blue stain for blood smears and malarial parasites, in 1891. Known as *Romanovsky stain.*

Epidemic arthritic erythema
. . . See under *Haverhill fever.*

Epidemic keratoconjunctivitis, original description of
ERNST FUCHS, Austrian ophthalmologist, 1851-1930, was the first to describe epidemic keratoconjunctivitis, in 1889.

Epidemic myositis, first description of
. . . See under *Epidemic pleurodynia.*

Epidemic pleurodynia, first description of

EJNAR OLUF SØRENSEN SYLVEST, Norwegian physician, 1880-19??, gave the first description of epidemic pleurodynia, in 1930. Known as *Bornholm disease* (in allusion to the name of an island), *epidemic myositis,* etc.

Epidemiology, founder of modern

GUILLAUME DE BAILLOU, French physician, 1538-1616, is regarded as the founder of modern epidemiology. He is also credited with the introduction of the term *rheumatism* and with giving the first clear description of whooping cough.

Epidermis, lowest layers of; stratum germinativum epidermidis

MARCELLO MALPIGHI, Italian anatomist, 1628 - 1694, described the deep layers of the epidermis in 1665. The term *malpighian layer* is applied especially to the germinative layer or the layer of columnar cells which rests on the basement membrane and gives rise to the other layers.

Epidermolysis bullosa, eponymic description of

JOHANNES K. A. E. GOLDSCHEIDER, German neurologist, 1858-1935, gave a complete description of epidermolysis bullosa in 1882. Called *Goldscheider's disease.*

Epidermolysis bullosa, eponymic description of

HEINRICH KOEBNER, German dermatologist, 1838-1904, described epidermolysis bullosa, a skin disease of infants characterized by the development of vesicles, bullae, and epidermal cysts. Published in 1886. Known as *Koebner's disease.*

Epidermolysis bullosa, original description of

WILLIAM TILBURY FOX, English dermatologist, 1836-1879, gave the original description of epidermolysis bullosa, in 1879.

Epidermophytosis cruris, fungous origin of

. . . See under *Tinea cruris.*

Epididymis, early description of

NATHANIEL HIGHMORE, English physician and anatomist, 1613-1685, gave a good description of the epididymis, in 1651.

Epididymitis, gonorrheal, operation for

FRANCIS RANDAL HAGNER, American surgeon, 1873 - 1940, introduced an "open operation" for the relief of gonorrheal epididymitis. Published in 1906.

Epigenesis, proof of theory of

CASPAR FRIEDRICH WOLFF, German anatomist, 1733-1794, showed that the chick's intestine is formed by the rolling of a layer of the blastoderm, thus proving his theory of epigenesis. Published in 1768.

Epilepsy and anemia of medulla oblongata

MARSHALL HALL, English physician and physiologist, 1790-1857, suggested that epilepsy is caused by anemia of the medulla oblongata. Recorded in 1851.

Epilepsy and anemia, relationship between

MARSHALL HALL, English physician and physiologist, 1790-1857, was the first to call attention to the relationship between anemia and epilepsy. Recorded in 1851.

Epilepsy, cortical form of; eponymic description

ALEKSEI YAKOVLEVICH KOZHEVNIKOV, Russian neurologist, 1836-1902, described a form of epilepsy of cortical origin. Recorded in 1893-4. Known as *Kozhevnikov's epilepsy*.

Epilepsy, early mention of

HIPPOCRATES, Greek physician, 460-377 B.C., gave the first known recorded description of epilepsy in children. He referred to it, and to other convulsive disorders, as the sacred disease.

Epilepsy, electroencephalography in study of

FREDERICK LUCIEN GOLLA, English physician, 1878-19??, with S. GRAHAM and W. GREY WALTER, introduced the use of the electroencephalograph in the study of epilepsy and demonstrated the changes observed in this disease. Published in 1937.

Epilepsy, familial myoclonus, eponymic description of

HEINRICH UNVERRICHT, German physician, 1853-1912, was the first to describe familial myoclonus epilepsy, a condition marked by clonus of muscle groups and mental deterioration. Published in 1891. Known as *Unverricht's disease*.

Epilepsy, hemiplegic or Jacksonian, eponymic description of

JOHN HUGHLINGS JACKSON, English neurologist, 1835-1911, gave a classic description of hemiplegic or focal epilepsy, in a paper titled "Unilateral epileptiform seizures, attended by temporary defect of sight." Published in 1863. Known as *Jacksonian epilepsy*.

Epilepsy, hemiplegic or Jacksonian, first mention of

L. FRANÇOIS BRAVAIS, French physician, 179?-18??, gave the first known description of hemiplegic epilepsy, later presented more fully by J. H. JACKSON. Published in 1827.

Epilepsy, introduction of term

AVICENNA, Persian physician and philosopher, 980-1037, is credited with introducing the word *epilepsy (epilepsis), circa* 1005.

Epilepsy, ligation of vertebral arteries in

WILLIAM ALEXANDER, English surgeon, 1844-1919, attempted to relieve epilepsy by ligating the vertebral arteries. Published in 1889.

Epilepsy, medulla as causative seat of

JACOB LUDWIG CONRAD SCHROEDER VAN DER KOLK, German pathologist, 1797-1862, confirmed that the medulla is the causative seat of epilepsy. Recorded in 1859.

Epilepsy, phenobarbital in treatment of

ALFRED HAUPTMANN, German neurologist, 1881-1948, introduced phenobarbital in the treatment of epilepsy. Recorded in 1912.

Epilepsy, removal of cervical sympathetic ganglia in

WILLIAM ALEXANDER, English surgeon, 1844-1919, was the first to excise the superior cervical sympathetic ganglia in an attempt to treat epilepsy. Published in 1889.

Epilepsy resulting from skull fracture

ARETAEUS THE CAPPADOCIAN, Greek physician in Rome, *circa* 81-138, was the first to record a case of epilepsy due to a depressed fracture of the skull. Exact date not available.

Epilepsy, unilateral, early description of

RICHARD BRIGHT, English physician, 1789-1858, described unilateral epilepsy, in 1836. This was described earlier by L. F. BRAVAIS, and later by J. H. JACKSON.

Epileptic convulsion, tetanic nature of

WILLIAM RICHARD GOWERS, English neurologist, 1845 - 1915, is credited with being the first to note the tetanic nature of epileptic convulsions. Recorded in 1881.

Epileptiform movements, correlation of, with lesions in cerebral cortex

JOHN HUGHLINGS JACKSON, English neurologist, 1835-1911, studied localized epileptiform movements and correlated them with lesions of the motor area of the cerebral cortex. Reported in 1875.

Epinephrine, chemical formula of

THOMAS BELL ALDRICH, American physiologist, 1861 - 19??, deter-

mined the chemical formula of epinephrine. Recorded in 1901.

Epinephrine, crystalline, isolation of

THOMAS BELL ALDRICH, American physiologist, 1861 - 19??, isolated epinephrine in crystalline form. Recorded in 1901.

Epinephrine hypersensitiveness test in hyperthyroidism

EMIL GOETSCH, American surgeon, 1883-   , developed a test to differentiate hyperthyroidism from functional nervous disorders by the use of a subcutaneous injection of epinephrine. A positive reaction is marked by an increase in blood pressure and pulse rate by at least 10 points. Reported in 1918.

Epinephrine, isolation and naming of

JOHN JACOB ABEL, Baltimore pharmacologist and physiologist, 1857-1938, studied, isolated, and named the "blood-pressure-raising constituent of the suprarenal capsule" epinephrine. Report published in 1897.

Epinephrine, isolation of, in crystalline form

JOKICHI TAKAMINE, Japanese chemist working in the United States, 1854-1922, was first to isolate epinephrine in crystalline form, in 1901.

Epiploic foramen, eponymic description of

JACOBUS BENIGNUS WINSLOW, Danish anatomist in France, 1669-1760, described the epiploic foramen which connects the two sacs of the peritoneum. Recorded in 1732. Known as *foramen of Winslow*.

Episiotomy, first, in America

VALENTINE H. TALIAFERRO, American surgeon, 1831-1888, is credited with performing the first episiotomy in America, on December 2, 1851. Published in 1852.

Epistaxis, cure of, by pulling head upward

OTTO NAEGELI, Swiss physician, 1871-1938, described a maneuver to stop nosebleed by pulling the head upward with the physician's hands under the occiput and the jaw of the patient. Recorded in 1907. Known as *Naegeli's maneuver*.

Epistaxis, renal

. . . See under *Renal epistaxis, early description of*

Epithelioma adenoides cysticum

. . . See under *Adenoid cystic epithelioma.*

Epithelioma, introduction of term

ADOLPH HANNOVER, Danish pathologist, 1814-1894, is credited with introducing the term *epithelioma*, circa 1843. Recorded in 1852.

Epithelium is true lining of body cavities and covering of body surfaces

FRIEDRICH G. J. HENLE, German anatomist, 1809 - 1885, was the first to recognize that epithelial tissue is the true covering of body surfaces and the lining of body cavities and tubes. Reported in 1837.

Epithelium

. . . See also under specific kind of epithelium, as *columnar epithelium,* etc.

Epoophoron, eponymic description of

JOHANN CHRISTIAN ROSENMÜLLER, German anatomist, 1771-1826, described the epoophoron or parovarium, in 1802. Known as *organ* or *body of Rosenmüller.*

Epsom salt, description of

NEHEMIAH GREW, English anatomist, 1641-1712, wrote a treatise on Epsom Salt in 1695. The salt is chiefly magnesium sulfate, and derives its name from the mineral springs at Epsom, where the medicinal properties were noted as early as 1618.

Erb-Duchenne paralysis, eponymic description of

GUILLAUME BENJAMIN AMAND DUCHENNE, French neurologist, 1806-1875, described the upper-arm type of brachial paralysis involving the upper roots of the brachial plexus, due to destruction of the fifth and sixth cervical roots. Published in 1872. The condition was also described by WILHELM HEINRICH ERB, German physician, 1840-1921, in 1873. Known as *Erb-Duchenne* or *Duchenne-Erb paralysis.*

Erb-Duchenne paralysis, pre-eponymic description of

WILLIAM SMELLIE, English obstetrician, 1697-1763, is credited with describing the condition now known as Erb-Duchenne paralysis in a posthumous publication which appeared in 1768.

Erb's sign for tetany

. . . See under *Tetany, increased irritability of motor nerves in.*

Ergograph for study of muscle contraction

ANGELO MOSSO, Italian physiologist, 1846-1910, invented an ergograph for recording and measuring the force and frequency of the flexion of fingers and of muscles in general. Recorded in 1888.

Ergometrine, isolation of

HAROLD W. DUDLEY, English physiologist and biochemist, 1887-1935, with JOHN C. MOIR, isolated ergometrine, in 1935.

Ergonovine, isolation of

. . . See under *Ergometrine.*

Ergot, first mention of

ADAM LONITZER, English apothecary, 1532-15??, is credited with being the first to describe the action of ergot, in 1561.

Ergot, first use of, in labor

ARMAND PAULITZKY, French accoucheur, 17??-17??, was probably the first to use ergot in the management of labor, in 1785.

Ergot in induction of labor, in America

JOHN STEARNS, American physician, 1770-1848, is credited with being first to use ergot to induce labor, in the United States. Recorded in 1808.

Ergotamine, isolation of

KARL SPIRO, German biochemist, 1867-1932, with AUGUST STOLL, isolated ergotamine. Recorded in 1921.

Ergotoxine, isolation of

GEORGE BARGER, English chemist, 1878-1939, with F. H. CARR and H. H. DALE, isolated ergotoxine. Recorded in 1906.

Erichsen's disease

. . . See under *Railway spine or brain.*

Erlenmeyer flask, invention of

EMIL ERLENMEYER, German chemist, 1825-1909, devised a conical flask which allows the contents to be shaken without danger of spilling and which is easily cleaned, *circa* 1863.

Erysipelas, demonstration of streptococcus in

FRIEDRICH FEHLEISEN, German physician in the United States, 1854-1924, demonstrated the presence of streptococci in the erysipelatous skin, in 1882. He also induced the disease in man and in animals by inoculation of pure cultures of streptococci. The organism is known as *Streptococcus pyogenes* and *Fehleisen's streptococcus.*

Erysipelas, first adequate modern description of

WILLIAM CULLEN, Scottish physician, 1710-1790, is credited with being the first to give a clear account of erysipelas, *circa* 1760.

Erysipelas, recognition of contagiousness of

WILLIAM CHARLES WELLS, English physician, 1757-1817, is credited with recognizing the contagiousness of erysipelas, *circa* 1800.

**Erysipelas toxin in treatment
of sarcoma**

. . . See under *Sarcoma, use of
erysipelas toxin in treatment of.*

**Erysipelas, treatment of,
with antitoxin**

KONRAD E. BIRKHAUG, American
bacteriologist, 1892-   , reported
on the treatment of erysipelas with
antistreptococcic serum, in 1926.

***Erysipeloid,* introduction
of term**

ANTON JULIUS FRIEDRICH ROSEN-
BACH, German physician and bacteriologist, 1842-1923, is credited
with introducing the term *erysipeloid* to describe a dermatitis caused
by *Erysipelothrix rhusiopathiae.*
Published in 1887.

Erysipeloid or erythema serpens

. . . See under *Erythema serpens.*

**Erysipeloid, original
description of**

WILLIAM TILBURY FOX, English
dermatologist, 1836-1879, gave an
original description of erysipeloid,
a dermatitis caused by infection
with *Erysipelothrix rhusiopathiae,*
in 1873.

**Erythema elevatum diutinum,
early description of—1887**

GEORGE STEVENSON MIDDLETON,
Scottish physician, 1853-1928, described *erythema elevatum diutinum,* a skin disease marked by firm,
persistent, painless nodules, first
noted on the hands of a rheumatic
patient. Published in 1887.

**Erythema elevatum diutinum,
early description of—1889**

JUDSON SYKES BURY, English physician, 1852-1944, described a case

of erythema marked by firm, persistent nodular elevations, known
as *Bury's disease* and *erythema
elevatum diutinum.* Published in
1889.

Erythema gluteale

. . . See under *Jacquet's disease.*

**Erythema induratum; tubercu-
losis indurativa**

ANTOINE P. E. BAZIN, French dermatologist, 1807 - 1878, described
erythema induratum in 1861.

**Erythema infectiosum, early
description of**

GEORG STICKER, German physician and epidemiologist, 1860-19??,
described erythema infectiosum, in
1899. Known as *Sticker's disease.*

**Erythema multiforme exudativum,
early description of**

FERDINAND VON HEBRA, Austrian
dermatologist, 1816 - 1880, described erythema multiforme exudativum, in 1860. Known as *Hebra's disease.*

**Erythema occurring after injection
of arsphenamine preparations**

. . . See under *Arsphenamine erythema.*

Erythema serpens or erysipeloid

WILLIAM MORRANT BAKER, London surgeon, 1839-1896, described
an infective dermatitis usually
starting from a wound and remain-
ing localized. Known as *erythema
serpens* or *erysipeloid.* Reported in
1873.

**Erythredema polyneuropathy;
infantile acrodynia**

PAUL SELTER, German pediatrician, 1866-1941, gave the first clear

description of infantile acrodynia, a disease of infants marked by swelling and a bluish-red discoloration of the hands and feet. Published in 1903. Known as *pink disease, Swift's disease, trophodermatoneurosis,* etc.

Erythroblastic anemia, familial, in Mediterranean peoples

THOMAS BENTON COOLEY, American physician, 1871 - 1945, with E. R. WITWER and O. P. LEE, reported familial erythroblastic anemia in children in the Mediterranean area, in 1927. Known as *thalassemia* and as *Cooley's ane-*

Erythroblastosis fetalis due to
mia.

Rh incompatibility

PHILIP LEVINE, American pathologist, 1900-   , with L. BURNHAM, E. M. KATZIN, and P. VOGEL, described erythroblastosis fetalis due to Rh incompatibility between the mother and child. Published in 1941.

Erythrocytes, elliptical

. . . See under *Elliptocytes.*

Erythrocytes, refractile bodies in, in cases of poisoning

ROBERT HEINZ, German physician and pharmacologist, 1865 - 1924, described certain refractile inclusion bodies seen in erythrocytes in cases of poisoning, as with phenylhydrazine, and after splenectomy. Recorded in 1890. The inclusions were also described by PAUL EHRLICH, in 1892. Known as *Heinz-Ehrlich bodies.*

Erythrocytes, separation of, from plasma; followed by reinjection

. . . See under *Plasmapheresis.*

Erythromelalgia, early description of—1872

SILAS WEIR MITCHELL, American physician, 1829-1914, gave an accurate description of erythromelalgia, in 1872. Known as *Mitchell's disease.*

Erythromelalgia, early description of—1892

CARL A. C. J. GERHARDT, German physician, 1833 - 1902, described erythromelalgia in 1892. Known as *Gerhardt's disease.*

Erythromycin, discovery of

JAMES MYRLIN McGUIRE, American scientist, 1909-   , with R. L. BUNCH, R. C. ANDERSON, H. E. BOAZ, E. H. FLYNN, H. M. POWELL, and J. W. SMITH, discovered erythromycin or ilotycin. Recorded in 1952.

Erythrophil substance of cell nuclei

. . . See under *Red-staining nuclear substance of cells.*

Escherichia coli, first description of

THEODOR ESCHERICH, German physician, 1857-1911, was the first to describe *Bacterium coli,* now known as *Escherichia coli.* Published in 1886.

Esophageal dilator, invention of—1939

DONOVAN C. BROWNE, American physician, 1898-   , in collaboration with GORDON McHARDY (American physician, 1910-   ), invented an esophageal dilator, in 1939.

**Esophageal stricture, use
of string in**

. . . See under *String operation.*

**Esophageal tumor, first
operation for**

ALBRECHT THEODOR VON MIDDEL-
DORPF, Breslau surgeon, 1824-
1868, is credited with performing
the first operation for a tumor of
the esophagus, in 1857.

Esophagoplasty, first attempt at

JOHANN VON MIKULICZ-RADECKI,
Rumanian surgeon in Austria,
1850-1905, was the first to perform
esophagoplasty in a case involving
resection of the upper part of the
esophagus for cancer. Recorded in
1886.

**Esophagoscope, electric,
first use of**

JOHANN VON MIKULICZ-RADECKI,
Rumanian surgeon in Austria,
1850-1905, was the first to make
use of the electric esophagoscope.
Recorded in 1881.

**Esophagoscope, electric,
invention of**

JOSEPH LEITER, Austrian physician,
1824-1892, is credited with inventing the electric esophagoscope, in
1880.

**Esophagoscope, first clinical
use of**

ADOLF KUSSMAUL, German physician, 1822-1902, was the first to
use the esophagoscope clinically,
circa 1867. Reported in 1900, by
GUSTAV KILLIAN.

**Esophagoscope, radium therapy
by use of**

JEAN GUISEZ, French physician,
1872-19??, with JEAN JULES BAR-

CAT, introduced the use of the esophagoscope in radium therapy.
Published in 1909.

**Esophagoscopy, develop-
ment of**

CHEVALIER JACKSON, American
surgeon, 1865-   , devised techniques and instruments for use in
esophagoscopy, thus laying the
foundation of modern esophagol-
ogy.

**Esophagotomy, first recorded,
for relief of stricture**

JOHN WATSON, American surgeon,
1807-1863, is credited with performing the first recorded operation
of esophagotomy for the relief of
esophageal stricture. Recorded in
1844.

Esophagus, first excision of

CHRISTIAN ALBERT THEODOR BILL-
ROTH, Austrian surgeon, 1829-
1894, was the first to excise the
esophagus in man. Reported in
1872.

**Esophagus, first successful
resection of thoracic
portion of**

FRANZ TOREK, American surgeon,
1861-1938, performed the first successful resection of the thoracic portion of the esophagus for the treatment of carcinoma. Published in
1913.

**Esophagus, plastic surgery
of—1886**

JOHANN VON MIKULICZ-RADECKI,
Rumanian surgeon in Austria,
1850-1905, reported a case of resection and plastic reconstruction
of the esophagus, in 1886.

Esophagus, rupture of, report on

HERMANN BOERHAAVE, Dutch physician, 1668-1738, described a case involving rupture of the esophagus. Reported in 1724.

Essential renal hematuria

. . . See under *Renal epistaxis, early description of.*

Essential thrombopenia

. . . See under *Thrombopenic purpura.*

Esthiomene, first description of

PIERRE CHARLES HUGUIER, French surgeon, 1804-1873, was the first to describe esthiomene, a chronic ulceration of the vulva due to lymphogranuloma venereum. Published in 1849.

Estradiol, isolation of

DONALD WILLIAM MACCORQUODALE, St. Louis chemist, 1898- , with S. A. THAYER and E. A. DOISY, isolated estradiol from the liquor folliculi of the hog's ovaries. Reported in 1936.

Estrin, introduction of term

CHARLES WILLIAM BELLERBY, English physician, 19??- , with A. S. PARKES, introduced the term *estrin* to designate the estrogenic hormone extracted by fat solvents from the ovary and placenta. Recorded in 1926.

Estriol from placental tissue, isolation of

JOHN SYMONDS LYON BROWNE, Canadian biochemist, 1904- , isolated estriol from placental tissue. Recorded in 1933.

Estrogenic hormone in treatment of amenorrhea

CARL KAUFMANN, German physi-

cian, 1900- , was the first to use estrogenic hormone in the treatment of amenorrhea. Published in 1932.

Estrogenic hormones in male urine

ERNST LAQUEUR, Dutch physician, 1901- , with E. DINGEMANSE, P. C. HART, and S. E. DE JONGH, reported the finding of estrogenic activity in the urine of males. Published in 1927.

Estrogenic hormones, use of, in ovariectomized patients

CARL KAUFMANN, German physician, 1900- , was the first to use estrogenic hormone successfully on ovariectomized women. Recorded in 1932.

Estrone, crystalline, first isolation of

EDWARD ADELBERT DOISY, American physiologist and biochemist, 1893- , with C. D. VELER and S. A. THAYER, prepared crystalline estrone, in 1930.

Estrone, isolation of, from urine of pregnant women

EDWARD A. DOISY, American physiologist and biochemist, 1893- , with SIDNEY A. THAYER (American physician, 1902-), and CLEMENT D. VELER, isolated estrone from the urine of pregnant women, in 1929.

Estrus, vaginal smear test for

CHARLES RUPERT STOCKARD, American biochemist, 1879-1939, and GEORGE NICHOLAS PAPANICOLAOU (Greek anatomist and physician in the United States, 1883-), developed a vaginal smear test for estrus. The method helped to demonstrate the histologic changes taking place in the vagina during the menstrual cycle. Recorded in 1917.

Ether anesthesia by way of rectum

NIKOLAI IVANOVICH PIROGOFF, Russian surgeon, 1810-1881, was the first to use ether per rectum to induce anesthesia. Recorded in 1847. It is said that the French surgeon P. J. ROUX suggested such use of ether earlier in the same year.

**Ether anesthesia, early use
    of—1842**

CRAWFORD WILLIAMSON LONG, American physician, 1815-1878, was probably the first to use ether as an anesthetic, in March, 1842, at Jefferson, Georgia. However, no record of the procedure appeared until 1849.

**Ether anesthesia, early use
    of—1846**

HENRY JACOB BIGELOW, American surgeon, 1818-1890, reported the use of ether as an anesthetic on Nov. 3, 1846.

**Ether anesthesia, early use
    of—1846**

WILLIAM THOMAS GREEN MORTON, American dentist, 1819-1868, discovered the anesthetic properties of ether, independently of C. W. LONG, and used it for the first time in tooth extraction on October 16, 1846.

**Ether anesthesia in obstetrics,
    advocacy of**

WALTER CHANNING, American physician, 1786-1876, advocated the use of ether anesthesia in obtetrics. Recorded in 1848.

**Ether anesthesia, introduction
    of, in Europe**

ROBERT LISTON, Scottish surgeon in England, 1794-1847, is credited with the introduction of ether anesthesia in England and the Continent. He used the anesthetic on Dec. 21, 1846.

**Ether, first definite discovery
    of—1540**

VALERIUS CORDUS, German botanist and chemist, 1515-1544, is credited with preparing ethyl ether in 1540.

**Ethopropazine in treatment
    of parkinsonism**

. . . See under *Parkinsonism*.

**Ethyl chloride anesthesia,
    introduction of**

JOHANN FERDINAND MARTIN HEYFELDER, German surgeon, 1798-1869, introduced ethyl chloride in anesthesia, in 1848.

**Ethylene, introduction of,
    in anesthesia**

ARNO BENEDICT LUCKHARDT, American surgeon, 1885-19??, with JAY BAILEY CARTER, introduced ethylene as an anesthetic. Published in 1923.

Ethylhydrocupreine in pneumococcal infections

. . . See under *Optochin*, etc.

**Eucupine, as local anesthetic,
    introduction of**

JULIUS MORGENROTH, German physician, 1871-1924, with E. BUMKE, discovered the high potency of eucupine as a local anesthetic. Published in 1918.

Eugenics, founder of

FRANCIS GALTON, English geneticist, 1822-1911, is regarded as the
founder of eugenics. He founded
the *Eugenics Laboratory* in 1904.

Eugenics, introduction of term

FRANCIS GALTON, English geneticist, 1822-1911, is credited with
introducing the term *eugenics,* in
1883.

**Eustachian tube, first cathe-
terization of**

EDMÉ GILLIS GUYOT, French feld-
sher and postmaster, 1706-1786, is
credited with being the first to catheterize the auditory tube, by way of
the mouth. Recorded in 1724.

**Eustachian tube, first catheteri-
zation of, through nose**

ARCHIBALD CLELAND, English surgeon, 1709-1774, devised a tube
with which he cathetrized the auditory tube by way of the nose. Published in 1744.

Eustachian tube

. . . See also under *Auditory tube.*

Evipal (evipan), introduction of

HELMUT WEESE, German physician, 1897-1954, with W.
SCHARPFF, introduced hexobarbital
(evipal, evipan) in medical usage.
Recorded in 1932.

Evolution, doctrine of—1864

HERBERT SPENCER, English naturalist and philosopher, 1820-1903,
propounded the doctrine of evolution several years before Darwin.
Published 1864-7.

**Evolution, theory of, by
natural selection**

CHARLES R. DARWIN, English naturalist, 1809-1882, propounded a
theory of evolution in accordance
with which higher organisms are
developed from lower ones by the
influence of natural selection. Promulgated in his text *On the Origin
of Species,* published in 1859.

Ewing's tumor or sarcoma

. . . See under *Endothelial myeloma.*

**Exanthema subitum; fourth
disease**

CLEMENT DUKES, English physician, 1845-1925, described a disease of children characterized by
remittent fever followed by a rash
on the trunk. Called *Dukes' disease, fourth disease, roseola infantum* and *parascarlatina.* Recorded
in 1900.

**Excitatory process of heart,
electrical phenomena
involved in**

. . . See under *Electrical phenomena.*

Excito-secretory system of nerves

HENRY FRASER CAMPBELL, American physician, 1824-1891, proposed
the theory that the sympathetic
nervous system is the excito-secretory mechanism which activates the
glands. He coined the term *excito-
secretory.* Published in 1857.

**Exfoliative dermatitis, epidemic,
first description of**

THOMAS DIXON SAVILL, English
physician, 1856-1910, is believed to
have been first to describe epidemic
exfoliative dermatitis, in 1891.
Known as *Savill's disease.*

**Exophthalmic goiter, cervical
sympathectomy for—1900**

MATHIEU JABOULAY, French surgeon, 1860-1913, performed cervi-

cal sympathectomy for exophthalmic goiter. Published in 1900.

Exophthalmic goiter, description of, in 1802

GIUSEPPE FLAJANI, Italian surgeon and anatomist, 1741-1808, gave the first known description of exophthalmic goiter in 1802. Known as *Flajani's disease*.

Exophthalmic goiter, description of, in 1815

CALEB HILLIER PARRY, English physician, 1755-1822, is credited with observing exophthalmic goiter in 1786 and making a brief note of it in 1815. A more detailed report was published posthumously in 1825. Known as *Parry's disease*.

Exophthalmic goiter, description of, in 1835

ROBERT JAMES GRAVES, Irish physician, 1797-1853, gave the first satisfactory description of exophthalmic goiter in 1835. Known as *Graves's disease*.

Exophthalmic goiter, description of, in 1840

KARL ADOLPH VON BASEDOW, German physician, 1799-1854, gave a classic description of exophthalmic goiter in 1840. He pointed out tachycardia, heat flushes, sweating, and goiter as the outstanding manifestations. Known as *Basedow's disease* or *syndrome*.

Exophthalmic goiter, eye bruit in

DAVID RIESMAN, American physician, 1867-1940, described a bruit which can be heard by placing the stethoscope over the closed eye in exophthalmic goiter. Published in 1916. Known as *Riesman's eyeball sign* in exophthalmic goiter.

Exophthalmic goiter, eye signs in

. . . See under *Eye signs of exophthalmic goiter*.

Exophthalmic goiter, increased metabolism in—1893

FRIEDRICH VON MÜLLER, German physician, 1858-1941, showed that exophthalmic goiter is invariably associated with an increase in metabolic rate. Recorded in 1893.

Exophthalmic goiter, increased metabolism in—1895

ADOLF MAGNUS-LEVY, German physician in the United States, 1865-1955, demonstrated that the metabolic rate is increased in exophthalmic goiter, a finding recorded previously by FRIEDRICH VON MÜLLER. Published in 1895.

Exophthalmic goiter, iodine in preoperative treatment of

HENRY STANLEY PLUMMER, American physician, 1874-1937, advocated the use of iodine in the preoperative treatment of exophthlamic goiter. Published in 1923.

Exophthalmic goiter produced experimentally

WALTER BRADFORD CANNON, American physiologist, 1871-1945, with C. A. L. BINGER and R. FITZ, produced hyperthyroidism or exophthalmic goiter experimentally. Reported in 1915.

Exophthalmic goiter, thiobarbital in treatment of

EDWIN BENNETT ASTWOOD, American physician, 1909-   , introduced the use of thiobarbital in the treatment of exophthalmic goiter. Published in 1945.

Exophthalmic goiter, tremor in

PIERRE MARIE, French neurologist, 1853-1940, was the first to record tremor as a sign of exophthalmic goiter. Published in 1883.

Exosmosis, coining of term

RENÉ J. H. DUTROCHET, French physiologist, 1776-1847, originated the term *exosmosis,* in 1827.

Extension apparatus for treating fracture of femur

GURDON BUCK, American surgeon, 1807-1877, devised an extension apparatus comprising weights and pulleys for treatment of fractured femur. Reported in 1860. Known as *Buck's extension.*

External iliac artery, early ligation of—1808

ASTLEY P. COOPER, English surgeon, 1768-1841, ligated the external iliac artery in 1808, in a case of aneurysm. The limb was dissected 18 years later.

External iliac artery, early ligation of—1809

JOHN ABERNETHY, English surgeon, 1764-1831, was the first to ligate the external iliac artery in a case of aneurysm, reportedly in 1796. The operation, known as *Abernethy's operation,* was recorded in 1809.

External iliac artery, early ligation of—1811

JOHN S. DORSEY, American surgeon, 1783-1818, ligated the external iliac artery successfully, in 1811, in treating a case of inguinal aneurysm.

External iliac artery, early ligation of—1815

GUILLAUME DUPUYTREN, French surgeon, 1777-1835, performed a ligation of the external iliac artery in 1815.

External jugular vein, sinus of

LORENZ (LAURENTIUS) HEISTER, German surgeon and anatomist, 1683-1758, described a sinus of the external jugular vein. Published in 1720. Known as *Heister's diverticulum.*

External respiratory nerve, description of

. . . See under *Long thoracic nerve.*

Exteroceptor, introduction of term

CHARLES SCOTT SHERRINGTON, English neurophysiologist, 1857-1952, introduced the term *exteroceptor,* to describe a receptor for stimuli from the external surface of the body, in 1906.

Extraperitoneal shortening of round ligaments for correction of displaced uterus

. . . See under *Uterus, operation for displacement of,* etc.

Extrapleural pneumolysis

. . . See under *Pulmonary tuberculosis, removal of apex in.*

Extrasystoles, experimental production of

JOHN ALEXANDER MACWILLIAM, Aberdeen physician, 1857-1937, demonstrated that extrasystoles can be produced experimentally by the injection of poisons into the blood stream. Reported in 1887.

Extrovert, introduction of term, in psychiatric sense

CARL GUSTAV JUNG, Swiss psychiatrist, 1875-19??, introduced the term *extrovert* as used in psychiatry. He classified all individuals into either extroverts or introverts. Reported *circa* 1900.

Exudate and transudate, differentiation between

SEBASTIANO RIVALTA, Italian veterinary surgeon, 1852-1893, developed a method for differentiating between an exudate and a transudate by allowing a drop to sink in a solution of acetic acid. If the sample drop sinks and leaves a trail of turbidity, the fluid is an exudate. Date not available. Known as *Rivalta's test*.

Exudative retinopathy

. . . See under *Retinitis exudativa*.

Eye, cilia on inner surface of ciliary body of

. . . See under *Cilia on inner surface of ciliary body*.

Eye compared to camera obscura

RENÉ DESCARTES, French scientist and philosopher, 1596-1650, compared the eye to the camera obscura (a camera consisting of a dark chamber provided with an opening or lens through which an image is projected in natural colors onto an opposite surface). Reported in 1637.

Eye crises in tabes dorsalis

PIETER KLAZES PEL, Dutch physician, 1852-1919, described ophthalmic crises occurring in tabes dorsalis. Published in 1898. Known as *Pel's crises*.

Eye, crystalline lens of; early recognition—1675

ANTONJ VAN LEEUWENHOEK, Dutch naturalist, 1632-1723, is credited with an early recognition of the structure of the crystalline lens, in 1675.

Eye, crystalline lens of

. . . See also under *Lens*.

Eye disease and general disease of body, relation between

CARL FRIEDRICH RICHARD FÖRSTER, German physician, 1825-1902, drew attention to the relationship between disease of the eye and general disease of the body. Recorded in 1877.

Eye disease in relation to general organic disease

HERMANN SCHMIDT-RIMPLER, German physician, 1838-1915, pointed out the relationship between eye disease and general organic disease. Recorded in 1898.

Eye diseases, early atlas of

. . . See under *Atlas of diseases of eye, early edition*.

Eye examination for schoolchildren, advocate of, in Germany—1883

HERMANN L. COHN, German ophthalmologist, 1838-1906, was the earliest advocate of routine eye examination for schoolchildren. Recorded in 1883.

Eye examination for schoolchildren, advocate of, in Germany—1898

HERMANN SCHMIDT-RIMPLER, German physician, 1838-1915, was an early advocate of routine eye examination for schoolchildren. Recorded in 1898.

Eye examination, lateral illumination in

RICHARD LIEBREICH, German ophthalmologist, 1830-1917, was the first to use lateral illumination in inspection of the eye. Published in 1855.

Eye examination through candle flame

ERNST WILHELM VON BRÜCKE, Austrian physiologist, 1819-1892, invented a method for examining the fundus of the eye. The eye was illuminated by a candle flame, and the examiner looked into a tube passing through the flame. Recorded in 1845.

Eye, excision of, for cancer

GEORG BARTISCH, German ophthalmologist, 1535-1606, is credited with being the first to excise the eye in a case of cancer. Recorded in 1583.

Eye, fibrous sheath of; eponymic description

JACQUES RENÉ TENON, French surgeon, 1724-1816, described the fibrous capsule which covers the posterior two-thirds of the eyeball and serves as a synovial sac. Published in 1806. Known as *Tenon's capsule.*

Eye hospital in Europe, establishment of first

GEORG JOSEPH BEER, Austrian ophthalmologist, 1763-1821, is credited with establishing the first eye hospital in Europe, in 1786.

Eye, lymph space between Tenon's capsule and

JACQUES RENÉ TENON, French surgeon, 1724-1816, described the lymph space between the fibrous capsule of the eye and the eyeball. Published in 1806. Known as *Tenon's space.*

Eye, metallic particles in, instrument for locating

. . . See under *Metallic particles in eye.*

Eye, motor anomalies of; early classification

GEORGE THOMAS STEVENS, American ophthalmologist, 1832-1921, developed an early classification of the motor anomalies of the ocular muscles. Published in 1886.

Eye muscles originate from margin of optic canal, observation that

JULIUS CAESAR ARANTIUS, Italian physician, 1530-1589, was the first to prove that some of the external muscles of the eye originate from the margin of the optic foramen. Reported in 1571.

Eye, pathologic movements of

ALFRED KARL GRAEFE, German ophthalmologist, 1830-1899, described many pathologic movements of the eye, in 1858.

Eye, posterior scleral protuberance of

. . . See under *Posterior scleral protuberance.*

Eye, pyriform scleral fissure of, in early fetal life

. . . See under *Pyriform scleral fissure,* etc.

Eye, rotation of, around line of sight

FRANS C. DONDERS, Dutch physician, 1818-1889, declared that the rotation of the eye around the line of sight is involuntary. Reported in 1847. Called *Donders' law.*

Eye signs of exophthalmic goiter, description of

FRIEDRICH W. E. A. VON GRAEFE, German ophthalmologist, 1828-1870, was first to describe the eye signs often seen in exophthalmic goiter. Reported in 1864.

Eye strain as cause of headache, early observation on

SILAS WEIR MITCHELL, American neurologist, 1829-1914, noted the relation of excessive use of the eyes to headache. Published in 1874.

Eyelid, posterior tarsal glands of

EMILIJ FRANZEVIC VON WOLFRING, Polish ophthalmologist, 1832-1906, described the small glands in the subconjunctival tissue on the pos-terior aspect of the tarsal plates of the eyelids, in 1868. Known as *Wolfring's glands.* Known also as *accessory lacrimal glands.*

Eyelid, sebaceous follicles of

. . . See under *Glands between tar-sus and conjunctiva of eyelid.*

Eyelid, upper, lag of, in looking downward, as sign in exophthalmic goiter

FRIEDRICH W. E. A. VON GRAEFE, German ophthalmologist, 1828-1870, described the lag of the up-per eyelid in following the down-ward movement of the pupil, as noted in exophthalmic goiter. Re-ported in 1864. Known as *von Graefe's sign.*

Eyeshield made of watch crystal, for sound eye

. . . See under *Watch crystal eye-shield.*

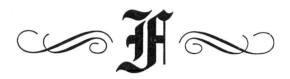

Facial angle as criterion of race

PIETER CAMPER, Dutch anatomist, 1722-1789, described the concept of "facial angle," mainly with reference to the slope of the forehead, as a criterion of race. Reported *circa* 1760.

Facial canal

. . . See under *Facial nerve, canal for.*

Facial expressions of emotion, study of

GUILLAUME B. A. DUCHENNE, French neurologist, 1806-1875, made an early study of the mechanism involved in the facial expression of emotion, in 1862.

Facial features in relation to to character

. . . See under *Physiognomy.*

Facial hemiatrophy, early record of—1825

CALEB HILLIER PARRY, English physician, 1755-1822, described possibly the first recorded cases of facial hemiatrophy, in his *Collected Works,* in 1825.

Facial hemiatrophy, eponymic description of

MORITZ HEINRICH ROMBERG, German neurologist, 1795-1873, de-scribed a progressive facial hemiatrophy along the course of the trigeminal nerve. Published in 1846. Known as *Romberg's disease.*

Facial hemiplegia, early description of

NICOLAUS A. FRIEDREICH, German physician, 1761-1836, described facial paralysis. Published in 1797.

Facial nerve, anastomosis of, with hypoglossal

. . . See under *Anastomosis of facial with hypoglossal,* etc.

Facial nerve, canal for, early description of—1561

GABRIEL FALLOPIUS, Italian anatomist, 1523-1562, described the facial canal, the canal for the facial nerve, in 1561. Known as *fallopian aqueduct, canal,* or *isthmus.*

Facial nerve, pars intermedia

. . . See under *Nerve, intermedius, of Wrisberg.*

Facial nerves, first clear description of function of

HERBERT MAYO, English physician, 1796-1852, gave the first clear description of the function of the facial nerves. Published in 1822.

**Facial neuralgia, excision of maxil-
lary nerve for relief of**

. . . See under *Maxillary nerve, excision of*, etc.

**Facial paralysis, eponymic
description of**

CHARLES BELL, Scottish physician, 1774-1842, was the first to
describe facial paralysis resulting
from a lesion of the facial nerve.
Recorded in 1821. Known as
Bell's palsy.

**Facial paralysis, treatment of,
by anastomosis with spinal
accessory nerve**

HARVEY W. CUSHING, Boston surgeon, 1869 - 1939, successfully
treated facial paralysis by effecting
an anastomosis between the facial
nerve and the spinal accessory
nerve. Reported in 1903.

**Falciform process of fascia
lata, description of**

ALLAN BURNS, Scottish physician
and anatomist, 1781 - 1813, described the falciform process of the
fascia lata, in 1811.

**Fallopian tubes, eponymic
description of**

. . . See under *Uterine tubes, classic
description of*.

**Familial centrolobar sclerosis,
eponymic description of**

LUDWIG MERZBACHER, German
physician in Argentina, 1875-19??,
described a congenital and familial
disease characterized by speech
disturbances, incoordination, intellectual retardation, etc., and due to
atrophy of the white matter of the
brain. Published in 1908. The condition was described earlier by

FRIEDRICH PELIZAEUS (German
neurologist, 1850-1917), in 1885.
Known as *Merzbacher - Pelizaeus
disease* and *aplasia axialis extracorticalis congenita*.

**Familial hemolytic jaundice,
eponymic description of**

ANATOLE MARIE EMILE CHAUF-
FARD, French physician, 1855-
1932, described familial hemolytic
jaundice, in 1899. OSCAR MIN-
KOWSKI, Lithuanian pathologist in
Germany, 1858-1931, described the
same condition in 1900. Known as
Chauffard-Minkowski disease.

**Familial splenic anemia,
eponymic description of**

PHILIPPE C. E. GAUCHER, French
physician, 1854-1918, described a
type of splenic anemia marked by
familial incidence and by the presence in the spleen of cells containing the lipoid kerasin. Reported in
1882. Known as *Gaucher's disease*
and as *cerebroside lipoidosis*. The
cells containing the lipoid kerasin
are known as *Gaucher's cells*.

Faradic electricity, early use of

GUILLAUME BENJAMIN AMAND
DUCHENNE, French neurologist,
1806-1875, introduced the use of
faradic currents in the practice of
medicine, in 1830. His text on electrotherapy appeared in 1855.

**Faradization of human cortex,
first demonstration of**

ROBERTS BARTHOLOW, American
physician, 1831-1904, was the first
to apply electrodes to the human
cortex and to demonstrate contra-
lateral muscular contractions. Reported in 1874.

Fascia dentata or dentate gyrus

PIERRE TARIN, French anatomist, 1708 - 1761, described a serrated process of gray matter under the hippocampus major, *circa* 1738. Known as *gyrus dentatus, fascia dentata,* and *Tarin's fascia.*

Fascia lata attached to pubic crest, description of

WILLIAM COWPER, English surgeon, 1666 - 1709, described that part of the fascia lata which is attached to the crest of the pubes, in 1698. Known as *Cowper's ligament.*

Fascia of abdomen, deep layer of superficial

ANTONIO SCARPA, Italian anatomist and surgeon, 175?-1832, described a portion of the deep layer of the superficial fascia of the anterior abdominal wall, in 1809. Named *Scarpa's fascia* in 1854, by JOHN STRUTHERS.

Fascia of abdomen

. . . See also under *Superficial fascia.*

Fascia, rectovesical, early description of

. . . See under *Rectovesical fascia.*

Fascia, superficial, superficial layer of, over lower portion of abdomen

. . . See under *Superficial fascia,* etc.

Fascia transversalis, early description of

ASTLEY P. COOPER, English surgeon, 1768-1841, gave a description of the fascia transversalis, lying between the transversalis muscle and the peritoneum. Published in 1804.

Fasciculus cerebellospinalis, description of

PAUL EMIL FLECHSIG, German neurologist, 1847 - 1929, described the tract of ascending fibers, in the lateral surface of the spinal cord, known as *fasciculus cerebellospinalis, tractus spinocerebralis dorsalis,* and as *Flechsig's tract.* Reported in 1876.

Fasciculus cuneatus

. . . See under *Cuneate fasciculus of spinal cord.*

Fasciculus dorsolateralis, of Lissauer

. . . See under *Dorsolateral tract; marginal tract.*

Fasciculus gracilis, early description of—1860

FRIEDRICH GOLL, Swiss anatomist, 1829-1903, described the fasciculus gracilis, the median portion of the dorsal funiculus of the spinal cord, in 1860. Published in 1868.

Fasciculus intermediolateralis

. . . See under *Rubrospinal tract.*

Fasciculus retroflexus, eponymic description of

THEODOR HERMANN MEYNERT, German neurologist and psychiatrist in Austria, 1833 - 1892, described a small bundle of nerve fibers extending between the habenula of the thalamus and the interpeduncular space. Published in 1867. Known as *Meynert's fasciculus* or *bundle* and as the *habenulopeduncular tract.*

Fat embolism, pulmonary

. . . See under *Pulmonary fat embolism.*

Fat pad in cheek, description of

MARIE F. X. BICHAT, French anatomist and physiologist, 1771-1802, gave the first description of the fat pad (sucking pad) of the cheek. Reported in his text in 1802.

Fatigue, study of causes of—1890

ANGELO MOSSO, Italian physiologist, 1846-1910, studied the causes of fatigue and demonstrated that fatigue results from the toxic products of muscular contraction. Published in 1890.

Fats are compounds of fatty acids and glycerol, discovery that

MICHEL E. CHEVREUL, French chemist, 1786-1889, was the first to demonstrate that fats are composed of fatty acids and glycerol. Reported in 1823.

Favus, causative agent of, discovery of—1839

JOHANN LUCAS SCHÖNLEIN, German physician, 1793-1864, discovered the cause of favus to be a fungus now known as *Achorion schoenleini* or *Trichophyton schoenleini*. Recorded in 1839.

Favus, causative agent of, discovery of—1841

DAVID GRUBY, French dermatologist, 1810 - 1898, discovered and described the fungi causing favus. Reported in 1841. The organisms involved are *Trichophyton violaceum, Trichophyton (Achorion) schoenleini,* and *Microsporum gypseum.* The infection is known also as *tinea favosa, tinea lupinosa, porrigo sentulata,* etc.

Feeding by stomach tube, introduction of

JOHN HUNTER, Scottish surgeon, 1728-1793, is said to have introduced the method of artificial feeding by means of a flexible stomach tube. Reported in 1793.

Feeling-type personality, introduction of concept of

CARL GUSTAV JUNG, Swiss psychiatrist, 1875 - 19??, introduced the concept of a feeling-type personality in which actions, attitudes, and reactions are directed by feeling or emotion, rather than by thought or deliberation. *Circa* 1908.

Fehling's solution, reagent, test

HERMANN VON FEHLING, German chemist, 1812 - 1885, invented a solution used in testing for sugar, especially in the urine. Published 1848.

Female pelvis, classification of, modern

WILLIAM EDGAR CALDWELL, American obstetrician, 1880-1943, proposed a modern classification of the varieties of the female pelvis with regard to form and measurements, in collaboration with HOWARD CARMAN MOLOY (American gynecologist, 1903-1953). Known as the *Caldwell-Moloy classification.* Reported in 1933.

Femoral artery, first successful ligation of

HENRY U. ONDERDONK, American surgeon, 17??-183?, was the first to ligate successfully the femoral artery. Performed Jan. 17, 1813. Recorded in 1814.

Femoral head, artificial, of acrylic resin

JEAN JUDET, American orthopedist, 1905- , with ROBERT LOUIS JUDET, used acrylic in the construction of an artificial femoral head in arthroplasty of the hip joint. Recorded in 1950.

Femoral hernia, early description of

PIERRE AUGUSTIN BECLARD, French anatomist, 1785-1825, described femoral hernia in 1827.

Femoral triangle, eponymic description of

ANTONIO SCARPA, Italian anatomist and surgeon, 175?-1832, described the femoral triangle formed by the inguinal ligament, the sartorius muscle, and the adductor longus muscle. Published in 1809. Known as *Scarpa's triangle*.

Femur, fracture of internal condyle of

ALFRED STIEDA, German surgeon, 1869-1945, described fracture of the medial condyle of the femur, *circa* 1905. Known as *Stieda's fracture*.

Femur, head of; first recorded excision

ANTHONY WHITE, English surgeon, 1782-1849, is credited with performing the first recorded excision of the head of the femur for disease of the hip joint, in 1821. Published in 1838.

Femur, head of; first recorded excision in America

HENRY JACOB BIGELOW, American surgeon, 1818-1890, is credited with performing the first excision of the head of the femur in America. Recorded in 1852.

Femur, intertrochanteric osteotomy of

JOHN RHEA BARTON, American surgeon, 1794-1871, devised an operation involving intertrochanteric osteotomy. Reported in 1826.

Fenestra rotunda and fenestra ovalis

CECILIO FOLLI, Italian anatomist, 1615-1660, described the fenestra rotunda and the fenestra ovalis of the ear. Published in 1645.

Fenestration in treatment of partial deafness

ADOLF PASSOW, German otologist, 1859-1926, was the first to attempt the formation of an opening into the labyrinth of the ear to improve hearing in otosclerosis. Published in 1897.

Ferments, early appreciation of physiologic importance of

JEAN BAPTISTE VAN HELMONT, Belgian physiologist and chemist, 1577-1644, was the first to recognize the physiologic importance of ferments. Published posthumously in 1648.

Fertilization, mechanism of

WILHELM A. O. HERTWIG, German embryologist, 1849-1922, demonstrated that in the process of fertilization the spermatozoon enters the ovum and the male and female pronuclei unite. Published in 1875.

Fetal circulation, first adequate description of

WILLIAM HUNTER, Scottish surgeon, anatomist, and obstetrician, 1718-1783, is credited with being the first to give a clear and accurate account of the fetal circulation. Published in 1774.

Fetal heart sounds, auscultation of
JEAN ALEXANDRE LEJUMEAU, French obstetrician, 1787-1877, introduced the method of auscultation of the fetal heart as a diagnostic procedure, although others had sporadically practiced it before. Recorded in 1822.

Fetal membranes, rupture of, to induce labor
FRANÇOIS MAURICEAU, French obstetrician, 1637-1709, is credited with being first to describe the rupture of the fetal membranes as a means of inducing labor. Recorded in 1668.

Fetters in mental hospitals, abandonment of use of
VINCENZO CHIARUGI, Italian physician, 1759-1820, is believed to have been the first to discontinue the use of fetters in European mental hospitals, in 1793.

Fetus, respiration in, effected through placenta
JOHN MAYOW, English physiologist, 1643-1679, demonstrated that fetal respiration is effected through the placenta. Recorded in 1674.

Fever, effect of, on psychoses
JULIUS WAGNER VON JAUREGG, Austrian physician, 1857-1940, was the first to suggest the use of fever in the treatment of psychoses. First studies recorded in 1887.

Fevers, early monograph on
DANIEL SENNERT, German physician, 1572-1637, wrote an important early monograph on fevers, in 1627.

Fibers extending across right atrium of heart
HANS CHIARI, German pathologist, 1851-1916, described delicate fibers which sometimes extend across the right atrium of the heart, from the crista terminalis to the openings of the inferior vena cava. Reported in 1897. Known as *Chiari's network*.

Fibrils in dentin and cementum of tooth, description of
VICTOR VON EBNER, Austrian histologist, 1842-1925, described threadlike fibrils in the cementum and dentin of teeth. Reported in 1890. Known as *Ebner's fibrils.*

Fibrin foam, development of
F. DOUGLAS INGRAHAM, American surgeon, 1898-   , developed fibrin foam, a fibrin product used as a hemostatic in neurosurgery. Reported in 1944.

Fibrin glue in skin grafting, introduction of
MACHTELD ELISABETH SANO, American pathologist, 1903-   , introduced the use of fibrin glue in skin grafting. Published in 1943.

Fibrin, introduction of term
ALEXANDER SCHMIDT, German physiologist, 1831-1894, recognized that the protein of the plasma plays a part in coagulation through the formation of fibers. He introduced the term *fibrin* in 1866.

Fibrinogen, part of, in blood clotting; discovery of
WILLIAM HEWSON, English sur-

geon, 1739-1774, is credited with discovering that fibrinogen is essential and responsible for the clotting of blood, in 1768. Reported in 1770. Hewson did not use the term *fibrinogen,* but called the substance "coagulable lymph."

Fibroma of ovary with ascites and hydrothorax, syndrome of

JOE VINCENT MEIGS, Boston gynecologist, 1892-   , described a syndrome of fibroma of the ovary accompanied by ascites and hydrothorax, in 1934. Known as *Meigs's syndrome.*

Fibrous cavernitis

. . . See under *Penis, fibrosis of corpora cavernosa of.*

Fibrous myositis, early description of

AUGUST VON FRORIEP, German anatomist, 1849-1917, described a type of myositis marked by the formation of connective tissue in the muscle substance. Known as *Froriep's induration.* Recorded circa 1888.

Fibula, fracture of lower end of, eponymic description of

GUILLAUME DUPUYTREN, French surgeon, 1777-1835, gave a comprehensive description of fracture of the lower end of the fibula with rupture of the lateral ligament and disclocation. Reported in 1819. Known as *Dupuytren's fracture.*

Fibula, fracture of lower end of

. . . See under *Pott's fracture of the fibula.*

Fifth cranial nerve, sensory and motor function of

CHARLES BELL, Scottish physician, 1774-1842, showed that the fifth cranial nerve has both sensory and motor functions. Reported in 1821.

Fight-flight mechanism, first description of

WALTER BRADFORD CANNON, American physiologist, 1871-1945, demonstrated that under emotional stress the sympathetic system and the adrenal medulla produced "visceral adjustments adapted to the preservation of the organism." This is known as the *fight-flight mechanism.* Reported in 1915.

Filaria bancrofti, introduction of name

THOMAS SPENCER COBBOLD, Engglish parasitologist, 1828-1886, introduced the name *Filaria bancrofti* about 1877, in honor of JOSEPH BANCROFT, English physician in Australia, 1836-1894. The organism is also known as *Wuchereria bancrofti.*

Filaria hominis, discovery of

PATRICK MANSON, Scottish parasitologist, 1844-1922, is credited with discovering the organism *Filaria hominis.* Recorded in 1898.

Filarial infection, complete cycle of

GEORGE CARMICHAEL LOW, English physician, 1872-1952, demonstrated the complete cycle of filarial infection, from man to mosquito to man. Recorded in 1900.

Filatov-Dukes disease

. . . See under *Rubeola scarlatinosa.*

Filial regression, theory of

FRANCIS GALTON, English geneticist, 1822-1911, proposed the theory of filial regression in accordance with which offspring of parents who are unusual in some way tend to regress to the average for the group. Reported in 1869.

Filter for purifying water in the field, for troops

. . . See under *Water purification in field.*

Filter of unglazed porcelain

CHARLES E. CHAMBERLAND, French bacteriologist, 1851-1908, devised an unglazed porcelain filter, made of kaolin and sand, which allows the separation of bacteria-free filtrates. Known as *Pasteur-Chamberland filter.* Introduced in 1884.

Filtrable virus as cause of disease in animals

FRIEDRICH AUGUST JOHANNES LOEFFLER, German bacteriologist, 1852-1915, with PAUL FROSCH, recognized the cause of foot-and-mouth disease, thus demonstrating for the first time that a filtrable virus may be the agent of animal disease. Published in 1897.

Fingernails, alternate flushing and blanching of

HEINRICH IRENAEUS QUINCKE, German physician, 1842-1922, described the phenomenon of alternate blanching and flushing of the fingernails, observed in aortic insufficiency. Recorded in 1868. Known as *Quincke's sign* or *pulse.*

Fingernails, transverse lines on, in exhausting diseases

. . . See under *Lines, transverse, on fingernails.*

Fingerprints, early classification of—1823

JOHANNES EVANGELISTA VON PUR-

KINJE, Bohemian physiologist, 1787-1869, demonstrated the importance of fingerprints and devised the first classification. Recorded in 1823.

Fingerprints as method of identification, early suggestion regarding—1892

FRANCIS GALTON, English geneticist, 1822-1911, proposed the use of fingerprints as a means of identification, in 1892.

Fingers, contracture of; Dupuytren's contracture

. . . See under *Hand, contracture of.*

Fingertips, tactile corpuscles in

. . . See under *Tactile nerve endings in tips of fingers and toes.*

First aid, first book on

STEPHEN BRADWELL, English physician, 15??-1644, is credited with writing the first book on first aid. Published in 1633.

First-aid kit for use on battlefield, introduction of

JOHANN FRIEDRICH A. VON ESMARCH, German military surgeon, 1823-1908, introduced the use of a first-aid package on the battlefield, in 1869.

First anatomic lecture in the American Colonies

THOMAS CADWALADER, American physician, 1708-1779, gave what was probably the first anatomic lecture in the American Colonies, in 1730.

First medical monograph published in the American Colonies

"An essay on the West India drygripes," a monograph on lead poisoning or colic, written by THOMAS CADWALADER (American physician, 1708-1779) was probably the first medical monograph published in the American Colonies. It appeared in 1745.

Fission, multiplication of bacteria by

FERDINAND JULIUS COHN, German bacteriologist, 1828-1898, discovered that bacteria can multiply by fission. Reported *circa* 1872.

Fissure extending from central fissure to occipital lobe

ADOLF PANSCH, German anatomist, 1841-1887, described a brain fissure which extends from the lower end of the central fissure to the occipital lobe. Recorded in 1866. Known as *Pansch's fissure.*

Fissure of Rolando, eponymic description of

LUIGI ROLANDO, Italian anatomist, 1773-1831, described a fissure between the parietal and frontal lobes, in 1825. It was named *fissure of Rolando* by FRANÇOIS LEURET, in 1839.

Fissure of Sylvius; lateral cerebral fissure

FRANCISCUS SYLVIUS (Franciscus de le Boë), Dutch physician, 1614-1672, described the fissure which separates the anterior lobe of the cerebrum from the middle lobe. Recorded in 1641.

Fixing fluid of Zenker

FRIEDRICH ALBERT ZENKER, German pathologist, 1825-1898, devised a fixing fluid consisting chiefly of mercuric chloride and potassium dichromate. Recorded in 1894.

Flaccid paralysis, arthrodesis for relief of disability due to

. . . See under *Arthrodesis.*

Flagellate form of malarial parasites

. . . See under *Malarial parasites, mode of conjugation of.*

Flap amputation, first record of

JAMES YONGE, English surgeon, 1646-1721, described the first flap amputation. Recorded in 1679.

Flaxedil, introduction of

. . . See under *Gallamine triethiodide.*

Flour, unbolted, advocacy of

. . . See under *Graham flour.*

Fluid, absorption of, by blood vessels

FRANÇOIS MAGENDIE, French physiologist, 1783 - 1855, established that fluids are absorbed by blood vessels as well as by lymphatics. Published in 1821.

Fluorescein in neurosurgery, clinical use of

GEORGE EUGENE MOORE, American neurosurgeon, 1920-   , introduced the use of fluorescein in the localization of brain tumors. Published in 1948.

Foam cells

. . . See under *Mikulicz's cells,* etc.

Focal infection in teeth, first recognition of

EDWARD CARL ROSENOW, American bacteriologist, 1875-19??, was the first to point out that focal infection may reside in the teeth. Published in 1921.

**Focal infection, introduction
of doctrine of**

FRANK BILLINGS, American physician, 1854 - 1932, introduced the doctrine of focal infection. Reported in 1912 and 1916.

Folic acid, erythrocyte maturation influence of

TOM DOUGLAS SPIES, American physician, 1902-   , with C. F. VILTER, M. B. KOCH, and M. H. CALDWELL, demonstrated that folic acid is a factor in the maturation of erythrocytes. Recorded in 1945.

Folic acid, first recognition of

LUCY WILLS, English physician, 18??-19??, is credited with being first to recognize the hemopoietic effect of folic acid. Published, in a report on the curative effect of yeast extract, in 1931.

Folic acid, isolation of

ALBERT GARLAND HOGAN, American biochemist, 1884-   , with ERNEST MILFORD PARROTT, isolated vitamin B-c or folic acid. Published in 1940.

**Folic acid, isolation and
synthesis of**

ROBERT CRANE ANGIER, American scientist, 1917-   , with associates, isolated, determined the structure of, and finally synthesized folic acid. Recorded in 1946.

**Folliculitis decalvans, eponymic
description of**

CHARLES EUGENE QUINQUAUD, French physician, 1841-1894, described folliculitis decalvans, a chronic form of folliculitis of the scalp resulting in patchy baldness.

Recorded in 1888. Known as *Quinquaud's disease.*

Fomites, introduction of term

GIROLAMO FRACASTORO, Italian pathologist, 1483-1553, introduced the term *fomites* to describe clothing, utensils, and other articles of a sick person that may transmit the disease. Reported in 1546.

Fontana's spaces or canal

. . . See under *Pectinate ligament, spaces between the fibers of.*

**Fontanel, posterior, early
description of**

GIULIO CASSERIO, Italian anatomist, 1561-1616, gave one of the earliest descriptions of the posterior fontanel. Recorded in 1600.

Food analysis, pioneer work in

. . . See under *Analyses of foods and fertilizers.*

**Food, digested, is carried to
liver in portal blood**

FRANÇOIS MAGENDIE, French physiologist, 1783-1855, demonstrated that digested food is carried to the liver by way of the portal circulation. Published in 1844.

Food, specific dynamic action of

. . . See under *Specific dynamic action of foodstuffs.*

Food-stuffs, first classification of

JUSTUS VON LIEBIG, German chemist, 1803-1873, provided the first classification of the processes of nutrition and of the organic foodstuffs. Recorded in 1842.

**Foot and mouth disease in animals,
causative virus of**

. . . See under *Virus, filtrable, as cause of disease in animals.*

Foot, Pirogoff's amputation of

NIKOLAI IVANOVICH PIROGOFF, Russian surgeon, 1810-1881, introduced an osteoplastic operation for the amputation of the foot in which part of the calcaneus bone is retained. Recorded in 1854.

Foramen for palatine nerve

ANTONIO SCARPA, Italian anatomist and surgeon, 175?-1832, described two foramina situated behind the middle incisors, transmitting the nasopalatine nerves. Recorded in 1799. Known as *Scarpa's foramen* or *foramina*.

Foramen of Bochdalek

. . . See under *Hiatus pleuroperitonealis*.

Foramen of Magendie, eponymic description of

FRANÇOIS MAGENDIE, French physiologist, 1783-1855, described an opening in the membranous roof of the fourth ventricle which forms a passage between the fourth ventricle and the subarachnoid space. Published in 1842.

Foramen of Monroe

. . . See under *Interventricular foramen of human brain*.

Foramen of Morgagni

. . . See under *Diaphragm, congenital defects in*.

Foramen of Vesalius at base of skull

ANDREAS VESALIUS, Belgian anatomist, 1514-1564, described a foramen occurring at the base of the skull at the inner side of the foramen ovale. Recorded in 1543. Known as *Vesalius' foramen*.

Foramen of Winslow

. . . See under *Epiploic foramen*, etc.

Foramen ovale of heart, early description of, in 1571

JULIUS CAESAR ARANTIUS, Italian physician, 1530 - 1589, described the foramen ovale in his comprehensive text on embryology, published in 1571.

Foramen ovale of heart, early description of—1575

LEONARDO BOTALLUS, Italian physician, 1530-16??, gave one of the early descriptions of the foramen ovale of the heart, *circa* 1575.

Foramen ovale of heart, vestigial, description of

PIERRE GASSENDI, French physician, 1592-1655, showed the existence of a vestigial foramen ovale in the adult. Recorded in 1640.

Forceps, obstetric, invention of first practical

. . . See under *Obstetrical forceps*, etc.

Forcipressure, introduction of

. . . See under *Hemostatic forceps*.

Foreign proteins, test for, based on protective ferment

. . . See under *Serum reaction based on presence of protective ferment in body*.

Formaldehyde in tissue fixation first use of

F. BLUM, German physician, 18??-19??, was the first to use formaldehyde for tissue fixation. Recorded in 1893.

Fossa navicularis **vestibuli vaginae, introduction of term**

FRANÇOIS MAURICEAU, French obstetrician, 1637 - 1709, is credited with the introduction of the term *fossa navicularis* into the vocabulary of obstetrics. Recorded in 1668.

Fossa navicularis of urethra, valve or fold in

. . . See under *Urethra, valve in fossa navicularis of.*

Fossa of Rosenmuller

. . . See under *Pharynx, lateral recess of.*

Fothergill's disease

. . . See under *Trigeminal neuralgia, eponymic description of.*

Fourchette, **introduction of term**

FRANÇOIS MAURICEAU, French obstetrician, 1637 - 1709, is credited with introducing the term *fourchette* into the vocabulary of obstetrics. Recorded in 1668.

Fourth cranial nerves, discovery of

. . . See under *Trochlear nerves.*

Fourth disease; parascarlatina; Dukes' disease

. . . See under *Rubeola scarlatinosa* and *Exanthema subitum.*

Fourth ventricle, puncture of, makes animal diabetic

CLAUDE BERNARD, French physiologist, 1813 - 1878, showed that puncture of the floor of the fourth ventricle made dogs diabetic. Reported in 1849.

Fowler's position, introduction of

GEORGE RYERSON FOWLER, American surgeon, 1848-1906, introduced a position for the patient in which the head of the bed is elevated about 18 to 20 inches. Recorded in 1900.

Fowler's solution, introduction of

. . . See under *Solution of potassium arsenite.*

Fractional sterilization, introduction of

JOHN TYNDALL, English physicist, 1820-1893, introduced the method of fractional sterilization, in 1877. The procedure is known as *Tyndallization.*

Fractional test meal examination

MARTIN EMIL REHFUSS, American physician, 1887 - 19??, devised a method of fractional test meal examination in which portions of a standard test meal are removed from the stomach at certain intervals by means of a stomach tube. Recorded in 1914. Known as the *Rehfuss method.*

Fracture, treatment of, by traction exerted on wires passed through the bone

MARTIN KIRSCHNER, German surgeon, 1879 - 1942, introduced a method for treating fractures by exerting traction on pins or wires passed through the bone. Recorded in 1909. Known as *Kirschner's traction.*

Fracture, treatment of, with metal band

FREDERICK WILLIAM PARHAM, American surgeon, 1856-1927, with E. D. MARTIN, introduced the use of a steel or aluminum band to hold together the ends of a broken bone, until union is established. Published in 1913. Known as *Parham-Martin band*.

Frame used in tuberculosis of spine, fractures of thigh, etc.

EDWARD HICKLING BRADFORD, American orthopedic surgeon, 1848-1926, devised a frame made of gas-pipe and canvas for handling children with tuberculosis of the spine. It was later modified for use in fracture of the thigh, joint disease, etc. Reported in 1890. Known as a *Bradford frame*.

Frédet-Ramstedt operation

. . . See under *Pyloric stenosis, congenital,* etc.

Freezing tissue for microscopic examination, method of

JULIUS FRIEDRICH COHNHEIM, German pathologist, 1839 - 1884, was the first to use the method of freezing tissue for microscopic study. Date not available.

Fresh air, early advocacy of

BENJAMIN FRANKLIN, American statesman and scientist, 1706-1790, was an early advocate of fresh air as an adjunct to hygiene.

Fresh fruit in diet of sailors, introduction of

GILBERT BLANE, Scottish physician, 1749-1834, introduced the use of lemons and limes in the diet of sailors of the British navy, to prevent scurvy. Reported in 1785.

Friedel Pick's disease

. . . See under *Liver, pseudocirrhosis of, with pericarditis.*

Friedreich's disease

. . . See under *Paramyoclonus multiplex.*

Frog lymph hearts, discovery of

JOHANNES MÜLLER, German anatomist and physiologist, 1801-1858, discovered the lymph hearts of the frog. Published in 1833.

Frog, rheoscopic

. . . See under *Rheoscopic frog, original description of.*

Frog's egg, segmentation of; observations on

JEAN LOUIS PRÉVOST, French physician, 1790-1850, with JEAN B. A. DUMAS, observed and gave the first description of the segmentation of the frog's egg. Recorded in 1827.

Frogs, fatherless, successful raising of

JACQUES LOEB, American biologist, 1859 - 1924, successfully raised frogs from unfertilized eggs to maturity. Reported in 1908.

Fröhlich's syndrome, pre-eponymic description of

BERNHARD MOHR, German physician, 181?-18??, was the first to describe pituitary obesity with infantilism, later to be known as *Fröhlich's syndrome*. Published in 1840.

Fröhlich's syndrome

. . . See also under *Adiposogenital dystrophy.*

Frommel's disease

. . . See under *Uterus, atrophy of, in prolonged lactation.*

Frontal lobes, destruction of, causes character changes

LEONARDO BIANCHI, Italian psychiatrist and neurologist, 1848-1927, demonstrated that bilateral destruction of the frontal lobes in monkeys caused changes of character. Published in 1920.

Frontal lobes, infiltration of, for relief of pain

FELIX MANDL, Austrian surgeon, 1892-   , introduced infiltration of the frontal lobes for the relief of intractable pain. Recorded in 1950.

Frontal lobotomy, early record of

G. BURCKHARDT, German surgeon, 18??-19??, performed frontal lobotomy on four mental patients, in 1890. Recorded in 1891.

Frontal lobotomy in treatment of mental disorders

ANTONIO C. A. F. EGAS MONIZ, Portuguese neurologist, 1874-19??, described a method of frontal (prefrontal) lobotomy for the relief of certain mental disorders. Reported in 1936.

Frontopontine bundle of brain, classic description of

FRIEDRICH ARNOLD, German anatomist, 1803 - 1890, described the frontopontine tract or bundle, a tract of fibers arising from the pons varolii and extending anteriorly to form part of the cerebral peduncle. Reported in 1838.

Frozen sections, first use of

PIETER DE RIEMER, Scandinavian anatomist, 1760-1831, is believed to have been the first to prepare frozen anatomical sections. Recorded in 1818.

Frozen sections in Russia

NIKOLAI IVANOVICH PIROGOFF, Russian surgeon, 1810 - 1881, is credited with introducing frozen section technique into Russia, *circa* 1852.

Fulguration of urinary bladder tumors by way of the urethra

. . . See under *Transurethral fulguration.*

Functional and organic heart disease, distinction between

JEAN N. CORVISART DES MARETS, French physician, 1755-1821, distinguished between organic and functional heart disease. Published in 1806.

Fundamental units of protoplasm are granular particles, theory holding that

RICHARD ALTMANN, German histologist, 1852-1900, propounded a theory which holds that the fundamental units of protoplasm are granular particles. It is known as *Altmann's theory.* Reported *circa* 1890.

Funiculus of Rolando

. . . See under *Medulla oblongata, funiculus of.*

Funnel with perforated plate supporting filter paper

EDUARD BUCHNER, German chemist, 1860-1917, invented a funnel having a perforated plate on which filter paper is placed. Introduced in 1889. Known as *Buchner funnel* or *filter.*

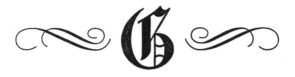

**Gallamine triethiodide,
introduction of**

DANIEL BOVET, French pharmacologist, 19??-   , with S. COURVOISIER, R. DUCROT, and R. HORCLOIS, introduced the curariform substance gallamine triethiodide, also known as *flaxedil*. Published in 1946.

**Gallbladder, glands or tubular
structures in wall of**

HUBERT VON LUSCHKA, German anatomist, 1820 - 1875, described atypical bile ducts in the wall of the gallbladder. Recorded in 1858. Known as *Luschka's glands*.

**Gallbladder, non-surgical
drainage of**

SAMUEL JAMES MELTZER, American physician, 1851-1920, was the first to suggest non-surgical drainage of the gallbladder. Recorded in 1917.

Gallbladder radiography, introduction of successful

See under *Cholecystography*, etc.

**Gallstone, first removal of,
from living subject**

WILHELM FABRY (Fabricius Hildanus), German surgeon, 1560-1634, is credited with being the first to remove a gallstone from a living patient. Operation performed in 1618.

Gallstones, first roentgenographic study of

J. CHAPPUIS, French physician, 185?-19??, with H. CHAUVEL, recorded the first roentgenographic studies of biliary concretions. Published in 1896.

**Gallstones, roentgenographic
visualization of**

A. BUXBAUM, Austrian physician, 1860 - 1933, demonstrated gallstones by means of roentgenography, in 1898.

**Galvanic electricity, first
successful use of**

GUSTAF SAMUEL CRUSELL, Swedish physician, 1810-1858, was the first to use galvanism successfully as a therapeutic measure. He treated a case of urethral stricture. Recorded in 1841-43.

**Galvanocautery in laryngeal
surgery**

FRIEDRICH EDUARD RUDOLPH VOLTOLINI, German otolaryngologist, 1819-1889, is credited with being the first to apply galvanocautery in laryngeal surgery. Recorded in 1867.

Galvanocautery in major surgery, introduction of

ALBRECHT THEODOR VON MIDDEL-DORPF, Breslau surgeon, 1824-1868, is credited with introducing improved galvanocautery in use in major surgery. Published in 1854.

Galvanocautery in prostatic obstruction

ENRICO BOTTINI, Italian surgeon, 1837-1903, devised a method for cutting a channel through the enlarged prostate, in cases of obstruction, by the use of galvanocautery. Reported in 1874. The operation was by the intraurethral route.

Galvanocautery, invention of modern

CHARLES GABRIEL PRAVAZ, French physician, 1791-1853, is credited with inventing the basic procedures of modern galvanocautery. Recorded in 1853.

Galvanometer for use in electro-cardiography, invention of

WILLEM EINTHOVEN, Dutch physiologist, 1860 - 1927, invented a sensitive instrument for measuring feeble electric currents. It consists, essentially, of a special metal thread stretched between the poles of a magnet, the thread moving laterally when current is passed through it. Reported in 1900.

Gamma globulin, discovery of

OTTO PORGES, Austrian physician, 1879-19??, with K. SPIRO, discovered gamma globulin, in 1903.

Ganglia of auricular septum of frog's heart

FRIEDRICH H. BIDDER, German anatomist, 1810 - 1894, described two ganglia found in the auricular septum of the frog's heart. Reported in 1842.

Ganglion, carotid, eponymic description of

AUGUST CARL BOCK, German anatomist, 1782 - 1833, described the carotid ganglion, the ganglion in the lower portion of the cavernous sinus. Published in 1833. Known as *Bock's ganglion*.

Ganglion, celiac, early description of

FRED BYRON ROBINSON, American surgeon and anatomist, 1857-1910, described the celiac ganglion (or ganglia) of the abdomen, which he called the "abdominal brain." Published in 1899.

Ganglion, cervico-uterine, eponymic description of

FERDINAND FRANKENHÄUSER, German gynecologist, 1826 - 1894, described the cervico-uterine ganglion, a ganglion near the cervix of the uterus. Recorded in 1867. Known as *Frankenhäuser's ganglion*.

Ganglion formed by lower cervical and first thoracic ganglia

JOHANN ERNST NEUBAUER, German anatomist, 1742 - 1777, described a large ganglion formed by the union of the first thoracic and lower cervical ganglia. Recorded in 1776. Known as *Neubauer's ganglion*.

Ganglion, gasserian

. . . See under *Gasserian ganglion*.

Ganglion impar

. . . See under *Coccygeal ganglion*.

Ganglion of Auerbach's plexus

LEOPOLD AUERBACH, German anatomist, 1828-1897, described ganglion cells situated in the plexus of autonomic nerve fibers between the muscular coats of the intestine. Reported in 1862 and 1863. Known as *Auerbach's ganglion*.

Ganglion of glossopharyngeal nerve at jugular foramen

JOHANN EHRENRITTER, Austrian anatomist, 17??-1790, described a ganglion of the glossopharyngeal nerve near the jugular foramen. Known as *Ehrenritter's ganglion* and *ganglion superius*. Recorded *circa* 1775.

Ganglion of great splanchnic nerve, eponymic description of

JOHANN GEORG C. F. M. LOBSTEIN, German surgeon and pathologist, 1777-1835, described a ganglion or enlargement of the great splanchnic nerve, above the diaphragm. Recorded in 1823. Known as *Lobstein's ganglion*.

Ganglion of lowest occipital segment in human embryo

. . . See under *Ganglion, rudimentary, of dorsal root of hypoglossal nerve*.

Ganglion of vestibular nerve

ANTONIO SCARPA, Italian anatomist and surgeon, 175?-1832, described a ganglion of the vestibular nerve, at its junction with the facial, in 1779. Known as *Scarpa's ganglion*.

Ganglion on extensor tendons of hand

OLOF OF ACREL, Swedish surgeon, 1717-1806, described a ganglion occurring on the extensor tendons of the wrist or hand. Published in 1780.

Ganglion, otic, classic description of

FRIEDRICH ARNOLD, German anatomist, 1803-1890, described the otic ganglion, a ganglion situated below the foramen ovale which sends fibers to the tympanic muscles and tensor palati. Reported in 1828. Known as *Arnold's ganglion*.

Ganglion, petrous, original description of

CARL SAMUEL ANDERSCH, German anatomist, 1732-1777, described the petrous ganglion, a ganglion on the glossopharyngeal nerve near the lower border of the petrous bone. Published in 1797.

Ganglion, rudimentary, of dorsal root of hypoglossal nerve

AUGUST VON FRORIEP, German anatomist, 1849-1917, described a vestigial dorsal root ganglion of the hypoglossal nerve. Reported in 1885.

Gärtner's bacillus

. . . See under *Salmonella enteritidis, description of*.

Gartner's duct, eponymic description of

HERMANN T. GARTNER, Danish anatomist, 1785-1827, described a cord or tube occurring occasionally as a remnant of the Wolffian duct, and extending from the epoophoron to the vagina, through the broad ligament. It was possibly noted by MALPIGHI as early as 1681, but was reported in some detail by Gartner in 1822. Known also as *ductus epoophori longitudinalis*.

**Gas burner with adjustable
air inlet at base**

. . . See under *Bunsen burner*.

Gas gangrene bacillus

. . . See under *Bacillus aerogenes
capsulatus*.

***Gas*, introduction of term**

JEAN BAPTISTE VAN HELMONT, Belgian physiologist and chemist,
1577 - 1644, introduced the term
gas, to describe the fluid (apparently carbon dioxide) produced by
a ferment. Recorded in 1648.

**Gases, diffusion of, law
pertaining to**

THOMAS GRAHAM, Scottish chemist, 1805-1869, studied the physical
laws governing the diffusion of
gases and promulgated his law
which states that the rates of diffusion of gases are inversely proportional to the square roots of their
relative densities. Reported in
1832. Known as *Grahams's law*.

Gases, liquefaction of, method for

. . . See under *Liquefaction of gases*.

**Gases, respiratory, apparatus
for analyzing**

. . . See under *Respiratory gases*,
etc.

Gaskell's bridge

. . . See under *Atrioventricular
bundle, early description of*.

**Gasserian ganglion, excision of,
in trigeminal neuralgia**

. . . See under *Semilunar ganglion*,
etc.

***Gasserian ganglion*, naming of**

ANTON BALTHASAR RAYMUND
HIRSCH, Austrian anatomist, 1743-

18??, introduced the term *gasserian
ganglion* (originally *Gasserian*), in
1765, in honor of JOHANN LAUREN-
TIUS GASSER, Austrian anatomist,
1702-1777.

Gastrectomy, first recorded

. . . See under *Pylorectomy*.

**Gastrectomy, first successful,
in America**

JOHN MONTGOMERY BALDY, American gynecologist, 1860 - 1934, is
credited with performing the first
gastrectomy in America, in 1893.
There is a possibility that the first
excision of the stomach in the United States was performed in 1887 by
AUGUSTUS CHARLES BERNAYS.
Baldy himself referred to this claim.

**Gastric fistula, first operation
for relief of**

ALBRECHT THEODOR VON MIDDEL-
DORPF, Breslau surgeon, 1824-1868,
is credited with performing the
first operation for the relief of a
gastric fistula, in 1859.

**Gastric fistula, study of
digestion in**

. . . See under *Digestion, process
of, in living subject*.

Gastric glands, cells of—1870

RUDOLF P. H. HEIDENHAIN, German physiologist, 1834 - 1897, described certain "delomorphous and
adelomorphous" cells in the glands
of the stomach. Reported in 1870.
Known as *Heidenhain's cells*.

**Gastric juice, chronic hyper-
secretion of**

. . . See under *Gastrosuccorrhea*,
etc.

Gastric juice, human, first isolation of

EDWARD STEVENS, English physician, 17??-18??, is credited with being first to isolate human gastric juice and to demonstrate digestion *in vitro*. Recorded in 1777. RÉAUMUR had previously isolated gastric juice from a pet buzzard.

Gastric juice, hydrochloric acid in, discovery of

WILLIAM PROUT, English physiologist, 1785-1850, discovered the presence of hydrochloric acid in the gastric juice, in 1824.

Gastric juice, psychic secretion of, early report on

FRIEDRICH H. BIDDER, German anatomist, 1810 - 1894, described psychic secretion of gastric juice and the presence in it of hydrochloric acid. Reported in 1852.

Gastric juice, solvent action of, due to acid

JOHN RICHARDSON YOUNG, American physician, 1782-1804, recognized that the solvent action of the gastric juice is due to some form of acid but concluded that it was phosphoric acid. Published in 1803.

Gastric juice, solvent action of, on foods

RENÉ ANTOINE FERCHAULT DE RÉAUMUR, French physiologist, 1683-1757, obtained gastric juice from a buzzard and showed that the juice had a solvent effect on foods. Published in 1752.

Gastric lavage in diagnosis of tuberculosis in infants

HENRI MEUNIER, French physician, 1864-19??, introduced the method of gastric lavage for the diagnosis of tuberculosis in children and infants. Recorded in 1898.

Gastric outline by means of x-rays and lead contrast medium

... See under *Stomach, first roentgenographic outline of.*

Gastric ulcer, early description of—1830

JEAN CRUVEILHIER, French pathologist, 1791-1874, described several cases of gastric ulcer, in 1830. Known to the French as "la maladie de Cruveilhier."

Gastric ulcer, first clear description of symptoms of

MATTHEW BAILLIE, English physician, 1761-1823, gave the first adequate description of the symptoms and morbid anatomy of gastric ulcer. Recorded in 1793.

Gastric ulcer, first recorded case of

MARCELLO DONATI, Italian physician, 1538-1602, is credited with recording a case of gastric ulcer in 1586.

Gastric ulcer, niche in, description of

MARTIN HAUDEK, Austrian roentgenologist, 1880-1931, is credited with being first to describe the characteristic niche of gastric ulcer, as seen in roentgenograms. Reported in 1910. Known as *Haudek's niche.*

Gastric ulcer, perforated, first recorded case of

CHRISTOPHER RAWLINSON, English physician, 168?-1752, presented the first recorded case of a perforated gastric ulcer. Published in 1727.

Gastric ulcer, perforated, first successful suture of

LUDWIG HEUSNER, German surgeon, 1846-1916, was the first to suture successfully a perforation of a gastric ulcer, in 1892. Reported by HERMANN KRIEGE, in 1892.

Gastrin, early description of

JOHN SYDNEY EDKINS, English physiologist, 1863-1940, is credited with being the first to describe gastrin or gastric secretin. Published in 1905.

Gastrin, more definite description of

ANDREW CONWAY IVY, American physiologist, 1893- , with JAMES IRVING FARRELL, demonstrated the presence of gastrin, a hormone found in the pyloric mucosa which on injection stimulates gastric secretion. Recorded in 1925.

Gastrodiaphany, introduction of

MAX EINHORN, American physician, 1862-1953, introduced the method of gastrodiaphany, the examination of the stomach by means of a light passed down the esophagus, in 1889.

Gastroduodenal nasal tube, invention of—1921

ABRAHAM LOUIS LEVIN, American physician, 1880-1940, invented a nasal gastroduodenal tube for use in gastrointestinal operations. Recorded in 1921. Known as the *Levin tube*.

Gastroduodenostomy, early performance of—1892

MATHIEU JABOULAY, French surgeon, 1860-1913, was probably the first to perform gastroduodenostomy, in 1892.

Gastroduodenostomy, early performance of—1902

JOHN M. T. FINNEY, American surgeon, 1863-1942, devised an operation for gastroduodenostomy, in 1902. Known as *Finney's operation*.

Gastroenterostomy tube, double-barreled

WILLIAM OSLER ABBOTT, Philadelphia physician, 1902-1943, in cooperation with ARTHUR JOY RAWSON, American scientist, 1896- , devised a double-barreled gastroenterostomy tube for use in postoperative care. Report published in May, 1937. The tube is known eponimically as the *Abbott-Rawson tube*.

Gastrophotography, introduction of

OTTO PORGES, Austrian physician, 1879-19??, is credited with introducing methods of gastric photography in medicine. Recorded in 1929.

Gastroptosis, operation for, involving plication of gastrohepatic ligament

HENRY DORRANCE BEYEA, American surgeon, 1867-1924, devised an operation for gastroptosis in which the stomach is suspended by plication of the gastrohepatic and gastrophrenic ligaments. Report published in 1903.

Gastroptosis

. . . See also under *Enteroptosis*, etc.

**Gastroscope, flexible, intro-
duction of**

RUDOLF SCHINDLER, German-
American surgeon, 1888- , invented and introduced the flexible
gastroscope. Reported in 1932.

**Gastrostomy, early performance
of—1846**

CHARLES EMMANUEL SEDILLOT,
French surgeon, 1804-1883, performed gastrostomy in 1846. It is
believed to be the first such operation on record.

**Gastrostomy, first record of,
in America**

FRANCIS F. MAURY, American surgeon, 1840-1879, is credited with
performing the first operation of
gastrostomy in the United States.
Published in 1870.

**Gastrostomy, first record of,
in Britain**

JOHN COOPER FORSTER, English
surgeon, 1824-1896, recorded the
first operation of gastrostomy in
England. Published in 1858.

**Gastrosuccorrhea; Reichmann's
disease**

MIKOLAJ REICHMANN, Polish physician, 1851-1918, gave the first
description of gastrosuccorrhea, a
condition marked by chronic hyper-
secretion of gastric juice. Published
in 1882.

**Gastrula, two-layered,
concept of**

ERNST HEINRICH PHILIPP AUGUST
HAECKEL, German biologist, 1834-
1919, proposed a theory of a two-
layered gastrula from which all
multicellular organisms originate.
Published in 1874.

Gatch bed

... See under *Bed, surgical, for supporting patient in semisitting posture.*

**Gaucher's disease; cerebroside
lipoidosis**

... See under *Familial splenic anemia, eponymic description of.*

Geiger counter, invention of

HANS GEIGER, German physicist,
1882-1945, invented an instrument
for the detection of radiation. It
consists essentially of an electrode
in a hollow metallic cylinder filled
with gas which, when ionized by
radiation, permits current to flow,
the current actuating a counting device. Introduced in 1912.

Geisböck's disease

... See under *Polycythemia hyper-
tonica.*

Geissler tube, invention of

HEINRICH GEISSLER, German physicist, 1814-1879, invented a glass
tube containing a rarefied gas and
two electrodes, the gas becoming
luminous when the current is on.
The color of the glow depends on
the kind of gas. Introduced in 1863.

**Genes, transmutation of,
by roentgen rays**

HERMANN JOSEPH MULLER, American geneticist, 1890- , studied the
artificial transmutation of genes by
means of roentgen rays. Published
reports appeared in 1927-29. Received the Nobel prize in 1946.

**Genetics, statistical, founder
of school of**

FRANCIS GALTON, English geneticist, 1822-1911, is credited with

being the founder of the statistical school of genetics.

Geneva Convention, first, organization of

JEAN HENRI DUNANT, Swiss philanthropist, 1828-1910, is credited with the organization of the first Geneva Convention, in 1864. The International Red Cross Society was founded by the Geneva Convention.

Gentian violet, bactericidal action of

JOHN WOOLMAN CHURCHMAN, American physician, 1877 - 1937, discovered the specific bactericidal action of gentian violet with regard to staphylococci. Recorded in 1912 and 1925.

Gentian violet in treatment of burns, introduction of

ROBERT HENRY ALDRICH, Boston surgeon, 1902-   , is credited with introducing gential violet in the treatment of burns. Recorded in 1933.

Geriatrics, first exclusive book on—1724

JOHN FLOYER, English physician, 1649-1734, wrote what is considered the first book devoted entirely to geriatrics. It was published under the title *Medicina Gerocomica*, in 1724.

Gerlach's valve

. . . See under *Appendix, valve at opening of.*

Germ plasm, immortality of; introduction of concept

AUGUST FRIEDRICH LEOPOLD WEISMANN, German biologist, 1834-1914, is credited with formulating the doctrine of the immortality of the germ plasm. Recorded in 1892.

Germ theory of disease, early suggestion of—1546

GIROLAMO FRACASTORO, Italian pathologist, 1483-1553, suggested the germ theory of infection as early as 1546.

Germ theory of disease, establishment of—1861

LOUIS PASTEUR, French scientist and bacteriologist, 1822-1895, through his experiments with fermentation, demonstrated that certain diseases are caused by living organisms. He also refuted the doctrine of spontaneous generation. Recorded in 1861.

Germ theory of disease, proof of—1865

CASIMIR JOSEPH DAVAINE, French physician, 1812-1882, was one of the first to prove the germ theory of disease, by demonstrating that anthrax, a specific disease, is caused by the anthrax bacillus, a specific organism. Recorded in 1865.

German measles

. . . See under *Rubella.*

Germanin in treatment of trypanosomiasis

. . . See under *Trypanosomiasis.*

Germinal epithelium, eponymic description of

HEINRICH WILHELM GOTTFRIED WALDEYER-HARTZ, German anatomist, 1836-1921, described the germinal epithelium in 1870. Known as *Waldeyer's epithelium.*

Germinal spot of animal egg, discovery of

JEAN J. M. C. V. COSTE, French embryologist, 1807-1873, discovered and described the germinal spot of the animal ovum. Reported in 1837.

Germ-layer theory, fondation of

CASPAR FRIEDRICH WOLFF, German anatomist, 1733-1794, rejected the embryonic preformation theory and substituted the "layer theory" which laid the foundation of the germ-layer theory, propounded later by HEINRICH C. PANDER and CARL ERNST VON BAER. Published in 1759.

Germ-layer theory, origination of

KARL ERNST VON BAER, German embryologist born in Estonia, 1792-1876, enunciated the germ-layer theory in 1817, on the basis of research in collaboration with C. H. PANDER, German anatomist. The germ-layer theory holds that the embryo develops three primary germ layers from which all organs and tissues are derived. Baer originally concieved four layers, skin, muscular, vascular, and mucous.

Giant cells of percentral convolution, early description of

WILLIAM BEVAN LEWIS, English pathologist, 1847-1929, described the giant cells found in the precentral convolution of the brain, in 1878.

Giant cells of tubercle

. . . See under *Tubercle, giant cell of tuberculous.*

Giant follicular lymphadenopathy—1925

NATHAN E. BRILL, American physician, 1860-1925, was the first to describe giant follicular hyperplasia involving the spleen and lymph nodes, called also giant follicular lymphadenopathy. Reported with G. BAEHR and N. ROSENTHAL in 1925. Known as *Brill-Symmers disease.*

Giant follicular lymphadenopathy—1927

DOUGLAS SYMMERS, American physician, 1879-19??, described giant follicular lymphadenopathy in a paper titled "follicular lymphadenopathy with splenomegaly," in 1927. He published another paper on giant follicular lymphadenopathy in 1938. Known as *Brill-Symmers disease.*

Giant pyramidal cells of cerebral cortex, discovery of

VLADIMIR A. BETZ, Russian anatomist, 1834-1894, discovered and described the giant pyramidal cells of the cerebral cortex. Report published in 1874. Known as *cells of Betz.* The cells were first illustrated by BEVAN-LEWIS, in 1878.

Gigantism due to hyperpituitarism, eponymic description of

PIERRE EMILE LAUNOIS, French physician, 1856-1914, with M. CLERET, described gigantism resulting from excessive pituitary secretion. Published in 1910. Known as *Launois' syndrome* and *Launois-Cleret syndrome.*

Gigli's saw

. . . See under *Wire saw, invention of.*

Gilchrist's disease

... See under *Blastomycosis, North American,* etc.

Gill slits, structures homologous with, in mammals

MARTIN HEINRICH RATHKE, German anatomist, 1783-1860, discovered certain structures in avian and mammalian embryos which are homologous with the gill slits of fishes. Published in 1832.

Gimbernat's ligament

... See under *Lacunar ligament.*

Gingival glands

... See under *Serres' glands in infants.*

Glacial acetic acid and potassium bichromate, use of

JOHANNES EVANGELISTA VON PURKINJE, Bohemian physiologist, 1787-1869, introduced the use of glacial acetic acid and potassium bichromate in histological procedures, *circa* 1834.

Gland, sublingual, eponymic description of

AUGUSTUS QUIRINUS RIVINUS, German anatomist and botanist, 1652-1723, described the sublingual gland, *circa* 1680. Published in 1691. Known as *Rivinus' gland.*

Gland

... See also under name of particular gland, as *Pituitary gland,* and under *Glands.*

Glanders bacillus, discovery of

FRIEDRICH AUGUST JOHANNES LOEFFLER, German bacteriologist, 1852-1915, discovered the glanders bacillus in 1882.

Glanders, diagnostic reaction for

ISIDORE STRAUS, French physician, 1845-1896, devised a reaction test for the diagnosis of glanders. In this test material suspected of containing virulent glanders bacilli is injected into the peritoneal cavity of a male guinea pig. If the material is active, scrotal lesions develop. Recorded in 1889. Known as *Straus's reaction.*

Glanders, early description of

PHILIBERT CHABERT, French veterinarian, 1737-1814, is credited with an excellent description of glanders. Published in 1779.

Glanders in horse is communicable to man, proof that

JOHN ELLIOTSON, English surgeon, 1786-1868, demonstrated that glanders in the horse is communicable to man. Recorded in 1830.

Glanders is not a form of tuberculosis, proof that

PIERRE FRANÇOIS OLIVE RAYER, French dermatologist, 1793-1867, is said to have been first to describe glanders in man and to prove that glanders is not a form of tuberculosis. Recorded in 1837.

Glanders, mallein test for, invention of

VICTOR BABES, Rumanian microbiologist, 1854-1926, devised a mallein test for glanders. It is an intradermal test and is used to detect both latent and chronic conditions. Reported in 1891.

Glands between tarsus and conjunctiva of eyelid

HEINRICH MEIBOM, German physician and anatomist, 1638-1700,

described the glands situated between the tarsus and conjunctiva of the eyelid. Published in 1666. Known as *Meibomian glands*. GIULIO CASSERIO (Italian anatomist, 1561-1616) is said to have noted the glands in 1609.

Glands, enlarged supraclavicular, in tuberculous children

ROBERT WILLIAM PHILIP, Scottish physician, 1857-1912, described enlarged supraclavicular glands occurring in tuberculous children. Published in 1912. Known as *Philip's glands*.

Glands, mucous, of cervix of uterus; Nabothian glands

MARTIN NABOTH, German anatomist, 1675-1721, described the mucous follicles or glands of the cervix uteri near the external os. Published in 1707. Known as *Nabothian follicles* or *glands*.

Glands near tip of tongue, description of, in 1826

PHILIPPE FREDERIC BLANDIN, French surgeon, 1798-1849, described the mixed glands near the tip of the tongue. Reported in 1826. Known as *Blandin's glands* and as *Nuhn's glands,* in allusion to ANTON NUHN who described the same glands in 1845.

Glands near tip of tongue, description of, in 1845

ANTON NUHN, German anatomist, 1814-1889, described the mixed glands near the tip of the tongue. Reported in 1845. Known as *Nuhn's glands* and as *Blandin's glands,* in allusion to PHILIPPE FREDERIC BLANDIN who described the glands in 1826.

Glands of male urethra, eponymic description of

ALEXIS LITTRÉ, French surgeon and anatomist, 1658-1726, was the first to describe the mucous glands of the male urethra, in 1700. Known as *Littré's glands*.

Glands, sublingual, smaller ducts of

AUGUSTUS QUIRINUS RIVINUS, German anatomist and botanist, 1652-1723, described the smaller ducts of the sublingual glands. Published in 1691. Called the *Rivinian ducts*.

Glandular fever

. . . See under *Infectious mononucleosis*.

Glandular secretion, law of

RUDOLF P. H. HEIDENHAIN, German physiologist, 1834-1897, formulated the so-called law of glandular secretion, which states that secretion always involves a change of structure in the gland. Promulgated in 1866.

Glass drainage tube in intestinal operations

FRANK THOMAS PAUL, English surgeon, 1851-1941, devised a glass drainage tube for use in intestinal operations. Recorded in 1895. A similar tube was invented about the same time by SAMUEL J. MIXTER. Known as *Paul's tube, Paul-Mixter's tube*.

Glass tube, use of, in draining ventricles in hydrocephalus

EDWARD WYLLYS ANDREWS, Chicago surgeon, 1856-1927, described an improved technique in which glass tubes were used for subdural drainage of the lateral ventricles in internal hydrocephalus. Reported in 1911.

Glauber's salt

. . . See under *Sodium sulfate, introduction of.*

Glaucoma, glaucosan for relief of

. . . See under *Glaucosan in glaucoma.*

Glaucoma, hardness of eye in, early notice of

RICHARD BANISTER, English oculist, 15??-16??, observed the hardness of the eyeball in glaucoma. Published in 1622.

Glaucoma, increased intraocular pressure in, discovery of

WILLIAM MACKENZIE, Scottish ophthalmologist, 1791-1868, was probably the first to associate increased intraocular pressure with glaucoma. Published in 1830.

Glaucoma, iridencleisis for

. . . See under *Iridencleisis.*

Glaucoma, physostigmine in treatment of

. . . See under *Physostigmine in treatment of glaucoma.*

Glaucoma, sclerocorneal trephining for relief of

ROBERT HENRY ELLIOTT, English ophthalmologist, 1864-1936, devised an operation for relief of glaucoma by sclerocorneal trephining. Reported in 1909.

Glaucosan in glaucoma, introduction of

CARL HAMBURGER, German ophthalmologist, 1870-1944, introduced glaucosan for the relief of glaucoma. Published in 1926.

Glenoid fossa, abnormal shallowness of, first observation on

VINCENZO GIUFFRIDA-RUGGERI, Italian anthropologist, 1872-1922, observed the incompleteness or abnormal shallowness of the glenoid fossa. Reported in 1897. Known as *Giuffrida-Ruggeri's stigma.*

Globulin in cerebrospinal fluid, test for excess of

PIERO BOVERI, Italian neurologist, 1879-1932, devised a test for detecting excess of globulin in cerebrospinal fluid by the use of a solution of potassium permanganate. Introduced in 1909.

Glomerular filtration rate in man, first measurement of

POUL BRANDT REHBERG, Danish physiologist, 18??-19??, was the first to measure the glomerular filtration rate in man. Published in 1926.

Glomerulonephritis, early description of—1870

THEODOR ALBRECHT EDWIN KLEBS, German bacteriologist, 1834-1913, described glomerulonephritis in 1870. Known as *Klebs's disease.*

Glossitis in pernicious anemia

WILLIAM HUNTER, English physician, 1861-1937, described glossitis associated with pernicious anemia, marked by smooth atrophy, in 1900. Known as *Hunter's glossitis.*

**Glossopharyngeal and vagus
nerves, ascending
roots of**

. . . See under *Vagus and glossopharyngeal nerves.*

**Glucose in diabetic urine,
identification of**

MICHEL E. CHEVREUL, French
chemist, 1786-1889, investigated
the sugar in diabetic urine and
proved it to be glucose. Reported
in 1815.

Glutathione, isolation of

FREDERICK G. HOPKINS, English
biochemist, 1861-1947, isolated
glutathione, the co-enzyme of gly-
oxalase, in 1921.

Gluteal artery, first ligation of

JOHN BELL, Scottish surgeon and
anatomist, 1763-1820, is credited
with performing the first recorded
ligation of the gluteal artery. Published in 1801.

Glutin, discovery of

. . . See under *Chondrin and glutin.*

**Glycine in myasthenia
gravis**

. . . See under *Myasthenia gravis.*

**Glycocoll in myasthenia
gravis**

. . . See under *Myasthenia gravis.*

**Glycogen, catalytic metabolism
of, process involved in**

CARL FERDINAND CORI, American
biochemist and physiologist, 1896-
, and GERTY THERESA CORI,
American biochemist, 1896- , investigated and described the processes involved in the catalytic

metabolism of glycogen. They received the Nobel prize, with B. A.
HOUSSAY, in 1947.

**Glycogen production by
liver, discovery of**

CLAUDE BERNARD, French physiologist, 1813-1878, discovered the
glycogenic function of the liver.
Recorded in 1848.

**Glycogenic thesaurismosis,
early description of**

. . . See under *Glycogenosis.*

**Glycogenosis, early
description of—1931**

EDGAR VON GIERKE, German pathologist, 1877-1945, described a
metabolic disease of childhood
marked by abnormal storage of glycogen in the liver, hypoglycemia,
etc. Reported in 1931. Known also
as *von Gierke's disease, glycogenic
thesaurismosis, glycogneic hepato-
nephromegaly,* etc.

**Glycogens, catalytic
transformation of**

CARL FERDINAND CORI, American
physiologist and biochemist, 1896-
, with his wife, GERTY THERESA
CORI, demonstrated the course of
the catalytic transformations of
glycogen in the body. Published in
1947.

**Glycosuria, experimental,
introduction of—1886**

JOSEPH VON MERING, German physician, 1849-1908, is credited with
having produced glycosuria experimentally by the use of phlorhizin,
in 1886.

Goethe's bone

. . . See under *Intermaxillary bone.*

Goiter, endemic, prevention of, by iodine

GASPARD ADOLPH CHATIN, French physician, 1813-1901, demonstrated that iodine can prevent the development of endemic goiter and cretinism. Published in 1850.

Goiter, use of calcined sponge in treatment of

THOMAS PROSSER, English physician, 1724-1792, dispensed calcined sponge as a remedy for goiter. Recorded in 1769.

Goiter, use of seaweed in

ROGER OF PALERMO, Italian surgeon, *circa* 1140-1210, advocated the use of seaweed in the treatment of goiter. Recorded in 1170.

Goiter

. . . See also under *Exophthalmic goiter, Hyperthyroidism,* etc.

Gold chloride method for nerve endings

ERNST FISCHER, German histologist, 184?-19??, was the first to record the demonstration of nerve endings by means of the gold chloride method. Published in 1876.

Gold radon seed, invention of

. . . See under *Radon tube.*

Gold, use of, in tuberculosis

. . . See under *Tuberculosis, introduction of sanocrysin in treatment of.*

Golden Square Hospital in London, founding of

MORELL MACKENZIE, English laryngologist, 1837-1892, founded the Golden Square Hospital in London, the first hospital in the world devoted entirely to diseases of the throat, in 1863.

Golgi apparatus, original description of

CAMILLO GOLGI, Italian histologist, 1844-1926, described a network of fibers or canals in the cytoplasm of many cells. Reported in 1885. Known as *Golgi apparatus* or *network.*

Golgi's cells

. . . See under *Astrocytes; Golgi's cells.*

Gonococcal ophthalmia, silver nitrate in

ÉTIENNE FRANÇOIS JULLIARD, French physician, 1804-1882, introduced the use of silver nitrate in the treatment of blennorrheal (gonococcal) ophthalmia. Recorded in 1835.

Gonococcus as cause of ulcerative endocarditis

WILLIAM SYDNEY THAYER, Baltimore physician, 1864-1932, with GEORGE ALBERT BLUMER, demonstrated that the gonococcus may be the cause of ulcerative endocarditis. Recorded in 1896.

Gonococcus, discovery of

. . . See under *Gonorrhea, discovery of gonococcus in.*

Gonococcus, first cultivation of

LEO LEISTIKOW, German bacteriologist, 1847-1917, is credited with being the first to successfully cultivate the gonococcus. Recorded in 1882.

Gonococcus in acute cystitis, demonstration of

ERNST WERTHEIM, Austrian gynecologist, 1864-1920, demonstrated the presence of the gonococcus in some cases of acute cystitis in women. Recorded in 1896.

Gonorrhea, complement-fixation test for

RUDOLF MÜLLER, Austrian dermatologist, 1877-1934, with MAURICE OPPENHEIM, developed a complement-fixation test for the diagnosis of gonorrhea. Published in 1906. Known as *Müller-Oppenheim reaction.*

Gonorrhea, differentiation of, from other venereal diseases

PHILLIPPE RICORD, French urologist and dermatologist, 1800-1889, differentiated gonorrhea from syphilis and other venereal diseases. Reported in 1838.

Gonorrhea, discovery of gonococcus in

ALBERT L. S. NEISSER, German physician, 1855-1916, discovered the gonococcus in 1879.

Gonorrhea, latent, and sterility in women

EMIL NOEGGERATH, American gynecologist and obstetrician, 1827-1895, drew attention to the importance of latent gonorrhea in women with regard to sterility. Recorded in 1876.

Gonorrhea, two-glass urine test for

HENRY THOMPSON, English surgeon and urologist, 1820-1904, introduced the two-glass urine test for gonorrhea, *circa* 1860.

Gonorrheal discharge is pus, recognition that

SEBASTIANUS PETRITIUS, Italian physician, *circa* 1550-1625, is believed to have been the first to recognize that the discharge from the penis in gonorrhea is pus, not semen, in 1591.

Gout and rheumatism, distinction between

THOMAS SYDENHAM, English physician, 1624-1689, clearly differentiated between rheumatism and gout. Published in 1683.

Gouty concretions, composition of

WILLIAM HYDE WOLLASTON, English physician and physicist, 1766-1828, discovered urates in gouty concretions. Reported in 1797.

Graafian follicle, early description of

REGNIER DE GRAAF, Dutch anatomist, 1641-1673, gave the first description of the structure now known as Graafian follicle. He also demonstrated ovulation. Published in 1672.

Graafian follicle, introduction of term

ALBRECHT VON HALLER, Swiss anatomist, 1708-1777, introduced the term *graafian follicle, circa* 1730, in allusion to REGNIER DE GRAAF, Dutch anatomist, 1641-1673, who gave a classic description of the structure in 1672.

Graafian follicles, real function of

KARL ERNST VON BAER, German embryologist born in Estonia, 1792-1876, was the first to point out that the graafian follicles are not the eggs from which organisms develop, as was held at the time, but that they contain the true ova. Reported in 1827.

Graham flour, introduction of

SYLVESTER GRAHAM, American dietitian and reformer, 1794-1851, introduced the use of unbolted or whole-wheat flour about 1836. GRAHAM was an advocate of temperance and vegetarianism, believing that meat was the cause of abnormal cravings.

Graham Steell murmur

. . . See under *Pulmonary valve insufficiency, murmur of.*

Graham-Cole test, introduction of

. . . See under *Cholecystography, introduction of successful.*

Graham's law, promulgation of

. . . See under *Gases, diffusion of, law pertaining to.*

Grain itch, discovery of cause of

LYMAN T. RAWLES, American physician, 1877-19??, is credited with the discovery of *Pediculoides ventricosus,* the causative agent of grain itch. Recorded in 1909.

Gramicidin, discovery of

RENÉ JULES DUBOS, French bacteriologist in the United States, 1901- , discovered gramicidin, a component of tyrothricin, in 1939.

Gram's stain, introduction of

HANS C. J. GRAM, Danish bacteriologist, 1853-1938, devised an arbitrary staining method by which microorganisms can be divided into two classes, the *gram-positive* and *gram-negative.* The organisms are first stained with gentian violet, then treated with Gram's iodine, washed, and stained with safranin. The gram-positive organisms retain the gentian violet stain; the gram-negative organisms take the safranin stain. The method was introduced in 1884.

Grancher's system for boarding out children

. . . See under *Children from tuberculous households,* etc.

Granular cell myoblastoma

ALEKSEI IVANOVICH ABRIKOSOV (or ABRIKOSSOFF), Russian pathologist, 1875-19??, described a tumor of striated muscle made of groups of cells which are like or resemble primitive myoblasts. It is also known as *Abrikosov's tumor.* Date not available.

Granules in white blood cells, staining of

. . . See under *Leukocytes, staining of granules of.*

Granulosa cell tumor, original description of

CLEMENS VON KAHLDEN, German pathologist, 1859 - 1903, was the first to describe granulosa cell tumor, in 1895.

Granulosis rubra nasi, description of—1894

JOHN JAMES PRINGLE, English dermatologist, 1855 - 1922, was the first to describe granulosis rubra nasi, but not under this name, in 1894.

Granulosis rubra nasi, description of—1901

JOSEF JADASSOHN, German dermatologist, 1863 - 1936, described granulosis rubra nasi, a disorder of the skin of the nose associated with hyperhidrosis and marked by redness and scattered reddish specks. Reported in 1901. The name *granulosis rubra nasi* was applied to the condition by Jadassohn.

Granulosis rubra nasi, introduction of term

JOSEF JADASSOHN, German dermatologist, 1863-1936, introduced the term *granulosis rubra nasi*, in 1901.

Granville's hammer, invention of

... See under *Hammer for administering vibratory massage*.

Gratiolet's optic radiation

... See under *Optic radiation, description of*.

Gravitation, law of

ISAAC NEWTON, English scientist, 1642-1727, made his first observations on the law of gravitation in 1666. It was accepted as proved in 1682.

Grawitz's tumor

... See under *Hypernephroma, early investigation of*.

Gray's Anatomy, first appearance of

HENRY GRAY, English anatomist, 1825-1861, produced the first edition of his now famous text, under the title *Anatomy, Descriptive and Surgical*, in 1858. The first American edition appeared in 1859.

Greek medical terms, translation of, into Latin

... See under *Translation of Greek medical terms*, etc.

Griesinger's disease

... See under *Chlorosis, Egyptian, is due to ancylostomiasis*.

Grocco's triangle

... See under *Paravertebral triangle*.

Groove at lower border of chest corresponding to insertion of diaphragm

EDWARD HARRISON, English physician, 1766-1838, described a groove or depression near the lower border of the chest, corresponding to the attachment of the diaphragm, seen especially in children with rickets. Known as *Harrison's groove*. Introduced *circa* 1798.

Growth hormone of hypophysis, discovery of

HERBERT M. EVANS, American physician, 1882-   , is credited with discovering the growth hormone in the anterior lobe of the pituitary. First report in 1921.

Growth of new tissue takes place by division of preexisting cells

ROBERT REMAK, German physiologist and neurologist, 1815 - 1865, was the first to announce that growth of new tissue begins by division of pre-existing cells. Recorded in 1852.

Growth quotient, law of constant

MAX RUBNER, German physiologist, 1854-1932, discovered the law of constant growth quotient, which means that the energy used for growth is a constant fraction of the total energy used by the organism. Published in 1902. Known as *Rubner's law*.

Gruber's hernia

... See under *Hernia, internal mesogastric*.

Guanidine, use of, in myasthenia gravis
. . . See under *Myasthenia gravis, use of guanidine in.*

Guarnieri's bodies
. . . See under *Smallpox, inclusion bodies in lesions of.*

Gubernaculum testis, eponymic description of
JOHN HUNTER, Scottish surgeon, 1728-1793, described a fetal cord extending between the bottom of the scrotum and the lower end of the epididymis, present during the descent of the testis. Published in 1762. Known as *Hunter's gubernaculum.*

Gubler's paralysis
. . . See under *Hemiplegia, alternate, early description of—1856.*

Guerin's valve or fold
. . . See under *Urethra, valve in fossa navicularis of.*

Guillotine for excising tonsils, invention of
JOSEPH FRANÇOIS BENOIT CHARRIÈRE, French surgeon and instrument maker, 1803-1876, devised a guillotine-type instrument for excising the tonsils. Introduced *circa* 1842.

Gull's disease, eponymic description of
. . . See under *Thyroid gland, atrophy of, with myxedema.*

Gull-Sutton's disease, eponymic description of
. . . See under *Arteriocapillary fibrosis.*

Gunning's splint
. . . See under *Jaw, fracture of, splint for.*

Gunn's dots
. . . See under *Macula lutea, white dots seen above.*

Gunshot wounds, first adequate account of
HIERONYMUS BRUNSCHWIG, German surgeon, 1450-1533, gave the first detailed description of gunshot wounds, in 1497.

Gwathmey's method of general anesthesia
. . . See under *Anesthesia, general, by rectal injection of ether and oil.*

Gymnastics and massage in therapeutics
PER HENRIK LING, Swedish physician, 1776-1839, is credited with introducing gymnastics and massage into therapeutics. He was instrumental in the establishment of a school for the training of teachers in gymnastics, in 1813. His work on gymnastics was published in 1840.

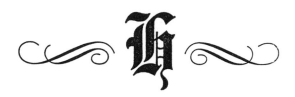

Habenulopeduncular tract, eponymic description of

THEODOR HERMANN MEYNERT, German neurologist and psychiatrist in Austria, 1833 - 1892, described a small bundle of nerve fibers extending between the habenula of the thalamus and the interpeduncular space. Published in 1867. Known as *Meynert's fasciculus* or *fasciculus retroflexus*.

Haemocytometer, construction of first

LOUIS CHARLES MALASSEZ, French physiologist, 1842-1909, is credited with making the first haemocytometer. Recorded in 1874.

Haemocytometer, introduction of term

WILLIAM RICHARD GOWERS, English neurologist, 1845 - 1915, is credited with the introduction of the term *haemocytometer* to designate the instrument devised by LOUIS CHARLES MALASSEZ in 1874. Recorded in 1877.

Hair catheter, invention of

JACQUES G. T. MAISONNEUVE, French surgeon, 1809 - 1897, devised a hair cathether in 1845.

Hair follicle, outer layer of cells in inner root sheath of

FRIEDRICH G. J. HENLE, German anatomist, 1809 - 1885, described the outer layer of cells in the inner root sheath of a hair follicle, between Huxley's layer and the outer root sheath. Reported in 1840. Known as *Henle's layer*.

Hair follicles, Huxley's layer of root sheath of

THOMAS HENRY HUXLEY, English biologist, 1825 - 1895, described a layer of the inner root sheath of a hair follicle, situated between the inner sheath cuticle and Henle's layer. Recorded in 1845. Known as *Huxley's layer*.

Hallucinations can be induced artificially, demonstration that

HUGO CARL LIEPMANN, German neurologist, 1863 - 1925, demonstrated, in 1906, that hallucinations can be induced by artificial means. Liepmann made the observation in a study of alcoholic delirium.

Hamburger phenomenon

... See under *Albumin and chloride shift between plasma and erythrocytes*.

Hammer for administering vibratory massage in nervous disorders

JOSEPH M. GRANVILLE, English physician, 1833 - 1900, devised a "hammer" for the administration of vibratory massage in treating functional and organic nervous disorders. Reported in 1882.

Hammond's disease

. . . See under *Athetosis, eponymic description of.*

Hand, contracture of; Dupuytren's contracture

GUILLAUME DUPUYTREN, French surgeon, 1777 - 1835, described a painless, chronic contracture of the hand due to a disorder of the palmar fascia, resulting in flexion of the fingers, especially of the third and fourth. The term is also applied, sometimes, to a similar contracture of the plantar fascia. Published in 1831.

Hand paralysis following injury of brachial plexus

AUGUSTA DEJERINE - KLUMPKE, French neurologist, 1859 - 1927, gave the first clear description of paralysis and atrophy of the muscles of the hand resulting from a lesion in the brachial plexus. Published in 1885. Known as *Klumpke's paralysis.*

Hand-Schüller-Christian disease—1893

ALFRED HAND, American physician, 1868-1949, gave the earliest description of the disease now known as *Hand-Schüller-Christian disease,* in 1893. He referred to it as a condition marked by polyuria and tuberculosis.

Hand-Schüller-Christian disease—1915

ARTUR SCHÜLLER, Austrian neurologist, 1874-19??, described the condition in 1915, remarking on the defects in the membranous bones.

Hand-Schüller-Christian disease—1919

HENRY A. CHRISTIAN, American physician, 1876-1951, gave a more complete description of the disease in 1919. It is marked by exophthalmos, diabetes insipidus, and defects in the membranous bones. The condition is known also as chronic idiopathic xanthomatosis.

Hand-Schüller-Christian disease and xanthomatosis

RUSSELL STURGIS ROWLAND, American physician, 1874 - 1938, studied cases of the Hand-Schüller-Christian syndrome and concluded that the disease is due to xanthomatosis. Published in 1928.

Hand-Schüller-Christian disease, first description of

. . . See under *Craniohypophysial xanthomatosis.*

Hanot's disease

. . . See under *Biliary cirrhosis; hypertrophic biliary cirrhosis.*

Harley's disease

. . . See under *Hemoglobinuria, paroxysmal or intermittent.*

Harrington's solution

. . . See under *Solution, disinfectant, for hand sterilization.*

Hasner's fold

. . . See under *Lacrimal fold, eponymic description of.*

Hassall's corpuscles

. . . See under *Thymus, concentrically striated bodies in.*

Haudek's niche

. . . See under *Gastric ulcer, niche in.*

Haverhill fever, first description of

EDWIN HEMPHILL PLACE, American physician, 1880-19??, with L. E. SUTTON and OTTO WILLNER, first reported the so-called Haverhill fever, a disease which appeared in Haverhill, Mass., in 1926. The investigators isolated an organism found to be identical with *Streptothrix muris ratti* and *Streptobacillus moniliformis*. Published in 1926. The condition is now known as rat-bite fever. Known also as *erythema arthriticum epidemicum* or *epidemic arthritic erythema*.

Haversian canals

. . . See under *Bone, canals of, containing blood and lymph vessels.*

Haversian glands

. . . See under *Synovial membranes, folds or pads on.*

Hay fever, early recognition of—1819

JOHN BOSTOCK, English physician, 1773-1846, described a "case of periodical affection of the eyes and chest," in 1819. BOSTOCK called the condition *catarrhus aestivus*. Hay fever is sometimes still called *Bostock's catarrh*.

Hayem's corpuscle

. . . See under *Achromacyte, early description of.*

Headache caused by astigmatism

. . . See under *Astigmatism as cause of headache, etc.*

Headache caused by eye strain

. . . See under *Eye strain as cause of headache, etc.*

Headache induced by histamine

. . . See under *Histamine headache, etc.*

Head's areas

. . . See under *Hyperalgesia of skin in visceral disease.*

Health examinations, periodic, first proposal of

LEMUEL SHATTUCK, Boston schoolmaster, 1793-1859, with N. P. BANKS and J. ABBOTT, prepared a general plan for the promotion of public health in Massachusetts in which the idea of periodic health examinations was first proposed. Published in 1850.

Hearing, resonance theory of

HERMANN L. F. VON HELMHOLTZ, German physiologist and physicist, 1821-1894, promulgated a resonance theory of hearing which holds that the motion of the stapes sets up vibrations in the perilymph resulting in secondary vibrations in the basilar membrane, each basilar fiber responding sympathetically to a definite frequency. Reported in 1862.

Heart, accelerator nerves of, discovery of

. . . See under *Accelerator nerves of heart.*

Heart, action currents of

. . . See under *Action currents of heart.*

Heart action is muscular contraction, early recognition of fact that

LEONARDO DA VINCI, Italian artist and scientist, 1452-1519, was probably the first to recognize that the action of the heart is a muscular contraction. Exact date not available.

Heart action, neurogenic theory of

... See under *Neurogenic theory of action of heart.*

Heart action, restoration of, by intracardiac injection

REINHARD VON DEN VELDEN, German physician, 1880-1941, was the first to attempt intracardiac injection to restore heart action after complete cessation. Recorded in 1919.

Heart as center of vascular system, early recognition of

ARISTOTLE, Greek scientist and philosopher, 384-322 B.C., recognized the heart as the center of the vascular system. It is believed that he did not differentiate between arteries and veins. Exact date not available.

Heart, beaded muscular fibers in subendocardial layer of

JOHANNES EVANGELISTA VON PURKINJE, Bohemian physiologist, 1787-1869, described certain beaded muscular fibers found in the form of a network in the subendocardial tissue of the ventricles of the heart and believed to serve as conductors of stimuli from the atria to the ventricles. Published in 1839. Known as *Purkinje's fibers* or *network*.

Heart beat, slowing of, by pressure in inferior carotid triangle

JOHANN N. CZERMAK, Bohemian physiologist, 1828-1873, discovered the fact that pressure exerted on a point in the inferior carotid triangle of the neck causes a slowing of the heart beat. Reported *circa* 1865. The pressure at this point stimulates the vagus.

Heart block, characteristic syndrome of—1761

GIOVANNI BATTISTA MORGAGNI, Italian anatomist and pathologist, 1682-1771, gave the first classic description of heart block, in 1761.

Heart block, characteristic syndrome of—1792

THOMAS SPENS, Scottish physician, 1764-1842, described a typical case of heart block marked by bradycardia and attacks of syncope. Report was published in 1792. The condition was previously described by GIOVANNI BATTISTA MORGAGNI, in 1761, and later by ROBERT ADAMS, in 1826, and WILLIAM STOKES, in 1846. The syndrome is known as the *Spens syndrome* and the *Stokes-Adams syndrome*.

Heart block, characteristic syndrome of—1826

ROBERT ADAMS, Irish physician, 1791-1875, presented a classic picture of heart block characterized by syncope with or without convulsive seizures, in 1826. The condition is known by the eponyms *Stokes-Adams syndrome* and *Spens syndrome*.

Heart block, characteristic syndrome of—1846

WILLIAM STOKES, Irish physician,

1804-1878, described a characteristic case of heart block, in 1846. The condition was previously given a classic description by ROBERT ADAMS, in 1826, and by SPENS in 1792. It is known as the *Stokes-Adams syndrome* and the *Spens syndrome*.

Heart block, introduction of term

WALTER H. GASKELL, English physiologist and anatomist, 1847-1914, is credited with introducing the term *heart block, circa* 1881.

Heart, capillaries in muscle fibers of

ARTHUR VINCENT MEIGS, American physician, 1850-1912, described capillaries between the muscle fibers of the heart. Recorded in 1891. Known as *Meig's capillaries*.

Heart, catheterization of; development of method for

WERNER THEODOR OTTO FORSS-MANN, German physician, 1904- , described a method for catheterizing the heart by passing a thin catheter through a vein in the arm. Forssmann performed the operation on himself. Recorded in 1929.

Heart, contraction current of, in frog

RUDOLPH ALBERT VON KÖLLIKER, Swiss histologist, 1817-1905, with HEINRICH MÜLLER (German anatomist, 1820-1864), demonstrated that the frog's heart produces an electric current at each contraction. Recorded in 1856.

Heart disease, congenital, marked by a tetralogy

ETIENNE L. A. FALLOT, French physician, 1850-1911, described a type of congenital heart disease marked by dextroposition of the aorta (so that it receives blood from both ventricles), pulmonary atresia or stenosis, hypertrophy of the right ventricle, and ventricular septal defects. Published in 1888. Known as the *tetralogy of Fallot*.

Heart disease, organic and functional, distinction between

. . . See under *Functional and organic heart disease*.

Heart, downward displacement of

GAETANO RUMMO, Italian physician, 1853-1917, described a downward displacement of the heart, in 1898. Known as *Rummo's disease* and *cardioptosis*.

Heart failure, low-sodium diet in

HENRY ALFRED SCHROEDER, American physician, 1906- , demonstrated the importance of a low salt diet in congestive heart disease. Published in 1941.

Heart, fatty infiltration of

ERNST VIKTOR VON LEYDEN, German physician, 1832-1910, was the first to describe fatty infiltration of the heart. Published in 1882.

Heart, fatty or fibrous degeneration of

RICHARD QUAIN, English physician, 1816-1898, described a fatty or fibrous degeneration of the muscle of the heart, in 1849. Known as *Quain's fatty degeneration*.

Heart, first successful suture of

LUDWIG REHN, German surgeon,

1849-1930, is credited with being the first to suture a wound of the human heart successfully. Recorded in 1896.

Heart fluoroscopy, early reference to

FRANCIS HENRY WILLIAMS, Boston physician, 1852-1936, advocated the use of the fluoroscope in determining the outline of the heart. Recorded in 1896.

Heart, hypertrophy and dilitation of, distinction between

... See under *Hypertrophy and dilation of heart,* etc.

Heart hypertrophy in aortic insufficiency is a compensatory condition, observation that

DOMINIC JOHN CORRIGAN, Irish physician, 1802-1880, pointed out that hypertrophy of the heart in aortic disease is not a disease in itself but a compensatory mechanism or condition. Reported in 1832.

Heart in myxedema, first record of

HERMANN ZONDEK, German physician in Israel, 1887- , was the first to describe the heart changes occurring in myxedema. Published in 1918.

Heart, increasing blood supply of, by grafting muscular tissue

CLAUDE S. BECK, American surgeon, 1894- , with VLADIMIR L. TICHY, American surgeon, 1899- , devised operations for increasing the blood supply to the heart by suturing muscular tissue to the abraded surface of the organ and thus providing a collateral circula-

tion. Recorded in 1935. The operation is known as cardiomyopexy.

Heart, increasing blood supply of, by uniting parietal pericardium with surface of heart

CLAUDE S. BECK, American surgeon, 1894- , with VLADIMIR L. TICHY, American surgeon, 1899- , devised an operation for increasing the blood supply to the heart by uniting the parietal pericardium with the surface of the heart. Reported in 1935. Known as cardiopericardiopexy.

Heart, inhibitory substance recovered from, after vagus stimulation

OTTO LOEWI, German pharmacologist in the United States, 1873-19??, demonstrated that an inhibitory substance could be isolated from the heart after vagus stimulation. Reported in 1921.

Heart, intrinsic ganglia of

ROBERT REMAK, German physiologist and neurologist, 1815-1865, described a group of nerve cells in the heart, near the superior vena cava. Recorded in 1844. Known as *Remak's ganglion* or *ganglia.*

Heart, irritable; neurocirculatory asthenia; effort syndrome

... See under *Irritable heart.*

Heart, mammalian, isolation of, in perfusion chamber

HENRY NEWELL MARTIN, American physiologist, 1848-1896, was first to isolate the mammalian heart in a perfusion chamber, in 1881.

Heart murmurs, mechanism of; early description

ALLAN BURNS, Scottish physician

and anatomist, 1781-1813, described the mechanism of heart murmurs, in 1809.

Heart, muscular structure of

NIELS STENSEN, Danish anatomist, 1638-1686, proved that the heart is composed primarily of muscle. Published in 1664.

Heart, noninflammatory fibrotic disease of

DAVID RIESMAN, American physician, 1867-1940, described a noninflammatory degenerative fibrosis of the myocardium, in 1920. Known as *Riesman's myocardosis.*

Heart rate and blood pressure, relationship between

ÉTIENNE JULES MAREY, French physiologist, 1830-1904, was the first to recognize the relationship between the heart rate and the blood pressure. Recorded in 1861.

Heart, special nerves of

WALTER HOLBROOK GASKELL, English physiologist and anatomist, 1847-1914, described the accelerator nerves of the heart and demonstrated that impulses from the ganglia in the sinus venosus influence the rhythm of the heart but do not originate the beat. Recorded in 1882. Known as *Gaskell's nerves.*

Heart, special nerves of

IVAN PETROVICH PAVLOV, Russian physiologist, 1849-1936, discovered (independently of Gaskell) the accelerator and vasoconstrictor nerves of the heart, *circa* 1884.

Heart, Starling's law of the

ERNEST HENRY STARLING, English physiologist, 1866-1927, stated that the output of the heart per beat is proportional to the extent of the diastolic filling. Published in 1918.

Heart, third sound of

WILLIAM SYDNEY THAYER, Baltimore physician, 1864-1932, is credited with being first to call attention to the third sound of the heart. Published in 1908.

Heart, vascular plexuses of

FREDERIK RUYSCH, Dutch anatomist, 1638-1731, was first to describe the vascular plexuses of the heart. Recorded in his *Thesaurus Anatomicus,* published 1701-1716.

Heart, wounded, method of suturing with deep stay suture

DANIEL COLLIER ELKIN, American surgeon, 1893- , devised a method for suturing a wounded heart by use of a deep stay suture, to control bleeding until the edges of the wound are approximated. Reported in 1932.

Heat cramps caused by loss of base, chlorides, etc.

JOHN HAROLD TALBOTT, New York physician, 1902- , demonstrated that heat cramps are due to the loss of water, base, and chlorides in the perspiration. Recorded in 1933.

Hebephrenia, early description of

KARL LUDWIG KAHLBAUM, German psychiatrist, 1828-1899, described hebephrenia, in 1863.

Heberden's nodes

... See under *Osteoarthritis, nodes on interphalangeal joints in.*

Hebra's disease

... See under *Erythema multiforme exudativum, early description of.*

Hegar's sign

. . . See under *Uterus, softening of lower segment of, in pregnancy.*

Heidenhain's cells

. . . See under *Gastric glands, cells of.*

Heister's valve

. . . See under *Cystic duct, spiral valve of.*

***Helicotrema,* introduction of term**

GILBERT BRESCHET, French anatomist, 1784-1845, introduced the term *helicotrema* to designate the structure of the cochlea. Recorded in 1834.

Helium, isolation of, in a mixture with argon

WILLIAM RAMSAY, English scientist, 1852-1916, isolated helium in a mixture with argon by treating pitchblende with sulfuric acid, in 1895.

Helium, spectroscopic discovery of—1868

EDWARD FRANKLAND, English chemist, 1825-1899, with JOSEPH NORMAN LOCKYER, English astronomer, 1836-1920, discovered a bright yellow line in the solar spectrum near the D line of sodium. The line was attributed by the observers to a hypothetical element to which they gave the name helium, in 1868.

Helium, use of, in respiratory disease

ALVAN LEROY BARACH, American physician, 1895-   , introduced helium in therapeutics, in the treatment of respiratory disease. Published in 1934.

Helmholtz's theory of color vision

. . . See under *Color vision, Helmholtz theory of.*

Helweg's bundle

. . . See under *Nerves, tract of, in cervical region.*

***Hematoblast,* introduction of term**

GEORGES HAYEM, French physician, 1841-1933, introduced the term *hematoblast,* said to have been applied at first only to a blood platelet. The term is now applied to a primitive mass or cell from which an erythrocyte is developed. Originated in 1877.

Hematomyelia, central, eponymic description of

LAZAR SALOMOVITCH MINOR, Russian neurologist, 1855-19??, described central hematomyelia, an escape of blood within the spinal cord, in 1892. Known as *Minor's disease.*

Hematuria, paroxysmal, early description of

CHARLES STEWART, English surgeon, 17??-18??, described a case of paroxysmal hematuria, in 1794.

Hemiballism, nuclear degeneration causing

JULES BERNARD LUYS, French neurologist, 1828-1897, described the subthalamic nucleus whose degeneration causes hemiballism. Recorded in 1865.

Hemin crystals in test for blood

LUDWIG T. S. TEICHMANN, German histologist, 1825-1895, devised a test for blood in which a positive reaction is expressed by the formation of hemin crystals. Recorded in 1853. Known as *Teichmann's crystals.*

Hemin, synthesis of

HANS FISCHER, German chemist, 1881-1945, did fundamental research in the field of heme compounds. His most notable achievement was the synthesis of hemin. Received the Nobel prize in 1930.

Hemiplegia, alternate, early description of—1856

ADOLPHE GUBLER, French physician, 1821-1879, described alternate or crossed hemiplegia, a form which affects parts on opposite sides of the body, in 1856. Known as *Gubler's paralysis, Weber-Gubler syndrome, Millard-Gubler paralysis,* etc.

Hemiplegia, alternate, involving lateral rectus muscle on one side and paralysis of limbs on other side

AGUSTE L. J. MILLARD, French physician, 1830-1915, described the superior type of alternate hemiplegia involving, in the reported case, paralysis of the lateral rectus muscle on the side of the lesion and paralysis of the limbs on the other side. In other cases the peripheral facial muscles on the side of the lesion are involved. Published in 1864. Known as *Millard-Gubler syndrome.* etc.

Hemiplegia, alternate, involving oculomotor nerve on one side and paralysis of limbs on other side

HERMANN DAVID WEBER, English physician, 1823-1918, described a superior type of alternate hemiplegia involving, in several cases reported, paralysis of the oculomotor nerve on one side and spastic paralysis of the limbs on the opposite side of the lesion. Published in 1863. Known as *Weber's paralysis, Weber-Gubler syndrome, Millard-Gubler syndrome,* etc.

Hemiplegia, spastic, of extremities, eponymic description of

CARL WERNICKE, German neurologist, 1848-1905, described a form of spastic hemiplegia of the extremities in which some groups of muscles are affected less than other groups. Recorded in 1889. The same condition was described by LUDWIG MANN (German neurologist, 1866-1936) in 1896. Known as *Wernicke-Mann type* of palsy or paralysis.

Hemisporosis, early description of

HENRI GOUGEROT, French physician, 1881-19??, with CARAVEN, described hemisporosis. Published in 1909.

Hemochromatosis, first description of

ARMAND TROUSSEAU, French physician, 1801-1867, was the first to describe hemochromatosis, in 1865. Known as *Trousseau's disease.*

Hemochromatosis, introduction of term

FRIEDRICH DANIEL VON RECKLINGHAUSEN, German pathologist, 1833-1910, introduced the name *hemochromatosis,* in 1889.

Hemocytometer

... See under *Haemocytometer.*

Hemodynamometer, mercury, introduction of

JEAN LÈONARD MARIE POISEUILLE, French physiologist, 1799-1869, is credited with constructing the first mercury manometer or hemodynamometer. Published in 1828.

Hemoglobin, colorimetric determination of

JOHN SCOTT HALDANE, Scottish physiologist, 1860-1936, devised a colorimetric method for the determination of hemoglobin. He also established a standard scale. Introduced *circa* 1901.

Hemoglobin, combining power of

CARL GUSTAV VON HÜFNER, German physiologist, 1840-1908, measured the combining power of hemoglobin and showed that one gram combines with 1.34 c.c. of oxygen. Recorded in 1894.

Hemoglobin determination by Tallqvist method

THEODOR WALDEMAR TALLQVIST, Finnish physician, 1871-1927, devised a simple but only approximately correct method for hemoglobin determination. A blood blot is compared with a series of lithographed color standards showing tints of various concentrations of hemoglobin. Published in 1900. Known as *Tallqvist's scale* or *method*.

Hemoglobin, discovery of

OTTO FUNKE, German physician, 1828-1879, is credited with the discovery of hemoglobin, in 1851.

Hemoglobin, isolation of, in crystalline form

OTTO FUNKE, German physician, 1828-1879, isolated hemoglobin in crystalline form in 1853. This was also accomplished in the same year by ERNST F. I. HOPPE-SEYLER, German physiological chemist, 1825-1895.

Hemoglobin, introduction of term

ERNST F. I. HOPPE-SEYLER, German physiological chemist, 1825-1895, is credited with the introduction of the term *haemoglobin,* about 1862.

Hemoglobinometer, early invention of—1878

WILLIAM RICHARD GOWERS, English neurologist, 1845-1915, is credited with inventing the first practical hemoglobinometer, in 1878.

Hemoglobinometer, early invention of—1901

JOHN SCOTT HALDANE, Scottish physiologist, 1860-1936, modified the hemoglobinometer invented by W. R. GOWERS. Recorded in 1901.

Hemoglobinuria, epidemic, eponymic description of

FRANZ CARL LUDWIG VON WINCKEL, German physician, 1837-1911, described hemoglobinuria of the newborn, accompanied by cyanosis, jaundice, and nervous symptoms. Recorded in 1879. Known as *Winckel's disease.*

Hemoglobinuria following physical exertion

. . . See under *March hemoglobinuria.*

Hemoglobinuria, paroxysmal or intermittent, eponymic description of

GEORGE HARLEY, English physi-

cian, 1829-1896, described a disorder marked by transitory hemoglobinuria following prolonged exertion or exposure to cold and by
the presence in the blood of a special hemolysin which is active only
at low temperatures. Reported in
1865. Known as *Harley's disease.*

Hemolytic jaundice of newborn

DOMENICO PANAROLI, Italian physician, 16??-1657, described hemolytic jaundice of the newborn, in
1652.

Hemolytic jaundice with anemia

. . . See under *Acquired hemolytic
jaundice with anemia.*

Hemophilia, early mention of

Earliest known mention of hemophilia is made in the Talmud (completed in the 5th or 6th century).
An infant known to have, or suspected of having, hemophilia was
exempted from the ritual of circum-
cision. The condition was later described by ALBUCASIM, celebrated
Spanish-Arabian physician of the
10th century.

Hemophilia, first complete
description of—1803

JOHN CONRAD OTTO, American
physician, 1774-1844, gave the first
full description of hemophilia,
pointing out that females are not
affected but can transmit the disease to the male. Published in 1803.

Hemophilia, first full clinical
description of—1855

JOHANN LUDWIG GRANDIDIER, German physician, 1810-187?, gave the
first full clinical picture of hemophilia, in 1855.

Hemophilia, introduction
of term

JOHANN LUCAS SCHÖNLEIN, German physician, 1793-1864, is credited with the introduction of the
term *hemophilia.* Recorded in 1828.

Hemophilia, Nasse's law of

CHRISTIAN FRIEDRICH NASSE, German physician, 1778-1851, stressed
the fact, noted previously, that
women can transmit hemophilia but
are themselves immune to it. Published in 1820.

Hemophilia, snake venom
in treatment of

ROBERT GWYN MACFARLANE,
English physician, 189?-   , with
BURGESS BARNETT, introduced the
use of snake venom in the treatment
of hemophilia. Published in 1934.

Hemophilus ducreyi,
discovery of

. . . See under *Chancroid, causative
organism of.*

Hemophilus duplex, isolation of

KARL T. P. P. AXENFELD, German
ophthalmologist, 1867-1930, and
VICTOR MORAX, French ophthalmologist, 1866-1935, isolated
Hemophilus duplex almost simultaneously, in 1896, but quite independently. The organism is also
known as the *Moraxella lacunata*
and *Morax-Axenfeld bacillus.* The
conjunctivitis caused by the organism is known as *Morax-Axenfeld
conjunctivitis.*

Hemophilus influenzae,
discovery of

. . . See under *Influenza bacillus.*

Hemophilus influenzae, isolation of

RICHARD EDWIN SHOPE, American physician, 1901- , isolated *Hemophilus influenzae*. Recorded in 1931.

Hemophilus pertussis, discovery of

JULES J. B. V. BORDET, Belgian bacteriologist and pathologist, 1870-19??, with OCTAVE GENGOU, French bacteriologist, 1875-19??, discovered *Hemophilus pertussis*. Reported in 1906.

Hemorrhagic diathesis of Willebrand

. . . See under *Pseudohemophilia, hereditary.*

Hemorrhagic disease of newborn, early report

FRANCIS MINOT, American physician, 1821-1899, described hemorrhagic disease of the newborn, with an analysis of 46 cases. Published in 1852.

Hemorrhagic telangiectasis, hereditary

. . . See under *Telangiectasis, hereditary hemorrhagic.*

Hemostatic forceps, introduction of, in surgery

ARISTIDE AUGUSTE STANISLAUS VERNEUIL, French surgeon and anatomist, 1823-1895, is credited with introducing forcipressure in surgery, in 1875.

Hemotachometer, invention of

KARL VIERORDT, German physiologist, 1818-1884, invented a hemotachometer with which he measured the rate of the blood flow in various arteries. He also studied the influence of various factors, as pulse rate, upon the rate of flow. Published in 1858.

Henderson-Paterson bodies

. . . See under *Molluscum contagiosum, inclusion bodies in.*

Henke's space

. . . See under *Spinal column and pharynx, space between.*

Henke's triangle

. . . See under *Triangle formed by border of rectus muscle and inguinal fold.*

Henle's layer

. . . See under *Hair follicle, outer layer of cells in inner root sheath of.*

Henle's loop

. . . See under *Uriniferous tubule, U-shaped turn in.*

Henle's membrane

. . . See under *Artery, fenestrated membrane of.*

Henle's spine

. . . See under *Suprameatal spine, original description of.*

Henle's warts

. . . See under *Cornea, outgrowth of cells at periphery of.*

Henoch's purpura

. . . See under *Purpura, nonthrombopenic, marked by acute intestinal symptoms.*

Hensen's duct or canal

. . . See under *Membranous labyrinth, small canal leading from.*

Heparin, clinical use of, as anticoagulant

DONALD WALTER GORDON MUR-

RAY, American surgeon, 1896-   ,
with L. B. JAQUES, T. S. PERRETT,
and C. H. BEST, used heparin clinically in treating thrombosis of veins
following injury. Recorded in 1937.

Heparin in blood transfusion

PER JOHANNES HEDENIUS, Swedish
physician, 1906-   , introduced
the use of heparin as an anticoagulant in blood transfusion. Recorded
in 1936.

Heparin, introduction of term

LUTHER EMMETT HOLT, American
pediatrician, 1855-1924, and WIL-
LIAM HENRY HOWELL, American
physiologist, 1860-1945, introduced the term *heparin,* in 1918.
See also under *Heparin, isolation
of.*

Heparin, isolation of

JAY MCLEAN, American physiologist, 1890-19??, working in Howell's laboratory, in Baltimore, was
the first to isolate the anticoagulant
substance now called heparin, in
1916. The name *heparin* was applied by HOLT and HOWELL, after
further investigation, in 1918.

Hepatic artery, aneurysm of

HEINRICH IRENAEUS QUINCKE,
German physician, 1842-1922, observed an aneurysm of the hepatic
artery, in 1870. Published in 1871.

Hepatic artery, successful ligation of

HANS KEHR, German surgeon,
1862-1916, is said to have successfully ligated the hepatic artery. Recorded in 1903.

Hepatization of lungs in pneumonia, early note on

MATTHEW BAILLIE, English physician, 1761-1823, described hepati-
zation of the lungs in pneumonia, in
his text published in 1793.

Hepatotomy, first use of

ROBERT LAWSON TAIT, English
surgeon and gynecologist, 1845-
1899, is credited with introducing
hepatotomy. Published in 1881.

Herbal, earliest, printed in English

RYCHARDE BANCKES, 16th century
English physician, was the author
of the first herbal printed in English, in 1525.

Herbal, most comprehensive, of 16th century

LEONHARD FUCHS, German botanist, 1501-1566, wrote the most comprehensive work of the 16th century in the field of herbs and vegetable drugs. Published in 1542.

Hereditary cerebellar sclerosis

PIERRE MARIE, French neurologist,
1853-1940, described hereditary
cerebellar sclerosis, marked by
ataxia, speech defects, nystagmus,
etc. Recorded in 1893. Known as
Marie's ataxia. Also called *hereditary cerebellar ataxia.*

Hereditary deforming chondrodysplasia

. . . See under *Dyschondroplasia,
eponymic description of.*

Hereditary edema of the legs, earliest description of—1891

MAX NONNE, German neurologist,
1861-19??, is credited with giving
the earliest description of hereditary edema of the legs, in 1891.
Known as *Milroy's disease* and
Meige's disease.

Hereditary edema of the legs, eponymic description of—1892

WILLIAM FORSYTH MILROY, American physician, 1855-1942, recorded an "undescribed variety of hereditary edema" of the legs, in 1892. It is said that WILLIAM OSLER introduced the name. Known as *Milroy's disease.*

Hereditary edema of the legs, eponymic description of—1899

HENRI MEIGE, French physician, 1866-1940, described chronic hereditary trophedema *(trophoedeme chronique hereditaire),* in 1899. Known as *Meige's disease* and *Milroy's disease.*

Hereditary hemorrhagic telangiectasis

. . . See under *Telangiectasis, hereditary hemorrhagic.*

Hereditary spinal sclerosis; Friedreich's ataxia

NIKOLAUS FRIEDREICH, German neurologist, 1825-1882, described a hereditary disease, usually beginning early in life, characterized by sclerosis of the dorsal and lateral columns of the spinal cord. Reported in 1863.

Hereditary spinocerebellar ataxia, original description of

SANGER BROWN, American psychiatrist, 1852-1928, described a hereditary type of spinocerebellar ataxia. Known as *Sanger Brown's ataxia.* Date not available.

Heredity, hypothesis for explanation of, resembling side-chain theory

JOHN GEORGE ADAMI, English pathologist working in Canada, 1862-1926, offered a hypothesis concerning heredity, especially with reference to the inheritance of acquired characteristics, which resembles Ehrlich's side-chain theory of immunity. Published in 1901.

Heredity, role of chromosomes in

. . . See under *Chromosomes as agents of heredity,* etc.

Hernia, congenital, first description of

PERCIVALL POTT, English surgeon, 1714-1788, gave the first recorded description of congenital hernia, in 1756.

Hernia, femoral, complete; eponymic description of

FRANZ CASPAR HESSELBACH, German surgeon and anatomist, 1759-1816, gave a clear description of a complete femoral hernia, in 1798. Known as *Hesselbach's femoral hernia.*

Hernia, femoral, early description of

GUY DE CHAULIAC, French surgeon, 1300-1368, is credited with giving the earliest known description of femoral hernia, in 1363.

Hernia in which only part of intestinal lumen is involved

AUGUST GOTTLIEB RICHTER, German surgeon, 1742-1812, described a type of intestinal hernia in which only part of the lumen was involved. Published in 1778. Known as *Richter's hernia.*

Hernia, inguinal, external and internal, early differentiation of

LORENZ (LAURENTIUS) HEISTER, German surgeon and anatomist, 1683-1758, is credited with differentiating between direct and indirect inguinal hernias, in 1724.

Hernia, inguinal, external and internal, early differentiation of

FRANZ CASPAR HESSELBACH, German surgeon and anatomist, 1759-1816, differentiated between the two types of inguinal hernia and termed them *external* and *internal, circa* 1814.

Hernia, inguinal, with diverticulum through cribriform fascia

FRANZ CASPAR HESSELBACH, German surgeon and anatomist, 1759-1816, described inguinal hernia with a diverticulum through the cribriform fascia, *circa* 1810. Known as *Hesselbach's hernia.*

Hernia, internal mesogastric, description of

WENZEL LEOPOLD GRUBER, Bohemian anatomist in Russia, 1814-1890, described internal mesogastric hernia, in 1863. Known as *Gruber's hernia.*

Hernia, lumbar, in Petit's triangle

JEAN LOUIS PETIT, French surgeon, 1674-1750, described a lumbar hernia through a space bounded by the external oblique and latissimus dorsi muscles and the iliac crest. Published in 1774. The hernia was described earlier, in 1731, by R. J. C. DE GARENGEOT, but it is known as *Petit's hernia.*

Hernia of a diverticulum

ALEXIS LITTRÉ, French surgeon and anatomist, 1658-1726, was the first to describe herniation of a diverticulum (Meckel's diverticulum), in 1719. Known as *Littré's hernia.* The condition was described more fully, in 1778, by AUGUST GOTTLIEB RICHTER, German surgeon, 1742-1812.

Hernia of intestine between vitelline duct and abdominal wall

JEAN BAPTISTE BARTH, German physician, 1806-1877, described herniation of loops of small intestine between a persistent vitelline duct and the abdominal wall. Published in 1836. Known as *Barth's hernia.*

Hernia, retrocecal, first description of

LÉON RIEUX, French surgeon, *circa* 1815-1880, described a hernia consisting of an intestinal protrusion behind the cecum. Recorded in 1853. Known as *Rieux's hernia.*

Hernia, retroperitoneal, through duodenojejunal fossa

WENZEL TREITZ, Austrian physician and anatomist, 1819-1872, described a retroperitoneal hernia with a protrusion through the duodenojenjunal fossa. Published in 1857. Known as *Treitz's hernia.*

Hernia, sliding or slipped

ANTONIO SCARPA, Italian anatomist and surgeon, 175?-1832, described a type of slipping or sliding hernia in which a part of the colon is drawn in the hernial sac by the peritoneum to which it is attached. Recorded in 1821. Known as *Scarpa's hernia.*

Hernia, strangulated, first description of operation for

PIERRE FRANCO, French surgeon, 1500-1561, is credited with having given the first description of an operation for the relief of strangulated hernia, in 1556.

Herpangina, original description of

JOHN ZAHORSKY, American pediatrician, 1871-19??, was the first to describe herpangina, an infectious disease characterized by fever and ulcerations in the faucial area. Published in 1920.

Herpes zoster due to lesion of spinal ganglia

FRIEDRICH WILHELM FELIX VON BÄRENSPRUNG, German dermatologist, 1822-1864, was the first to suggest that the cause of herpes zoster is a lesion of the spinal ganglia. Recorded in 1861.

Herpes zoster, infectiousness of

LOUIS THÉOPHILE JOSEPH LANDOUZY, French physician, 1845-1917, was the first to recognize the infectiousness of herpes zoster. Recorded in 1884.

Herpes zoster, infectiousness of; first demonstration

KARL KUNDRATITZ, German physician, 1890- , was the first to demonstrate the infectiousness of herpes zoster. Published in 1925.

Herpes zoster, pathology of, early recognition

HENRY HEAD, English neurologist, 1861-1940, with ALFRED W. CAMPBELL, studied herpes zoster and established that the disease is an inflammation of the posterior nerve ganglia and roots (caused by the virus *Briareus varicellae*). Reported in 1900.

Herrick's anemia

. . . See under *Anemia, sickle-cell, first clear description of.*

Herxheimer's reaction

. . . See under *Syphilitic symptoms, exacerbation of.*

Hesselbach's hernia

. . . See under *Hernia, inguinal, with diverticulum through cribriform fascia.*

Hesselbach's triangle

. . . See under *Triangle, anatomic, limited by rectus muscle, etc.*

Heterophoria, glass rods for measuring degree of

ERNEST EDMUND MADDOX, English ophthalmologist, 1860-1933, devised an instrument, consisting of parallel cylindrical glass rods, for testing and measuring the degree of heterophoria. Recorded in 1898. Known as the *Maddox rod* or *rods*.

Heubner's disease

. . . See under *Syphilitic endarteritis of cerebral vessels.*

Hexamethonium bromide, introduction of

WILLIAM DRUMMOND MACDONALD PATON, English pharmacologist, 19??- , with ELEANOR ZAIMIS, introduced hexamethonium bromide, the ganglion-blocking substance. Published in 1949.

Hexestrol, isolation of

N. R. CAMPBELL, English scientist, 19??- , with E. C. DODDS and

W. Lawson, isolated hexestrol, a synthetic estrogen, in 1938.

Hexosephosphoric esters in ossification

Robert Robison, English biochemist, 1883-1941, pointed out the importance of the hexosephosphoric esters in the process of ossification. Published in 1923.

Hiatus pleuroperitonealis; foramen of Bochdalek

Vincent Alexander Bochdalek, Bohemian anatomist, 1801-1883, described an opening in the fetal diaphragm which may become the site of congenital diaphragmatic hernia. Called *foramen of Bochdalek*. Introduced *circa* 1850.

Hidradenitis suppurativa

. . . See under *Hydradenitis destruens suppurativa*.

Hidrocystoma, first description of

Andrew Rose Robinson, American dermatologist, 1845-1924, is credited with giving the first description of hidrocystoma, a sweat gland retention cyst, in 1884. Known as *Robinson's disease*.

High altitude disease or erythremia

. . . See under *Mountain sickness, chronic*.

High altitude sickness due to anoxemia

Paul Bert, French physician, 1833-1886, demonstrated that the symptoms of high altitude or mountain sickness are due to anoxemia. Published in 1878.

High frequency currents, first use of, in diathermy and coagulation

Karl Franz Nagelschmidt, German physician, 1875-1952, is credited with being first to introduce the use of high frequency electric currents and radiation in both coagulation and diathermy. Recorded in 1909.

High frequency currents in electrotherapy, introduction of

Jacques Arsène d'Arsonval, French physicist and physiologist, 1851-1940, introduced the use of high frequency alternating currents of high voltage and low amperage. Recorded in 1892. The treatment is known as d'arsonvalization.

Hip, dislocation of, toward anterior superior iliac spine

Giovanni Battista Monteggia, Italian surgeon, 1762-1815, described a dislocation in the hip joint in which the head of the femur is displaced toward the anterior superior iliac spine, *circa* 1810. Known as *Monteggia's dislocation*.

Hip joint, congenital dislocation of; first clear description

Guillaume Dupuytren, French surgeon, 1777-1835, gave the first clear description of congenital dislocation of the femur in the hip joint. Published in 1826.

Hip joint, first excision at, in America

Henry Jacob Bigelow, American surgeon, 1818-1890, is credited with performing the first excision of the head of the femur in America. Recorded in 1852.

Hip joint, first successful amputation at, in the United States

Walter Brashear, Maryland

surgeon, 1776-1860, is credited with performing the first successful amputation at the hip joint in the United States, in 1806. Recorded in 1853. The operation was performed at Bardstown, Ky.

Hippuric acid, determination of structure of

JUSTUS VON LIEBIG, German chemist, 1803-1873, was first to determine the constitution of hippuric acid, in 1839.

Hippuric acid, differentiation of, from benzoic acid

JUSTUS VON LIEBIG, German chemist, 1803-1873, was the first to distinguish between hippuric acid and benzoic acid, in 1829.

Hippuric acid, earliest detection of—1768

HILAIRE MARIE ROUELLE, French pharmacologist, 1718-1779, is credited with being first to detect the presence of hippuric acid in the urine, in 1768. It is so named because first isolated from the urine of horses (Gr. *hippos,* horse) and other herbivorous animals.

Hippuric acid, first clear discovery of

FRIEDRICH WÖHLER, German chemist, 1800-1882, first discovered hippuric acid in 1824, but did not follow it up till 1842 when he confirmed the discovery and demonstrated that ingested benzoic acid is excreted as hippuric acid, in the urine. This observation is considered the starting point of modern chemistry of metabolism.

Hippuric acid liver function test

ARMAND JAMES QUICK, American physician, 1894-   , with H. N. OTTENSTEIN and H. WELTCHEK, described an intravenous hippuric acid liver function test. Published in 1938.

Hippuric acid, synthesis of

V. DESSAIGNESS, English chemist, 1818-18??, was the first to synthesize hippuric acid, from benzoyl chloride and zinc glycocollide, in 1853.

Hirschsprung's disease

. . . See under *Megacolon, congenital, etc.*

Hirsutism and diabetes in female

EMILE CHARLES ACHARD, French physician, 1860-1941, with JOSEPH THIERS, described a syndrome of hirsutism in the female associated with diabetes. Recorded in 1921. Known as *Achard-Thiers syndrome.*

Histamine action on peripheral vessels

HENRY HALLETT DALE, English physiologist, 1875-19??, with ALFRED NEWTON RICHARDS, demonstrated that the action of histamine is located in the smaller arterioles and the capillaries. Recorded in 1918.

Histamine headache, original description of

BAYARD TAYLOR HORTON, American physician, 1895-   , described a type of vascular headache resulting from administration of histamine. Reported in 1939. Known as *Horton's syndrome.*

Histamine headache

. . . See also under *Histaminic cephalalgia.*

Histamine, isolation of, from ergot

GEORGE BARGER, English scientist, 1878-1939, with HENRY H. DALE, isolated histamine from ergot, in 1910.

Histamine, isolation of, from intestinal mucosa

GEORGE BARGER, English scientist, 1878-1939, with HENRY H. DALE, isolated histamine from animal intestinal mucosa, in 1911.

Histamine, release of, in anaphylaxis

CARL ALBERT DRAGSTEDT, American physician, 1895-   , with ERICH GEBAUER-FUELNEGG, demonstrated the release of histamine into the circulation as the result of an anaphylactic reaction. Published in 1932.

Histamine-like substance, postulation of

THOMAS LEWIS, English cardiologist, 1881-1945, with RONALD THOMSON GRANT, suggested the existence of a histamine-like substance which is the cause of anaphylactic symptoms. Published in 1924.

Histaminic cephalalgia, early description of

CALEB HILLIER PARRY, English physician, 1755-1822, described a form of headache now known as histaminic cephalalgia. Published in 1792.

Histidine, discovery of

ALBRECHT KOSSEL, German physiologist, 1853-1927, discovered histidine as a decomposition product in sturgeon testes, *circa* 1896. Published in 1899.

Histidine, structure of—1904

HERMANN PAULY, German physiologist, 1870-19??, is credited with determining the structure of histidine, in 1904.

Histology, founder of modern

MARIE F. X. BICHAT, French anatomist and physiologist, 1771-1802, renowned for his contributions to descriptive anatomy, is considered the founder of modern histology.

Histoplasmosis, original description of

SAMUEL TAYLOR DARLING, American physician, 1872-1925, described a disease of the reticuloendothelial system marked by fever, anemia, enlargement of the liver, etc., and caused by infection with *Histoplasma capsulatum.* Published in 1906. Known also as *reticuloendothelial cytomycosis* and as *Darling's histoplasmosis.*

History of medicine, first American work on

PETER MIDDLETON, American physician, 17??-1781, wrote the first American book on the history of medicine. Published in 1769.

History of medicine, first book on, by Englishman

JOHN FREIND, English medical historian, 1675-1728, wrote the first book on the history of medicine produced by an Englishman. Published in 1725-26.

History of medicine, first important book on

SYMPHORIEN CHAMPIER, French physician, 1472-1539, wrote the first important book on the history of medicine. Published in 1506.

History of medicine, first large book on

DANIEL LE CLERC, Swiss physician, 1652-1728, is credited with writing the first large book on the history of medicine. Published in 1729.

Hodgkin's disease and aleukemic leukemia, differentiation between

CARL STERNBERG, German pathologist, 1872-1935, was the first to differentiate between Hodgkin's disease and aleukemic leukemia. Published in 1898.

Hodgkin's disease and lymphosarcoma, differentiation between

JULIUS DRESCHFELD, English physician, 1845-1907, was probably the first to differentiate between Hodgkin's disease and lymphosarcoma. Published in 1892.

Hodgkin's disease, eponymic description of

THOMAS HODGKIN, English physician, 1798-1866, described a progressive, painless, and fatal enlargement of the lymph nodes, spleen, and other lymphoid tissue. Reported in 1832. Known also as *malignant granuloma, infectious granuloma, lymphosarcoma, pseudoleukemia,* etc.

Hodgkin's disease, giant polynuclear cells in

DOROTHY REED (Mrs. Mendenhall), American pathologist, 1874-19??, described the giant ploynuclear cells found in the lymph nodes in Hodgkin's disease. Recorded in 1902. Known as *Dorothy Reed cells, Sternberg-Reed cells.* CARL

STERNBERG, German pathologist, 1872-1935, described the cells in 1898.

Hodgkin's disease, introduction of term

SAMUEL WILKS, English physician, 1824-1911, is credited with introducing the eponymic term *Hodgkin's disease,* in 1865.

Hodgkin's disease, nitrogen mustards in treatment of

ALFRED GILMAN, American scientist, 1908-   , with FREDERICK STANLEY PHILIPS, introduced the nitrogen mustards in the treatment of Hodgkin's disease. Published in 1946.

Hodgson's disease

. . . See under *Aorta, dilatation of proximal part of.*

Hoffmann's Anodyne

. . . See under *Compound Spirit of Ether.*

Hoffmann's atrophy

. . . See under *Progressive muscular atrophy; Hoffmann's atrophy.*

Hoffmann's drops

. . . See under *Spirit of Ether.*

Holger Nielsen resuscitation technique

. . . See under *Artificial respiration, arm-lift method of.*

Hollow cone method of amputation, development of

EDWARD ALANSON, English surgeon, 1747-1823, developed a method of amputation in which the skin and muscles are cut in a circular manner so as to leave a stump shaped like a hollow cone. Published in 1779.

Home's lobe or gland

. . . See under *Prostate, subsidiary lobe of.*

Homogentisic acid in urine, discovery of

CARL WILHELM BOEDEKER, German physician, 1816-1879, was the first to find homogentisic acid in urine. Published in 1859.

Homologues and analogues, differentiation between

RICHARD OWEN, English physician, 1804-1892, is credited with formulating the distinction between organs of similar structure and development (homologues) and organs of similar function but different origin and structure (analogues). Published in 1843.

Hook for decapitating fetus in difficult labor

CHARLES PAJOT, French obstetrician, 1816-1896, devised a hook for severing the fetal head in difficult labor. Recorded in 1865. Known as *Pajot's hook.*

Hookworm disease, causative agent of

. . . See under *Ancylostomiasis, causative agent of.*

Hookworm disease in Puerto Rico

. . . See under *Ancylostomiasis, prevalence of, in Puerto Rico.*

Hookworm disease, oil of chenopodium in

WILHELM AUGUST PAUL SCHÜFFNER, German pathologist, 1867-1949, with HERMAN VERVOORT, introduced the use of oil of chenopodium in the treatment of ancylostomiasis, in 1900. Published in 1912.

Hookworm in cat, discovery of

JOSEPH LEIDY, American physician, 1823-1891, discovered the hookworm in a cat. He also suggested the possibility that the hookworm is responsible for pernicious anemia in man. Recorded in 1886.

Hookworm infestation

. . . See also under *Ancylostomiasis.*

Hormone, introduction of term

ERNEST HENRY STARLING, English physiologist, 1866-1927, was the first to use the term *hormone* in the modern sense. Recorded in 1905. The word is said to have been suggested by W. B. HARDY.

Horner's syndrome, eponymic description of

JOHANN FRIEDRICH HORNER, Swiss ophthalmologist, 1831-1886, described a syndrome resulting from paralysis of the cervical sympathetic nerves, marked by ptosis of the upper eyelid, enophthalmos, miosis, anhidrosis, etc. Recorded in 1869.

Horner's syndrome, pre-eponymic description of—1727

FRANÇOIS POURFOIR DU PETIT, French physician, 1664-1741, produced a syndrome in animals similar to Horner's syndrome in man. Recorded in 1727.

Horner's syndrome, pre-eponymic description of—1839

E. S. HARE, English physician, 1805-1869, gave a brief description of the condition later to be called the Horner syndrome. Recorded in 1839.

Horner's syndrome, pre-eponymic description of—1858

CLAUDE BERNARD, French physiologist, 1813-1878, described the condition now known as Horner's syndrome, in 1858.

Horner's teeth

. . . See under *Incisor teeth with grooves.*

Horse, anatomy of, first book on

ANDREW SNAPE, English anatomist, 1646-1711, is credited with writing the first book on the anatomy of the horse, in English. Published in 1683.

Houston's valves

. . . See under *Rectal valves, eponymic description of.*

Howell's bodies

. . . See under *Red blood cells, nuclear particles in.*

Huguier's canal

. . . See under *Temporal bone, canal in, for chorda tympani nerve.*

Human ovum, fertilized, 7½ days old

JOHN ROCK, American gynecologist and obstetrician, 1890-   , with ARTHUR TREMAIN HERTIG, described a fertilized human ovum aged 7½ days. Recorded in 1942. Known as *Rock-Hertig* ovum.

Human ovum, fertilized, 13-14 days old

THOMAS HASTIE BRYCE, Scottish physician, 1862-1946, with JOHN HAMMOND TEACHER, demonstrated a human embryo aged 13 to 14

days. Recorded in 1908. Known as *Bryce-Teacher* ovum.

Humerus, excision of head of

CHARLES WHITE, English surgeon, 1728-1813, is credited with being the first to excise the head of the humerus, in 1769.

Hunger pain, introduction of term

BERKELEY G. A. MOYNIHAN, English surgeon, 1865-1936, is credited with introducing the expression *hunger pain,* in 1901, to describe the pain felt by patients with duodenal ulcer several hours after a meal.

Hunger pains are caused by cramplike contractions of stomach, demonstration that

WALTER BRADFORD CANNON, American physiologist, 1871-1945, demonstrated by means of x-rays that hunger pains are caused by cramplike contractions of the stomach. Reported in 1912.

Hunter's canal

. . . See under *Canal of Hunter.*

Hunter's glossitis

. . . See under *Glossitis in pernicious anemia.*

Huntington's chorea

. . . See under *Chorea, chronic hereditary, in adults; eponymic description of.*

Hunt's syndrome of facial paralysis, herpes, etc.

JAMES R. HUNT, American neurologist, 1874-1937, described a syndrome associated with disease of the geniculate ganglion of the seventh nerve, marked by herpes, earache, and, sometimes, facial paralysis. Published in 1907. Known as *Hunt's syndrome.*

Hurler's disease
. . . See under *Lipochrondrodystrophy.*

Huschke's valve
. . . See under *Lacrimal fold, eponymic description of.*

Hutchinson's disease
. . . See under *Serpiginous angioma, eponymic description of.*

Hutchinson's prurigo
. . . See under *Summer prurigo, eponymic description of.*

Hutchinson's teeth
. . . See under *Teeth, notched, seen in congenital syphilis.*

Hutchison's tumor
. . . See under *Adrenal gland sarcoma with skull metastases.*

Huxley's layer
. . . See under *Hair follicles, Huxley's layer of root sheath of.*

Hyaloid canal of eye, description of
JULES GERMAIN CLOQUET, French anatomist, 1790-1883, was the first to describe the central canal of the vitreous, known as the hyaloid canal. Reported *circa* 1821.

Hyaluronidase; spreading factor; Duran-Reynals' factor
. . . See under *Spreading factor.*

Hydatid cysts and tapeworms, relation between
KARL GEORG FRIEDRICH RUDOLF LEUCKART, German physician, 1823-1898, demonstrated the relation between hydatid cysts and small tapeworms, in the dog. Published 1863-76.

Hydatid disease, precipitin reaction test for
CHARLES AUGUSTE FLEIG, French physiologist, 1883-1912, with MARCEL LISBONNE, developed a precipitin reaction test for the diagnosis of hydatid disease. Recorded in 1907.

Hydatid of Morgagni, eponymic description of
GIOVANNI BATTISTA MORGAGNI, Italian anatomist and pathologist, 1682-1771, described the cystic remnant of the Müllerian duct which is attached, in the case of the male, to the head of the epididymis, or, in the case of the female, to the oviduct. Recorded between 1706 and 1717. The hydatid of the male is known also as *appendix testis.*

Hyde's disease
. . . See under *Prurigo nodularis,* etc.

Hydradenitis destruens suppurativa, first description of
JONATHAN HUTCHINSON, English surgeon, 1828-1913, gave the first description of hydradenitis destruens suppurativa (hidradenitis suppurativa), later known as *Pollitzer's disease.* Recorded in 1879.

Hydroa, original description of
. . . See under *Dermatitis herpetiformis.*

Hydrocele, cervical, eponymic description of
JEAN PIERRE MAUNOIR, Swiss surgeon, 1768-1861, described a con-

genital lymphatic cyst of the neck, in 1825. Known as *cervical hydrocele* and *Maunoir's hydrocele*.

Hydrocele, early description of

PERCIVALL POTT, English surgeon, 1714-1788, gave a classic description of hydrocele or "watery rupture." Published in 1762.

**Hydrocele, operation for, by
    complete eversion of
    tunica vaginalis**

EDWARD WYLLYS ANDREWS, Chicago surgeon, 1856-1927, devised an operation for the radical cure of hydrocele by complete eversion of the tunica vaginalis. It is known as the *bottle operation,* and was reported in 1907.

**Hydrocephalus, acute, first
    description of**

JOHN CHEYNE, Scottish physician, 1777-1836, is believed to have been the first to describe acute hydrocephalus. Recorded *circa* 1808.

**Hydrocephalus, experimental,
    production of**

WALTER E. DANDY, Baltimore neurosurgeon, 1886-1946, produced hydrocephalus experimentally, in 1913.

**Hydrocephalus, surgical
    treatment of**

WALTER EDWARD DANDY, Baltimore neurosurgeon, 1886-1946, treated communicating hydrocephalus by extirpation of the choroid plexus of the lateral ventricles. Published in 1918.

**Hydrochloric acid in gastric
    juice, discovery of**

WILLIAM PROUT, English physiologist, 1785-1850, discovered the presence of hydrochloric acid in the gastric juice, in 1824.

**Hydrochloric acid in gastric juice,
    test for**

GUSTAV TÖPFER, German physician, 1858-1918, devised a test for hydrochloric acid in gastric juice. Recorded in 1894.

**Hydrogen ion concentration,
    symbol of**

. . . See under *pH.*

Hydrogen, isolation of

HENRY CAVENDISH, English scientist, 1731-1810, isolated hydrogen in 1766. Published in 1784.

Hydrogen peroxide, discovery of

LOUIS JACQUES THÉNARD, French chemist, 1777-1857, is credited with discovering hydrogen peroxide, in 1818.

**Hydrometer scale for determin-
    ing specific gravity**

ANTOINE BAUMÉ, French chemist, 1728-1805, devised a hydrometer scale for determining the specific gravity of liquids. Reported in 1769.

Hydronephrosis, early description and naming of

PIERRE FRANÇOIS OLIVE RAYER, French dermatologist, 1793-1867, is credited with describing and naming hydronephrosis, *circa* 1839.

**Hydronephrosis, surgical
    treatment of**

FRIEDRICH TRENDELENBURG, German surgeon, 1844-1924, was the first to use surgical measures for the relief of hydronephrosis. Recorded in 1890. Operation performed in 1886.

Hydronephrosis, surgical treatment of; first successful

ERNST GEORG FERDINAND VON KÜSTER, German surgeon, 1839-1930, is credited with the first successful surgical treatment of hydronephrosis. Published in 1892.

Hydrophobia, presence of virus in nerve tissue and the blood in

LOUIS PASTEUR, French scientist and bacteriologist, 1822-1895, with C. CHAMBERLAND and P. P. E. ROUX, demonstrated the presence of rabies virus in the blood and nerve tissue of rabid animals. Recorded in 1884.

Hydrophobia, presence of virus in saliva in

GEORG GOTTFRIED ZINKE, German physician, 1771-1849, successfully transmitted rabies from a rabid dog to a healthy dog by injection of saliva, thus demonstrating the presence of virus in the saliva. Recorded in 1804.

Hydrophobia, use of attenuated vaccine in prophylaxis against

LOUIS PASTEUR, French scientist and bacteriologist, 1822-1895, was the first to use attenuated vaccine as a prophylactic against rabies, in 1885.

Hydropic degeneration of island of Langerhans

. . . See under *Islands of Langerhans,* etc.

Hygiene, early modern work on

ANDREW BOORDE, English physician, 149?-15??, wrote the earliest of the modern works on hygiene. Published in 1547.

Hygiene in jails, early advocate of

STEPHEN HALES, English clergyman and physiologist, 1677-1761, invented a ventilator for use in jails, mines, etc., thus contributing greatly to the improvement of hygienic conditions in jails. Recorded in 1743.

Hygiene in schools, early advocate of

HERMANN L. COHN, German ophthalmologist, 1838-1906, was an early advocate of systematized hygiene in schools. In 1883 he proposed regular eye examinations for schoolchildren. The plan was put into practice in 1885.

Hygiene, personal, early work on

LUIGI CORNARO, Italian physician, 1467-1566, wrote one of the earliest works on personal hygiene. Published in 1558.

Hygiene, public, first extensive work on

JOHANN PETER FRANK, German physician, 1745-1821, "Father of Public Hygiene," wrote the first extensive systematic work on public hygiene. Published in nine volumes between 1779 and 1827.

Hyoscine, early investigation of

HORATIO CHARLES WOOD, Philadelphia physician, 1841-1920, was probably the first to discover the pharmacologic properties of hyoscine. Published in 1885.

Hyoscine, isolation of

ALBERT LADENBURG, German chemist, 1842-1911, is credited with being first to isolate hyoscine or scopolamine. Recorded in 1881.

Hyoscyamine in eye examination

. . . See under *Atropine and hyoscyamine in eye examination.*

Hyperalgesia of skin in visceral disease

HENRY HEAD, English physician, 1861-1940, described areas of hyperalgesia of the skin associated with disease of internal organs. Published in 1893. Known as *Head's areas.*

Hyperchlorhydria, eponymic description of

MICHAEL JOSEPH ROSSBACH, German physician, 1842-1894, described a form of nervous dyspepsia marked by hyperchlorhydria. Recorded in 1884. Known as *Rossbach's disease.*

Hyperchlorhydria, mucous spirals in

. . . See under *Spiral mucous bodies in gastric secretion in hyperchlorhydria.*

Hyperemesis gravidarum, early description of

PAUL DU BOIS, French obstetrician, 1795-1871, described pernicious vomiting of pregnancy. Published in 1852.

Hyperemia in treatment of inflammation

AUGUST K. G. BIER, German surgeon, 1861-1949, described a method for treating inflammation by the use of active and passive hyperemia. First reported in 1892.

Hyperemia, introduction of term

GABRIEL ANDRAL, French physician, 1797-1876, is credited with the introduction of the term *hyperemia,* about 1827.

Hypermetropia, definition of

. . . See under *Hyperopia, description and definition of.*

Hypernephroma, early investigation of

PAUL ALBERT GRAWITZ, German pathologist, 1850-1932, did original work on hypernephroma, a tumor whose structure resembles that of the adrenal gland cortex. Recorded in 1884. Known as *Grawitz's tumor.*

Hypernephroma, introduction of term

OTTO LUBARSCH, German pathologist, 1860-1933, is credited with introducing the term *hypernephroma,* in 1894.

Hyperopia, description and definition of

FRANS C. DONDERS, Dutch physician, 1818-1889, defined the condition of hyperopia (hypermetropia), in 1864.

Hypersensitiveness, local, production of

CARL W. PRAUSNITZ (also known as CARL P. GILES), German bacteriologist, 1876-19??, with HEINZ KÜSTNER (German gynecologist, 1897-   ), demonstrated the transferability of local hypersensitivity by the intradermal injection of serum of an allergic person into a normal person. Reported in 1921. Known as the *Prausnitz-Küstner reaction.*

Hypertelorism; craniofacial dysostosis; description of—1912

OCTAVE CROUZON, French neurologist, 1874-1938, described craniofacial dysostosis or hypertelorism, in 1912. Known as *Crouzon's disease.*

Hypertelorism; craniofacial dysostosis; description of—1924

DAVID M. GREIG, Scottish physician, 1864-1936, described craniofacial dysostosis or hyertelorism, in 1924. Called *Greig's hypertelorism* and *ocular hypertelorism.*

Hypertension, experimental, early work on

HARRY GOLDBLATT, American pathologist, 1891- , in collaboration with J. Lynch, R. F. Hanzal, and W. W. Summerville, produced experimental hypertension in dogs by constricting the renal arteries. First report published in 1934.

Hypertension, resection of splanchnic nerves for

MAX MINOR PEET, American neurosurgeon, 1885-1949, excised the greater and lesser splanchnic nerves and the lower thoracic ganglia for the relief of hypertension. Preliminary report published in 1935.

Hypertension, rice diet in treatment of

WALTER KEMPNER, American physician, 1903- , introduced a rice diet for the treatment of hypertension and kidney disease. Recorded in 1944.

Hypertension, salt-free diet in treatment of

. . . See under *Salt-free diet,* etc.

Hypertension, sympathectomy in treatment of

. . . See under *Sympathectomy.*

Hypertension, thiocyanates in treatment of

GUSTAV TREUPEL, German physician, 1867-1926, with A. EDINGER, introduced thiocyanates in the treatment of hypertension. Recorded in 1900.

Hyperthyroidism, acetonitril test for

. . . See under *Acetonitril.*

Hyperthyroidism, experimental production of

. . . See under *Exophthalmic goiter produced experimentally.*

Hyperthyroidism, test for, by injection of epinephrine

. . . See under *Epinephrine hypersensitiveness test in hyperthyroidism.*

Hyperthyroidism

. . . See also under *Exophthalmic goiter.*

Hypertrophic pulmonary osteoarthropathy, first description of

EUGEN BAMBERGER, Austrian physician, 1822-1888, described hypertrophic pulmonary osteoarthropathy in 1889. The condition was described in 1890 by PIERRE MARIE, the French neurologist. Known as *Marie-Bamberger disease.*

Hypertrophy and dilatation of heart, distinction between

JEAN N. CORVISART DES MARETS, French physician, 1755-1821, distinguished between hypertrophy and dilatation of the heart, in 1806.

Hyperventilation syndrome, early description of

CHARLES KORAN MAYTUM, American physician, 1895-　　, described a case of tetany resulting from fuctional dyspnea with hyperventilation. Published in 1933.

Hypnotism, first recorded experiment in

ATHANASIUS KIRCHER, German scholar and mathematician, 1602-1680, is credited with the first recorded experiment in hypnotism. Published in 1680.

Hypnotism, introduction of term

JAMES BRAID, Scottish physician, 1795-1860, coined the word *hypnotism.* Reported in 1843.

Hypnotism, practical application of, in treating neuroses

HIPPOLYTE BERNHEIM, French physician, 1840-1919, was the first to apply hypnotism to the treatment of neuroses. Recorded in 1884. He wrote a book on hypnotic suggestion, in 1891.

Hypochondria due to moisture in air

GEORGE CHEYNE, English physician, 1671-1743, believed that hypochondria is due to excess moisture in the air and to variability of the weather. Recorded in 1733.

Hypodermic injection in treatment of disease

ALEXANDER WOOD, Scottish physician, 1817-1884, is credited with being one of the first to use hypodermic injection in the treatment of disease, in 1853. Published in 1855.

Hypodermic injection in treatment of neuralgia, first use of

FRANCIS RYND, Irish physician,

1801-1861, was the first to devise a crude form of hypodermic needle and associated apparatus for injection of medicinal fluid in treatment of neuralgia. Recorded in 1845.

Hypodermic syringe, metal, invention of

CHARLES GABRIEL PRAVAZ, French physician, 1791-1853, is credited with inventing the first practical metal syringe provided with a hollow needle. He used it primarily to inject aneurysms. Recorded in 1853.

Hypoglossal nerves, occasional anastomosis between

JOSEPH HYRTL, Hungarian anatomist, 1810-1894, discovered an occasionally occurring anastomosis between the right and left hypoglossal nerves in the geniohyoid muscle. Recorded in 1842. Known as *Hyrtl's loop.*

Hypohemia intertropicalis or oppilação is due to ancylostomiasis

OTTO EDUARD HEINRICH WUCHERER, German physician, 1820-1873, recognized that the Brazilian disease known as oppilação or hypohemia intertropicalis was due to ancylostomiasis. Published in 1866.

Hypophysectomy causes atrophy of sex organs

SAMUEL JAMES CROWE, American physician, 1883-19??, with HARVEY CUSHING and JOHN HOMANS, demonstrated that excision of the pituitary gland results in atrophy of the genital organs. Published in 1910.

Hypophysectomy, first successful experimental

VICTOR ALEXANDER HADEN HORS-

LEY, English surgeon, 1857-1916, performed the first successful experimental hypophysectomy in dogs. One animal survived six months. Published in 1886.

Hypophysial cachexia, eponymic description of

MORRIS SIMMONDS, German physician, 1855-1925, described a condition of hypopituitary cachexia marked by premature senility, due to atrophy of the pituitary body. Recorded in 1914. Known as *Simmonds' disease*.

Hypothalamus and pituitary, nerve pathways between

STEPHEN WALTER RANSON, Chicago neuroanatomist, 1880-1942, established the existence of nerve pathways between the hypothalamus and the pituitary. Recorded in 1935, with H. KABAT and H. W. MAGOUN.

Hypothalamus, first experimental work on

JOHANN PAUL KARPLUS, Austrian physiologist, 1866-1936, with ALOIS KREIDL (Austrian physiologist, 1864-1928), recorded the first experimental work on the hypothalamus, in 1909.

Hypothalamus, functional significance of, early recognition

BYRON BRAMWELL, English physician, 1847-1931, recognized and described the functional part played by the hypothalamus, in 1888.

Hyrtl's loop

... See under *Hypoglossal nerves, occasional anastomosis between.*

Hysterectomy, abdominal, early successful

WILHELM ALEXANDER FREUND,

German surgeon, 1833-1918, devised an operation of abdominal hysterectomy, which he performed successfully in a case of cancer. Published in 1878.

Hysterectomy, abdominal, first successful

WALTER BURNHAM, American surgeon, 1808-1883, is credited with being the first to perform a successful hysterectomy by the abdominal route, on May 25, 1853.

Hysterectomy, vaginal, early successful

VINCENT CZERNY, German surgeon, 1842-1916, is believed to have been the first to perform a total hysterectomy by the vaginal route. Recorded in 1879.

Hysteria, early description of

THOMAS WILLIS, English physician and anatomist, 1621-1675, gave a classic description of hysteria. Recorded in 1671.

Hysterical chorea, early description of

ETIENNE JULES BERGERON, French physician, 1817-1900, described hysterical chorea. His pupil R. BERLAND named the condition *Bergeron's disease*, in a paper published in 1880.

Hysteromyomectomy, first successful

... See under *Uterine fibromyoma, first excision of.*

Hysterosalpingography, manometer used in

... See under *Instrument for measuring pressure during injection of radiopaque material*, etc.

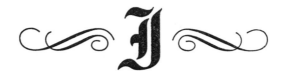

Ice bag for application to the spine

JOHN CHAPMAN, English physician, 1821-1894, devised an elongated ice bag suitable for application to the spine. Introduced *circa* 1865.

Ichthyol, introduction of, in dermatology

PAUL GERSON UNNA, German dermatologist, 1850-1929, was first to use ichthyol in treating skin disorders. Recorded in 1886.

Ichthyosis hystrix, original description of

JOHN MACHIN, English physician, 16??-1751, was the first to describe ichthyosis hystrix, a form of ichthyosis with "dry and warty knobs." Recorded in 1733.

Id, ego, and superego, introduction of concepts of

SIGMUND FREUD, Austrian psychiatrist, 1856-1939, introduced the hypothetical division of the mind into the *id, ego,* and *superego.* Recorded *circa* 1905.

Identification of persons by measuring selected parts of body

ALPHONSE BERTILLON, French criminologist, 1853-1914, devised a method of identifying persons by compiling measurements of selected parts of the body. Introduced in 1886. Known as the Bertillon system, now superseded by the fingerprint method.

Idiopathic steatorrhea

. . . See under *Sprue, nontropical.*

Idiots, early classification of —1866

JOHN L. H. DOWN, London physician, 1828-1896, presented observations on an ethnic classification of idiots, in 1866.

Ignipuncture in treating detachment of retina

. . . See under *Retina, detachment of,* etc.

Ileitis, regional, first description of

BURRILL B. CROHN, American physician, 1884-   , with LEON GINZBURG and G. D. OPPENHEIMER, described regional ileitis as a clinical and pathologic entity, in 1932. Known as *Crohn's disease.*

Ileocecal fold, bloodless; fold of Treves

FREDERICK TREVES, English surgeon, 1853-1923, described a relatively bloodless ileocecal fold of peritoneum associated with the appendix. Recorded in 1885. Known as *bloodless fold of Treves.*

Ileocecal valve, early description of—1588

GASPARD BAUHIN, Swiss anatomist, 1560-1624, gave a good account of the ileocecal valve. Recorded in 1588.

Ileocecal valve, early description of—1652

NICHOLAS TULP, Dutch physician and anatomist, 1593-1674, described the ileocecal valve, *circa* 1640. Published in 1652.

Ileum, congenital atresia of, first recorded cases of

JAMES CALDER, Scottish surgeon, 170?-17??, gave the first description of two infants born with congenital atresia of the ileum. Published in 1733.

Ileum, diverticulum of

. . . See under *Diverticulum of ileum derived from persistent yolk stalk.*

Ileum, kink in terminal part of

WILLIAM ARBUTHNOT LANE, Scottish surgeon in England, 1856-1943, described an inconstant band of fibers or a membrane in the small intestine which helps to support the full secum. The kinking of this band may cause an obstruction in the last part of the ileum, known as *Lane's kink.* The condition was first observed by Lane in 1903; published in 1910. The band is known as *Lane's band.*

Iliac and femoral arteries, ligation of, for aneurysm

. . . See under *Aneurysm, ligation of iliac and femoral arteries in.*

Iliacosubfascial fossa, description of

ALFRED VON BIESIADECKI, Polish physician, 1839-1888, described a fossa beneath the iliac fascia, in 1878. Known as *Biesiadecki's fossa.*

Illuminating gas, poisonous effect of, is due to affinity for hemoglobin

YANDELL HENDERSON, American physiologist, 1873-1944, demonstrated that the poisonous effect of illuminating gas is due to the affinity of its carbon monoxide for hemoglobin. Reported in 1916.

Images, three pairs of, seen in pupil

. . . See under *Pupil, three sets of images seen in.*

Immunity, antibacterial, mechanism involved in

ELIE METCHNIKOFF, Russian physiologist in France, 1845-1916, reported a classical study of the mechanism involved in specific antibacterial immunity, in 1901. He received the Nobel prize in 1908.

Immunity may be produced by injection of dead organisms

DANIEL ELMER SALMON, American pathologist, 1850-1914, demonstrated that immunity may be secured by the use of dead virus or filtered products of specific microorganisms. Recorded in 1886.

Immunity, Pasteur's theory of

LOUIS PASTEUR, French scientist and bacteriologist, 1822-1895, explained immunity following an attack of a disease by the assumption that a certain material needed for the growth of the organism is exhausted by the disease. Recorded in 1880.

Immunity, side-chain theory of

. . . See under *Side-chain theory of immunity.*

Immunochemistry and structure of proteins

LINUS CARL PAULING, American chemist, 1901- , did basic research in immunochemistry, the structure of crystals, proteins, etc., and the nature of chemical bonds. Received Nobel prize in 1954.

Impetigo circumpilaris infantilis, first description of

MAX BOCKHART, German physician, 184?-19??, was the first to describe impetigo circumpilaris infantilis, in 1887. Known as *Bockhart's impetigo.*

Impetigo contagiosa, original description of

WILLIAM TILBURY FOX, English dermatologist, 1836-1879, gave the original description of impetigo contagiosa. Recorded in 1864.

Impetigo herpetiformis, early description of — 1872

FERDINAND VON HEBRA, Austrian dermatologist, 1816-1880, described impetigo herpetiformis, in 1872.

Impetigo herpetiformis, early description of — 1887

MORITZ KAPOSI, Hungarian derm-

atologist, 1837-1902, described impetigo herpetiformis, a condition affecting most frequently pregnant women and marked by the appearance of groups of pustules. Reported in 1887.

Impotence, treatment of, by occlusion of vas deferens

EUGEN STEINACH, Austrian surgeon, 1861-1944, devised an operation for the treatment of impotence in which the ductus deferens is occluded. Published in 1920. Known as *Steinach's operation* or *method.*

Impregnation after destruction of spinal cord

FRIEDRICH LEOPOLD GOLTZ, German physiologist, 1834-1902, with ERNST JULIUS RICHARD EWALD (German physiologist, 1855-1921), demonstrated that it was possible to impregnate a dog after its spinal cord had been severed. Recorded in 1896.

Incisive bone

. . . See under *Intermaxillary bone.*

Incisor teeth with grooves

WILLIAM EDMONDS HORNER, American anatomist, 1793-1853, described incisor teeth marked by grooves, due to deficiency of enamel. Recorded in 1829. Known as *Horner's teeth.*

Incisura tympanica

. . . See under *Tympanic sulcus, notch at upper border of.*

Incubator for prematurely born infants

ÉTIENNE STÉPHANE TARNIER, French obstetrician, 1828-1897, devised an incubator for the care of prematurely born infants. It was warmed by a kerosene flame and used at the Paris *La Maternité* in 1884.

Incubator for prematurely born infants

KARL SIEGMUND FRANZ CREDÉ, German gynecologist, 1819-1892, devised an incubator for the care of prematurely born infants, in 1888. Known as *Credé's incubator.*

Incus, discovery of

ALESSANDRO ACHILLINI, Italian anatomist, 1463-1512, is credited with being the discoverer of the incus of the middle ear. Exact date not available.

Indefatigability of nerve tissue

HENRY PICKERING BOWDITCH, American physiologist, 1840-1911, demonstrated that mammalian nerve tissue cannot be exhausted by continued stimulation. Published in 1890. Known as *Bowditch's law.* The indefatigability of nerve was demonstrated earlier, in 1884, by NIKOLAI IGOREVICH WEDENSKY.

Index Medicus, monthly, founding of

The monthly *Index Medicus* was founded by JOHN SHAW BILLINGS, American Army medical officer and librarian, 1838-1913, and ROBERT FLETCHER, American surgeon and bibliographer, 1823-1912. First volume appeared in 1879.

Index of malignancy, definition of

ALBERT C. BRODERS, American pathologist, 1885-19??, proposed an index of malignancy based on the finding that the more undifferentiated or embryonic the cells of a tumor are, the more malignant is the tumor. Reported *circa* 1920.

Index-Catalogue of the Library of the Surgeon General

The compilation of the *Index-Catalogue* of the Library of the Surgeon General was begun in 1880, under the direction of JOHN SHAW BILLINGS, American Army medical officer and librarian, 1838-1913.

India ink in microscopical examination

ROBERT BURRI, Swiss bacteriologist, 1867-19??, introduced the use of India ink for staining specimens to be examined microscopically. Reported in 1909. Known as *Burri's method.*

Indican, isolation of, from urine

MAX JAFFE, German biochemist, 1841-1911, is credited with isolating indican from the urine, in 1877.

Indole formation, peptone solution used in test for

. . . See under *Solution of peptone and sodium chloride,* etc.

Induction coil, Ruhmkorff's

HEINRICH DANIEL RUHMKORFF, German instrument maker in Paris, 1803-1877, constructed an effective induction coil having a hammer-type circuit breaker and a secondary coil made of a long, thin wire, in 1851.

Infantile acrodynia

. . . See under *Erythredema polyneuropathy.*

Infantile splenomegaly

. . . See under *Splenic anemia of infants.*

Infantilism of Lorain type

PAUL JOSEPH LORAIN, French physician, 1827-1875, described the persistence of infantile traits in adolescent and adult life, marked by physical, sexual, and mental underdevelopment. Published in a letter serving as a preface to a thesis by FANEAU DE LA COUR, in 1871. Known as *Lorain syndrome.*

Infantilism, thyroid or dysthyroidal

EDOUARD BRISSAUD, French physician, 1852-1909, described the condition known as thyroid or dysthyroidal infantilism. Published in 1907.

Infants, caloric requirements of, early determination of

OTTO J. L. HEUBNER, German pediatrician, 1843-1926, with MAX RUBNER (German physiologist, 1854-1932), determined the caloric requirements of infants and introduced caloric feeding. Published in 1897.

Infectious jaundice, discovery of causative agent of

. . . See under *Leptospira icterohaemorrhagiae.*

Infectious mononucleosis, early description of — 1885

NIL F. FILATOV, Russian pediatrician, 1846-1902, described infectious mononucleosis in 1885. He called it idiopathic adenitis. Known as *Filatov's disease.*

Infectious mononucleosis, early description of — 1889

EMIL PFEIFFER, German physician, 1846-1921, described infectious mononucleosis in 1889. He called it "drüsenfieber" or glandular fever.

Infectious mononucleosis, introduction of term

THOMAS PECK SPRUNT, Baltimore physician, 1884-   , is credited with introducing the term *infectious mononucleosis.* Recorded in 1920.

Infectious mononucleosis, Paul-Bunnell test for

JOHN RODMAN PAUL, American physician, 1893-   , with WALLS WILLARD BUNNELL, developed a test for infectious mononucleosis, based on the presence in the patient's blood of antibodies for the red blood cells of sheep. Recorded in 1932.

Inferior horns of lateral ventricles of brain, good description of

JULIUS CAESAR ARANTIUS, Italian physician, 1530-1589, gave the first clear description of the inferior horns of the lateral ventricles of the brain. Probable date 1571.

Inferior temporal sulcus of cerebral hempisphere

SHOBAL V. CLEVENGER, American neurologist, 1843-1920, gave the first description of the inferior temporal sulcus of the cerebral hemisphere. Recorded *circa* 1880.

Infiltration anesthesia, development of

CARL LUDWIG SCHLEICH, German surgeon, 1859-1922, is credited with developing infiltration anesthesia which was introduced by HALSTED. Reported in 1894 and 1895.

Inflammation, accumulation of leukocytes in

JULIUS FRIEDRICH COHNHEIM, German pathologist, 1839-1884, promulgated the theory that inflammation is accompanied by an accumulation of leukocytes which pass through the capillary walls. Published in 1867.

Inflammation, Metchnikoff's theory of

ELIE METCHNIKOFF, Russian physiologist in France, 1845-1916, presented a classic description of the mechanism involved in inflammation; published in 1892.

Influenza B virus, isolation of

THOMAS FRANCIS, American immunologist, 1900-   , isolated the influenza B virus. Recorded in 1940.

Influenza bacillus, discovery of

RICHARD FRIEDRICH JOHANNES PFEIFFER, German bacteriologist 1858-19??, discovered the influenza bacillus, *Hemophilus influenzae*, in 1892. He believed it to be the causative agent of influenza. Known as *Pfeiffer's bacillus*.

Influenza C virus, isolation of

RICHARD MORELAND TAYLOR, American immunologist, 1887-19??, isolated influenza C virus. Published in 1949.

Influenza, popularization of term, in English

JOHN PRINGLE, Scottish physician, 1707-1782, is credited with making the term *influenza* popular in the English language. He did not, however, originate the word.

Influenza, transmission of, from animal to man

WILSON SMITH, English physician, 1897-   , with CHARLES HERBERT STUART-HARRIS, successfully transferred influenza from an animal (ferret) to man. Published in 1936.

Influenza, transmission of, from man to animal

. . . See under *Influenza, virus from patients affected with.*

Influenza virus, cultivation of

FRANK MACFARLANE BURNET, Australian physician, 1899-   , cultivated the virus of epidemic influenza on the developing egg. Published in 1935.

Influenza, virus from patients affected with

WILSON SMITH, English physician, 1897-   , with C. H. ANDREWES and P. P. LAIDLAW, successfully infected laboratory animals with material obtained from the throat of influenza patients. Recorded in 1933.

Infraclavicular fossa, eponymic description of

JOSEPH JACOB VON MOHRENHEIM, Austrian surgeon, 173?-1799, described the infraclavicular fossa bounded by the clavicle, pectoralis major, deltoid, and pectoralis minor. Reported *circa* 1755. Known as *Mohrenheim's fossa*.

Inguinal colostomy above inguinal ligament

HERBERT WILLIAM ALLINGHAM, English surgeon, 1862-1904, introduced an operation for the performance of inguinal colostomy one-half inch above the inguinal ligament. He pointed out its advantage over the lumbar operation, with special reference to prevention of the passage of feces below the artificial anus. Report published in 1887. Known as *Allingham's operation*.

Inguinal hernia, Bassini's operation for

EDOARDO BASSINI, Italian surgeon, 1844-1924, devised one of the early modern operations for inguinal hernia. It includes the excision of the sac and the suturing of the conjoined tendon to the inguinal ligament. Recorded in 1889.

Inguinal hernia, operation for, by imbrication or lap joint method

EDWARD WYLLYS ANDREWS, Chicago surgeon, 1856-1927, devised a plastic operation for the repair of inguinal hernia by the imbrication or lap joint method. Reported in 1895. Known as the *Andrews operation* and as the *Wyllys Andrews method*.

Inguinal hernia, repair of, by transplantation of rectus muscle

JOSEPH COLT BLOODGOOD, Baltimore surgeon, 1867-1935, devised an operation for the radical cure of inguinal hernia in which the rectus muscle is transplanted and the conjoined tendon is obliterated. Reported in 1918.

Inguinal ligament, early description of — 1543

ANDREAS VESALIUS, Belgian anatomist, 1514-1564, described the inguinal ligament in his work published in 1543. The structure is occasionally referred to as *Vesalius's ligament*.

Inguinal ligament, first good description of

GABRIEL FALLOPIUS, Italian anatomist, 1523-1562, gave the first adequate description of the inguinal ligament. Recorded in 1584.

Inguinal ligament, practical description of, with relation to hernia

FRANÇOIS POUPART, French surgeon, 1616-1708, described the inguinal ligament in its relation to hernia, thus giving it new significance. Known as *Poupart's ligament*. Published in 1695.

Inguinal ring, external, yellow fibers of

ALLEN THOMSON, Scottish anatomist, 1809-1884, described yellow fibers occurring occasionally in the inner half of the subcutaneous inguinal ring, *circa* 1850. Known as *Thomson's fascia*.

Inhalation device for administration of anesthetics by drop method

OSCAR HUNTINGTON ALLIS, American surgeon, 1836-1921, invented an inhalation device for the administration of anesthetics by the drop method. Reported in 1874.

Inheritance, law of filial regression in

FRANCIS GALTON, English geneticist, 1822-1911, propounded the law of filial regression in accordance with which offspring of parents with unusual characteristics tend to regress to the average for the group. Recorded in 1869.

Inheritance, Mendel's law of

GREGOR JOHANN MENDEL, Aus-GREGOR JOHANN MENDEL, Austrian monk and botanist, 1822-1884, discovered certain principles governing the inheritance of some characteristics. In accordance with are not intermediate between the parents in the quality of characteristics, but inherit fully from either one or the other. Recorded in 1866. Known as *Mendel's* or *Mendelian law*.

Inhibitory respiratory center

... See under *Pneumotaxic center, eponymic description of*.

Inion, introduction of, as craniometric point

PIERRE PAUL BROCA, French surgeon and anthropologist, 1824-1880, defined *inion* as a craniometric point. Exact date not available.

Ink blot intelligence test

HERMANN RORSCHACH, Swiss psychiatrist, 1884-1922, devised a test for intelligence and emotional elements of personality based on the interpretation of 10 ink blots. Published in 1921. Known as *Rorschach test*.

Innominate artery, early ligation of — 1818

VALENTINE MOTT, American surgeon, 1785-1865, recorded a case in which he ligated the innominate artery, in 1818.

Insane, abandonment of chains and fetters for

VINCENZO CHIARUGI, Italian physician, 1759-1820, is credited with being the first in Europe to abandon the use of chains and fetters in the treatment of the insane. His work, advocating various reforms, was published in 1793.

Insane, humane treatment of

... See under *No-restraint method of treating insane*.

Insane, treatment of, in France

JEAN E. D. ESQUIROL, French psychiatrist, 1772-1840, greatly influenced the treatment of the insane in France. He wrote the first modern textbook of psychiatry. Published in 1838.

Insanity, moral, introduction of concept of

JAMES COWLES PRICHARD, Scottish physician, 1786-1848, introduced the concept of moral insanity, in 1835.

Insanity, moralistic theory of

WILHELM GRIESINGER, German neurologist, 1817-1868, disposed of the moralistic theory of insanity, a theory proposed by JOHANN C. A. HEINROTH. His text on the pathology and treatment of mental disease appeared in 1845.

Insanity

... See also under name of particular form of disorder, as *Manic-depressive, Psychasthenia*, etc.

Instrument for collecting urine from each kidney separately — 1904

GEORGES LUYS, French urologist, 1870-19??, devised a segregator, an instrument with which to collect urine from each kidney separately. Reported in 1904. Known as *Luy's segregator*.

Instrument for detecting bullets in tissues

. . . See under *Bullets in tissues, instrument for detecting*.

Instrument for dilating cervix

. . . See under *Cervical dilator made of steel*.

Instrument for measuring alcohol in breath

. . . See under *Drunkometer, invention of*.

Instrument for measuring pressure during injection of radiopaque material into uterus

JULIUS JARCHO, American gynecologist and obstetrician, 1882- , invented a manometer to measure the pressure during injection of radiopaque material into the uterus in hysterosalpingography. The instrument is also used in pyelography and in testing the patency of the uterine tubes. Known as *Jarcho's pressometer*. Date not available.

Instrument for measuring velocity of blood in circulation

JAN DOGIEL, Russian physiologist, 1830-1905, invented an instrument for measuring the velocity of the blood flow in circulation, in 1867. Called *stromuhr*. In the same year, a similar instrument was invented independently by Karl Friedrich W. Ludwig, German physiologist, 1816-1895.

Instrument

. . . See also under name of particular instrument, as under *Manometer*.

Insula of cerebral hemisphere

JOHANN CHRISTIAN REIL, Dutch physiologist, 1759-1813, described a triangular area which forms the floor of the lateral cerebral fossa. Recorded in 1796. Known as *island of Reil*.

Insulin, crude form of; first isolation

GEORG LUDWIG ZUELZER, German physician, 1870-1949, isolated a pancreatic extract containing insulin. The extract had unpredictable reactions which led to its abandonment. Recorded in 1908.

Insulin, crystalline, first production of

JOHN JACOB ABEL, Baltimore pharmacologist and physiologist, 1857-1938, was the first to obtain insulin in crystalline form. Recorded in 1926.

Insulin, discovery of

FREDERICK GRANT BANTING (Canadian physician, 1891-1941), in association with CHARLES HERBERT BEST (Canadian physiologist, 1899-   ) and JOHN JAMES RICKARD MACLEOD (Scottish physiologist in America, 1876-1935), discovered insulin. Reported in 1922. Banting and Macleod received the Nobel prize in 1923.

Insulin, early improved form of

JAMES BERTRAM COLLIP, Canadian physician and biochemist, 1892- , was the first to improve the original crude insulin by isolating it in at least a semipure form. Recorded in 1923.

Insulin, introduction of term

JEAN DE MEYER, French physiologist, 1878- , is believed to have been the first to use the term *insuline, circa* 1909.

Insulin, protamine, introduction of

HANS CHRISTIAN HAGEDORN, Danish scientist, 1888- , with B. N. JENSEN, N. B. KRARUP, and I. WODSTRUP, introduced protamine insulin. Reported in 1936.

Insulin shock treatment of mental disorders

. . . See under *Schizophrenia, insulin shock treatment of.*

Insulin-producing cells of pancreas

. . . See under *Islands of Langerhans, discovery of.*

Insulin

lar form of insulin, as *Protamine-zinc insulin.*

Integrative action of nervous system

. . . See under *Nervous system, integrative action of.*

Intelligence quotient

. . . See under *Intelligence test, development of.*

Intelligence test, development of

ALFRED BINET, French psychologist, 1857-1911, and THEODORE SIMON, French psychologist, 1873-19??, developed an intelligence test in which the intellectual power of the subject is estimated by comparison with the intellectual power of normal subjects at various ages. The "mental age" thus derived is divided by the chronological age of the subject to give the *I.Q.* or intelligence quotient. Developed in 1905-1908. Published in 1911.

Intelligence test, nonverbal, for subjects with speech difficulty

ETHEL L. CORNELL, American psychologist, 1892- , and WARREN W. COXE, American psychologist, 1886- , devised a nonverbal intelligence test which is useful in testing subjects having language or speech difficulty. Known as *Cornell-Coxe Performance Ability Scale.* Exact date not available.

Interauricular septum, ganglionic cells in

KARL FRIEDRICH W. LUDWIG, German physiologist, 1816-1895, discovered the ganglionic cells of the interauricular septum, in the frog, in 1848.

Intercostal muscles, function of, in respiration

HENRY NEWELL MARTIN, American physiologist, 1848-1896, with EDWARD MUSSEY HARTWELL, established the function of the intercostal muscles in respiration. Published in 1879-80.

Intercostal nerves do not originate in cerebrum

FRANÇOIS POURFOIR DU PETIT, French physician, 1664-1741, disproved the prevalent belief that the intercostal nerves originate in the cerebrum. Published in 1727.

Intercostal nerves, early description of

THOMAS WILLIS, English physician and anatomist, 1621-1675, described the intercostal nerves. Published posthumously in 1684.

Intermaxillary bone, discovery of

JOHANN WOLFGANG VON GOETHE, German poet and anatomist, 1749-1832, described a bone in the middle front part of the upper jaw, separate in fetal life. Reported in 1786. Known as *Goethe's bone* and as *incisive bone*.

Intermediate disk of striated muscle

WILHELM KRAUSE, German anatomist, 1833-1910, described the so-called intermediate disk of striated muscle, *circa* 1860. Known as *Krause's membrane, Dobie's line,* etc.

Intermediolaterial cell column of spinal cord; Clarke's column

JACOB A. L. CLARKE, English physician, 1817-1880, discovered and described the intermediolateral column of cells of the spinal cord. It is situated in the posterior gray column, extending longitudinally from the 7th and 8th cervical masses to the level of the 2nd lumbar nerve. Reported in 1851. Known also as the *dorsal nucleus of Clarke*.

Intermenstrual pain or mittelschmerz, early description of

WILLIAM OVEREND PRIESTLEY, Scottish gynecologist, 1829-1901, described *mittelschmerz* or intermenstrual pain. Published in 1872.

Intermittent claudication, earliest report on

BENJAMIN C. BRODIE, English surgeon, 1783-1862, is believed to have been the first to describe intermittent claudication in man, in 1846.

Intermittent claudication, early description of — 1858

JEAN MARTIN CHARCOT, French neurologist, 1825-1893, gave one of the earliest accounts of intermittent claudication, in 1958.

Internal iliac artery, first successful ligation of

WILLIAM STEVENS, Scottish surgeon, 1786-1868, is credited with being the first to ligate the internal iliac artery successfully, Dec. 27, 1812. Recorded in 1814. The patient lived ten years after the operation.

Internal maxillary artery, early description of

GUIDO GUIDI, Italian physician and anatomist, 1500-1569, described the internal maxillary artery, *circa* 1559. Published in a posthumous work, in 1611. Known as the *Vidian artery*.

Internal secretion, early concept of

THÉOPHILE DE BORDEU, French physician, 1722-1776, recorded the earliest concept of internal secretion. He believed that every organ, tissue, and cell produces some substance which it discharges into the blood, thus affecting other parts and structures of the body. Published in 1775.

Internal secretion, first demonstration of

ARNOLD ADOLPH BERTHOLD, German physician, 1803-1861, was the first to demonstrate the existence of an internal secretion by transplanting cock's testes to another part of the fowl's body and thereby preventing atrophy of the comb. Recorded in 1849.

Internal secretion, hormonal control of

WILLIAM MADDOCK BAYLISS, English physician, 1860-1924, and ERNEST HENRY STARLING, English physiologist, 1866-1927, promulgated the theory of the hormonal control of internal secretion. Published in 1904.

Internal secretion, introduction of expression

CLAUDE BERNARD, French physiologist, 1813-1878, is credited with originating the expression "internal secretion" and with initiating the study of endocrinology. Recorded in 1855.

International Red Cross Society, founding of

. . . See under *Geneva Convention.*

Interoceptor, introduction of term

CHARLES SCOTT SHERRINGTON, English neurophysiologist, 1857-1952, introduced the term *interoceptor,* to describe a receptor of stimuli from the gastrointestinal tract. Published in 1906.

Interpeduncular fossa, eponymic description of

PIERRE TARIN, French anatomist, 1708-1761, described a depression on the underside of the mesencephalon, between the cerebral peduncles, *circa* 1740. Known as *Tarin's fossa.*

Interscapulothoracic amputation of arm

PAUL BERGER, French surgeon, 1845-1908, devised the interscapulothoracic or interthoracicoscapular operation for the amputation of the arm at the shoulder girdle. Recorded in 1883. Known as the *Berger amputation.*

Interstitial pregnancy

. . . See under *Pregnancy, interstitial,* etc.

Interventricular foramen of human brain

ALEXANDER MONRO, *secundus,* Scottish anatomist, 1733-1817, described the interventricular foramen of the human brain, the opening between the lateral and third ventricles, in 1783. Known as *foramen of Monro.* It is said that Monro made the discovery in 1753, at the age of 20.

Intervertebral disk injury as cause of "sciatica"

JOEL ERNEST GOLDTHWAIT, American physician, 1866-19??, suggested that intervertebral disk injury may be the cause of "sciatica," "lumbago," "paraplegia," etc. Reported in 1911.

Intervertebral disk injury as cause of "sciatica," demonstration of

GEORGE STEVENSON MIDDLETON, Scottish physician, 1853-1928, reported a case of injury of the spinal cord and symptoms of "sciatica" due to rupture of an intervertebral disk during muscular effort. Published in 1911.

Intestinal anastomosis,
  catgut ring in
. . . See under *Catgut ring*.

Intestinal bacterial flora,
  discovery of
JOSEPH LEIDY, American physician, 1823-1891, is said to have discovered the bacterial flora of the intestine. Published in 1849.

Intestinal distention, apparatus
  for decompression of
OWEN HARDING WANGENSTEEN, American surgeon, 1898- , devised an apparatus for the relief of distention in cases of intestinal obstruction by suction siphonage through a nasal catheter. Recorded in 1932. Known as *Wangensteen's tube* or *apparatus*.

Intestinal drainage tube with
  double channel
THOMAS GRIER MILLER, American physician, 1886-19??, with WILLIAM OSLER ABBOTT, American physician, 1902-1943, devised a double-lumen intestinal drainage tube, used mainly for relief of distention. Recorded in 1934. Known as the *Miller-Abbott tube*.

Intestinal glands, early
  description of — 1731
DOMENICO M. G. GALEAZZI, Italian physician, 1686-1775, described the simple tubular depressions in the mucosa of the small intestine, in 1731. Known as *Galeati's glands* and as *Lieberkühn's glands*.

Intestinal glands, early
  description of — 1745
JOHANN N. LIEBERKÜHN, German anatomist, 1711-1756, described

the simple tubular depressions in the mucosa of the small intestine, in 1745. Known as *Lieberkühn's glands* and as *Galeati's glands*.

Intestinal lymphatics,
  discovery of
OLOF RUDBECK, Swedish anatomist, 1630-1702, is credited with discovering the lymphatic system of the intestine and its connection with the thoracic duct, in 1651. Recorded in 1653.

Intestinal lymphatics,
  discovery of
THOMAS BARTHOLIN, Danish anatomist, 1616-1680, discovered the intestinal lymphatics and claimed to have anticipated Rudbeck. He was probably the first to recognize the significance of the lymphatics, whether or not he was the original discoverer. Recorded in 1653.

Intestinal lipodystrophy,
  introduction of term
GEORGE HOYT WHIPPLE, American pathologist, 1878-19??, described intestinal lipodystrophy and introduced the term, in 1907.

Intestinal obstruction, lumbar
  colostomy for relief of
. . . See under *Lumbar colostomy*.

Intestinal resection for cancer,
  first recorded
JEAN FRANÇOIS REYBARD, French surgeon, 1790-1863, performed the first recorded intestinal resection for cancer. Published in 1844.

Intestinal worms and their
  eradication, early book on
ALEXANDER OF TRALLES, Byzantine physician and author, 525-605,

was the author of a master work titled *The Art of Medicine,* consisting of twelve volumes. He was also the author of an original work on intestinal worms and methods for their eradication. The exact date of this is not available. Some observers consider him the first parasitologist.

Intestine, autonomic nerve fibers between muscular coats of

... See under *Auerbach's plexus.*

Intenstine, small, circular folds in; eponymic description of

THEODOR KERCKRING, German anatomist in Holland, 1640-1693, described the transverse mucous folds of the small intestine. Recorded in 1670. Known as *valvulae conniventes* (closing valves) and *Kerckring's folds* or *valves.*

Intestine

... See also under *Intestinal,* and under name of particular part of the intestine, as *Duodenal, Duodenum,* etc.

Intoximeter, invention of

... See under *Drunkometer, invention of.*

Intracerebral protection test

... See under *Yellow fever, mouse test for.*

Intracranial hemorrhage in newborn, operation for

HARVEY W. CUSHING, Boston surgeon, 1869-1939, performed the first successful operation for intracranial hemorrhage in the newborn, in 1905.

Intracranial pressure, increased, pain reflex in

FERDINAND ADALBERT KEHRER,

German neurologist, 1883-19??, described an auriculopalpebral reflex consisting of closure of the eyelids in response to certain stimuli when the intracranial pressure is increased. Known as *Kehrer's reflex* and *Kisch's reflex.* Exact date not available.

Intracranial pressure, lowering of, with hypertonic solutions

LEWIS HILL WEED, American anatomist, 1886-1952, introduced the use of hypertonic salt solution, by ingestion or by injection, for the relief of high intracranial pressure. Published in 1919.

Intraocular endometrial transplants in study of menstruation

... See under *Menstruation, study of,* etc.

Intratracheal insufflation, method of anesthesia by

... See under *Anesthesia by intratracheal insufflation.*

Intravenous injection in man, first recorded successful

JOHANN DANIEL MAJOR, German physician, 1634-1693, is credited with being the first to inject a medicinal substance successfully into the vein of a human being. Recorded in 1662.

Intravenous urography, introduction of

MOSES SWICK, German-American urologist, 1900-   , is credited with the introduction of intravenous urography. Published in 1929.

Intravital staining, Ehrlich's method of

PAUL EHRLICH, German bacteriologist and pathologist, 1854-1915, introduced a method of intravital staining using methylene blue. Published in 1886.

Intravital staining of bones by food

JOHN BELCHIER, English surgeon, 1706-1785, succeeded in staining the bones of living fowls by feeding them madder-soaked bran. This method constituted an early form of vital staining and aided in the study of osteogenesis. Published in 1738.

Introvert, introduction of term, in psychiatric sense

CARL GUSTAV JUNG, Swiss psychiatrist, 1875-19??, introduced the term *introvert* into psychiatric terminology. Jung classified all persons as either introverts or extroverts. Reported *circa* 1900.

Intubation, laryngeal, in croup

JOSEPH P. O'DWYER, American otolaryngologist, 1841-1898, devised the first satisfactory metal tube and method for laryngeal intubation in croup. Recorded in 1885. Known as *O'Dwyer tube*.

Intuitional-type personality, introduction of concept of

CARL GUSTAV JUNG, Swiss psychiatrist, 1875-19??, introduced the concept of an intuitional-type personality in which actions and attitudes are directed by unconscious or vaguely conscious stimuli, i.e., by "intuition." Presented *circa* 1908.

Intussusception, first successful operation for, in adult

CORNELIUS HENRIK VELSE, Dutch surgeon, 1704-17??, is said to have performed the first successful operation for intussusception in an adult. Recorded in 1742.

Intussusception, first successful operation for, in infant

JONATHAN HUTCHINSON, English surgeon, 1828-1913, is credited with performing the first successful operation for intussusception in an infant, in 1871.

Inulin clearance test for kidney function

ALF SVEN ALVING, American physician, 1902-   , with BENJAMIN F. MILLER, introduced the inulin clearance test as a criterion of kidney function. Recorded in 1940.

Iodine, discovery and isolation of

BERNARD COURTOIS, French chemist, 1777-1838, discovered iodine and isolated it from seaweed, in 1812.

Iodine in exophthalmic goiter

. . . See under *Exophthalmic goiter*.

Iodine in thyroid gland, presence of

EUGEN BAUMANN, German physician and biochemist, 1846-1896, proved the presence of iodine in the thyroid, in chemical combination. Reported in 1895.

Iodine in treatment of goiter — 1819

JOHN ELLIOTSON, English surgeon, 1786-1868, used iodine in the treatment of goiter at St. Thomas's Hospital, in 1819.

Iodine in treatment of goiter, early suggestion of

WILLIAM PROUT, English chemist,

1785-1850, stated that he had recommended the use of iodine in the treatment of goiter to JOHN ELLIOTSON, who used it in 1819.

Iodine, internally, in thyroid disorders, first use of

JEAN FRANÇOIS COINDET, French physician, 1774-1834, is believed to have been the first to use iodine internally in the treatment of thyroid disorders. Reported in 1820.

Iodized oil for x-ray visualization, introduction of

CARLOS HEUSER, Argentine surgeon, 1879-1934, is credited with introducing iodized oil as an x-ray contrast medium, for visualization of the uterine cavity. Described in 1928.

Iodized salt, suggestion of, for prevention of goiter

JEAN B. J. D. BOUSSINGAULT, French physician and physiological chemist, 1802-1887, suggested the use of iodized salt in the diet for the prevention of goiter. Reported in 1833.

Iodoform, discovery of

GEORGES SIMON SÉRULLAS, French chemist, 1774-1832, discovered idoform, in 1822.

Iodoform dressings in surgery, first use of

ALBERT VON MOSETIG-MOORHOF, Austrian surgeon, 1838-1907, is credited with devising iodoform dressings for use in surgery. Published in 1882.

Ion, Introduction of term

MICHAEL FARADAY, English chemist and physicist, 1791-1867, introduced the term *ion*, on the basis of the Greek *ienai*, to go, in allusion to the movement of the ions in the electrolyte. Reported in 1833.

Ipecac in Europe, introduction of

WILLEM PISO, (GUILLAUME LE POIS), Dutch naturalist, 1611-1678, is credited with introducing ipecac in Europe, *circa* 1648. Published in 1658.

Iridectomy in treatment of glaucoma, early practice of

GEORG JOSEPH BEER, Austrian ophthalmologist, 1763-1821, was an advocate of iridectomy as early as 1798.

Iridectomy in treatment of glaucoma, in France

LOUIS A. DESMARRES, French ophthalmologist, 1810-1882, is credited with having introduced iridectomy for the treatment of glaucoma in France, *circa* 1850.

Iridectomy in treatment of glaucoma, in Germany

FRIEDRICH W. E. A. VON GRAEFE, German ophthalmologist, 1828-1870, is credited with introducing iridectomy for the treatment of glaucoma in Germany. Recorded in 1857.

Iridencleisis for relief of glaucoma

SÖREN HOLTH, French ophthalmologist, 1863-1937, introduced the operation of iridencleisis for the relief of glaucoma. Published in 1907.

Iridenleisis, Langenbeck's operation of

CONRAD JOHANN MARTIN LANGEN-

BECK, German ophthalmologist, 1776-1851, devised an operation of iridencleisis for the construction of an artificial pupil by implanting a slip of iris in a corneal incision. Published in 1811.

Iris, pectinate ligament of

... See under *Pectinate ligament of iris.*

Iris, muscle of, consists of smooth fibers

RUDOLPH ALBERT VON KÖLLIKER, German anatomist, 1817-1905, demonstrated that the contracting structure of the iris consists of smooth muscle. Reported *circa* 1848.

Iritis, introduction of term

JOHANN ADAM SCHMIDT, German ophthalmologist, 1759-1809, introduced the term *iritis,* in 1801.

Iron deficiency anemia, introduction of concept of

GUSTAV VON BUNGE, German physician, 1844-1920, introduced the concept of iron deficiency anemia in a monograph on iron therapy, published in 1895.

Iron, intravenous administration of

JOSEPH ABRAHAM NISSIM, English physician, 19??-   , reported the intravenous administration of iron preparations, in 1947.

Iron lung, invention of

PHILIP DRINKER, American industrial hygienist, 1894-   , invented the so-called "iron lung." Recorded in 1929.

Irradiation of oils by ultraviolet rays

ALFRED FABIAN HESS, American physician, 1875-1933, was the first to show that irradiation of certain oils and foods with ultraviolet rays imparts to these substances antirachitic properties. Recorded in 1929.

Irrigation method with sodium hypochlorite through envelope of oiled silk

JOHN BUNYAN, English surgeon, 1907-   , with WILLIAM STANNARD, devised a method for treating burns by sealing a waterproof and airtight envelop of oiled silk to the burned area and irrigating with a 5 per cent solution of sodium hypochlorite through special openings in the envelope. Reported in 1940.

Irritability of living tissue, introduction of concept

FRANCIS GLISSON, English physician, 1597-1677, introduced the concept of irritability, as a property of living tissue, *circa* 1675.

Irritable heart, early description of — 1870

ARTHUR B. R. MYERS, English physician, 1838-1921, described the effort syndrome or irritable heart in a paper "On the etiology and prevalence of disease of the heart among soldiers," in 1870.

Irritable heart, early description of — 1871

JACOB MENDES DA COSTA, American surgeon, 1833-1900, gave one of the earliest descriptions of the condition known as *irritable heart, soldier's heart, Da Costa's syndrome,* etc. Reported in 1871.

Ischias, introduction of term

DOMENICO COTUGNO, Italian anatomist, 1736-1822, is credited with the introduction of the term *ischias,* in 1764.

Island of Reil

. . . See under *Insula of cerebral hemisphere.*

Islands of Langerhans, discovery of

PAUL LANGERHANS, German physician, 1847-1888, discovered irregular islands of cells in the pancreas which produce insulin. Reported in 1869. Known as *islet of pancreas* and *islets or islands of Langerhans.*

Islands of Langerhans, hydropic degeneration of

FREDERICK MADISON ALLEN, American physician, 1879-19??, discovered the nature of hydropic degeneration of the pancreatic islands of Langerhans. Reported in 1912.

Islands of Langerhans, relation of, to diabetes

MOSES BARRON, American physician and pathologist, 1883-   , studied the relation of the islands of Langerhans to diabetes. This work is said to have led to the discovery of insulin. Recorded in 1920.

Isoagglutination, early recognition of danger of

LUDVIG HEKTOEN, American pathologist, 1863-1951, was possibly the first to call attention to the danger of isoagglutination in transfusion of blood. Reported in 1907.

Isoagglutinins in human blood, discovery of — 1900

KARL LANDSTEINER, American pathologist, 1868-1943, discovered isoagglutinins in human blood serum, in 1900.

Isoagglutinogens in human blood cells, discovery of — 1900

KARL LANDSTEINER, American pathologist, 1868-1943, discovered isoagglutinogens in human blood cells, in 1900.

Isomorphism, discovery of phenomenon of

ERNST EILHARD MITSCHERLICH, German chemist, 1794-1863, discovered and described isomorphism, in 1819.

Isotopes in leukemia

. . . See under *Radioactive isotopes in leukemia.*

Itch mite as causative agent of scabies

. . . See under *Scabies, relation of itch mite to.*

Iter chordae anterius

. . . See under *Temporal bone, canal in, for chorda tympani nerve.*

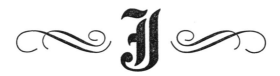

Jackson's membrane, eponymic description of

JABEZ NORTH JACKSON, American surgeon, 1868-1935, described a thin membrane sometimes seen covering the first part of the large intestine. Reported in 1909. Known also as *Jackson's veil.*

Jacob's membrane

. . . See under *Rods and cones, layer of; eponymic description*

Jacob's ulcer

. . . See under *Rodent ulcer of eyelid.*

Jacobson's nerve

. . . See under *Tympanic nerve, early description of.*

Jacobson's plexus

. . . See under *Tympanic plexus, eponymic description of.*

Jacquet's disease, dermatitis, or erythema

LUCIEN JACQUET, French dermatologist, 1860-1915, described a dermatitis in the diaper area of infants. Recorded in 1889. Known also as *erythema gluteale.*

Jadassohn's disease

. . . See under *Maculopapular erythroderma, eponymic description of.*

Jakob's disease

. . . See under *Spastic pseudosclerosis, eponymic description of.*

Janet's disease

. . . See under *Psychasthenia, eponymic description of.*

Japanese beriberi, origin of

. . . See under *Beriberi, Japanese, etc.*

Jarcho's pressometer

. . . See under *Instrument for measuring pressure during injection of radiopaque material into uterus.*

Jarisch-Herxheimer reaction

. . . See under *Syphilitic symptoms, exacerbation of.*

Jarjavay's muscle

. . . See under *Depressor urethrae muscle, eponymic description of.*

Jarvis's snare

. . . See under *Snare for removing polyps from nose and throat.*

Jaundice, acquired hemolytic, with anemia

. . . See under *Acquired hemolytic jaundice with anemia.*

Jaundice, leptospiral, eponymic description of

ADOLPH WEIL, German physician,

1848-1916, described an acute infectious disease marked by jaundice, fever, nephritis, etc., and caused by the spirochete *Leptospira icterohaemorrhagiae*. Known as *Weil's disease, leptospirosis icterohaemorrhagica,* etc. Recorded in 1886. The condition is also known as *Fiedler's disease,* in allusion to CARL L. A. FIEDLER, German Physician, 1835-1921, who described it at about the same time.

Jaundice, pulse characteristic of

JULES EDOUARD A. MONNERET, French physician, 1810-1868, was the first to note the characteristic soft, slow, and full pulse observed in jaundice. Recorded in 1852. Known as *Monneret's pulse.*

Jaundice, spirochetal, eponymic description of — 1883

LOUIS T. J. LANDOUZY, French physician, 1845-1917, described spirochetal jaundice, in 1883. Known as *Landouzy's disease;* also called *Fiedler's disease* and *Weil's disease.*

Jaundice

. . . See also under specific type of jaundice, as *Infectious jaundice.*

Jaw, fracture of, splint for

THOMAS B. GUNNING, American dentist, 1813-1889, devised a metal splint, resembling a double dental plate with an opening in front, for treating fracture of the jaws. Reported in 1866. Known as *Gunning's splint.*

Jaw, upper, first excision of

HORATIO GATES JAMESON, Baltimore surgeon, 1788-1855, is credited with the first recorded excision of the superior maxilla. Performed November 11, 1820.

Jaworski's corpuscles

. . . See under *Spiral mucous bodies in gastric secretion in hyperchlorhydria.*

Jansen's disease

. . . See under *Retinochoroiditis juxtapapillaris, eponymic description of.*

Jockey-strap itch, fungous origin of

. . . See under *Tinea cruris.*

Journal of Anatomy and Physiology, founding of

GEORGE MURRAY HUMPHRY, English surgeon, 1820-1896, is credited with being the founder of the *Journal of Anatomy and Physiology,* in 1867.

Junod's boot

. . . See under *Boot for producing vacuum around a limb,* etc.

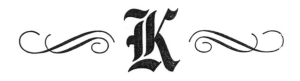

Kahn test, original description of

REUBEN LEON KAHN, American bacteriologist, 1887- , developed a quantitative precipitation test for the diagnosis of syphilis. First report published in 1922.

Kala-azar, experimental transmission of, by sandfly

C. S. SWAMINATH, Indian physician, 19??- , with H. E. SHORTT and L. A. P. ANDERSON, successfully transmitted kala-azar to man by the bite of the sandfly *Phlebotomus argentipes*. Published in 1942.

Kala-azar, first definite mention of

JOHN JAMES CLARKE, English physician in India, 1827-1895, gave the first definite account of kala-azar. Published in 1882.

Kala-azar, small bodies found in spleen and liver of patients with

WILLIAM B. LEISHMAN, British Army surgeon, 1865-1926, described small round bodies found in the spleen and liver of patients affected with kala-azar. These are the intracellular forms of the parasite causing the disease. Reported May 30, 1903. The same bodies were described by CHARLES DONO-

VAN, Irish physician, 1863-1951, in a report published July 11, 1903. Called *Leishman-Donovan bodies*. It is said that Leishman noted the bodies in 1900.

Kala-azar, tartar emetic in treatment of

OLIVEIRA GASPAR DE VIANNA, Brazalian physician, 1885-1914, was the first to use antimony potassium tartrate in the treatment of South American leishmaniasis. Recorded in 1912 and 1914.

Kaposi's disease

. . . See under *Xeroderma pigmentosum, eponymic description of*.

Kaposi's sarcoma

. . . See under *Sarcoma, multiple idiopathic hemorrhagic, eponymic description of*.

Karyo-, introduction of prefix

LEOPOLD AUERBACH, German anatomist, 1828-1897, is credited with introducing the term *karyo-*, a prefix used to indicate the nucleus of a cell. First used in 1874 in the word *karyolysis. Karyo-* is based on the Greek *karyon*, nucleus or nut.

Karyokinesis and cell division, classic description of

WALTHER FLEMMING, German anatomist, 1843-1905, gave a classic description of the phenomena involved in division of the nucleus in mitosis. Published in 1882.

Karyokinesis, introduction of term

The typical changes involved in cell division were named karyokinesis by W. SCHLEICHER in 1878, on the basis of the Greek *karyon* (nut or nucleus) and *kinesis* (movement). WALTHER FLEMMING called the process *mitosis,* in 1880, on the basis of the Greek *mitos,* a thread, in allusion to the formation of a threadlike structure in one of the stages.

Karolysis, introduction of term

. . . See under *Karyo-, introduction of prefix.*

Karyoplasm, introduction of term

WALTHER FLEMMING, German anatomist, 1843-1905, introduced the term *karyoplasm* to describe the protoplasm of the nucleus of a cell. It is based on the Greek *karyon* (nucleus) and *plasma* (plasm). *Circa* 1878.

Kehrer's reflex

. . . See under *Intracranial pressure, increased, pain reflex in.*

Keloid, distinction between true and Alibert's form of

THOMAS ADDISON, English physician, 1793-1860, described two forms of keloid, the "true" keloid and Alibert's keloid. Recorded in 1854.

Keloid, early accurate description of

JEAN LOUIS ALIBERT, French dermatologist, 1766-1837, gave the first clear description of keloid in his *Note sur la keloide,* published in 1816. The condition was noted earlier, in 1790, by Retz.

Keloid, growth resembling a

CAESAR HENRY HAWKINS, English surgeon, 1798-1884, described a growth which resembles a keloid but is merely a hypertrophied scar. Recorded in 1833. Known as *Hawkins' keloid.*

Kenny treatment of poliomyelitis

ELIZABETH KENNY, Australian nurse in the United States, 1886-1952, developed a treatment for anterior poliomyelitis in which hot, moist packs are used in the acute stage, with passive exercise started early and followed as soon as possible by active exercise. Published in 1937.

Keratitis, introduction of term

JAMES WARDROP, English surgeon, 1782-1869, is credited with being the first to use the term *keratitis.* Introduced *circa* 1808.

Keratoconus, early description of — 1868

FRIEDRICH W. E. A. VON GRAEFE, German ophthalmologist, 1828-1870, described a cone-shaped deformity of the cornea, known as keratoconus, in 1868.

Keratoplasty, modern, introduction of

ARTHUR VON HIPPEL, German ophthalmologist, 1841-1917, developed a technique for keratoplasty which is the basis of the modern operation. Recorded in 1888.

Keratoscope, invention of

ANTONIO PLÁCIDO DA COSTA, Portuguese ophthalmologist, 1848-1916, invented and introduced the use of the keratoscope. Reported in 1882. Known as *Plácido's disk*.

Keratosis blennorrhagica, early description of

JEAN BAPTISTE EMIL VIDAL, French dermatologist, 1825-1893, described keratosis blennorrhagica, a condition characterized by the formation of thickened horny growths on the skin. Published in 1893.

Keratosis follicularis, early description of — 1860

HENRI CHARLES LUTZ, French physician, *circa* 1819-1882, is credited with being the first to describe keratosis follicularis, in 1860.

Keratosis follicularis, early description of — 1889

JEAN F. DARIER, French dermatologist, 1856-1938, described keratosis follicularis, characterized by papules containing crusts which can be squeezed out, in 1889. Known as *Darier's disease*.

Keratosis follicularis, early description of — 1889

JAMES CLARKE WHITE, American dermatologist, 1833-1916, gave a clear description of keratosis follicularis, in 1889. Known as *White's disease*.

Keratosis pilaris, eponymic description of

PAUL TAENZER, German dermatologist, 1858-1919, described ulerythema ophryogenes or keratosis pilaris, a skin disease marked by the formation of a hard nodule around each hair follicle. Published in 1889. Known as *Taenzer's disease*.

Kerckring's folds or valves

. . . See under *Intestine, small, circular folds in.*

Kerckring's ossicle

. . . See under *Occipital bone, ossification center which becomes basilar process of.*

Kernicterus, first description of

JOHANNES ORTH, German physician, 1847-1923, was the first to describe kernicterus, a severe form of icterus of the newborn marked by erythroblastosis fetalis and degenerative changes in the nuclei of the brain. Published in 1875.

Kernig's sign in meningitis

. . . See under *Meningitis, Kernig's sign in.*

Kidney, arteriosclerotic atrophy of

WILLIAM WITHEY GULL, English physician, 1816-1890, with HENRY GAWEN SUTTON, gave the first accurate description of arteriosclerotic atrophy of the kidney. Published in 1872. Known as *Gull-Sutton disease*.

Kidney, artificial, production of

WILLEM JOHAN KOLFF, Dutch physician, 1911-   , and associates, devised a so-called artificial kidney, a dialyzer having an extensive surface. Reported in 1944.

Kidney, corpuscle of; malpighian corpuscle of kidney

MARCELLO MALPIGHI, Italian anatomist, 1628-1694, described the tuft of blood vessels surrounded by the expanded initial part of the uriniferous tubule. Recorded in 1666. Known as *renal corpuscle* and *malpighian corpuscle* of the kidney.

Kidney decortication, first performance of

. . . See under *Renal decortication.*

Kidney diseases, first treatise on

FRANCISCO DIAZ, Spanish surgeon, 16th century, wrote the first treatise on the diseases of the kidney, bladder, and urethra. Published in 1588.

Kidney extract having pressor activity

ROBERT ADOLF ARMAND TIGERSTEDT, Finnish physiologist, 1853-1923, with P. G. BERGMAN, discovered a pressor substance in crude extracts of kidney, later identified as renin. Published in 1898.

Kidney, first excision of, in America

ERASTUS BRADLEY WOLCOTT, American surgeon, 1804-1880, performed the first recorded excision of the kidney in the United States. Reported by C. L. STODDARD, in 1861.

Kidney, first excision of, in Europe

GUSTAV SIMON, German surgeon, 1824-1876, is credited with being the first in Europe to excise a kidney. Recorded in 1870.

Kidney fixation, early operation for

. . . See under *Nephropexy.*

Kidney function tests, phenolsulfonphthalein in

. . . See under *Phenolsulfonphthalein excretion by kidney.*

Kidney, glomerular tuft of; eponymic description

MARCELLO MALPIGHI, Italian anatomist, 1628-1694, described the unit of kidney structure consisting of a capillary tuft surrounded by the expanded initial part of the uriniferous tubule. Reported in 1666. Known as *malpighian body* or *corpuscle* of kidney.

Kidney, papillary ducts of

LORENZO BELLINI, Italian anatomist, 1643-1704, described the tubes formed by the union of several collecting tubules and emptying into the pelvis of the kidney. Recorded in 1662. Known as *Bellini's ducts.*

Kidney, perirenal insufflation of oxygen in study of

H. H. CARELLI, Argentinian physician, 18??-19??, with ALFREDO SORDELLI, introduced the method of perirenal insufflation of oxygen in roentgenographic studies of the kidney. Published in 1921.

Kidney, pyramid of; eponymic description

MARCELLO MALPIGHI, Italian anatomist, 1628-1694, described the conical masses of tissue which make up the medullary part of the kidney. Recorded in 1666. Known as *renal pyramid* and *malpighian pyramid.*

Kidney, stellate veins of; eponymic description

PHILIPPE VERHEYEN, Flemish anatomist, 1648-1710, described a stellate plexus of veins situated beneath the capsule of the kidney. Recorded in 1693. Known as *Verheyen's stars, venae stellatae renis,* and *stellate veins.*

Kidney stones, experimental production of

FELIX MANDL, Austrian surgeon, 1892-   , produced renal stones artificially in guinea pigs by intermittent obstruction of the urine and by injection of parathyroid extract. Published in 1933.

Kidney, transplantation of, from one animal to another

ALEXIS CARREL, French surgeon, 1873-1944, successfully transplanted a kidney from one animal to another. Reported in 1908.

Kidney, transplantation of, in man

RICHARD HAROLD LAWLER, American surgeon, 1895-   , with J. W. WEST, P. H. McNULTY, E. J. CLANCY, and R. P. MURPHY, successfully performed a homotransplantation of the kidney in the human. Recorded in 1950.

Kidney tubules, reabsorption of water by

ERNEST HENRY STARLING, English physiologist, 1866-1927, with E. B. VERNAY, demonstrated that the kidney tubules reabsorb water. Published in 1925.

Kielland obstetric forceps

. . . See under *Obstetric forceps with articulation allowing blades to move over each other.*

Kienböck's atrophy

. . . See under *Atrophy of bone*

associated with inflammatory conditions of the extremities.

Kienböck's disease

. . . See under *Semilunar bone, chronic osteitis of.*

Kienböck's disease of the spinal cord

. . . See under *Syringomyelia, traumatic, eponymic description of.*

Kiernan's spaces

. . . See under *Liver, interlobular spaces of; eponymic description.*

Kiesselbach's area or triangle

. . . See under *Nasal septum, thin and vascular area of,* etc.

Kilian's pelvis

. . . See under *Pelvis spinosa,* and under *Pelvis, spondylolisthetic.*

Kinematization of stumps

. . . See under *Kineplastic amputation.*

Kineplastic amputation, first practice of

ANTONIO CECI, Italian orthopedic surgeon, 1852-1920, is credited with being the first to utilize the kineplastic method of amputation suggested and devised by VANGHETTI. Recorded in 1906.

Kineplastic amputation, introduction of

GIULIANO VANGHETTI, Italian orthopedic surgeon, 1861-1940, introduced kineplastic amputation in which the muscles above the amputation are used to form a stump which can best be utilized with an artificial limb. Recorded in 1898.

Known as kinematization of stumps.

Kingsbury-Clark albumin standards, introduction of

... See under *Albumin standards.*

Kirschner's traction

... See under *Fracture, treatment of, by traction exerted on wires passed through the bone.*

Kirschner's wires or nails

... See under *Wires or nails for passing through bone,* etc.

Kisch's reflex

... See under *Intracranial pressure, increased, pain reflex in.*

Kjeldahl's method for nitrogen determination

... See under *Nitrogen content of organic compounds,* etc.

Klebsiella pneumoniae, isolation of

CARL FRIEDLANDER, German pathologist, 1847-1887, isolated *Klebsiella pneumoniae (Friedlander's bacillus),* in 1883.

Klebs's disease

... See under *Glomerulonephritis, early description of.*

Klippel-Feil syndrome

... See under *Cervical vertebrae, congenital fusion of.*

Klippel's disease

... See under *Arthritic general pseudoparalysis, eponymic description of.*

Klumpke's paralysis

... See under *Hand paralysis following injury of brachial plexus.*

Knee, calcification of medial lateral ligament of

AUGUSTO PELLEGRINI, Italian surgeon, 1875-19??, described an abnormal calcification of the medial lateral ligament of the knee, following trauma. First recorded in 1905. The condition was described in 1908 by ALFRED STIEDA, German surgeon, 1869-1945. Known as *Pellegrini-Stieda disease.*

Knee, internal derangement of

WILLIAM HEY, English surgeon, 1736-1819, described a so-called internal derangement of the knee joint, a condition characterized by abnormal mobility and partial dislocation, usually due to injury of the medial semilunar cartilage. Published in 1803.

Knee jerk, absence of, in tabes dorsalis

CARL FRIEDRICH O. WESTPHAL, German neurologist, 1833-1890, demonstrated the value of the patellar tendon reflex in diagnosis, especially its absence in locomotor ataxia. Reported in 1875. The absence of the knee jerk is known as *Westphal's sign.* The diagnostic value of the sign was also discovered, in the same year, by WILHELM H. ERB, German neurologist, 1840-1921.

Knee jerk can be accentuated by sensory stimulation

SILAS WEIR MITCHELL, American neurologist, 1829-1914, demonstrated that the force of the knee jerk can be augmented by sensory stimulation. Recorded in 1886.

Knee, operation on

... See under name of condition involved, as *Ankylosis.*

Koch's bacillus, discovery of
. . . See under *Tubercle bacillus, discovery of.*

Koch-Weeks bacillus
. . . See under *Pinkeye, causative organism of.*

Koebner's disease
. . . See under *Epidermolysis bullosa, eponymic description of.*

Köhler's tarsal scaphoiditis
. . . See under *Tarsal navicular bone, osteochondrosis of.*

Kolmer's test
. . . See under *Syphilis, Kolmer's modification of Wassermann's test for.*

Koplik spots, discovery of
. . . See under *Measles, Koplik spots in.*

Korsakoff's psychosis or syndrome
SERGEI SERGEYEVICH KORSAKOFF, Russian neurologist, 1853-1900, described a psychosis, usually due to chronic alcoholism, marked by disturbance of orientation, polyneuritis, retrograde amnesia, hallucinations, etc. Report published in 1887. Known as *Korsakoff's psychosis* or *syndrome.*

Kozhevnikov's epilepsy
. . . See under *Epilepsy, cortical form of,* etc.

Krabbe's disease
. . . See under *Diffuse infantile familial cerebral sclerosis.*

Kraurosis volvae, early description of—1879
AUGUST BREISKY, German gyne-cologist, 1832-1889, described kraurosis of the vulva, in 1879.

Kraurosis vulvae, early description of—1899
EMILE ARNOUX, French gynecologist, 1871-19??, studied and described kraurosis vulvae. Published in 1899.

Krause's glands
. . . See under *Lacrimal glands, accessory, of upper eyelid.*

Krompecher's tumor
. . . See under *Rodent ulcer, eponymic description of.*

Krukenberg's tumor
. . . See under *Carcinoma of ovary, marked by signet-ring-like cells.*

Krypton, discovery of—1898
WILLIAM RAMSAY, English scientist, 1852-1916, with M. W. TRAVERS, discovered krypton ("the hidden one"), in 1898.

Kundrat's disease
. . . See under *Lymphosarcoma, eponymic description of.*

Kupffer's cells
. . . See under *Liver, stellate cells in sinusoids of.*

Kussmaul's aphasia
. . . See under *Speech, voluntary abstaining from, as seen in psychoses.*

Kussmaul's disease
. . . See under *Periarteritis nodosa, eponymic description of.*

Kussmaul's respiration
. . . See under *Diabetic coma, labored breathing of.*

Kwashiorkor, introduction of term

CICELY DELPHINE WILLIAMS, English physician, 18??- , introduced the term *kwashiorkor,* meaning "red boy," to describe a nutritional disease of children occurring in South Africa. Published in 1935. The first known description of the condition was published in 1926, by L. NORMET.

Kymograph, invention of

KARL FRIEDRICH W. LUDWIG, German physiologist, 1816-1895, invented the kymograph by modifying POISEUILLE'S hemodynamometer to which he added a revolving cylinder and a float provided with a writing point. Published in 1847.

Kymography of heart, introduction of

AUGUSTUS WARREN CRANE, American physician, 1868-1937, is credited with introducing kymography of the heart in clinical cardiology. Published in 1916.

Kyphoscoliotic pelvis, early description of

CARL C. T. LITZMANN, German gynecologist and obstetrician, 1815-1890, described the kyphoscoliotic type of female pelvis, irregularly contracted due to rickets, in 1853.

Kyphosis, angle at base of skull in

CONRAD THEODOR ACKERMANN, German physician, 1825-1896, described the angle at the base of the skull characteristic of kyphosis and certain other conditions. Recorded in 1882. Known as *Ackermann's angle.*

Kyphosis dorsalis juvenilis, eponymic description of

HOLGER WERFEL SCHEUERMANN, Danish orthopedist, 1877-19??, described osteochondrosis of the vertebrae, in 1920. Known as *Scheuermann's kyphosis* and as *Kyphosis dorsalis juvenilis.*

Kyphosis, tuberculosis as cause of

JOHANN ZACHARIAS PLATNER, German physician, 1694-1747, is credited with calling attention to the tuberculous origin of some forms of kyphosis. Published in 1744.

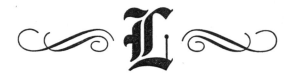

**Labarraque's solution,
introduction of**

ANTOINE G. LABARRAQUE, French
chemist and apothecary, 1777-
1850, compounded a solution of
chlorinated soda, for use as a disinfectant. Recorded in 1825.
Known also as *sodium hypochlorite
solution.*

Labor, induction of premature

CARL WENZEL, German physician,
1769-1827, was probably the first
to induce premature labor in the
course of ethical medical practice,
in 1804. Recorded in 1818.

**Labor, induction of premature,
by dilatation of cervix**

LUIGI MARIA BOSSI, Italian gynecologist, 1859-1919, introduced the
method of forced dilatation of the
cervix as a means of inducing premature labor. Recorded in 1892.

**Labor, induction of premature,
by dilatation of cervix
with sponges**

KARL ALEXANDER FERDINAND
KLUGE, German obstetrician, 1782-
1844, is credited with introducing a
method for induction of premature
labor by dilatation of the cervix
with sponges. Exact date not available.

**Laboratory of experimental
hygiene, founding of**

MAX JOSEPH VON PETTENKOFER,
German chemist and hygienist,
1818-1901, is credited with founding the first laboratory of experimental hygiene, in the 1860's.

Labyrinth, discovery of fluid in

THEODORUS PYL, German anatomist, 1695-175?, was the first to describe the fluid of the labyrinth and
to discuss its function. Recorded
in 1742.

Labyrinth, early reference to

EMPEDOCLES OF AGRIGENTUM,
Greek philosopher and medical observer, 5th century B. C., noted the
labyrinth, *circa* 445 B. C. GALEN
and VESALIUS also noted it.

**Labyrinth, first good
description of**

ANTONIO SCARPA, Italian anatomist
and surgeon, 1747-1832, gave the
first satisfactory description of the
labyrinth of the ear. Recorded in
1789.

***Labyrinth,* introduction
of term**

GABRIEL FALLOPIUS, Italian anatomist, 1523-1562, is credited with
applying the term *labyrinth* to the
internal ear, *circa* 1550.

**Labyrinth, membranous,
discovery of**

ANTONIO SCARPA, Italian anatomist
and surgeon, 1747-1832, is credited
with the discovery of the membranous labyrinth of the ear. Recorded
in 1772.

**Lacrimal and salivary glands,
chronic enlargement of**

JOHANN VON MIKULICZ-RADECKI,
Rumanian surgeon in Germany,
1850-1905, described a chronic
hypertrophic enlargement of the
lacrimal and salivary glands, in
1892. Known as *Mikulicz's disease.*

**Lacrimal duct, first adequate
description of**

GIOVANNI BATTISTA CARCANO
LEONE, Italian anatomist, 1536-
1606, was the first to give a full and
clear description of the lacrimal
duct, including its exact anatomical
position. Recorded in 1574.

**Lacrimal duct, stenosis of;
treatment by dilatation**

DOMINIQUE ANEL, French surgeon,
circa 1679-1730, is known for his
original treatment of stenosis of the
lacrimal duct by dilatation with a
probe of his own invention, followed by an astringent injection.
Published in 1713.

Lacrimal fistula, cause of

GEORG ERNST STAHL, German
physiologist and chemist, 1660-
1734, was the first to give a clear
explanation of the cause of lacrimal
fistula. Recorded in 1702.

**Lacrimal fold, eponymic
description of**

JOSEF VON HASNER, Bohemian
ophthalmologist, 1819-1892, described a fold of mucous membrane
situated at the lower orifice of the
nasolacrimal duct. Recorded in
1850. Known as *Hasner's fold,
plica lacrimalis, Huschke's valve,*
and *Rosenmüller's valve.*

**Lacrimal gland, palpebral
portion of**

JOHANN CHRISTIAN ROSENMÜL-
LER, German anatomist, 1771-1826,
described the palpebral part of the
lacrimal gland, in 1797. Known as
Rosenmüller's gland.

**Lacrimal gland, suspensory
ligament of**

SAMUEL THOMAS SOEMMERRING,
German anatomist, 1755-1830,
gave a clear description of the suspensory ligament of the lacrimal
gland, in 1802. Known as *Soemmerring's ligament.*

**Lacrimal glands, accessory, of
upper eyelid**

CARL F. T. KRAUSE, German anatomist, 1797-1868, described accessory lacrimal glands situated in the
upper eyelids. Known as *Krause's
glands.* Exact date not available.

Lacteal vessels

. . . See under *Lymphatics, early
recognition of.*

Lactic acid bacillus, isolation of

JOSEPH LISTER, English surgeon,
1827-1912, is credited with isolating the lactic acid bacillus. Recorded in 1873.

**Lactic acid in muscular
contraction**

WALTER MORLEY FLETCHER, English physiologist, 1873-1933, with
FREDERICK GOWLAND HOPKINS,

explained the production of lactic acid in the process of muscular contraction. Published in 1907.

Lactobacillus acidophilus,
isolation of

ERNST MORO, German pediatrician, 1874-1951, is credited with the isolation of *Lactobacillus acidophilus,* in 1900.

Lactobacillus bulgaricus,
eponymic description of

LEON MASSOL, Swiss bacteriologist, 1837-1909, described the *Lactobacillus bulgaricus,* in 1897. Known as *Massol's bacillus.*

Lacunar ligament, early
description of—1779

ANTONIO DE GIMBERNAT, Spanish surgeon and anatomist, 1734-1816, demonstrated the lacunar ligament in 1768. He published a report in 1779. Known as *Gimbernat's ligament.*

Lacunas of Morgagni

. . . See under *Urethra, lacunas of.*

Lalouette's pyramid

. . . See under *Thyroid gland, pyramidal lobe of.*

Lambda, introduction of,
as craniometric point

PIERRE PAUL BROCA, French surgeon and anthropologist, 1824-1880, defined *lambda* as a craniometric point. Exact date not available.

Lamina, anterior elastic,
description of

WILLIAM BOWMAN, English ophthalmologist and anatomist, 1816-1892, described the membrane separating the corneal epithelium from the substantia propria, i.e., the anterior elastic lamina. Reported in 1847. Known as *Bowman's membrane.*

Laminography, first
description of

. . . See under *Tomography.*

Landmarks in topography of
abdomen and chest,
planes used as

. . . See under *Planes used as landmarks,* and under name of particular plane.

Landouzy-Dejerine atrophy

. . . See under *Atrophy of muscles of face and scapulohumeral region.*

Landouzy's sciatica

. . . See under *Sciatica with atrophy of muscles of leg.*

Landry's paralysis

. . . See under *Paralysis, acute ascending spinal.*

Lane's band or kink

. . . See under *Ileum, kink in terminal part of.*

Langer's lines

. . . See under *Skin, lines of tension of.*

Langhans' cells

. . . See under *Cytotrophoblast, eponymic description of.*

Langhans' layer

. . . See under *Cytotrophoblast, eponymic description of.*

Lardacein amyloid
degeneration

. . . See under *Amyloid degeneration with deposit of lardacein.*

Laryngeal growth, first removal of, with aid of laryngoscope

GEORG RICHARD LEWIN, German surgeon, 1820-1896, is credited with being the first to remove a laryngeal growth with the aid of a laryngoscope. Recorded in 1861.

Laryngeal mirror, early suggestion for use of

ROBERT LISTON, Scottish surgeon in England, 1794-1847, proposed the use of a special mirror to inspect the larynx. Published in 1837.

Laryngeal operation performed through mouth

FRIEDRICH EDUARD RUDOLPH VOLTOLINI, German otolaryngologist, 1819-1889, performed the first laryngeal operation through the mouth. Published in 1889.

Laryngeal polyp, first bloodless enucleation of

VIKTOR VON BRUNS, German surgeon, 1812-1883, performed the first bloodless enucleation of a laryngeal polyp. Recorded in 1862.

Laryngeal polyp, first successful excision of

CHARLES HENRI EHRMANN, French surgeon, 1792-1878, is credited with being the first to operate successfully for the removal of a laryngeal polyp. Recorded in 1844.

Laryngismus stridulus, early description of

JOHN CLARKE, English physician, 1761-1815, gave an early description of laryngismus stridulus, in 1815.

Laryngismus stridulus, eponymic description of

JOHANN HEINRICH KOPP, German physician, 1777-1858, described laryngismus stridulus, *circa* 1808. Kopp attributed the condition to an enlarged thymus. Known as *Kopp's thymic asthma* or *Kopp's asthma.*

Laryngismus stridulus, first description of

JOHN MILLAR, Scottish physician, 1733-1805, is believed to have given the earliest complete account of laryngismus stridulus, in 1769. Known as *Millar's asthma.*

Laryngitis sicca, chronic laryngitis, classic description of

LUDWIG TÜRCK, Austrian neurologist, 1810-1868, gave a classic description of chronic laryngitis under the name of laryngitis sicca. Recorded in 1866. Known as *Türck's trachoma.*

Laryngoscope, first clinical application of

JOHANN NEPOMUK CZERMAK, Bohemian physiologist, 1828-1873, and LUDWIG TÜRCK, Austrian neurologist and laryngologist, 1810-1868, independently of each other gave the laryngoscope its first clinical application, in 1858.

Laryngoscope, first crude form of

BENJAMIN GUY BABINGTON, English physician, 1794-1866, devised a crude form of laryngoscope, which he called "glottiscope." Demonstrated on March 18, 1829. Published in 1829.

Laryngoscope, first direct-vision form of

ALFRED KIRSTEIN, German physician, 1863-1922, devised the first direct-vision laryngoscope. Recorded in 1895.

Laryngoscope, invention of modern

MANUEL GARCIA, Spanish singing teacher in London, 1805-1906, invented the modern laryngoscope. Reported in 1855.

Laryngoscopy, suspension, introduction of

GUSTAV KILLIAN, German laryngologist, 1860-1921, introduced the method of suspension laryngoscopy (performed with the head of the patient hanging over the edge of the examination table), in 1912.

Larynx, cancer of, first successful operation for

JACOB DA SILVA SOLIS-COHEN, American surgeon, 1838-1927, is said to have performed the first successful operation for cancer of the larynx. Recorded in 1867. In 1873, CHRISTIAN ALBERT THEODOR BILLROTH, Austrian surgeon, 1829-1894, performed a complete excision of the larynx for cancer. The patient died a month after the operation.

Larynx, cocaine in work on

EDMUND JELINEK, Austrian surgeon, 1852-1928, is credited with being the first to use cocaine as an anesthetic in surgery of the larynx. Recorded in 1884.

Larynx, corniculate cartilages of

GIOVANNI DOMENICO SANTORINI, Italian anatomist, 1681-1739, described the small nodule at the tip of each arytenoid cartilage. Pub-

lished in 1724. Known as *Santorini's cartilages* and *corniculate cartilages.*

Larynx, cuneiform cartilage of

HEINRICH AUGUST WRISBERG, German anatomist, 1739-1808, described the cuneiform cartilage of the larynx, situated in the aryteno-epiglottidean fold. Published in 1764 and 1785. Known as *Wrisberg's cartilage, cartilages* or *corpuscles.*

Larynx, earliest preserved treatise devoted to

GIOVANNI BATTISTA CODRONCHI, Italian physician, 1547-1628, wrote a treatise on the diseases of the larynx. Published in 1597. The treatise is now the earliest existing work devoted entirely to the larynx.

Larynx, early description of

GIULIO CASSERIO, Italian anatomist, 1561-1616, gave one of the earliest descriptions of the larynx, *circa* 1600.

Larynx, early photography of

THOMAS RUSHMORE FRENCH, American laryngologist, 1849-1929, is credited with devising a special photographic camera with which he obtained the first good pictures of the larynx. Recorded in 1882 and 1884.

Larynx, internal malignancy of, first operation for

BERNHARD FRAENKEL, German physician, 1836-1911, is said to have been the first to remove an intralaryngeal malignant growth successfully. Published in 1887.

Larynx, local application to

HORACE GREEN, American laryngologist, 1802-1866, is credited with being the first to attempt local application of medicinal substances to the larynx. The degree of success attained is questioned by some. Recorded in 1846.

Larynx, miliary tuberculosis of, early description

EMILE ISAMBERT, French physician, 1827-1876, an authority on laryngeal tuberculosis, described miliary tuberculosis of the larynx, in 1871. *Isambert's disease* refers to miliary tuberculosis of the larynx and pharynx.

Larynx, Morgagni's ventricle of

. . . See under *Morgagni's ventricle of larynx.*

Larynx, paralysis of, respiratory and phonatory

FRANZ RIEGEL, German physician, 1843-1904, differentiated between phonatory and respiratory paralysis of the larynx. Recorded in 1875.

Lasègue's disease

. . . See under *Persecution mania, early description of.*

Lasègue's sign

. . . See under *Sciatica, Lasègue's sign in.*

Lassar's zinc oxide paste

. . . See under *Zinc oxide paste.*

Latent heat, definition of

JOSEPH BLACK, Scottish chemist, 1728-1799, defined the concept of "latent heat." Reported in 1754.

Lateral cerebral fissure

. . . See under *Fissure of Sylvius.*

Lateral illumination of eye

. . . See under *Eye examination, lateral illumination in.*

Lateral sinus thrombosis, pressure test for

GEORGE LORING TOBEY, JR., American otolaryngologist, 1881-1947, with J. B. AYER, developed a test for lateral sinus thrombosis which is based on changes in the pressure of the cerebrospinal fluid elicited by compression of one or both jugular veins. Published in 1925. Known as *Tobey-Ayer test.*

Lateral ventricles of brain, inferior horns of

. . . See under *Inferior horns of lateral ventricles.*

Lateral vestibular nucleus, description of

OTTO F. K. DEITERS, German anatomist, 1834-1863, described the mass of gray matter in the floor of the fourth ventricle which gives origin to the median root of the auditory nerve. Reported in book published in 1865. Known of *Deiter's nucleus.*

Laurence-Moon syndrome, eponymic description of

JOHN ZACHARIAH LAURENCE, English physician, 1830-1874, with ROBERT CHARLES MOON, described a syndrome marked by hypogenitalism, obesity, retinitis pigmentosa, etc. Published in 1866.

Laurence-Moon-Biedl syndrome, eponymic description of

ARTUR BIEDL, German physician, 1869-1933, described and elaborated on the syndrome previously described by LAURENCE and MOON. Recorded in 1922.

Lauth's canal

. . . See under *Sinus, venous, of sclera, eponymic description of.*

Law of filial regression

. . . See under *Inheritance, law of filial regression in.*

Law of specific irritability

. . . See under *Nerve, law of specific energies of.*

Lead colic, early description of

THOMAS CADWALADER, American physician, 1708-1779, described lead colic in "An essay on the West India dry-gripes," published in 1745.

Lead colic, early recognition as definite syndrome

FRANÇOIS CITOIS, French physician, 1572-1652, gave a comprehensive description of lead colic under the name of "Poitou colic," in 1616. This led to the acceptance of the condition as a definite syndrome. The term *Poitou* refers to a province in France.

Lead colic of Devonshire

JOHN HUXHAM, English physician, 1692-1768, gave a good account of lead colic under the name of "Devonshire colic," but attributed the cause to tartar, extracted in the process of making cider, rather than to lead. Recorded in 1739.

Lead colic of Devonshire, recognition of cause of

GEORGE BAKER, English physician in Devonshire, 1722-1809, was the first to prove that Devonshire colic was caused by lead derived from the lead lining of the Devonshire cider presses. As a result of Baker's findings, lead was eliminated from the cider presses. Recorded in 1767.

Lead palsy, early account of

THOMAS CADWALADER, American physician, 1708-1779, was probably the first to describe lead palsy and also gave a classic account of lead colic. BENJAMIN FRANKLIN later proved that the condition resulted from the consumption of Jamaica rum which had been distilled through lead pipes. Recorded in 1745.

Lead poisoning, blue gum line in

. . . See under *Blue line in gums in chronic lead poisoning.*

Lead poisoning due to drinking of cider

. . . See under *Lead colic of Devonshire.*

Lead poisoning, first recorded case of

PAUL OF AEGINA, Greek physician, 625-690, gave the first known description of lead poisoning. Exact date not available.

Lead poisoning, paralysis of fingers and wrist in

ERNST JULIUS REMAK, German neurologist, 1849-1911, described a paralysis of the extensor muscles of the fingers and wrist, as seen in lead poisoning. Recorded in 1875.

Lead, use of, in treating epithelioma

WILLIAM BLAIR BELL, English gynecologist, 1871-1936, advocated the use of colloidal lead in treating epithelioma. Reported in 1922.

Leber's disease

. . . See under *Optic nerve, axial, neuritis of.*

Lederer's anemia

. . . See under *Anemia, acute hemolytic, Lederer's.*

Leech, artificial

. . . See under *Cupping device or artificial leech.*

Leech, medicinal use of

NICANDER, Greek physician and poet, 185-135 B.C., is credited with being the first to mention the use of leeches in treatment of disease. Exact date not available.

Lee's ganglion

. . . See under *Uterus, cervical ganglion of.*

Leg amputation at knee joint; first in America

NATHAN SMITH, American surgeon, 1762-1829, is credited with being the first in the United States to perform an amputation of the leg at the knee joint. Recorded in 1825.

Legal medicine, first important work on

GIOVANNI BATTISTA CODRONCHI, Italian physician, 1547-1628, wrote the first important work on legal medicine, in 1597.

Legs, hereditary edema of

. . . See under *Hereditary edema of the legs.*

Leishman-Donovan bodies, eponymic description of

WILLIAM B. LEISHMAN, British Army surgeon, 1865-1926, described small round bodies found in the spleen and liver of patients affected with kala-azar. These are the intracellular forms of the parasite causing the disease. Reported

May 30, 1903. The same bodies were described by CHARLES DONOVAN, Irish physician, 1863-1951, in a report published July 11, 1903. Known as *Leishman-Donovan bodies.* It is said that Leishman first noted the bodies in 1900.

Leishman-Donovan bodies, pre-eponymic description of

DAVID DOUGLAS CUNNINGHAM, English physician in India, 1843-1914, noted "peculiar parasitic organisms" in the tissue of a specimen of Delhi boil. Recorded in 1885. The bodies described by Cunningham were undoubtedly identical with the Leishman-Donovan bodies.

Leishmania infantum, description and naming of

CHARLES JULES HENRI NICOLLE, French bacteriologist, 1866-1936, described the organism causing infantile kala-azar and named it *Leishmania infantum.* Published in 1909.

Leishmania tropica, early description of

PETER BOROVSKY, Russian physician, 1863-1932, gave the first description of the organism causing cutaneous leishmaniasis, later named *Leishmania tropica,* in 1898.

Leishmaniasis

. . . See under *Kala-azar.*

Leloir's disease

. . . See under *Lupus vulgaris erythematoides, eponymic description of.*

Lembert's suture

. . . See under *Serous surface ap-*

proximation in intestinal surgery, etc.

Lemniscus lateralis, section of, in treatment of pain

ACHILLE MARIO DOGLIOTTI, Italian surgeon, 19??- , was the first to cut the lemniscus lateralis in man for the relief of intractable pain. Recorded in 1938.

Lemon juice for seamen in English navy, early advocacy of—1753

JAMES LIND, Scottish physician, 1716-1794, a pioneer in the field of naval hygiene in England, urged the issue of lemon juice to the seamen of the English navy. Report published in 1753. It was through these efforts that scurvy was eventually eradicated.

Lemons and limes in scurvy, early advocacy of—1617

JOHN WOODALL, English surgeon, 1556-1643, urged the eating of lemons and limes as a preventive measure against scurvy. Recorded in 1617.

Lemons and limes

. . . See also under *Fresh fruit in diet of sailors.*

Lens, crystalline, change in curvature of

CHRISTOPH SCHEINER, German physicist, 1575-1650, is said to have demonstrated that the curvature of the crystalline lens changes during accommodation. Published in 1619.

Lens, fibrous structure of, early reference to

PIETER CAMPER, Dutch anatomist, 1722-1789, is believed to have made the first observation regarding the fibrous structure of the crystalline lens. Recorded in 1746.

Lens, oil immersion, introduction of

. . . See under *Oil immersion lens.*

Lens, suspensory ligament of

. . . See under *Suspensory ligament of lens.*

Lenses, achromatic, improved

. . . See under *Achromatic lenses, improved.*

Lenticulostriate artery in cerebral hemorrhage

JEAN MARTIN CHARCOT, French neurologist, 1825-1893, observed the frequency of involvement of the lenticulostriate branch of the middle cerebral artery in cerebral hemorrhage. The artery is often referred to as *Charcot's artery of cerebral hemorrhage.* Recorded in 1878.

Leontiasis ossea, first description of

MARCELLO MALPIGHI, Italian anatomist, 1628-1694, is credited with being the first to describe a bilateral symmetrical hypertrophy of the bones of the skull, causing a lion-like facial expression. Published posthumously in 1700.

Leprolin, preparation of

ERNEST REINHOLD ROST, English physician in India, 1872-19??, prepared leprolin, a vaccine used with little success in the treatment of leprosy. Recorded in 1904.

Leprology, founder of modern or scientific

DANIEL CORNELIS DANIELSSEN,

Norwegian physician, 1815-1894, is regarded as the founder of scientific or modern leprology. With CARL WILHELM BOECK (Norwegian physician, 1808-1875), he gave the first modern description of leprosy, in 1847.

Leprosy, causative agent of

GERHARD H. A. HANSEN, Norwegian physician, 1841-1912, is credited with discovering *Mycobacterium leprae,* the causative agent of leprosy, in 1871.

Leprosy, chaulmoogra oil in treatment of

FREDERIC JOHN MOUAT, English physician, 1816-1897, is credited with introducing chaulmoogra oil in Western medicine, in 1854. The oil was, however, known to the Chinese and others many centuries before.

Leprosy, diasone in treatment of

ERNEST MUIR, American physician, 1880-19??, introduced diasone in the treatment of leprosy. Recorded in 1944.

Leprosy, modern treatment of

DANIEL C. DANIELSSEN, Norwegian physician, 1815-1894, is considered to be the inaugurator of the modern therapy of leprosy.

Leprosy, nodular, early description of

ARETAEUS THE CAPPADOCIAN, Greek physician, 30-90 A.D., described nodular leprosy under the title "On elephas." Known as *elephantiasis Aretaei.* Exact date not available.

Leprosy, promin in treatment of

GUY HENRY FAGET, American physician, 1891-   , with associates, introduced the use of promin, a preparation having the properties of sulfanilamide, in the treatment of leprosy. Recorded in 1943.

Leptosome body build, description of

ERNST KRETSCHMER, German psychiatrist, 1888-   , described the leptosome body build, marked by a slender and light physique. Published in 1927.

Leptospira canicola, first isolation of

A. KLARENBEEK, Dutch physician, 18??-   , with WILHELM AUGUST PAUL SCHÜFFNER, isolated *Leptospira canicola* from the urine of a dog. Published in 1933.

Leptospira canicola, human infection with

C. M. DHONT, Dutch physician, 19??-   , with A. KLARENBEEK, W. A. P. SCHÜFFNER, and J. VOET, recorded the first case of human infection with *Leptospira canicola,* in 1934.

Leptospira icterohaemorrhagiae, discovery of

RYUKICHI INADA, Japanese bacteriologist, 1874-1950, with R. HOKI, Y. IDO, H. ITO, and R. KANEKO, discovered *Leptospira icterohaemorrhagiae,* the causative agent of spirochetal jaundice. Recorded in 1916.

Leptospira icterohaemorrhagiae, early observation of

ARTHUR MARSTON STIMSON, American physician, 1876-19??, described an organism under the name of *Spirochaeta interrogans* which was later proved to be identical with *Leptospira icterohaemorrhagiae*. Published in 1907.

Leptospiral jaundice, demonstration of causative agent of

RYUKICHI INADA, Japanese bacteriologist and physician, 1874-1950, with R. HOKI, Y. IDO, H. ITO, and R. KANEKO, demonstrated that *Leptospira icterohaemorrhagiae* is the organism causing Weil's disease. Recorded in 1916.

Leptospiral jaundice, development of serum therapy for

RYUKICHI INADA, Japanese bacteriologist, 1874-1950, with R. HOKI, Y. IDO, H. ITO, and R. KANEKO, developed a successful serum for use in leptospiral jaundice. Reported in 1916.

Leptospiral jaundice, eponymic description of

ADOLF WEIL, German physician, 1848-1916, gave a classic description of leptospiral jaundice, in 1886. Known as *Weil's disease.*

Leptospiral jaundice, organism of; first note

. . . See under *Leptospira icterohaemorrhagiae.*

Leptospirosis icterohemorrhagica

. . . See under *Leptospiral jaundice.*

Leptospirosis in dogs, organism of

. . . See under *Leptospira canicola.*

Leriche's operation

. . . See under *Periarterial sympathectomy for relief of paresthesia and vasomotor disturbances.*

Lesser circulation, first description of

. . . See under *Pulmonary circulation.*

Lethargic encephalitis, early description of

CAMILLO BOZZOLO, Italian physician, 1845-1920, described lethargic encephalitis, in 1895. Known as *Bozzolo's disease.*

Lethargic encephalitis, first satisfactory description of

CONSTANTIN VON ECONOMO, Austrian neurologist, 1876-1931, gave the first satisfactory description of lethargic encephalitis (epidemic encephalitis), in 1917. Called *von Economo's disease.*

Letterer-Siwe disease, eponymic description of

ERICH LETTERER, German pathologist, 1895- , described a form of xanthomatosis or nonlipid reticuloendothelial disorder, in 1924. The same condition was described later from a clinical point of view by STURE AUGUST SIWE, German pediatrician, 1897- , in 1933.

Leucine in urine, in yellow atrophy of liver

FRIEDRICH T. VON FRERICHS, German pathologist, 1819-1885, discovered the presence of leucine in the urine of patients with acute yellow atrophy of the liver. Reported in 1854.

Leukemia, bone marrow changes in

ERNST NEUMANN, German pathologist, 1834-1918, gave the first adequate description of the changes taking place in the bone marrow in cases of myelogenous leukemia, in 1870.

Leukemia, first adequate description of

JOHN HUGHES BENNETT, Scottish physician, 1812-1875, gave the first clear description of a case of leukemia, in 1845. Another case, observed in 1841, was also reported at this time.

Leukemia, introduction of term

RUDOLF LUDWIG KARL VIRCHOW, German pathologist, 1821-1902, introduced the term *leukemia,* in 1845, a few weeks after the condition was described clearly for the first time by JOHN HUGHES BENNETT.

Leukemia, remissions in, produced by radium treatment

THOMAS ORDWAY, American physician, 1877-19??, described cases of remission in leukemia produced by radium treatment. Published in 1917.

Leukemia, urethane in treatment of

EDITH PATERSON, English physician, 19??-   , with A. HADDOW, I. A. THOMAS, and J. M. WATKINSON, introduced urethane in the treatment of leukemia. Published in 1946.

Leukemia, use of x-rays in

. . . See under *X-rays, first use of, in leukemia.*

Leukocyte with divided nucleus in acute leukemia

HERMANN RIEDER, German pathologist, 1858-1932, described a kind of leukocyte occurring in acute leukemia and regarded as an abnormal myeloblast or lymphoblast. Published in 1892. Known as *Rieder's cell.*

Leukocytes, accumulation of, in inflammation

. . . See under *Inflammation, accumulation of leukocytes in.*

Leukocytes, ameboid movement of, first observations on

THOMAS WHARTON JONES, English physician, 1808-1891, is credited with discovering the ameboid movement of leukocytes, in 1853.

Leukocytes are derived from lymphatic glands

WILLIAM HEWSON, English physiologist, 1739-1774, stated that the leukocytes are derived from the lymphatic "glands" and the thymus. Recorded in 1774.

Leukocytes, basophilic granules of

EDMUND VON NEUSSER, Austrian physician, 1852-1912, described basophilic granules seen around the nucleus of some leukocytes, in 1889. Known as *Neusser's granules.*

Leukocytes, classification of, on basis of nuclei

JOSEPH ARNETH, German physician, 1873-19??, devised a classification of polymorphonuclear leukocytes on the basis of the lobulation of their nuclei, in 1904.

Leukocytes, endothelial, introduction of term

FRANKLIN BURR MALLORY, American pathologist, 1862-1941, introduced the term *endothelial leuko-*

cytes to describe the large wandering cells of the tissues and circulating blood which have marked phagocytic power. Published in 1898.

Leukocytes, staining of granules of

PAUL EHRLICH, German bacteriologist and pathologist, 1854-1915, introduced the use of aniline dyes in the staining of granules in white blood cells. Recorded in 1877.

Leukocytosis, first description of

WILLIAM ADDISON, English physician, 1802-1881, gave the first known description of leukocytosis, though not under this name, *circa* 1843.

Leukocytosis, introduction of term

RUDOLF LUDWIG KARL VIRCHOW, German pathologist, 1821-1902, is credited with the introduction of the term *leukocytosis,* in 1858.

Leukoencephalitis concentrica; concentric sclerosis

OTTO MARBURG, Austrian neurologist, 1874-1948, described leukoencephalitis concentrica (encephalomyelitis periaxialis scleroticans), in 1906.

Leukopenia, first recorded fatal case of

PHILIP KING BROWN, American physician, 1869-1940, with WILLIAM OPHÜLS (American physician, 1871-1933), recorded a case of severe leukopenia which terminated in death. Published in 1901.

Leukoplakia buccalis, description of

. . . See under *Psoriasis buccalis.*

Levator glandulae thyreoideae

SAMUEL THOMAS SOEMMERRING, German anatomist, 1755-1830, described the levator glandulae thyreoideae. Date not available.

Levin tube

. . . See under *Gastroduodenal nasal tube, invention of.*

Levret's forceps

. . . See under *Obstetric forceps with cephalic and pelvic curves.*

Lex regia

. . . See under *Cesarean section for women dying in late pregnancy.*

Leyden jar, invention of

The earliest form of electrical condenser, the Leyden jar, was invented at about the same time but independently, in 1745-46, by E. G. VON KLEIST of Pomerania and P. VAN MUSSCHENBROEK of the University of Leyden.

Leydig cells

. . . See under *Testis, interstitial cells of; earliest description.*

Libman-Sacks disease

. . . See under *Endocarditis, atypical verrucous.*

Lichen chronicus simplex, eponymic description of

JEAN BAPTISTE EMIL VIDAL, French dermatologist, 1825-1893, described lichen chronicus simplex or neurodermatitis. Published in 1886. Known as *Vidal's disease.*

Lichen nitidus, eponymic description of

FELIX PINKUS, German dermatologist, 1868-1947, described a rare skin disease marked by small flat papules and named it lichen nitidus. Observed in 1901; recorded in 1907. Known as *Pinkus' disease.*

Lichen ruber acuminatus

. . . See under *Pityriasis rubra pilaris.*

Lichen ruber moniliformis, early description of—1886

MORITZ KAPOSI, Hungarian dermatologist, 1837-1902, described lichen ruber moniliformis, a condition marked by an eruption of flat papules in linear formation, especially on the extremities. Recorded in 1886.

Lichen urticatus, first description of

THOMAS BATEMAN, English physician, 1778-1821, was the first to describe lichen urticatus, in 1813.

Lichtheim's disease

. . . See under *Aphasia, subcortical, in which patient is able to indicate the number of syllables in a word.*

Lie detector test; Marston deception test

WILLIAM MOULTON MARSTON, American psychologist, 1893-1947, developed a lie-detection test based on variation in systolic blood pressure, in 1934.

Lie detector test

. . . See also under *Polygraph.*

Lieutaud's trigone

. . . See under *Trigone of bladder, eponymic description of.*

Ligament, annular, of recti muscles of eye

JOHANN GOTTFRIED ZINN, German anatomist, 1727-1759, described the annular ligament situated at the edge of the optic foramen, giving origin to the four recti muscles of the eye. Recorded in 1755. Known as *Zinn's ligament, annulus zinnii,* etc.

Ligament, arcuate, of diaphragm, early description of

JULIUS CAESAR ARANTIUS, Italian physician, 1530-1589, described one of the arched ligaments which connect the diaphragm with the first lumbar vertebra and the lowest ribs. Published in 1571.

Ligament connecting incus with roof of tympanic cavity

FRIEDRICH ARNOLD, German anatomist, 1803-1890, described the ligament connecting the body of the incus to the roof of the tympanic cavity. Reported in 1828.

Ligament extending from duodenojejunal junction to crus of diaphragm

WENZEL TREITZ, Austrian physician and anatomist, 1819-1872, described a suspensory fold of peritoneum extending from the left crus of the diaphragm to the duodenojejunal junction. Published in 1857. Known as *Treitz's ligament.*

Ligament extending from linea alba to inguinal ligament

ABRAHAM COLLES, Irish surgeon, 1773-1843, described a ligament formed from a portion of the aponeurosis of the external oblique muscle which extends from the linea alba to the inguinal ligament. Published in 1811.

Ligament of lateral meniscus

HEINRICH AUGUST WRISBERG,

German anatomist, 1739-1808, described the lateral meniscus ligament, in 1764. Known as *Wrisberg's ligament*.

Ligamentum pectinatum, spaces between fibers of
. . . See under *Pectinate ligament,* etc.

Ligamentum popliteum obliquum, description of
. . . See under *Posterior ligament of knee joint*.

Ligation of traumatic aneurysm
DOMINIQUE ANEL, French surgeon, *circa* 1679-1730, treated a case of traumatic aneurysm by ligation, in 1710.

Ligation of
. . . See under name of structure or vessel involved.

Ligature instead of cautery in vascular surgery
AMBROISE PARÉ, French surgeon, 1510-1590, introduced the method of ligation in vascular surgery, instead of cautery. Published in 1545.

Ligatures, buckskin and kid, introduction of
PHILIP SYNG PHYSICK, American surgeon, 1768-1837, introduced the use of absorbable buckskin and kid ligatures. Published in 1816.

Light, corpuscular theory of
ISAAC NEWTON, English scientist, 1642-1727, propounded a corpuscular theory of light. Published in 1704.

Light rays are perceived by retina, early pronouncement that
ALHAZEN, Arabian mathematician, physicist, and optician, *circa* 965-1039, recognized the fact that light rays are perceived by the retina. Exact date not available.

Light therapy, systematic use of
JOHANN WOLFGANG DÖBEREINER, German physician, 1780-1849, is credited with introducing light therapy on a systematic basis. Published in 1816.

Light, wave theory of; establishment of
THOMAS YOUNG, English physician, 1773-1829, is credited with establishing the wave theory of light. Expounded in a treatise *On the Theory of Light and Colours,* published in 1802.

Lightning is electrical phenomenon, proof that
BENJAMIN FRANKLIN, American statesman and scientist, 1706-1790, proved, by means of a kite experiment, that lightning is an electrical phenomenon, in June 1752.

Lightning rod, invention of
BENJAMIN FRANKLIN, American statesman and scientist, 1706-1790, is credited with inventing the lightning rod. The first reference to it is made in a note dated November 1749. He recommended it publicly in 1753.

Ligneous phlegmon, eponymic description of
PAUL RECLUS, French surgeon, 1847-1914, described a condition marked by induration of the subcutaneous tissue of the neck, in 1896. Known as *Reclus's disease*.

Lilienthal's probe
. . . See under *Probe for detecting*

bullets and other metal objects in the body.

Limbs, replacement of lost, by crustaceans

RENÉ ANTOINE FERCHAULT DE RÉAUMUR, French physiologist, 1683-1757, demonstrated that crustaceans are able to replace lost limbs. Published in 1712.

Limbus fossae ovalis

. . . See under *Annulus ovalis.*

Lindau-von Hippel disease

. . . See under *Retina, angiomatosis of,* etc.

Line between mental point and glabella

PAUL TOPINARD, French anthropologist, 1830-1911, described a hypothetical line extending between the glabella and the mental point. Published in 1876. Known as *Topinard's line.*

Line extended along buccal cusps of teeth

FERDINAND VON SPEE, German embryologist, 1855-1937, described an imaginary line extending along the tops of the buccal cusps from the last molar to the first bicuspid, in 1902. Known as *Spee's curve.*

Line marking level of base of skull

. . . See under *Reid's base line at level of base of skull.*

Line passing through opisthion and orbitale

LOUIS J. M. DAUBENTON, French physician and naturalist, 1716-1799, described a hypothetical line passing through the opisthion and orbitale points. Known as *Daubenton's line.* Exact date not available.

Linea semicircularis; line of Douglas

JAMES DOUGLAS, Scottish anatomist and obstetrician, 1675-1742, described a crescentric line marking the termination of the posterior sheath of the rectus muscle. Reported in 1707.

Lineae atrophicae, eponymic description of

SAMUEL WILKS, English physician, 1824-1911, described the lineae atrophicae, reddish lines on the abdomen observed in Cushing's syndrome. Recorded in 1861. Known as *Wilks's lines.*

Lines, transverse, on fingernails, resulting from exhausting diseases

JOSEPH H. S. BEAU, French physician, 1806-1865, was first to describe the transverse lines or rings seen on the fingernails in some cases of wasting or exhausting disease. Reported in August 1846. Known as *Beau's lines.*

Lingual vein, identification of

ALBRECHT VON HALLER, Swiss physiologist and anatomist, 1708-1777, identified the lingual vein as a blood vessel, in 1727. Previously it was considered by many as a salivary duct.

Linitis plastica, original description of

WILLIAM BRINTON, English physician, 1823-1867, described a hypertrophy of the submucous connective tissue of the stomach, linitis plastica, in 1859. Known as *Brin-*

ton's disease, leather bottle stomach, cirrhotic gastritis, etc.

Lipiodol, introduction of, in roentgenography

JEAN ATHANASE SICARD, French
physician, 1872-1929, introduced
the use of lipiodol as a contrast
medium in roentgenography. Recorded in 1921.

Lipocaic hormone, first description of

LESTER REYNOLD DRAGSTEDT,
American biochemist, 1893-   ,
with J. VAN PROHASKA and H. P.
HARMS, reported observations on a
lipocaic hormone, a substance derived from the pancreas which aids
in the metabolism of fat. Published
in 1936.

Lipochondrodystrophy, eponymic description of

GERTRUD HURLER, German pediatrician, 187?-19??, described lipo-
chondrodystrophy, a lipoid disturbance affecting bones, skin, cartilage, etc., in 1920. Known as
Hurler's disease.

Lipodystrophia progressiva, original description of

ARTHUR SIMONS, German physician, 1877-19??, described a rare
condition of lipomatosis characterized by emaciation of the upper part
of the body and by a disfiguring
obesity of the lower half. It affects
mostly girls. Recorded in 1911.
The condition was also described
by R. J. A. BARRAQUER, Spanish
physician. Date not available.
Known eponimically as *Barraquer's
disease* and *Barraquer-Simons disease.*

Lipoid histiocytosis

. . . See under *Niemann-Pick disease.*

Lipoid nephrosis, introduction of term

FRITZ MUNK, German physician,
1879-19??, is credited with introducing the term *lipoid nephrosis* in
a treatise published in 1913.

Liporrhagia retinalis

. . . See under *Retina, traumatic
angiopathy of.*

Lipschütz ulcer

. . . See under *Ulcer, acute vulvar,
eponymic description of.*

Liquefaction of gases, method for

PIERRE E. M. BERTHELOT, French
chemist, 1827-1907, devised a
method for liquefying gases, especially carbon dioxide. Reported in
1850.

Liquids, Pascal's law of pressure exerted on

. . . See under *Pascal's law,* etc.

Lisfranc's tubercle

. . . See under *Scalene tubercle on
upper surface of first rib.*

Lissauer's paralysis; atypical general paralysis

HEINRICH LISSAUER, German neurologist, 1861-1891, described an
atypical general paralysis marked
by aphasia, convulsions, monoplegia, etc. Published posthumously
in 1901.

Lissauer's tract

. . . See under *Dorsolateral tract;
marginal tract.*

Lister's tubercle

... See under *Radius, dorsal tubercle of*.

Litholapaxy, introduction of, in America

JACOB RANDOLPH, American surgeon, 1796-1848, is credited with introducing the operation of litholapaxy in the United States, in 1831.

Lithotomy, lateral, early form of

MARIANO SANTO DI BARLETTA, Italian physician, 1490-1550, is credited with improving and popularizing an operation for removal of urinary calculi which is the forerunner of the modern lateral lithotomy. Recorded in 1535. The method is said to have been invented by JOHN DE ROMANI in 1520, and first used by Mariano Santo in 1531.

Lithotomy, lateral, introduction of modern

WILLIAM CHESELDEN, English surgeon, 1688-1752, introduced lateral lithotomy, in 1727. Recorded by ALEXANDER REID in 1748.

Lithotomy position; semi- prone position

JAMES MARION SIMS, American surgeon, 1813-1883, introduced a gynecological position in which the patient lies on the left side and chest, with the right thigh drawn up, *circa* 1854. Known as *Sims' position*.

Lithotomy, suprapubic, introduction of

PIERRE FRANCO, French surgeon, 1500-1561, introduced the method of suprapubic lithotomy, in 1556.

Lithotrite for crushing calculi in urinary bladder

HENRY JACOB BIGELOW, American surgeon, 1818-1890, devised a special kind of lithotrite for crushing calculi in the urinary bladder; the fragments were removed by means of another instrument. Reported in 1878. Known as *Bigelow's lithotrite*.

Lithotrite, introduction of term

JEAN CIVIALE, French physician, 1792-1867, is credited with introducing the term *lithotrite, circa* 1826.

Lithotrite, modern, first practical

CHARLES L. S. HEURTELOUP, French surgeon, 1793-1864, is credited with producing the best lithotrite of his time, in 1833.

Lithotrite, modern, first suggestion for

WILLEM GRUITHUSIEN, Dutch physician in Germany, 1776-1847, is credited with making the first attempt to construct and use a modern lithotrite, in 1813.

Lithotrite, modern, first use of

LEROY D'ETOILLES, French surgeon, 178?-1862, is said to have been the first to use a crude modern lithotrite, in 1822.

Lithotrite, modern, introduction of screw design in

JAMES HODGSON, English physician, 1790-1859, is said to have introduced the screw power design into the modern lithotrite, *circa* 1825.

Lithotrite, modern, popularization of

JEAN CIVIALE, French physician,

1792-1867, is credited with devising the best lithotrite of his time and with popularizing lithotripsy. Recorded in 1826.

Lithotrite, rack and pinion in, introduction of

WILLIAM FERGUSSON, English surgeon, 1808-1877, is said to have introduced the rack and pinion in the structure of the lithotrite, *circa* 1834.

Little's disease

. . . See under *Cerebral spastic paralysis, congenital; eponymic description of.*

Little's disease, pre-eponymic description of

JAKOB HEINE, German physician, 1800-1879, is credited with giving an early but incomplete description of congenital cerebral spastic paralysis *(Little's disease)*, in 1840.

Littre's glands

. . . See under *Glands of male urethra, eponymic description of.*

Littre's hernia

. . . See under *Hernia of a diverticulum.*

Littre's operation

. . . See under *Colostomy, first suggestion of, in intestinal obstruction.*

Liver, acute yellow atrophy of; eponymic description

CARL VON ROKITANSKY, Austrian pathologist, 1804-1878, gave a classic description of acute yellow atrophy of the liver. He also named the disease. Recorded in 1842. Known as *Rokitansky's disease.*

Liver, acute yellow atrophy of; original description

RICHARD BRIGHT, English physician, 1789-1858, gave the original description of acute yellow atrophy of the liver. Published in 1836.

Liver, atrophic cirrhosis of; eponymic description

RENÉ THÉOPHILE HYACINTHE LAENNEC, French physician, 1781-1826, described atrophic or chronic interstitial hepatitis. Recorded in 1819. Known as *Laennec's cirrhosis.*

Liver, blood supply of, first clear description of

FRANCIS GLISSON, English physician, 1597-1677, gave the first clear description of the blood supply of the liver, in his *De Hepate,* in 1654.

Liver, capsule of, eponymic description of

FRANCIS GLISSON, English physician, 1597-1677, gave the first clear description of the liver stroma, the sheath of connective tissue which accompanies the vessels and the bile ducts, in 1654. Known as *Glisson's capsule.*

Liver, cirrhosis of; first description

JOHN BROWNE, English physician, 1642-170?, was the first to describe cirrhosis of the liver. Recorded in 1685.

Liver, endarteritis of, with obstruction

HANS CHIARI, German pathologist, 1851-1916, described an obliterating endarteritis and venous thrombosis of the liver. Reported in 1898. Known as *Chiari's disease.*

Liver in pernicious anemia—1926

GEORGE RICHARDS MINOT, American physician, 1885-1950, with WILLIAM PARRY MURPHY, introduced a diet rich in liver, in the treatment of pernicious anemia. Recorded in 1926. Known as the *Minot-Murphy diet.* Received the Nobel prize, with W. P. MURPHY and G. H. WHIPPLE, in 1934.

Liver, interlobular spaces of; eponymic description

FRANCIS KIERNAN, English surgeon and anatomist, 1800-1874, described interlobular spaces in the liver. Published in 1833. Known as *Kiernan's spaces.*

Liver, pseudocirrhosis of, with pericarditis

FRIEDEL PICK, German physician, 1867-1926, described a condition characterized by enlargement of the liver, peritonitis, and ascites, occurring in patients who had pericarditis. Published in 1896. Known as *Friedel Pick's disease, mediastinopericarditis,* and *polyserositis.*

Liver puncture, biopsy by

EDWARD STANLEY, English surgeon, 1793-1862, performed a liver puncture biopsy. Recorded in 1833.

Liver puncture, biopsy by

LUIGI LUCATELLO, Italian surgeon, 1863-1926, performed a liver puncture biopsy. Recorded in 1895.

Liver, raw, in blood regeneration

FRIEDA SAUR ROBSCHEIT-ROBBINS, American scientist, 1893-   , with GEORGE HOYT WHIPPLE (American pathologist, 1878-19??), discovered the favorable effect of liver upon blood regeneration in anemia. This led to the diet of Minot and Murphy. Recorded in 1925.

Liver, stellate cells in sinusoids of

KARL WILHELM VON KUPFFER, German anatomist, 1829-1902, described large stellate cells in the lining of the sinusoids of the liver. Published in 1876. Known as *Kupffer's cells.*

Liver, tongue-shaped lobe of

BERNHARD MORITZ CARL LUDWIG RIEDEL, German surgeon, 1846-1916, described a tongue-shaped mass of liver attached to the right lobe. Recorded in 1888. Known as *Riedel's lobe.*

Lobstein's disease

. . . See under *Osteogenesis imperfecta, eponymic description of.*

Lobstein's ganglion

. . . See under *Ganglion of great splanchnic verve, eponymic description of.*

Local anesthesia in operations on nose, introduction of

EDMUND JELINEK, Austrian surgeon, 1852-1928, is credited with introducing the use of local anesthesia (cocaine) in operations on nose, pharynx, etc., in 1884.

Local anesthesia

. . . See also under *Anesthesia,* and under name of particular type of anesthesia.

Locke's solution, introduction of

FRANK SPILLER LOCKE, English physician, *floruit* not available, compounded a solution of sodium chloride, potassium chloride, calcium chloride, sodium bicarbonate, and dextrose in water. There are several variants of the formula. Recorded in 1894.

Lockwood's ligament
... See under *Suspensory ligament of eye*, etc.

Locomotor ataxia
... See under *Tabes dorsalis*.

Loewenthal's tract
... See under *Tectospinal tract, eponymic description of*.

London School of Tropical Medicine, founding of
PATRICK MANSON, Scottish parasitologist, 1844-1922, founded the London School of Tropical Medicine, in 1898.

Long thoracic nerve; external respiratory nerve
CHARLES BELL, Scottish physician, 1774-1842, described the posterior or long thoracic nerve, or external respiratory nerve, in 1821. Known as *Bell's nerve*.

Louis's angle
... See under *Sternum, angle formed by body and manubrium of*.

Lower jaw, first excision of
GUILLAUME DUPUYTREN, French surgeon, 1777-1835, performed the first recorded successful excision of the lower jaw, in 1812. Published in 1820.

Lower's tubercle
... See under *Tubercle, intervenous, of heart*.

Low-sodium diet in heart failure
... See under *Heart failure*.

Lubarsch's crystals
... See under *Testis, crystals found in epithelial cells of*.

Lucas sign in rickets
... See under *Rickets, distention of abdomen in early*.

Ludwig's angina
... See under *Mouth, inflammation of floor of*.

Ludwig's filtration theory
... See under *Urine formation, filtration and reabsorption theory of*.

Lugol's Solution
... See under *Solution of Iodine, Strong*; etc.

Lumbar colostomy for relief of intestinal obstruction, first performance of
JEAN ZULEMA AMUSSAT, French surgeon, 1796-1856, is believed to have been the first to perform lumbar colostomy for the relief of intestinal obstruction. Reported in 1839.

Lumbar puncture, introduction of—1891
HEINRICH IRENAEUS QUINCKE, German physician, 1842-1922, introduced the use of lumbar puncture, for diagnosis and treatment, independently of others (e.g., WALTER E. WYNTER), in 1891.

Lumbar puncture, introduction of—1891
WALTER ESSEX WYNTER, English physician, 1860-1945, reported the performance of lumbar puncture in four cases of tuberculous meningitis. Published in 1891.

Lumbar puncture

. . . See also under *Spinal puncture.*

**Lumbocostal triangle,
description of**

VICTOR BOCHDALEK, Prague anatomist, 1835-1868, described the lumbocostal triangle. Known as the *Bochdalek triangle.* Date not available.

Lumsden's center

. . . See under *Pneumotaxic center, eponymic description of.*

**Lung carcinoma, diagnosis of,
by x-rays — 1905**

MAX OTTEN, German physician, 1877-19??, is believed to have been the first to diagnose primary carcinoma of the lung by use of roentgen rays. Published in 1905.

Lung decortication in treatment of empyema

EDMOND DELORME, French surgeon, 1847-1929, introduced decortication of the lung as treatment for chronic empyema. Published in 1894.

**Lung, extirpation of, for
tuberculosis**

WILLIAM MACEWEN, Scottish surgeon, 1848-1924, excised the left lung of a tuberculous patient, on April 24, 1895. The patient was reported alive as late as 1940.

Lung, massive collapse of

WILLIAM PASTEUR, English physician, 1856-1943, was the first to describe massive collapse of the lung. Published in 1908.

**Lung, total removal of; first
reported case**

EVARTS AMBROSE GRAHAM, American surgeon, 1883-19??, with JACOB JESSE SINGER, successfully removed the entire lung for carcinoma of the bronchus. Recorded in 1933.

**Lungs of newborn will float
if respiration took place**

JAN SWAMMERDAM, Dutch physician and naturalist, 1637-1680, discovered that the lungs of newborn infants will float on water if respiration took place after birth. This is an important finding in medical jurisprudence. Recorded in 1667.

Lungs

. . . See also under name of particular condition affecting the lungs.

**Lupus erythematosus, eponymic
description of**

PIERRE LOUIS ALPHÉE CAZENAVE, French dermatologist, 1795-1877, described lupus erythematosus, in 1850. Known as *Cazenave's lupus.*

**Lupus erythematosus, first
complete description of**

LAURENT THEODORE BIETT, Swiss physician working in France, 1781-1840, gave the first adequate description of lupus erythematosus. Reported in 1828. Known as *Biett's disease.*

**Lupus, first use of radium
in treatment of**

. . . See under *Tuberculous disease of skin,* etc.

Lupus pernio, early description of

. . . See under *Sarcoidosis.*

**Lupus, use of calciferol in
treatment of—1943**

JACQUES CHARPY, French dermatologist, 19??- , introduced calciferol in the treatment of tuberculosis of the skin. First reported in 1943. Another report about the use of large doses of vitamin D-2 appeared in 1946.

Lupus, use of calciferol in treatment of—1945

GEOFFREY BARROW DOWLING, English physician, 1891-   , and EBENEZER WILLIAM PROSSER THOMAS, introduced the use of calciferol in the treatment of lupus independently of JACQUES CHARPY, whose work was obscured by wartime occupation of France. Published in 1945.

Lupus verrucosus, first description of

RENÉ T. H. LAENNEC, French physician, 1781-1826, is credited with giving the first description of lupus verrucosus. Recorded in 1819.

Lupus vulgaris erythematoides, eponymic description of

HENRI CAMILLE C. LELOIR, French dermatologist, 1855-1896, described lupus vulgaris erythematoides (erythematodes), in 1890. Known as *Leloir's disease*.

Luschka's bursa

. . . See under *Bursa, pharyngeal, in infants.*

Luschka's cartilage

. . . See under *Vocal cord, cartilaginous nodule in.*

Luschka's foramen

. . . See under *Ventricle of brain, fourth, lateral openings of.*

Luschka's glands

. . . See under *Gallbladder, glands or tubular structures in wall of.*

Lutembacher's complex

. . . See under *Mitral stenosis associated with defects of interatrial septum.*

Luys' nucleus

. . . See under *Subthalamic nucleus, eponymic description of.*

Luy's segregator

. . . See under *Instrument for collecting urine from each kidney separately—1904.*

Lymph canaliculi in connective tissue

FRIEDRICH DANIEL VON RECKLINGHAUSEN, German pathologist, 1833-1910, described small lymph channels in the connective tissue, regarded as the terminal branches of the lymphatic vessels. Recorded in 1862. Known as *Recklinghausen's canals*.

Lymph formation, theory of, by diffusion—1849

FRIEDRICH WILHELM NOLL, German physiologist, 17??-1862, proposed a theory which holds that lymph is formed by diffusion of fluids from the blood through the vessel walls. Published in 1849.

Lymph nodes near pancreas, discovery of

GASPARO ASELLI, Italian anatomist, 1581-1626, discovered a group of lymphatic nodes at the root of the mesentery near the pancreas. Exact date not available. Known as *Aselli's glands* and *Aselli's pancreas*.

Lymph nodes, subdiaphragmatic, description of

DIMITRU GEROTA, Rumanian surgeon, 1867-1939, described the lymphatic route from the mammary glands to the liver or subdiaphragmatic nodes by which cancer of the breast may spread. Reported in 1896. Known as *para-mammary route of Gerota.*

Lymph nodules in mucous membrane of small intestine

JOHANN CONRAD PEYER, Swiss anatomist and naturalist, 1653-1712, described elevated areas composed of lymph nodules in the mucous membrane of the small intestine, chiefly in the ileum. Noted in 1673; published in 1677. Known as *Peyer's patches* or *nodules, aggregate follicles, agminated nodules,* etc. It is believed that the patches had been noted by MARCO AURELIO SEVERINO in 1645.

Lymph spaces in coats of an artery

. . . See under *Artery, spaces in external coat of.*

Lymph vessels, tracing of, from periosteum to cortex

WILLIAM C. CRUIKSHANK, English surgeon, 1745-1800, traced lymph vessels from the periosteum to the cortex of the bone. Reported in 1786.

Lymphadenoma with periodic attacks of pyrexia

PIETER KLAZES PEL, Dutch physician, 1852-1919, described the condition of lymphadenoma characterized by periodic attacks of pyrexia. Recorded in 1885. The same condition was described by WILHELM EBSTEIN (German physician, 1836-

1912) in 1887. Known as *Pel-Ebstein disease.*

Lymphatic system, division of, into superficial and deep

WILLIAM HEWSON, English surgeon, 1739-1774, studied the lymphatics in animals and man, and divided the system into two groups, the superficial and the deep. Reported 1769-1774.

Lymphatics, early recognition of

GASPARO ASELLI, Italian physician and anatomist, 1581-1626, is credited with discovering the lymphatics, under the concept of lacteal vessels. Recorded in 1627.

Lymphatics, valves of; early description

FREDERIK RUYSCH, Dutch anatomist, 1638-1731, described the valves of the lymphatics, in 1665.

Lymphatics, valves of; early discovery

JAN SWAMMERDAM, Dutch physician and naturalist, 1637-1680, discovered the valves of the lymphatics. Recorded in 1664.

Lymphatism; lymphotoxemia; original report on

. . . See under *Status lymphaticus.*

Lymphocytic choriomeningitis, first description of

ARVID JOHAN WALLGREN, Swedish pediatrician, 1889-   , was the first to describe acute lymphocytic choriomeningitis. Published in 1924.

Lymphocytic choriomeningitis, isolation of virus of

CHARLES ARMSTRONG, American physician, 1886-19??, with RALPH

DOUGALL LILLIE, isolated the virus of benign lymphocytic choriomeningitis. Published in 1934.

Lymphocytozoon pallidum

. . . See under *Ross's bodies in syphilis.*

Lymphodermia perniciosa, early description of

MORITZ KAPOSI, Hungarian dermatologist, 1837-1902, described lymphodermia perniciosa, a condition marked by enlargement of the lymph nodes due to leukocythemia. Recorded in 1885.

Lymphogranuloma venereum, causative agent of, is a virus

SVEN CURT ALFRED HELLERSTRÖM, Swedish physician, 1901- , with ERIK WASSÉN, demonstrated that the causative agent of lymphogranuloma inguinale is a virus. Published in 1930.

Lymphogranuloma venereum, complement-fixation test for

CLARA M. MCKEE, American microbiologist, 19??- , with G. W. RAKE and M. F. SHAFFER, developed a method for the diagnosis of lymphogranuloma venereum by a complement-fixation test. Published in 1940.

Lymphogranuloma venereum, cultivation of virus of

JOSEPH T. TAMURA, American microbiologist, 1903- , cultivated the virus of lymphogranuloma inguinale and experimented with its use in therapeutic inoculation. Recorded in 1934.

Lymphogranuloma venereum, first description of

WILLIAM WALLACE, Irish physi-

cian, 1791-1837, is said to have been the first to describe lymphogranuloma venereum, in 1833.

Lymphogranuloma venereum, vesicular test for

CARLOS OTTOLINA, American physician, 19??- , developed a method for the diagnosis of lymphogranuloma inguinale by means of a vesicular test. Published in 1941.

Lymphogranuloma venereum, virus of; first observation of

JOSÉ ANTONIO GAY-PRIETO, Spanish dermatologist, 18??-19??, is credited with being the first to observe the causative organism of lymphogranuloma venereum. Recorded in 1927.

Lymphogranuloma venereum

. . . See also under *Venereal lymphogranuloma.*

Lymphoma, malignant, early description of

CHRISTIAN ALBERT THEODOR BILLROTH, Austrian surgeon, 1829-1894, described a malignant lymphoma, in 1861.

Lymphosarcoma, eponymic description of

HANS KUNDRAT, Austrian physician, 1845-1893, decribed lymphosarcoma and differentiated it from Hodgkin's disease and other diseases of the lymphatic system. Published in 1893. Lymphosarcoma is known as *Kundrat's disease.*

Lyophilization, introduction of

. . . See under *Sera, method of dehydrating.*

**Lysivane in treatment
of parkinsonism**

. . . See under *Parkinsonism*.

**Lysolecithin in normal blood,
discovery of**

BENGT LUDWIG BERGENHEM, Swedish surgeon, 1898-   , with ROBERT SANNO FAHRAEUS, discovered lysolecithin in normal blood. Published in 1936.

**Lysozyme, discovery of,
in body secretions**

ALEXANDER FLEMING, Scottish bacteriologist, 1881-1955, discovered a bacteriolytic enzyme in body secretions, such as saliva, tears, nasal discharge, etc., especially effective against *Micrococcus lysodeikticus*. Recorded in 1932.

Lyster bag

. . . See under *Water bag for sterilizing water in camps,* etc.

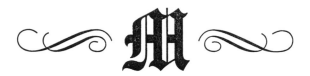

Macewen's triangle, original description of

WILLIAM MACEWEN, Scottish surgeon, 1848-1924, described a surgical triangle situated between the lower posterior edge of the root of the zygoma and the superior posterior edge of the external auditory meatus. Recorded in 1893. Known also as the *suprameatal triangle*.

Mackenrodt's ligament, eponymic description of

ALWIN KARL MACKENRODT, German gynecologist, 1859-1925, described a number of fibrous bands extending from the lower portion of the broad ligament to the supravaginal part of the cervix uteri. Recorded in 1895. Known as *cardinal ligament, uterosacral ligament,* and *cervicopelvic ligament*.

Macula lutea, earliest description of

EDME MARIOTTE, French scientist, 1620-1684, is credited with being first to describe the macula lutea, *circa* 1668.

Macula lutea, early description of

SAMUEL THOMAS SOEMMERRING, German anatomist, 1755-1830, gave the first full description of the macula lutea. Observations made in 1791; recorded 1795-98. Known as *Soemmerring's spot*.

Macula lutea, white dots seen above; Gunn's dots

ROBERT MARCUS GUNN, English ophthalmologist, 1850 - 1909, described certain white dots seen above or around the macula lutea on oblique or special illumination. Reported in 1883.

Maculopapular erythroderma, eponymic description of

JOSEF JADASSOHN, German dermatologist, 1863-1936, gave an accurate description of maculopapular erythroderma, in 1892. Known as *Jadassohn's disease*.

Maddox rod or rods

. . . See under *Heterophoria, glass rods for measuring degree of*.

Madelung's deformity

. . . See under *Wrist deformity caused by distortion of radius*.

Madura foot, early description of

GEORGE BALLINGALL, English surgeon, 1780-1855, gave an early description of maduromycosis or madura foot, probably in 1818. Known as *Ballingall's disease*.

Madura root, good description of

HENRY VANDYKE CARTER, English

physician in India, 1831-1897, gave the first adequate description of madura foot or maduromycosis, in 1861-74.

Madura foot

. . . See also under *Streptothrix madurae*.

Maggot cage, invention of

SAMUEL WILLIAM SIMMONS, American entomologist, 1907-   , devised a cage for the use in applying maggots to infected wounds. Published in 1932.

Maggots, early use of, on wounds

DOMINIQUE JEAN LARREY, French army surgeon, 1766-1842, is credited with being the first to recognize the therapeutic value of maggots in treating infected wounds. Recorded in 1812.

Maggots in treatment of osteomyelitis

WILLIAM S. BAER, American orthopedist, 1872-1931, described the treatment of chronic osteomyelitis with larvae of the bluebottle fly. Recorded in 1931.

Magnesium, indispensability of, in diet

HARRY DAYTON KRUSE, American biochemist, 1900-   , with E. R. ORENT and E. V. McCOLLUM, demonstrated that magnesium is essential to well-being. Recorded in 1932.

Magnesium, isolation of, in metallic state

ROBERT W. BUNSEN, German chemist, 1811-1899, was the first to obtain magnesium in the metallic state and to study its properties, *circa* 1849.

Magnesium salts, anesthetic effect of

JOHN AUER, American physician, 1875-1948, with SAMUEL J. MELTZER (American physiologist, 1851-1920) demonstrated the anesthetic properties of magnesium, in 1906.

Magnesium sulfate

. . . See under *Epsom Salt, description of*.

Magnet for removing metallic particles from eye—1605

WILHELM FABRY (Fabricius Hildanus), German surgeon, 1560-1634, used a magnet to extract iron and steel particles from the eye, *circa* 1605. The method is said to have been suggested to Fabry by his wife.

Magnet for removing metallic particles from eye—1902

OTTO HAAB, Swiss ophthalmologist, 1850-1931, invented a strong magnet used to extract magnetophilic particles from the eye. Reported in 1902. Known as *Haab's magnet*.

Magnetic field, effect of, on polarized light

. . . See under *Polarized light*.

Majocchi's disease

. . . See under *Purpura annularis telangiectodes*.

Maladie de Roger

. . . See under *Ventricles, communication between, abnormal*.

Malaria, atabrine (atebrine) in treatment of

WALTHER KIKUTH, German biochemist, 1896-   , introduced quinacrine hydrochloride (*atabrine, mepacrine,* etc.) in the treatment of malaria. Recorded in 1932.

Malaria carriers, demonstration of existence of

CHARLES F. CRAIG, American pathologist, 1872-1950, demonstrated the existence of malaria carriers, *circa* 1905.

Malaria, complete life cycle of parasite of bird

RONALD ROSS, English pathologist and parasitologist, 1857-1932, demonstrated the last link in the life cycle of the parasite of avian malaria when he discovered, on July 9, 1898, that mosquitoes which fed on infected birds and allowed the parasites to develop and localize in their salivary glands were able, upon stinging healthy birds, to transmit the disease. Published in 1898.

Malaria, control of, in Panama Canal zone

WILLIAM CRAWFORD GORGAS, American Army surgeon, 1854-1920, directed the antimalaria campaign in Panama during the building of the Panama Canal. In charge from 1904 to 1913.

Malaria, first lengthy account of

ADRIAN VAN DER SPIEGHEL, Belgian anatomist, 1578-1625, is credited with presenting the first full account of malaria. Published in 1624.

Malaria, first publication on cinchona in treatment of

PEDRO BARBA, Spanish physician, 1608-1671, wrote the first treatise on cinchona bark and its applica-

tion in the treatment of malaria. Published in 1642.

Malaria, introduction of term

FRANCESCO TORTI, Italian physician and pharmacologist, 1658-1741, is credited with the introduction of the term *malaria,* about 1690. Recorded in 1718. The term is based on the Italian *mala aria,* bad air, in allusion to the belief held at the time that the disease is caused by noxious exhalations of marshes. The word is said to have been introduced in the English language by Horace Walpole, in 1740.

Malaria is caused by a parasite, early suggestion that

JOHN KEARSLEY MITCHELL, American physician, 1793-1858, studied the theory that malaria is caused by a parasite. Published in 1849. The theory was suggested earlier, in 1844, by HENSINGER.

Malaria is transmitted by mosquitoes, early suggestion that

GIOVANNI MARIA LANCISI, Italian physician, 1654 - 1720, suggested that malaria is transmitted by mosquitoes but he assumed the causative agent to be a poison emanating from marshes. Recorded in 1717.

Malaria is transmitted by mosquitoes, proof that

RONALD ROSS, English pathologist, 1857-1932, was the first to prove that malaria is transmitted by mosquitoes. He demonstrated the *Plasmodium* in the stomach of a mosquito which fed on the blood of a malaria patient. Recorded in 1897.

Malaria, plasmoquine in treatment of

W. ROEHL, German parasitologist,

189?-   , introduced pamaquine naphthoate (*plasmoquine, plasmocide,* etc.) in the treatment of malaria. Reported in 1926.

Malaria, proguanil in treatment of

FRANCIS HENRY SWINTON CURD, English biochemist, 1909-1948, with D. G. DAVEY and F. L. ROSE, synthesized proguanil (*paludrine*) and tested it in the treatment of avian malaria. Recorded in 1945.

Malarial fever in treatment of paralytic dementia

JULIUS WAGNER VON JAUREGG, Austrian physician, 1857-1940, was the first to use fever therapy, inoculation with malarial parasites, in the treatment of dementia paralytica, in 1887. Having abandoned the method for about 30 years, Wagner reintroduced it in 1917. He received the Nobel prize in 1927.

Malarial parasite, differentiation of quartan from tertian

CAMILLO GOLGI, Italian histologist, 1844-1926, is credited with distinguishing between the quartan and tertian malarial parasites, in 1889.

Malarial parasite, early name of

CHARLES LOUIS ALPHONSE LAVERAN, French army physician and bacteriologist, 1845-1922, the man who discovered the malarial parasite, introduced the name *Oscillaria malariae* for the organism which he and ETTORE MARCHIAFAVA later designated *Plasmodium malariae.* Recorded in 1880.

Malarial parasite goes through sexual phase only in mosquito

GIOVANNI BATTISTA GRASSI, Italian

pathologist, 1854-1925, with AMICO BIGNAMI, Italian physician, 1862-1929, showed that the parasite causing malaria goes through the sexual phase of its life cycle only in the *Anopheles* mosquito. Published in 1899.

Malarial parasite, quartan, early description of

CAMILLO GOLGI, Italian histologist, 1844-1926, described the development of the quartan malarial parasite. Recorded in 1886.

Malarial parasites, first accurate description of

ETTORE MARCHIAFAVA, Italian pathologist, 1847-1935, gave the first accurate description of the malarial *Plasmodium,* in 1885.

Malarial parasites in blood cells, discovery of—1880

CHARLES LOUIS ALPHONSE LAVERAN, French army surgeon and bacteriologist, 1845-1922, discovered the malarial parasites in the blood cells of patients, in 1880. Report published in 1881.

Malarial parasites, mode of conjugation of

WILLIAM GEORGE MACCALLUM, Baltimore pathologist, 1874-1944, studied the mode of conjugation of the malarial parasites in birds and obtained the flagellate forms. Recorded in 1897.

Malarial parasites, sexual conjugation of

EUGENE LINDSAY OPIE, Baltimore pathologist, 1873-19??, proved sexual conjugation in malarial parasites. Published in 1898.

Malarial paroxysms are related to sporulation of parasites

CAMILLO GOLGI, Italian histologist and neurologist, 1844-1926, demonstrated that malarial paroxysms are concurrent with the sporulation of the parasites. Recorded in 1886.

Malassezia furfur; Malassezia tropica; Microsporon furfur

. . . See under *Pityriasis versicolor, causative organism of.*

Male sex hormone, androsterone, isolaton of

. . . See under *Androsterone.*

Male sex hormone, first active extract of—1927

LEMUEL CLYDE McGEE, American biochemist, 1902-   , is credited with being first to extract the active principle of the male sex hormone from the lipoid fraction of bull testes. Published in 1927.

Male sex hormone, first potent extract of—1929

CARL RICHARD MOORE, American zoologist, 1892-   , with T. F. GALLAGHER and F. C. KOCH, isolated the first potent testicular extract containing the male sex hormone (androsterone, testosterone). Published in 1929.

Male sex hormone, first use of

. . . See under *Testicular extract, early use of.*

Malignant granuloma

. . . See under *Hodgkin's disease, eponymic description of.*

Malingering, first treatise on

GIAMBATTISTA SILVATICO, Italian physician, 1550-1621, is credited with the writing of the first treatise on feigning illness, in 1595.

Mallein test for glanders

. . . See under *Glanders, mallein test for.*

Malleomyces pseudomallei

. . . See under *Pfeifferella whitmori.*

Malleus, anterior ligament of; early description—1600

GIULIO CASSERIO, Italian anatomist, 1561-1616, gave the first description of the anterior ligament of the malleus. Reported in 1600.

Malleus, anterior ligament of; early description—1869

HERMANN L. F. VON HELMHOLTZ, German physiologist and physicist, 1821-1894, described the anterior ligament of the malleus, in 1869. He considered the anterior and posterior ligaments as an "axial ligament" of the malleus.

Malleus, anterior process of; discovery of

CECILIO FOLLI, Italian anatomist, 1615-1660, described a delicate process arising from the anterior aspect of the neck of the malleus and attached to the petrous portion of the temporal bone. Reported in 1645. Known as the *Folian process.*

Malleus, discovery of

ALESSANDRO ACHILLINI, Italian anatomist, 1463-1512, is thought to be the discoverer of the malleus of the middle ear. Exact date unknown.

Mall's formula

. . . See under *Embryo, human, formula for estimating age of.*

Malocclusion of teeth, braces for

JOHN HUNTER, Scottish surgeon in England, 1728 - 1793, introduced the use of braces for the correction of dental malocclusion. Recorded in 1778.

Malocclusion of teeth, classification of

EDWARD HARTLEY ANGLE, American dentist, 1855-1930, devised a standard classification of the various types of malocclusion. Recorded in 1887. Known as *Angle's Classification of Malocclusion*.

Malocclusion of teeth, early methods for correction of

JOSEPH FOX, English surgeon and dentist, 1776-1816, was the first to formulate clear directions for the correction of malocclusion and other dental irregularities. Published in 1803.

Malpighian body

. . . See under *Kidney, glomerular tuft of.*

Malpighian corpuscle

. . . See under *Kidney, corpuscle of.* See also under *Spleen, corpuscle of.*

Malpighian layer

. . . See under *Epidermis, lowest layers of,* etc.

Malpighian pyramid

. . . See under *Kidney, pyramid of; eponymic description.*

Malta fever, agglutination test for

ALMROTH EDWARD WRIGHT, English pathologist and bacteriologist, 1861-1947, with D. SEMPLE, developed an agglutination test for Malta fever, i.e., for *Brucella melitensis* or *Micrococcus melitensis*. Recorded in 1897.

Malta fever, causative agent of

DAVID BRUCE, British pathologist and bacteriologist, 1855-1931, discovered the causative agent of Malta fever, *Micrococcus* or *Brucella melitensis*, in 1886.

Malta fever, differentiation of, from other fevers

JEFFERY ALLEN MARSTON, English physician, 1831-1911, is credited with differentiating Malta fever from other fevers. Recorded in 1863.

Malta fever organism is discharged in urine

A commission appointed in 1904 to investigate Malta fever discovered that the causative organism leaves the body of the patient mainly in the urine, and that it is capable of surviving outside of the body for a long time. Recorded *circa* 1905.

Malta fever organism, presence of, in blood from spleen

DAVID BRUCE, British pathologist and bacteriologist, 1855-1931, demonstrated the causative organism of Malta fever in blood aspirated from the spleen of a patient. Recorded in 1891.

Malta fever, reproduction of, in monkeys

DAVID BRUCE, British pathologist and bacteriologist, 1855-1931, cultivated the causative organism of Malta fever and reproduced the disease in monkeys by inoculation. Recorded in 1887.

Malthusianism

. . . See under *Population increases faster than food supply.*

Mammalian ovum, discovery of

. . . See under *Ovum of mammals.*

Mammalian ovum, segmentation of

. . . See under *Segmentation of mammalian ovum.*

Mammary cancer incidence in mice reduced by oophorectomy

LEO LOEB, American pathologist, 1869-19??, demonstrated that the incidence of hereditary mammary cancer in mice was reduced by oophorectomy. Published in 1919.

Mammillothalamic tract, eponymic description of

FÉLIX VICQ D'AZYR, French anatomist, 1748-1794, described a bundle of fibers extending from the mammillary body to the anterior nucleus of the thalamus. Published in 1781. Known as *bundle of Vicq d'azyr.*

Mandelic acid in urinary infections

MAX LEONARD ROSENHEIM, English physician, 1908-   , introduced the use of mandelic acid in the treatment of urinary infections. Recorded in 1935.

Mandible, bandage for use in fracture of

KASSON C. GIBSON, American dentist, 1849-1925, devised a special bandage for use in fracture of the mandible, to hold the fragments in place. Known as *Gibson's bandage.* Introduced *circa* 1895.

Mandible, wire splint in fracture of

. . . See under *Wire splint.*

Manic-depressive psychosis, early description of—1854

JEAN PIERRE FALRET, French psychiatrist, 1794-1870, presented an early description of manic-depressive psychosis, in 1854. Known also as *cyclic* or *circular insanity.*

Manic-depressive psychosis, introduction of concept of

EMIL KRAEPELIN, German psychiatrist, 1856-1926, is credited with introducing the psychiatric concept of manic-depressive psychosis, *circa* 1879.

Mann-Williamson ulcer

. . . See under *Ulcer, peptic, experimental production of.*

Manometer, early form of

STEPHEN HALES, English physiologist and clergyman, 1677-1761, devised a simple manometer the early form of which was a glass tube inserted into the artery of the subject. The pressure was estimated on the basis of the height of the blood column. The first experiments were performed in 1705.

Manometer, mercury, introduction of

. . . See under *Hemodynamometer, mercury,* etc.

Manometer

. . . See also under *Sphygmomanometer, Blood Pressure,* etc.

Manson's schistosomiasis

. . . See under *Schistosomiasis, intestinal.*

Mantoux's test

. . . See under *Tuberculin test, intradermal*.

Map of human cortex

KORBINIAN BRODMANN, German neurologist, 1868-1918, prepared a map of the human cortex designating 52 distinct regions. Published in 1908.

Mapharsen, introduction of, as antiluetic

ARTHUR LEWIS TATUM, American pharmacologist, 1884-19??, with GARRETT ARTHUR COOPER, introduced mapharsen, in 1934.

March foot, description of—1855

GUSTAV BREITHAUPT, German physician, 1812-18??, described march foot, in 1855.

March foot, description of—1887

JEAN EUGÈNE PAUZAT, French physician, 1842-1909, described march foot, in 1887.

March foot, description of—1921

CARL E. W. DEUTSCHLANDER, German surgeon, 1872-1942, gave a complete description of march foot, a condition marked by painful swelling of the forefoot and, usually, fracture of one or more metacarpal bones. It often follows foot strain incident to marching. Reported in 1921. Known as *Deutschlander's disease*.

March hemoglobinuria, first description of

RICHARD FLEISCHER, German physician, 1848-1909, gave the first description of hemoglobinuria following physical exertion, as in soldiers after a march. Published in 1881.

Marchi's method

. . . See under *Myelin sheaths, degenerating, staining of*.

Marfan's disease

. . . See under *Progressive spastic paraplegia in children with hereditary syphilis*.

Marfan's syndrome

. . . See under *Arachnodactyly with ectopia of crystalline lens*.

Marginal bundle, of Lissauer

. . . See under *Dorsolateral tract; marginal tract*.

Marie's ataxia

. . . See under *Hereditary cerebellar sclerosis*.

Marie's syndrome

. . . See *Acromegaly, classic description of*.

Marmorization of bone

. . . See under *Osteopetrosis*.

Marriages of consanguinity in relation to degeneration

JOHN L. H. DOWN, English physician, 1828-1896, wrote a treatise on the degeneration of race resulting from marriages of consanguinity. Published in 1866.

Marshall's vein

. . . See under *Vein, oblique, of Marshall*.

Martinotti's cells

. . . See under *Cells in cerebral cortex with ascending axons*.

Mask, surgical, introduction of

PAUL BERGER, French surgeon, 1845-1908, introduced the use of the gauze face mask, in October 1897.

Mass action, chemical, law of

PETER WAAGE, Norwegian chemist, 1833-1900, with C. M. GULDBERG, discovered the chemical law of mass action, in 1867.

Massive collapse of lung

. . . See under *Lung, massive collapse of.*

Mastoiditis, first clear description of

FRIEDRICH BEZOLD, German otologist, 1842-1908, is credited with the first adequate description of mastoiditis, in 1877.

Mastoiditis, first modern operation for

ANTON FRIEDRICH VON TRÖLTSCH, German otologist, 1829-1890, is credited with devising the first modern mastoid operation. Recorded in 1861.

Mastoiditis, first operation for, in England

JAMES HINTON, English surgeon, 1822-1875, performed the first operation for mastoiditis in England, in 1868.

Mastoiditis, first successful operation for

JEAN LOUIS PETIT, French surgeon, 1674-1750, is credited with performing the first successful operation for mastoiditis, in 1736.

Materia medica, founder of ancient

PEDANIOS DIOSCORIDES, Greek medical writer, first century A.D., prepared a work which Galen called the "most perfect treatise on materia medica." He is considered to be the founder of ancient materia medica.

Maternal and fetal circulations, recognition of separate nature of

WILLIAM HUNTER, Scottish surgeon and obstetrician, 1718-1783, is credited with discovering the separate nature of the maternal and fetal circulations, *circa* 1762. Reported in 1774.

Mauchart's ligaments

. . . See under *Odontoid ligaments, lateral.*

Maunoir's hydrocele

. . . See under *Hydrocele, cervical, eponymic description of.*

Mauthner's sheath; axilemma of Mauthner

. . . See under *Axilemma, eponymic description of.*

Maxillary nerve, excision of, for relief of facial neuralgia

JOHN MURRAY CARNOCHAN, American surgeon, 1817-1887, was the first to excise the maxillary nerve for relief of severe neuralgia of the face. Reported in 1858.

Maxillary sinus disease, relief of, by an auxiliary opening—1889

HENRI LUC, French laryngologist, 1855-1925, devised an operative procedure for the treatment of severe disorders of the maxillary sinus in which an additional opening is provided for the sinus in the anterior wall through a supradental fossa. Published in 1889. Known as the *Caldwell-Luc operation.*

Maxillary sinus disease, relief of, by an auxiliary opening—1893

GEORGE WALTER CALDWELL, American surgeon, 1866-1946, devised an operative procedure for the treatment of severe disorders of the maxillary sinus in which an auxiliary opening is provided for the sinus in the anterior wall through the canine fossa. Published in 1893. Known as *Caldwell-Luc operation.*

Maxillary sinus, early description of

GIULIO CASSERIO, Italian anatomist, 1561-1616, gave one of the earliest descriptions of the maxillary sinus. Recorded *circa* 1600.

Maxillary sinus, first operation for tumor in

JULES PLAIGNAUD, French surgeon, 1741-1806, is said to have performed the first successful operation for the excision of a tumor in the maxillary sinus, in 1789. Recorded in 1791.

Maxillary sinus, irrigation of, through natural orifice

ANSELME LOUIS BERNARD BERCHILLET JOURDAIN, French surgeon, 1734-1816, devised a method for washing the maxillary sinus through its passage in the middle meatus of the nose. Published in 1767.

Mazzini test for syphilis

. . . See under *Syphilis, microscopic flocculation test for.*

McBurney's incision

. . . See under *Appendectomy, incision for, in which muscles are separated by blunt dissection.*

McBurney's point

. . . See under *Appendicitis, point of special tenderness in.*

McDonald's solution

. . . See under *Solution for hand sterilization containing orthophenylphenate.*

McDowell's operation

. . . See under *Ovariectomy, early successful—1809.*

McLean's formula or index

. . . See under *Urea excretion index; McLean's formula.*

Measles, convalescent serum in; first use

F. CENCI, Italian physician, 1874-19??, was the first to use convalescent serum in the prophylaxis of measles. Recorded in 1907.

Measles, differentiation of, from scarlet fever

THOMAS SYDENHAM, English physician, 1624-1689, was one of the first to differentiate measles from scarlet fever. Recorded *circa* 1661.

Measles, experimental transmission of, in animals

ALBERT HENRI LOUIS JOSIAS, French physician, 1852-1906, transmitted measles to and in animals. Recorded in 1898.

Measles, experimental transmission of, in man

FRANCIS HOME, Scottish physician, 1719-1813, was the first to record experiments with transmission of measles, in man. Published in 1759.

Measles, Faroe Islands epidemic of

PETER LUDVIG PANUM, Danish physiologist, 1820-1885, made noteworthy studies of the epidemic of measles in the Faroe Islands, in 1846.

Measles, Koplik spots in

HENRY KOPLIK, New York pediatrician, 1858-1927, described the small red spots surrounded by a white area seen on the buccal mucous membrane in the prodromal stage of measles. Reported in 1896. Known as *Koplik's sign* or *spots*.

Measles, reproduction of, with blood taken from measles patients

LUDVIG HEKTOEN, American pathologist, 1863-1951, reproduced measles in man with blood taken from measles patients early in the disease. Reported in 1905.

Measles, transmission of, to monkeys

JOSEPH GOLDBERGER, American pathologist, 1874-1929, with J. F. ANDERSON, transmitted measles to monkeys, in 1910.

Measles, transmission of, to monkeys

JOHN F. ANDERSON, American physician, 1873-19??, with JOSEPH GOLDBERGER, successfully transmitted measles to monkeys. Recorded in 1911.

Measles virus, cultivation of—1938

HARRY PLOTZ, American physician

and bacteriologist, 1890-1947, successfully cultivated the measles virus in vitro. Recorded in 1938.

Meat diet, exclusive, in diabetes

ARNOLDO CANTANI, Italian physician, 1837-1893, suggested an exclusive meat diet for diabetics. Reported *circa* 1876. Known as *Cantani's diet*.

Mechanistic theory of life, promulgation of

JACQUES LOEB, American biologist, 1859-1924, proposed the mechanistic theory of life which holds that the male nucleus is not essential to the process of fertilization. The theory also holds that fertilization may be effected by chemical stimulation. Published in 1909.

Mecholyl chloride, introduction of

. . . See under *Methacholine chloride*, etc.

Meckel's cartilage

. . . See under *Cartilage of first branchial arch*, etc.

Meckel's cavity or cave

JOHANN FRIEDRICH MECKEL, German anatomist, 1714-1774, described a space or cavity between the two layers of the dura mater over the petrous portion of the temporal bone. It contains the trigeminal ganglion. Recorded in 1748.

Meckel's diverticulum

. . . See under *Diverticulum of ileum derived from persistent yolk stalk*.

Meckel's ganglion

. . . See under *Sphenopalatine ganglion, eponymic description of*.

**Medial lemniscus, connec-
tions of, with thalamus**

FREDERICK WALTER MOTT, English neurologist, 1853-1926, is credited with demonstrating the thalamic connections of the medial lemniscus or fillet. Recorded in 1886.

**Mediastinum testis, eponymic
description of**

NATHANIEL HIGHMORE, English
physician and anatomist, 1613-
1685, described the mediastinum
testis, the partial septum dividing
the testicle, in 1651. Known as
*body of Highmore, corpus highmo-
rianum.*

**Medical bibliography, first
attempt to produce a
systematic**

JAMES DOUGLAS, Scottish anatomist and obstetrician, 1675-1742,
made the first attempt to compile a
systematic bibliography of medical
literature, in 1715.

**Medical dictionary, first com-
plete, in United States**

ROBLEY DUNGLISON, American
physician and physiologist, 1798-
1869, was the author of the first
complete medical dictionary in the
United States. Published in 1833.

**Medical dictionary, first, to be
printed in the British Isles**

STEPHAN BLANKAART, Dutch physician, 1650-1702, wrote a medical
dictionary which was translated
into English and was the first one
to be published in the British Isles,
in 1684.

**Medical dictionary in re-
verse—from meaning
to word**

JAKOB EDWARD SCHMIDT, Ameri-

can physician and lexicographer,
1905-   , wrote the first medical
dictionary in which the *meanings*—
not the *words*—are listed in alphabetical order. This arrangement
enables the user to find a word on
the basis of its meaning, i.e., the
thought or concept it represents.
Titled *Reversicon: A Medical
Word Finder.* Published in 1958.

Medical dictionary of slang

. . . See under *Medical slang, first
dictionary of.*

**Medical document, oldest,
discovery of**

GEORG MORITZ EBERS, German
Egyptologist, 1837-1898, discovered a papyrus containing a record
of Egyptian medicine, in 1872. It
is the oldest medical document in
the world, *circa* 1502 B.C., and is
known as the *Ebers papyrus.*

**Medical ethics, early
discourse on**

SAMUEL BARD, American physician, 1742-1821, wrote a discourse
on the duties of a physician. Published in 1769.

Medical historian, first, of note

AULUS CORNELIUS CELSUS, Roman
physician and author, *circa* 53
B.C.-7 A.D., is considered to be
the first medical historian of importance. His *De Medicina* is the oldest medical document, with the ex-
ception of the writings of Hippocrates and the Ebers paryrus. The
manuscript was not discovered until 1443.

**Medical journal, first,
published in Paris**

NICOLAUS DE BLEGNY, French physician, 1652-1722, was the pub-

lisher of the first medical journal in Paris, in 1679.

Medical jurisprudence, early work on

FORTUNATO FELDI, Italian physician, 1550-1630, wrote an early work on medical jurisprudence, in 1602.

Medical literature, introduction of *Consilia* in

... See under *Clinical records, collections of*.

Medical slang, first dictionary of

JAKOB EDWARD SCHMIDT, American physician and lexicographer, 1905-   , wrote the first medical dictionary devoted to the slang and esoteric expressions of the medical and related professions. Titled *Dictionary of Medical Slang*. Published in 1959.

Medical statistics, pioneer in

JOHN GRAUNT, English haberdasher and train-band captain, 1620-1674, gave the first clear insight into the subject of life expectancy, in a work titled *Natural and Political Observations on the Bills of Mortality*. Published in 1661. Graunt recognized the principle of uniformity in large groups of vital and social facts. He prepared the earliest table of mortality.

Medionecrosis of aorta, classic description of

JAKOB ERDHEIM, Austrian physician, 1874-1937, gave a classic description of a condition marked by necrosis of the tunica media of the aorta, occasionally ending in rupture. Published in 1929.

Medulla oblongata, external arcuate fibers of

LUIGI ROLANDO, Italian anatomist, 1773-1831, described the external arcuate fibers of the medulla oblongata, in 1809. Known as *Rolando's fibers*.

Medulla oblongata, funiculus of

LUIGI ROLANDO, Italian anatomist, 1773-1831, described a longitudinal elevation on both sides of the lower part of the medulla oblongata. Recorded in 1809. Known as *Funiculus of Rolando*.

Medulla oblongata, solitary fasciculus of

BENEDICT STILLING, German anatomist, 1810-1879, described the solitary fasciculus of the medulla oblongata, in 1843. Known as *Stilling's bundle*.

Megacolon, congenital, eponymic description of

HARALD HIRSCHSPRUNG, Danish physician, 1830-1916, described congenital megacolon, congenital hypertrophic dilatation of the colon, in 1888. Known as *Hirschsprung's disease*.

Megakaryocytes in platelet formation

... See under *Blood platelets, megakaryocytes in formation of*.

Meglin's point

... See under *Point at which palatine nerve emerges from palatine foramen*.

Meibomian cyst; chalazion

The condition known as chalazion or *Meibomian cyst* was not discovered by HEINRICH MEIBOM, but was known to the physicians of antiquity. It was mentioned by both Hippocrates and Galen. The term is merely an allusion to the Meibomian glands, which Meibom described but did not discover. Introduced *circa* 1666.

Meibomian glands

... See under *Glands between tarsus and conjunctiva of eyelid.*

Meige's disease

... See under *Hereditary edema of the legs—1899.*

Meigs's capillaries

... See under *Heart, capillaries in muscle fibers of.*

Meigs's syndrome

... See under *Fibroma of ovary with ascites and hydrothorax.*

Meissner's corpuscles

... See under *Tactile nerve endings in tips of fingers and toes.*

Meissner's nerve plexus

... See under *Nerve plexus, submucous, of alimentary tract.*

Melanosis lenticularis progressiva

... See under *Xeroderma pigmentosum, eponymic description of.*

Melioidosis, eponymic description of

ALFRED WHITMORE, English surgeon in Indian Medical Service, 1876-1946, with C. S. KRISHNASWAMI, gave the first description of melioidosis, a glanders-like disease of rodents transmissible to man. Recorded in 1912. Known as *Whitmore's disease.*

Meltzer's method of intratracheal anesthesia

... See under *Anesthesia by intratracheal insufflation.*

Membrane, basement, discovery and naming of

... See under *Basement membrane.*

Membrane, Bowman's

... See under *Lamina, anterior elastic.*

Membrane, vestibular, of cochlea

ERNST REISSNER, German anatomist, 1824-1878, described the vestibular membrane of the cochlea. Recorded in 1851. Known as *Reissner's membrane.*

Membranous labyrinth, small canal leading from, to saccule

VIKTOR HENSEN, German pathologist, 1835-1924, described the *ductus reuniens,* a small canal extending from the saccule of the ear to the membranous labyrinth. Recorded in 1902. Known as *Hensen's duct* or *canal.*

Mendeleeff's law

... See under *Periodic law.*

Mendel's dorsal reflex of the foot

... See under *Toes, dorsal flexion of, when dorsum of foot is tapped.*

Mendel's law

... See under *Inheritance, Mendel's law of.*

Mendel's work, discovery of

HUGO MARIE DE VRIES, Amsterdam botanist, 1848-1935, discovered and confirmed Mendel's work and findings, *circa* 1899. Recorded 1901-3.

Ménière's syndrome; aural vertigo

PROSPER MÉNIÈRE, French otologist, 1799-1862, described a syndrome of deafness, tinnitus, and dizziness, often accompanied by nausea and vomiting, occurring in certain diseases of the internal ear. Published in 1861.

Ménière's syndrome, Charcot's completion of

JEAN MARTIN CHARCOT, French neurologist, 1825-1893, completed the description of the aural vertigo syndrome of Ménière. Recorded in 1874.

Ménière's syndrome, Dandy's operation for relief of

WALTER EDWARD DANDY, Baltimore surgeon, 1886-1946, devised an operation for the relief of Ménière's syndrome. Recorded in 1928.

Meningioma, early operation for removal of

WILLIAM WILLIAMS KEEN, American surgeon, 1837-1932, is credited with the successful removal of a meningioma, in 1888.

Meningitis, Kernig's sign of

VLADIMIR M. KERNIG, Russian neurologist, 1840-1917, discovered that extending the knee while the thigh is flexed at the hip is difficult or painful in case of meningitis. Observed in 1884; published in 1907. Known as *Kernig's sign.*

Meningitis, meningococcus, fulminating type of—1895

ARTHUR FRANCIS VOELCKER, English physician, 1861-1946, described a syndrome of acute collapse associated with hemorrhages in the adrenal glands and usually caused by a fulminating type of meningococcus meningitis. Recorded in 1895. Later called the *Waterhouse-Friderichsen syndrome.*

Meningitis, meningococcus, fulminating type of—1911

RUPERT WATERHOUSE, English physician, 1873-19??, described a syndrome of acute collapse associated with hemorrhages in the adrenal glands, usually observed in severe cases of meningococcus meningitis. Published in 1911. The condition was also described by CARL FRIDERICHSEN (Danish physician, 1886-19??), in 1918. Known as the *Waterhouse-Friderichsen syndrome.*

Meningitis, meningococcus, sulfonamide treatment of

HENRY STANLEY BANKS, English physician, 189?-   , was the first to use the sulfonamide drugs in the treatment of meningococcus meningitis. Recorded in 1939.

Meningitis, tuberculous, early description of

WILLIAM WOOD GERHARD, American physician, 1809-1872, gave the first accurate description of tuberculous meningitis, in 1833.

Meningococcus; *Neisseria meningitidis;* discovery of

ANTON WEICHSELBAUM, Austrian pathologist, 1845-1920, discovered the meningococcus (*Micrococcus meningitidis, Diplococcus intracellularis meningitidis,* etc.), the causative agent of cerebrospinal meningitis. Recorded in 1887. Known also as *Weichselbaum's coccus.*

Menstrual flow result of withdrawal of natural estrogen

EDGAR ALLEN, American anatomist, 1892-1943, with EDWARD

ADELBERT DOISY, American physiologist and biochemist, 1893-19??, demonstrated that the menstrual flow is a withdrawal expression of the endometrium in response to the cessation of estrogen activity in the body. Recorded in 1927.

Menstruation, study of, by intraocular endometrial transplants

JOSEPH ELDRIDGE MARKEE, American anatomist, 1904-   , studied the phenomenon of menstruation by observing the changes in intraocular transplants of endometrium. Also described rhythmic increases in circulation known as the *blush-and-blanch phenomena*. Exact date not available.

Mentagra barbae; Alibert's mentagra

. . . See under *Sycosis barbae, classic description of*.

Mental disorders, modern classification of

EMIL KRAEPELIN, German psychiatrist, 1856-1926, developed a modern classification of mental disorders, *circa* 1883.

Mental hospitals, abandonment of fetters in

VINCENZO CHIARUGI, Italian physician, 1759-1820, is believed to have been the first to discontinue the use of fetters in European mental hospitals, in 1793.

Mental processes, reaction time involved in

. . . See under *Reaction time*.

Mepacrine in treatment of malaria

. . . See under *Malaria*.

Meralgia paraesthetica, description of

MARTIN BERNHARDT, German neurologist, 1844-1915, described meralgia paresthetica, a condition marked by paresthesia in the outer surface of the thigh, or in the region supplied by the external cutaneous femoral nerve. Reported in 1878. Known as *Bernhardt's disease* or *paresthesia*.

Mercier's bar

. . . See under *Trigone of bladder, posterior bar of*.

Mercurial diuretic, first injection of

PAUL SAXL, German physician, 1880-1932, is credited with being first to use a mercurial diuretic (Novasurol) by injection in treating cardiac failure. Recorded in 1920.

Mercuric chloride in antisepsis, introduction of

ERNST VON BERGMANN, German surgeon, 1836-1907, introduced the use of corrosive sublimate in obtaining antisepsis. Recorded in 1887.

Mercuric chloride in treatment of syphilis

. . . See under *Syphilis, treatment of*, etc.

Mercurochrome, introduction of

HUGH HAMPTON YOUNG, Baltimore urologist, 1870-1945, with E. C. WHITE and E. O. SWARTZ, introduced the use of mercurochrome. Reported in 1919.

Mercury-vapor lamp for generation of ultra-violet rays

ERNST L. F. KROMAYER, German

dermatologist, 1862-1933, invented a water-cooled, mercury-vapor lamp provided with a quartz window which permits the passage of the ultraviolet rays. Introduced *circa* 1912. Known as *Kromayer's lamp.*

Merkel's corpuscles

... See under *Tactile nerve endings in submucosa of mouth and tongue.*

Merzbacher-Pelizaeus disease

... See under *Familial centrolobar sclerosis.*

Mesmerism

... See under *Animal magnetism, popularization of.*

Meson, prediction of existence of

HIDEKI YUKAWA, Japanese physicist, 1907-   , is credited with forecasting the existence of a subatomic particle carrying either a positive or a negative electric charge and having a mass intermediate in magnitude between that of a proton and an electron. Received the Nobel prize in 1949.

Mesonephric ridge, eponymic description of

CASPAR FRIEDRICH WOLFF, German anatomist, 1733-1794, described the lateral thickening of the urogenital ridge from which the mesonephros arises, *circa* 1765. Known as *Wolffian ridge.*

Mesonephros, duct of; eponymic description

CASPAR FRIEDRICH WOLFF, German anatomist, 1733-1794, described the duct of the mesonephros. Published in 1759. Known as *Wolffian duct.*

Mesonephros, eponymic description of

CASPAR FRIEDRICH WOLFF, German anatomist, 1733-1794, gave the first clear description of the mesonephros. Published in 1759. Known as *Wolffian body.*

Mesonephros, functional tubules of

CASPAR FRIEDRICH WOLFF, German anatomist, 1733-1794, described the twisting tubules which are the functional units of the mesonephros. Published in 1759. Known as *Wolffian tubules.*

Mesonephros, introduction of term

EDWIN RAY LANKESTER, English zoologist, 1847-1930, is credited with introducing the term *mesonephros,* about 1885.

Mesovarium, line of insertion of

... See under *Ovary, line of insertion of mesovarium in.*

Metabolism proportional to surface area of body

MAX RUBNER, German physiologist, 1854-1932, demonstrated that the total metabolism of the body is proportional to the surface area. Recorded in 1883.

Metacarpus, fracture of, special splint for

DAVID HAYES AGNEW, American surgeon, 1818-1892, invented a special splint for treating fracture of the metacarpus. He also devised a splint for fracture of the patella. Published in 1878.

Metachromatic granules found in bacteria

... See under *Babes-Ernst bodies or corpuscles.*

**Metallic particles in eye,
instrument for removing**

SAMUEL BERMAN, American electrical engineer, 1895-   , devised an apparatus for locating metallic particles in the eye. Date not available.

***Metanephros,* introduction
of term**

EDWIN RAY LANKESTER, English zoologist, 1847-1930, is credited with introducing the term *metanephros,* about 1885.

***Metaphase,* introduction of term**

. . . See under *Mitosis, three stages of.*

***Metastasis,* introduction of term**

JOSEPH CLAUDE ANTHELM RÉCAMIER, French gynecologist and obstetrician, 1774-1852, introduced the term *metastasis* to describe the spread of cancer. Recorded in 1829.

**Metastatic ophthalmia, classic
description of**

KARL THEODOR PAUL POLYKARPOS AXENFELD, German ophthalmologist, 1867-1930, gave a classic description of metastatic ophthalmia, in 1894.

**Metastatic ophthalmia, first
description of**

HEINRICH MECKEL VON HEMSBACH, German physician, 1822-1856, was the first to describe metastatic ophthalmia. Published in 1854.

**Metatarsalgia, anterior,
early description of**

LEWIS DURLACHER, English surgeon-chiropodist, 179?-18??, gave the first recorded description of anterior metatarsalgia, in "A treatise on corns, bunions, the diseases of nails, and the general management of the feet." Published in 1845.

**Metatarsalgia, anterior eponymic
description of**

THOMAS GEORGE MORTON, American surgeon, 1835-1903, gave the first adequate description of anterior metatarsalgia, "a peculiar and painful affection of the fourth metatarso-phalangeal articulation." Published in 1876. Known as *Morton's disease.*

**Metatarsus varus, congenital;
early description**

PHILIPP JAKOB WILHELM HENKE, German anatomist, 1834-1896, described congenital metatarsus varus, in 1863.

**Methacholine chloride,
introduction of**

RANDOLPH THOMAS MAJOR, American chemist, 1901-   , introduced methacholine chloride (mecholyl chloride), in 1932.

**Methemoglobinemia due to
nitrates in water**

HUNTER HALL COMLY, American physician, 1919-   , described methemoglobinemia in infants caused by the presence of nitrates in well water. Published in 1945.

**Methenamine, introduction of,
as urinary antiseptic**

ARTHUR NICOLAIER, German physician, 1862-19??, is credited with introducing methenamine as a urinary antiseptic, in 1894.

Methylene blue, introduction of, as a stain

PAUL EHRLICH, German bacteriologist and pathologist, 1854-1915, introduced methylene blue as a bacterial stain. Recorded in 1881.

Metopion, introduction of, as craniometric point

PIERRE PAUL BROCA, French surgeon and anthropologist, 1824-1880, defined *metopion* as a craniometric point. Date not available.

Metrazol, use of, in schizophrenia

... See under *Schizophrenia, treatment of, with metrazol.*

Metropathia hemorrhagica, first description of

ROBERT SCHROEDER, German gynecologist, 1884-19??, was the first to describe metropathia hemorrhagica, essential uterine bleeding, in 1919.

Meyer's line

... See under *Toe, great, normal line of.*

Meynert's cells, eponymic description of

THEODOR HERMANN MEYNERT, German neurologist and psychiatrist in Austria, 1833-1892, described solitary cells of pyramidal shape in the cerebral cortex near the calcarine fissure. Published in 1868.

Meynert's commissure, eponymic description of

THEODOR HERMANN MEYNERT, German neurologist and psychiatrist in Austria, 1833-1892, described a tract of nerve fibers crossing from the tuber cinereum to the opposite side. Recorded in 1867. Known as *Meynert's commissure.* Known also as *Meynert's radiation* and *fountain decussation.*

Meynert's fasciculus or bundle

... See under *Fasciculus retroflexus.*

Meynert's radiation

... See under *Meynert's commissure.*

Meynet's nodes or nodisities

... See under *Nodules in tendons and capsules of joints, in rheumatic conditions.*

Mibelli's disease No. 1

... See under *Angiokeratoma, eponymic description of.*

Mibelli's disease No. 2

... See under *Porokeratosis, eponymic description of.*

Michaelis's rhomboid, eponymic description of

GUSTAV ADOLPH MICHAELIS, German obstetrician, 1798-1848, described a diamond-shaped area just above the intergluteal cleft, formed by components of the sacrospinalis and gluteus maximus muscles and the dimples of the posterior superior spines of the ilia. Recorded in 1841. Known as *Michaelis's area* or *rhomboid.*

Microcephaly, early reference to

BARTHOLOMAEUS METLINGER, German pediatrician, 14??-1492, recorded the first known reference to microcephaly, in 1473.

Micrococcus albus; Staphylococcus epidermidis albus

WILLIAM HENRY WELCH, American pathologist, 1850-1934, discovered *Staphylococcus epidermidis albus* or *Micrococcus albus* and studied its relation to wound infection. Recorded in 1892.

Micrococcus catarrhalis, discovery of

RICHARD FRIEDRICH JOHANNES PFEIFFER, German bacteriologist, 1858-19??, is credited with discovering the *Micrococcus catarrhalis,* in 1896. Also known as *Neisseria catarrhalis.*

Microglia, discovery of and introduction of term

PIO DEL RIO HORTEGA, Spanish neurologist, 1882-1945, discovered the small neuroglia cells of the central nervous system and named them *microglia.* Recorded in 1921.

Microscope, compound, invention of

ZACHARIAS JANSEN, Dutch lens and spectacle maker, 16th century, is credited with inventing the compound microscope, about 1590.

Microscope condenser for concentrating light upon the object

ERNST KARL ABBE, German physicist and mathematician, 1840-1905, developed and introduced a system of lenses and mirror, attached to the lower end of a microscope, for concentrating light upon the object being observed. He described it in a paper published in 1886. The system of mirror and lenses is known as *Abbe's condenser.*

Microscope lenses, improved achromatic

. . . See under *Achromatic lenses, improved.*

Microscope ocular made of two planoconvex lenses

JESSE RAMSDEN, English astronomical-instrument maker, 1735-1800, devised a microscope eyepiece composed of two planoconvex lenses placed with the convexities apposed. *Circa* 1770. Known as *Ramsden ocular.*

Microscope, phase-contrast, invention of

. . . See under *Phase-contrast microscope.*

Microscope with achromatic lens, first construction of

GIOVANNI BATTISTA AMICI, Italian physicist and astronomer, 1784-1863, is believed to have been the first to construct a microscope having an achromatic lens. Reported in 1818.

Microsporon audouini

. . . See under *Microsporum audouini.*

Microsporon furfur; Malassezia tropica

. . . See under *Pityriasis versicolor, causative organism of.*

Microsporosis nigra

. . . See under *Tinea nigra,* etc.

Microsporum audouini, description of

DAVID GRUBY, French dermatologist, 1810-1898, described the organism *Microsporum audouini,* the causative agent of a form of tinea tonsurans, in 1843.

Microtome, early form of

JOHANNES EVANGELISTA VON PURKINJE, Bohemian physiologist, 1787-1869, is credited with devising and using the earliest form of microtome, *circa* 1830.

Microtome, first practical, introduction of

WILHELM HIS, *père*, Swiss anatomist and embryologist, 1831-1904, is credited with introducing the first satisfactory microtome, *circa* 1865.

Microtome, rotary, introduction of

CHARLES SEDGWICK MINOT, American physician, 1852-1914, is credited with the introduction of the rotary microtome, in 1886.

Microtome, sledge type, introduction of

CHARLES SEDGWICK MINOT, American physician, 1852-1914, introduced the sledge type or sliding microtome, in 1885.

Midbody of nuclear spindle, description of

EDWARD STRASBURGER, German histologist, 1844-1912, described the midbody or cell-plate, a mass of granules developed at the equator of the spindle during the anaphase of mitosis. It forms a dividing septum between the developing daughter cells. Reported *circa* 1884.

Middle ear, bag for inflating

ADAM POLITZER, Austrian otologist, 1835-1920, devised an apparatus or bag for use in inflating the middle ear. Recorded in 1863. Known as *Politzer bag*.

Middle ear, space in attic of

ALEXANDER PRUSSAK, Russian otologist, 1839-1907, described a membranous pouch in the attic of the middle ear, in 1867. Known as *Prussak's space* or *pouch*.

Midwifery, Father of Modern

HENDRIK VAN DEVENTER, Dutch obstetrician, 1651-1724, is regarded as the Father of Modern Midwifery. He is remembered for his studies of the female pelvis.

Migraine, first clear description of

JOHN FOTHERGILL, English physician, 1712-1780, is credited with giving the first accurate description of migraine, under the name of "sick headache." Recorded in 1778.

Migraine, periodic, with paralysis of oculomotor muscles

PAUL JULIUS MOBIUS, German neurologist, 1853-1907, described a form of periodic migraine associated with paralysis of the extraocular muscles of the eye. Published in 1884. Known as *Mobius' disease* and *periodic ophthalmoplegic migraine*.

Mikulicz's cells; foam cells

JOHANN VON MIKULICZ-RADECKI, Rumanian surgeon in Germany, 1850-1905, described large round or oval cells with a small pycnotic nucleus and vacuolated cytoplasm, occurring in rhinoscleroma. Published in 1876.

Mikulicz's disease

... See under *Lacrimal and salivary glands, chronic enlargement of*.

Mikulicz's drain, introduction of

JOHANN VON MIKULICZ-RADECKI, Rumanian surgeon in Germany, 1850-1905, introduced a drain consisting of a layer of gauze pushed into the wound cavity and packed with several thick wicks of gauze. Published in 1881.

Milian's erythema

. . . See under *Arsphenamine erythema, eponymic description of.*

Miliary, first use of term

GASPARD LAURENT BAYLE, French physician, 1774-1816, was the first to use the term *miliary*, probably in 1810.

Miliary tuberculosis, first reference to

MATTHEW BAILLIE, English physician, 1761-1823, was the first to call attention to a miliary type of tuberculosis, in his book on the morbid anatomy of some of the most important parts of the human body, published in 1793.

Military medicine, founder of

JOHN PRINGLE, Scottish physician, 1707-1782, is considered the founder of modern military medicine. He is also said to be the originator of the idea of a Red Cross. He wrote a book on the diseases of the army. Published in 1752.

Milk globules, casein coat surrounding

. . . See under *Casein coat surrounding milk globules.*

Millard-Gubler syndrome

. . . See under *Hemiplegia, alternate, involving lateral rectus muscle, etc.;* also, *Hemiplegia, alternate, early description of—1856.*

Millar's asthma

. . . See under *Laryngismus stridulus.*

Mills's disease

. . . See under *Progressive ascending paralysis or hemiplegia.*

Milroy's disease

. . . See under *Hereditary edema of the legs—1892.*

Mind is controlled by another person or an outside influence, feeling that one's

GATIAN DE CLERAMBAULT, French psychiatrist, 1872-1934, described a neurotic condition in which the patient believes that his mind is controlled by some outside influence or by another person. Known as *Clerambault-Kandinsky complex.* Introduced *circa* 1905.

Minor's disease

. . . See under *Hematomyelia, central, eponymic description of.*

Minor's tremor

. . . See under *Tremor, essential.*

Minot-Murphy diet

. . . See under *Liver in pernicious anemia.*

Minute particles, oscillating movement of

. . . See under *Brownian movement.*

Mirror for inspection of nasopharynx

. . . See under *Nasopharynx, examination of, by means of special mirror.*

Missing link concept, introduction of

EDWARD TYSON, English physician and anatomist, 1649-1708, is credited with introducing the concept of a missing link, in anthropology. He wrote the first important work on comparative morphology. Published in 1699.

Mitochondria, original description of

MARGARET R. LEWIS, American histologist, 18??-19??, with WARREN HARMON LEWIS, gave an original description of mitochondria. Recorded in 1914.

Mitosis, introduction of term

WALTHER FLEMMING, German anatomist, 1843-1905, introduced the term *mitosis*, in 1880, to describe the changes involved in the typical method of cell division. It is based on the Greek *mitos*, a thread, in allusion to the formation of a threadlike structure in one of the stages.

Mitosis, nuclear spindle in

. . . See under *Nuclear spindle in mitosis*.

Mitosis, three stages of; original description

EDUARD ADOLF STRASBURGER, German histologist, 1844-1912, gave the original description of the three stages of mitosis: the prophase, the metaphase, and the anaphase. Recorded *circa* 1884.

Mitral stenosis associated with defects of interatrial septum

RENÉ LUTEMBACHER, French cardiologist, 1884-19??, described a condition in which mitral stenosis is associated with interatrial septal defects. Recorded in 1916. Known as *Lutembacher's complex, syndrome,* or *disease*.

Mitral stenosis, congenital, first description of

PAUL LOUIS DUROZIEZ, French physician, 1826-1897, was the first to describe congenital mitral stenosis, in 1877. Known as *Duroziez's disease*.

Mitral stenosis, early description of—1674

JOHN MAYOW, English physician and physiologist, 1643-1679, was probably the first to describe mitral stenosis, in 1674.

Mitral stenosis, early recognition of—1809

ALLAN BURNS, Scottish physician and anatomist, 1781-1813, is remembered for his early recognition of mitral stenosis. Reported in 1809.

Mitral stenosis, presystolic murmur in

SULPICE ANTOINE FAUVEL, French physician, 1813-1884, is credited with giving the earliest description of the presystolic murmur in mitral stenosis. Recorded in 1843.

Mitral valve, ring of fibrocartilage serving as attachment to

ALBRECHT VON HALLER, Swiss physiologist and anatomist, 1708-1777, described the circle or ring of fibrocartilage to which the mitral valve is attached. Reported *circa* 1747. Known as *circulus callosus halleri*.

Mittelschmerz, early description of

. . . See under *Intermenstrual pain*.

Möbius' disease

. . . See under *Migraine, periodic, with paralysis of oculomotor muscles*.

Mohrenheim's fossa

... See under *Infraclavicular fossa, eponymic description of.*

Molar teeth, fifth cusp on

... See under *Cusp, fifth, on lingual surface of molar teeth.*

Molds, bactericidal action of; early recognition

JOHN TYNDALL, English physicist, 1820-1893, noted and described the bactericidal action of molds, in 1881.

Moll's glands

... See under *Ciliary glands, eponymic description of.*

Molluscum contagiosum, description of

THOMAS BATEMAN, English physician, 1778-1821, was the first to give an accurate account of molluscum contagiosum, in 1817.

Molluscum contagiosum, inclusion bodies in

WILLIAM HENDERSON, Scottish physician, 1810-1872, and ROBERT PATERSON, Scottish physician, 1814-1889, described inclusion bodies in molluscum contagiosum, independently, in 1841. Known as *Henderson-Paterson bodies* and *Paterson's bodies.*

Monakow's tract, fibers, or bundle

... See under *Rubrospinal tract.*

Monckeberg's arteriosclerosis

... See under *Arteriosclerosis affecting medium and small arteries.*

Monge's disease

... See under *Mountain sickness, chronic.*

Mongolism, clinical picture of; early description

JOHN L. H. DOWN, English physician, 1828-1896, described the clinical picture of mongolism, in 1866.

Mongolism, terminal phalanges in

FERDINAND SIEGERT, German pediatrician, 1865-1946, noted the shortness and curvature of the terminal phalanges of the little fingers in cases of mongolism. Reported in 1904. Known as *Siegert's sign.*

Monneret's pulse

... See under *Jaundice, pulse characteristic of.*

Monro's bursa

... See under *Olecranon, intratendinous bursa of.*

Monsters, classification of

ISIDORE GEOFFROY SAINT-HILAIRE, French zoologist, 1805-1861, devised a classification of human and animal monsters. Reported in his 3-volume work published in 1832-1837.

Monteggia's dislocation

... See under *Hip, dislocation of, toward anterior superior iliac spine.*

Montgomery's cups

... See under *Uterine mucosa, epithelial depressions in.*

Montgomery's glands or tubercles

... See under *Areola, enlargement of sebaceous glands of.*

Moral insanity or mania, eponymic description of

ISAAC RAY, American alienist, 1807-1881, described a form of insanity marked by impairment of the moral sense, in 1839. Known as *Ray's mania*.

Moranyl in treatment of trypanosomiasis

ERNEST FRANÇOIS AUGUSTE FOUR-NEAU, French chemist and pharmacologist, 1872-1949, introduced moranyl (a form of *suramin*) in the treatment of trypanosomiasis. Recorded in 1923.

Morax-Axenfeld bacillus, isolation of

. . . See under *Hemophilus duplex.*

Moraxella lacunata, isolation of

. . . See under *Hemophilus duplex.*

Morel ear

. . . See under *Ear with obliterated folds, as stigma of degeneracy.*

Morgagni's ventricle of larynx; ventriculus laryngis

GIOVANNI BATTISTA MORGAGNI, Italian anatomist and pathologist, 1682-1771, described an evagination of the mucous membrane of the larynx between the true and false vocal cords, extending nearly to the angle of the thyroid cartilage. Recorded between 1717 and 1719.

Morphine addiction, treatment of, with medicine said to contain strychnine and gold chloride

LESLIE E. KEELEY, American physician, 1832 - 1900, introduced a method for treating addiction to morphine, opium, and other habit-forming substances by the use of a remedy said to contain strychnine and gold chloride. Also used in treating alcoholics. Book published in 1881. Known as *Keeley cure* or *gold cure.*

Morphine, isolation of

FRIEDRICH WILHELM ADAM SER-TÜRNER, German pharmacologist, 1784-1841, isolated morphine in 1806.

Morphine, pre-anesthetic administration of

LÉON LABBÉ, French surgeon, 1832-1916, with E. GUYON, used morphine as a pre-anesthetic medication. Recorded in 1872.

Morphine prolongs chloroform anesthesia

CLAUDE BERNARD, French physiologist, 1813-1878, discovered that morphine prolongs and intensifies chloroform anesthesia. Recorded in 1864. It was LÉON LABBÉ who introduced morphine as a pre-anesthetic agent.

Morphology, introduction of term

JOHANN WOLFGANG VON GOETHE, German poet and anatomist, 1749-1832, is credited with the introduction of the term *morphology,* about 1788.

Morphology, founders of modern

KARL ERNST VON BAER, German embryologist, 1792-1876, and GEORGES LÉOPOLD CHRÉTIEN FRÉDÉRIC DAGOBERT CUVIER, French naturalist, 1769-1832, are regarded as the founders of modern morphology.

Mortality, early table of

. . . See under *Medical statistics, pioneer in.*

Morton's disease

. . . See under *Metatarsalgia, anterior, eponymic description of.*

Morvan's disease

... See under *Syringomyelia with atrophy and paralysis of hands and forearms.*

Mosetig-Moorhof bone wax

... See under *Bone wax, iodoform.*

Motor area, demonstration of existence of

... See under *Cerebral cortex, electric stimulation of.*

Motor area of cerebral cortex

LUIGI ROLANDO, Italian anatomist, 1773-1831, described the motor area in the cerebral cortex comprising both the precentral and the postcentral gyri. Known as *Rolando's area.* Recorded in 1824.

Motor area of cortex in dogs and monkeys, charting of

EDUARD HITZIG, German neurologist and psychiatrist, 1838-1907, experimented with electric stimulation of the cerebral cortex and clearly defined the limits of the cortical motor area in monkeys and dogs. Reported in 1874.

Motor function of anterior roots of spinal nerves, confirmation of

FRANÇOIS MAGENDIE, French physiologist, 1783-1855, confirmed the findings of Charles Bell that the anterior roots of the spinal nerves are motor in function. Reported in 1822. Known as *Bell-Magendie law.*

Motor function of anterior roots of spinal nerves, first demonstration of

CHARLES BELL, Scottish physician, 1774-1842, gave the earliest demonstration, in 1811, that the ante-rior roots of the spinal nerves are motor in function. Known as *Bell-Magendie law.*

Mountain sickness, chronic; Monge's disease

CARLOS MONGE, Peruvian physician, 1884-19??, described two forms of chronic mountain sickness developing in subjects who do not acclimatize adequately to the lower oxygen tension. Recorded in 1928. Known also as *high altitude disease* and *erythremia.*

Mountain sickness, description of

JOSE D'ACOSTA, Spanish missionary, 1539-1600, was the first to describe the signs and symptoms of mountain sickness, after his travels in Peru, in 1590. Known as *Acosta's disease.*

Mountain sickness due to anoxemia

... See under *High altitude sickness,* etc.

Mouth, inflammation of floor of; eponymic description

WILHELM FRIEDRICH VON LUDWIG, German surgeon, 1790-1865, described inflammation of the throat accompanied by cellulitis of the floor of the mouth. Published in 1836. Known as *Ludwig's angina.*

Mouth-breathing, recognition of bad effect of

GEORGE CATLIN, American ethnologist and painter, 1796-1872, was the first, in spite of his being a layman, to call attention to the undesirable effects of mouth-breathing. Published in 1861.

Much's granules

... See under *Tuberculous sputum, nonacid-fast granules in.*

Müllerian ducts

. . . See under *Embryonic ducts which in female develop into reproductive organs.*

Müller-Oppenheim reaction

. . . See under *Gonorrhea, complement-fixation test for.*

Müller's law

. . . See under *Nerve, law of specific energies of.*

Multiple myeloma, eponymic description of

CARL HUGO HUPPERT, Bohemian physician, 1832-1904, published a report on multiple myeloma on January 23, 1889. A week later, on January 30, 1889, another report on multiple myeloma was published by OTTO KAHLER, Austrian physician, 1849-1893.

Multiple myeloma, first description of

. . . See under *Myelomatosis.*

Multiple neuritis, alcoholic, original description of

JOHN C. LETTSOM, Virgin Islands physician, 1744-1815, is credited with being first to describe alcoholic multiple neuritis. Recorded 1779-1787.

Multiple sclerosis, early description of—1835

JEAN CRUVEILHIER, French pathologist, 1791-1874, gave an early and possibly first description of multiple or disseminated sclerosis, in 1835.

Multiple sclerosis, early description of—1849

FRIEDRICH T. VON FRERICHS, German pathologist, 1819-1885, is credited with giving the first scientific description of multiple sclerosis, in 1849.

Mumps, occurrence of orchitis in

ROBERT HAMILTON, Scottish physician, 1721-1793, gave the first modern description of orchitis as a complication of mumps. Paper read in 1773. Published in 1790.

Mumps virus, isolation of

CLAUD D. JOHNSON, American pathologist, 1882-19??, with ERNEST WILLIAM GOODPASTURE, isolated the virus causing mumps. Published in 1934.

Münchmeyer's disease

. . . See under *Myositis, progressive ossifying.*

Murmur, presystolic, at apex, in aortic regurgitation

AUSTIN FLINT, American physician, 1812-1886, described a presystolic murmur heard at the apex of the heart in aortic regurgitation. Reported in 1862. Known as *Flint's murmur.* Also called *Austin Flint murmur.*

Murmur

. . . See also under name of particular murmur, as *Pulmonary diastolic murmur.*

Murphy drip

. . . See under *Proctoclysis, continuous.*

Muscardine, parasitic nature of

. . . See under *Silkworm disease, parasitic nature of.*

Muscle activity and oxygen consumption

. . . See under *Oxygen is used in recovery phase of muscular activity.*

Muscle biopsy, early method for—1868

GUILLAUME B. A. DUCHENNE, French neurologist, 1806-1875, devised a technique for the removal and examination of small bits of muscle tissue from living subjects, in 1868.

Muscle, contractility of, as a property of the tissue

ALBRECHT VON HALLER, Swiss physiologist and anatomist, 1708-1777, demonstrated that muscle can be made to contract without the agency of nerve fibers. Reported in 1752.

Muscle contraction, heat production in

ARCHIBALD V. HILL, English biophysicist, 1886-19??, devised a technique to measure the heat production in a muscle during a single contraction cycle. Reported, with W. HARTREE, in 1920-1922. Received the Nobel prize in 1922.

Muscle contraction produces an electric current, proof that

RUDOLPH ALBERT VON KÖLLIKER, Swiss anatomist and histologist, 1817-1905, established the fact that contraction of muscles produces an electric current. Reported in 1856.

Muscle fiber develops from myoblast by division

MAXIMILIAN J. S. SCHULTZE, German anatomist and histologist, 1825-1874, demonstrated that each muscle fiber is developed from a single myoblast by division of its cell and nucleus. Recorded in 1861.

Muscle fibril, small mass in disk of

WILLIAM M. DOBIE, English anatomist, 1828-1915, described a small stainable mass in the middle of the transparent disk of a muscle fibril. Reported in 1859. Known as *Dobie's globule.*

Muscle, independent excitability of

CLAUDE BERNARD, French physiologist, 1813-1878, demonstrated the independent excitability of muscle by paralyzing the motor nerve endings with curare. Published in 1856.

Muscle of Horner

. . . See under *Tensor tarsi muscle* etc.

Muscle of Ludwig

. . . See under *Aryvocalis muscle,* etc.

Muscle of Müller

. . . See under *Ciliary muscle, inner circular part of; tarsal muscles of Müller;* and *orbital muscle of Müller.*

Muscle proteins are coagulable, demonstration that

WILHELM FRIEDRICH (WILLY) KUHNE, German physiologist, 1837-1900, established that muscle proteins are coagulable. Reported in 1859.

Muscle, smooth and striped, distinction between

GIORGIO BAGLIVI, Italian physician, 1668-1706, is believed to have been the first to distinguish between smooth and striped muscle, probably in 1700. Recorded in 1704.

Muscle, striped, early description of

. . . See under *Striated muscle,* etc.

Muscle, striped, early discovery of nature of—1675

ANTONJ VAN LEEUWENHOEK, Dutch naturalist, 1632-1723, is credited with recognizing the striped nature of voluntary muscle, in 1675.

Muscles are main source of animal heat, demonstration that

HERMANN L. F. VON HELMHOLTZ, German physiologist and physicist, 1821-1894, demonstrated that muscular contraction is the main source of animal heat. Reported in 1848.

Muscles, external intercostal, function of

GEORG ERHARD HAMBERGER, German physician, 1697-1755, demonstrated that the external intercostal muscles have an inspiratory function. Reported *circa* 1740.

Muscles, internal intercostal function of

GEORG ERHARD HAMBERGER, German physician, 1697-1755, demonstrated that the internal intercostal muscles aid in the process of expiration. Reported *circa* 1740.

Muscles, nitrogen metabolism of

LUDIMAR HERMANN, German physiologist, 1838-1914, studied the nitrogen metabolism involved in muscular work. Published in 1867.

Muscles, shortened, instrument for stretching

. . . See under *Apparatus for stretching shortened muscles.*

Muscular atrophy, hereditary familial spinal; eponymic description

GUIDO WERDNIG, Austrian neurologist, 186?-1929, described an infantile form of hereditary familial spinal muscular atrophy. Recorded in 1891. In the same year, the condition was also described by JOHANN HOFFMANN, German neurologist, 1857-1919. Known as *Werdnig-Hoffman syndrome* or *muscular atrophy.*

Muscular atrophy, lesions of spinal cord in

JEAN MARTIN CHARCOT, French neurologist, 1825-1893, with ALIX JOFFROY (French Physician, 1844-1908), discovered and described the lesions of the spinal cord in cases of muscular atrophy. Reported in 1869.

Muscular atrophy of scapulo-humeral region

EDME FÉLIX ALFRED VULPIAN, French physician, 1826-1887, described a form of progressive muscular atrophy involving the muscles of the scapulohumeral region, in 1860. Known as *Vulpian atrophy.*

Muscular atrophy, progressive myelopathic, early description of—1853

JEAN CRUVEILHIER, French pathologist, 1791-1874, gave an early description of progressive myelopathic muscular atrophy, now better known as *Duchenne-Aran* disease, in 1853. Known also as *Cruveilhier's disease.*

Musculocutaneous nerve, description of

GIULIO CASSERIO, Italian anatomist, 1561-1616, was the first to describe the musculocutaneous nerve. Recorded in 1627.

Mustard gas, discovery of

VICTOR MEYER, German scientist, 1848-1897, is credited with discovering mustard gas. Recorded in 1886.

Mutation theory, introduction of

HUGO MARIE DE VRIES, Amsterdam botanist, 1848-1935, is credited with introducing the theory of mutation which holds that new species arise through sudden changes in the offspring of normal parents. Recorded *circa* 1903.

Mutism, voluntary; Kussmaul's aphasia

. . . See under *Speech, voluntary abstaining from*, etc.

Myasthenia gravis, aminoacetic acid in treatment of

WALTER MEREDITH BOOTHBY, American surgeon, 1880-19??, introduced aminoacetic acid (also known as glycine and glycocoll) in the treatment of myasthenia gravis. Published in 1932.

Myasthenic gravis and hypertrophy of thymus

CARL WEIGERT, German pathologist and histologist, 1845-1904, is credited with drawing attention to the relation between hypertrophy of the thymus and myasthenia gravis. Recorded in 1901.

Myasthenia gravis and tumors of the thymus

ALFRED BLALOCK, Baltimore surgeon, 1899-   , with M. F. MASON, H. J. MORGAN, and S. S. RIVEN, treated myasthenia gravis

associated with tumors of the thymus by excision of the gland. Recorded in 1939.

Myasthenia gravis, early description of

SAMUEL WILKS, English physician, 1824-1911, is said to have been the first to describe a case of myasthenia gravis, in 1877.

Myasthenia gravis, ephedrine for relief of

HARRIET ISABEL EDGEWORTH, American biochemist, 1892-   , discovered the beneficial effect of ephedrine upon myasthenia gravis. Recorded in 1930.

Myasthenia gravis, physostigmine in treatment of

MARY BROADFOOT WALKER, English physician, 1896-   , introduced the use of physostigmine in the treatment of myasthenia gravis. Recorded in 1934.

Myasthenia gravis pseudoparalytica, early description of—1878

WILHELM H. ERB, German neurologist, 1840-1921, described myasthenia gravis pseudoparalytica, in 1878. Known as *Erb-Goldflam disease*.

Myasthenia gravis pseudoparalytica, early description of—1892

JOHANN IGNAZ HOPPE, Swiss physiologist, nineteenth century, described myasthenia gravis pseudoparalytica, in 1892.

Myasthenia gravis pseudoparalytica, early description of—1893

SAMUEL V. GOLDFLAM, Polish

neurologist, 1852-1932, described myasthenia gravis pseudoparalytica, in 1893. Known as *Erb-Goldflam disease* and *Hoppe-Goldflam symptom complex.*

Myasthenia gravis, thymectomy for relief of—1912

ERNST FERDINAND SAUERBRUCH, German surgeon, 1875-1951, advocated thymectomy for the relief of myasthenia gravis. Recorded by SCHUMACHER and ROTH in 1912.

Myasthenia gravis, thymectomy for relief of—1939

ALFRED BLALOCK, Baltimore surgeon, 1899- , with M. F. MASON, H. J. MORGAN, and S. S. RIVEN, treated myasthenia gravis by excision of the thymus gland. Recorded in 1939.

Myasthenia gravis, use of guanidine in

ANN STONE MINOT, American physiologist, 1894- , was the first to use guanidine in the treatment of myasthenia gravis. Published in 1938.

Mycobacterium leprae, discovery of

GERHARD H. A. HANSEN, Norwegian physician, 1841-1912, is credited with discovering the causative agent of leprosy, *Mycobacterium leprae,* in 1871.

Mycobacterium tuberculosis, discovery of

. . . See under *Tubercle bacillus, discovery of.*

Mycobacterium tuberculosis, first photograph of

GEORGE MILLER STERNBERG, American bacteriologist, 1838-

1915, was the first to photograph the *Mycobacterium tuberculosis.* Recorded in 1893.

Mycosis fungoides, classic description of

JEAN LOUIS ALIBERT, French dermatologist, 1766-1837, gave a comprehensive description of mycosis fungoides (pian fungoide) in 1806. It was reported in his *Description des maladies de la peau.* The condition is known as *Alibert's disease.*

Mycosis mucorina in man—1885

ARNOLD PALTAUF, Austrian physician, 1860-1893, is credited with reporting the first authentic case of mucosis mucorina in man. Published in 1885.

Mycosis of pharynx, first description of

BERNHARD FRAENKEL, German physician, 1836-1911, was the first to describe mycosis of the pharynx (mycosis pharyngis), in 1873.

Mydriasis, alternating, in neurasthenia

FRANZ RIEGEL, German physician, 1843-1904, described a form of alternating mydriasis observed in neurasthenic subjects. Published in 1900.

Myelin sheath stain by Weigert

CARL WEIGERT, German pathologist and histologist, 1845-1904, developed a myelin sheath stain, in 1882. Known as *Weigert's method* or *stain.* This is the best known of the many Weigert stains.

Myelin sheaths, degenerating, staining of

VITTORIO MARCHI, Italian neurohistologist, 1851-1908, demonstrated that decomposition products formed in degenerating myelin sheaths can be stained with osmic acid after specific preliminary treatment. This made it possible to trace a degenerating myelinated nerve fiber. Recorded in 1886. Known as *Marchi's method.*

Myelogenous leukemia, introduction of term

ERNST NEUMANN, German pathologist, 1834-1918, was the first to use the term *myelogenous leukemia,* in 1870.

Myelomatosis (multiple myeloma), first description of

WILLIAM MACINTYRE, English physician, 18??-1875, was the first to describe multiple myeloma or myelomatosis. Recorded in 1850.

Myenteric plexus, discovery of

. . . See under *Auerbach's plexus.*

Myoblastoma, granular cell

. . . See under *Granular cell myoblastoma.*

Myocarditis, introduction of term

JOSEPH FRIEDRICH SOBERNHEIM, German physician, 1803-1846, is credited with the introduction of the term *myocarditis,* about 1837.

Myocarditis, rheumatic, characteristic lesions of

KARL ALBERT LUDWIG ASCHOFF, German pathologist, 1866-1942, described the specific lesions of rheumatic myocarditis consisting of small areas of necrosis surrounded by lymphocytes and Aschoff cells, situated around the vessels in the myocardium. Recorded in 1904. Known as *Aschoff nodules* or *bodies.*

Myocardium, noninflammatory degenerative fibrosis of

. . . See under *Heart, noninflammatory fibrotic disease of.*

Myositis ossificans progressiva, early description of

JOHN FREKE, English physician, 1688-1756, described a case of myositis ossificans progressiva, in a report titled *A case of extraordinary exostoses on the back of a boy.* Published in 1740.

Myositis, progressive ossifying

ERNST MÜNCHMEYER, German physician, 1846-1880, described a diffuse progressive ossifying myositis. Published in 1869. Known as *Münchmeyer's disease.*

Myotonia and muscular atrophy, combined

CHARLES LOOMIS DANA, American neurologist, 1852-1935, was the first to give an adequate description of a condition marked by combined myotonia and muscular atrophy. Published in 1888.

Myotonia atrophica, introduction of term

GREGORI IVANOVICH ROSSOLIMO, Russian physician, 1860-1928, introduced the term *myotonia atrophica,* in 1902.

Myotonia congenita, early description of

ERNST VIKTOR VON LEYDEN, German physician, 1832-1910, gave an early, and possibly first, description of myotonia congenita. Recorded in 1876.

Myotonia congenita, eponymic description of

ASMUS JULIUS THOMAS THOMSEN, Danish physician, 1815-1896, described a congenital disease marked by tonic spasm of some of the muscles, on volitional movement or when the muscles are stimulated mechanically. Published in 1876. Known as *Thomsen's disease.*

Myotonograph, invention of

ADOLF FICK, German physiologist, 1829-1901, invented the myotonograph, an instrument for measuring and recording muscle tonus, *circa* 1864.

Myringotomy, first performance of

GORGAS "ELI" KONDELONI, French quack, 173?-1785, is said to have performed the first operation of myringotomy, in 1760.

Myringotomy for relief of auditory tube deafness

ASTLEY PASTON COOPER, English surgeon, 1768-1841, treated several cases of auditory tube deafness by incising the membrana tympani. Reported in 1801.

Myringotomy for relief of middle ear suppuration

JOHN CUNNINGHAM SAUNDERS, English surgeon, 1773-1810, was the first to advocate incision of the membrana tympani for the relief of acute middle ear suppuration. Published in 1806.

Myxadenitis labialis, classic description of

ERWIN VON BAELZ, German physician, 1849-1913, gave a classic description of the disease marked by the presence of painless papules on the mucous membranes of the lips. It is known as myxadenitis labialis, cheilitis glandularis apostematosa, and as *Baelz's disease.* Reported in 1890.

Myxedema and cretinism due to thyroid deficiency

VICTOR ALEXANDER HADEN HORSLEY, English surgeon, 1857-1916, demonstrated that myxedema, cretinism, and "cachexia strumipriva" are due to thyroid deficiency. Published in 1884.

Myxedema, experimental production of

JACQUES LOUIS REVERDIN, Swiss surgeon, 1842-1908, experimented with the production of myxedema in animals. Recorded in 1882. MORITZ SCHIFF had previously, in 1859, experimented with total removal of the gland. These early experiments invariably resulted in death of the animals.

Myxedema heart

. . . See under *Heart in myxedema, first record of.*

Myxoedema (myxedema), introduction of term

WILLIAM MILLER ORD, English surgeon, 1834-1902, is credited with coining and introducing the term *myxoedema* (later *myxedema*), in 1878.

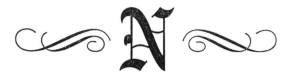

Nabothian cysts or ovules

MARTIN NABOTH, German anatomist, 1675-1721, described small retention cysts formed from the mucous glands in the cervix uteri. He at first mistook the cysts for ova, hence the term *ovula Nabothi*. Recorded in 1707.

Nabothian glands or follicles

. . . See under *Glands, mucous, of cervix of uterus*.

Naegele's obliquity; biparietal obliquity

FRANZ KARL NAEGELE, German obstetrician, 1778-1851, described a biparietal obliquity of the fetal head with relation to the superior pelvic strait, in 1819.

Naegele's pelvis

. . . See under *Pelvis contracted in one of oblique diameters*.

Naegeli's maneuver in epistaxis

. . . See under *Epistaxis, cure of, by pulling head upward*.

Nagana, arsenic in treatment of

DAVID LIVINGSTONE, Scottish explorer and physician, 1813-1873, was the first to use arsenic in the treatment of nagana, a disease of horses and cattle in Africa caused by *Trypanosoma brucei*. Recorded in 1858.

Nagana, causative agent of

DAVID BRUCE, British pathologist and bacteriologist, 1855-1931, demonstrated that nagana, a disease of horses and cattle in Central Africa, is due to the presence of a trypanosome (*Trypanosoma brucei*) which is transmitted to the animals by the bite of the tsetse fly. Reported in 1895. Known as *tsetse disease*.

Nanosomia pituitaria, introduction of term

JAKOB ERDHEIM, Austrian physician, 1874-1937, introduced the term *nanosomia pituitaria*, to describe pituitary dwarfism. Published in 1916.

Naphuride in treatment of trypanosomiasis

. . . See under *Trypanosomiasis*.

Narcolepsy, first full description of

JEAN BAPTISTE EDOUARD GÉLINEAU, French physician, 1859-192?, is credited with giving the first adequate description of narcolepsy. Recorded in 1880.

Narcosis, lipoid theory of

CHARLES ERNEST OVERTON, German pharmacologist, 1865-19??, introduced the lipoid theory of narcosis, in 1901.

**Narrow pelvis, bilateral
pelviotomy for relief of**
. . . See under *Dystocia, bilateral
pelviotomy for relief of*.

**Nasal concha, superior;
eponymic description**
GIOVANNI BATTISTA MORGAGNI,
Italian anatomist and pathologist,
1682-1771, described the superior
nasal concha, *circa* 1717. Known
as *Morgagni's concha*.

**Nasal secretion does not
originate in pituitary**
CONRAD VICTOR SCHNEIDER, German anatomist, 1614-1680, demonstrated that nasal mucus originates
in the nasal mucous membrane and
not in the pituitary, as had been
believed. Recorded in 1660.

**Nasal secretions originate in
pituitary body, rejection
of old theory that**
RICHARD LOWER, English physician, 1631-1691, was instrumental
in overthrowing the old Galenic
theory that nasal secretions take
origin in the pituitary gland, thus
obviating the fruitless attempts to
"purge the brain" in cases of
catarrh. Reported in 1672.

**Nasal septum, deviation of,
excision operation for**
EPHRAIM FLETCHER INGALS,
American surgeon, 1848-1918, introduced an operation of partial excision of the nasal septum for relief
of deviation. Recorded in 1882.

**Nasal septum, deviation of,
operation for, through
cruciate incision**
JOSEPH MORRIS ASCH, American
otolaryngologist, 1833-1902, de-

scribed an operation for the correction of deviated septum through a
cruciate incision over the deviation.
Reported in 1890.

**Nasal septum, thin and vascular
area of; often site of
hemorrhage**
WILHELM KIESSELBACH, German
laryngologist, 1839-1902, described
a thin and vascular part of the nasal
septum, often the site of hemorrhage, in 1884. Known as *Kiesselbach's area* or *triangle* and as *Little's area*.

**Nasal sinuses, first radiological
work on**
ARTHUR KUTTNER, German physician, 1862-1945, did the first important work on the radiography of
the nasal sinuses. Published in
1908.

**Nasal suppuration, surgical
treatment of**
LUDWIG GRÜNWALD, German rhinologist, 1863-19??, is credited with
being the first to use surgery in the
treatment of disease involving the
sphenoid and ethmoid bones and
for the relief of nasal suppuration.
Published in 1893.

Nasmyth's membrane
. . . See under *Enamel cuticle, primary;* also under *Dental capsule,
persistent*.

**Nasolacrimal duct, valve at
lower end of, descrip-
tion of**
GIOVANNI BATTISTA BIANCHI, Italian anatomist, 1681-1761, was the
first to describe the valve at the
lower end of the nasolacrimal duct.
Exact date not available.

Nasolambdoid line, eponymic description of

PAUL POIRIER, French surgeon, 1853-1907, described a topographical line extending from the nasofrontal angle to a point above the lambda, in 1880. Known as *Poirier's line*.

Nasopalatine nerve, early description of

DOMENICO COTUGNO, Italian anatomist, 1736-1822, described the nasopalatine nerve in 1760.

Nasopalatine nerve, ganglion of

JULES H. CLOQUET, French surgeon, 1787-1840, described a swelling of the nasopalatine nerve in the anterior palatine canal. Reported in 1818. Known as *Cloquet's ganglion*.

Nasopharyngeal diverticulum; Pertik's diverticulum

OTTÓ PERTIK, Hungarian pathologist, 1852-1913, described a condition of the lateral pharyngeal fossa marked by abnormal depth, considered a diverticulum of the nasopharyngeal space. Recorded in 1884.

Nasopharynx, examination of, by means of special mirror

JOHANN N. CZERMAK, Bohemian physiologist, 1828-1873, devised a small mirror suitable for inspecting the nasopharynx. Reported in 1858.

Nasse's law

. . . See under *Hemophilia, Nasse's law of*.

Naval hygiene, pioneer in English

JAMES LIND, Scottish physician, 1716-1794, wrote an essay on the most effectual means for preserving the health of seamen in the British navy. Published in 1757. Lind is regarded as the Father of Naval Hygiene in England. He advocated ventilation of ships, better food, the use of lemon juice, etc.

Navicular, carpal, osteoporosis of

GEORG KARL FELIX PREISER, German orthopedic surgeon, 1879-1913, described osteoporosis and atrophy of the carpal navicular bone due to trauma. Recorded in 1911. Known as *Preiser's disease*.

Neanderthal skull, first description of

HERMANN SCHAAFFHAUSEN, German anthropologist, 1816-1893, is credited with being first to describe the Neanderthal skull, in 1858.

Necator americanus, discovery of

. . . See under *Uncinaria americana*.

Neck, congenital lymphatic cyst of

. . . See under *Hydrocele, cervical, eponymic description of*.

Necrobiosis lipoidica diabeticorum—1929

ERICH URBACH, American dermatologist, 1893-1946, described necrobiosis lipoidica diabeticorum. Recorded in 1929. Known as *Oppenheim-Urbach disease*. Urbach is credited with introducing the name of the disease.

Necrobiosis lipoidica diabeticorum—1932

MORITZ OPPENHEIM, Vienna dermatologist, 1876-1949, described necrobiosis lipoidica diabeticorum, in 1932. Known as *Oppenheim-Urbach disease.*

Needle, surgical, cutting, with flat sides

WERNER HAGEDORN, German surgeon, 1831-1894, invented a surgical cutting needle with flat sides, the cutting edge being near the point. Introduced *circa* 1885.

Negri bodies, diagnostic of rabies

. . . See under *Rabies, inclusion bodies diagnostic of.*

Neisser-Wechsberg phenomenon

. . . See under *Complement deviation phenomenon.*

Nélaton's line in dislocation of hip

AUGUSTE NÉLATON, French surgeon, 1807-1873, described a line running from the anterior superior iliac spine to the tuberosity of the ischium. In dislocation of the femur, the tip of the greater trochanter is above this line. Known as *Nélaton's line.* Recorded in 1847.

Neoarsphenamine (neosalvarsan), introduction of

PAUL EHRLICH, German bacteriologist and pathologist, 1854-1915, introduced neosalvarsan in the treatment of syphilis. Recorded in 1912.

Neon, discovery of—1898

WILLIAM RAMSAY, English scientist, 1852-1916, with M. W. TRAVERS, discovered neon in 1898. It was isolated by fractionation of liquid air. The name means, in substance, "the new one."

Nephelometer, introduction of

THEODORE WILLIAM RICHARDS, American chemist, 1868-1928, with R. C. WELLS, devised a nephelometer, "an instrument for detecting and estimating opalescent precipitates." Recorded in 1904.

Nephritis, retinal changes in

. . . See under *Retinal changes in chronic nephritis.*

Nephropexy, early operation for

GEORGE MICHAEL EDEBOHLS, American surgeon, 1853-1908, is credited with performing nephropexy, in 1893. Report published under the title "Movable kidney; with a report of twelve cases treated by nephrorrhaphy."

Nephrorrhaphy

. . . See under *Nephropexy.*

Nephrosclerosis, arteriolar, description of

KARL THEODOR FAHR, German physician, 1877-1945, with FRANZ VOLHARD, German physician, 1872-1950, described arteriolar nephrosclerosis. Recorded in 1914.

Nephrosclerosis, malignant, description of

KARL THEODOR FAHR, German physician, 1877-1945, with FRANZ VOLHARD, German physician, 1872-1950, described malignant nephrosclerosis, *circa* 1916. Known as *Fahr-Volhard disease.*

Nephrosis, first complete description of

FRANZ VOLHARD, German physician, 1872-1950, with KARL THEODOR FAHR, gave the first complete description of "pure" nephrosis. Published in 1914.

Nernst lamp

. . . See under *Electric lamp having a filament of oxides of rare-earth metals.*

Nerve block anesthesia, introduction of

WILLIAM S. HALSTED, American surgeon, 1852-1922, is credited with introducing regional nerve block anesthesia by the use of cocaine. Reported in 1885.

Nerve cell degeneration; Nissl's degeneration

FRANZ NISSL, German neurologist, 1860-1919, described the degeneration of ganglion cells after the nerve fibers are severed. Recorded in 1892.

Nerve cells, Nissl bodies of

FRANZ NISSL, German neurologist, 1860-1919, described protein bodies staining with basic dyes which form the substance of the reticulum in the cytoplasm of a nerve cell. Recorded in 1894. Known also as *tigroid bodies* and *Nissl granules.*

Nerve, cut, loss of irritability of

JOHANN WILHELM RITTER, German physicist, 1776-1810, with EUSEBIO VALLI, demonstrated that section of a nerve results in an increase of irritability followed by loss of irritability, progressing toward the periphery. Date not available. Known as *Ritter-Valli law.*

Nerve degeneration, demonstration of

AUGUSTUS VOLNEY WALLER, English physiologist, 1816-1870, demonstrated nerve degeneration following section of the glosso-pharyngeal and hypoglossal nerves, in the frog. Recorded in 1850.

Nerve fiber survival, law of

AUGUSTUS VOLNEY WALLER, English physiologist, 1816-1870, demonstrated that a nerve fiber can survive only when it maintains continuity with its cell body. Recorded in 1850. Known as *Wallerian law of degeneration.*

Nerve fibers, connective tissue between, of a nerve trunk

FRIEDRICH G. J. HENLE, German anatomist, 1809-1885, described the endoneurium, the delicate connective tissue separating the nerve fibers of a nerve trunk. Reported in 1871. Known as *sheath of Henle.*

Nerve fibers, peripheral nonmedulated

ROBERT REMAK, German physiologist and neurologist, 1815-1865, discovered the peripheral non-medullated nerve fibers found chiefly in the sympathetic nerves. Published in 1838. Known as *fibers of Remak.*

Nerve impulse, chemical mediators of

OTTO LOEWI, American pharmacologist, 1873-19??, verified the theory, first suggested by T. R. ELLIOTT and others, that chemical mediators play a part in nerve impulse reactions. He demonstrated that stimulation of the vagus and the accelerator nerve produces slowing and acceleration of the heart through the liberation of substances identical with acetylcholine and epinephrine. First published in 1921.

Nerve impulse, chemical transmission of

THOMAS BENTON ELLIOTT, English physiologist, 1877-19??, was the first to propose the theory of chemical mediation of nerve impulses. He stated that on arrival at a smooth muscle cell, the nerve impulse liberates adrenin, which stimulates the muscle chemically. Published in 1904.

Nerve impulse, similarity of, to action of drugs

WALTER ERNEST DIXON, English physiologist and pharmacologist, 1871-1931, with PHILIP HAMILL, noted the simlarty between the effects of nerve stimulation and the action of certain drugs upon muscle tissue, especially with regard to the influence of muscarine on the heart. Published in 1909.

Nerve impulse speed, measurement of, by photography

JOHN SCOTT BURDON-SANDERSON, English physiologist, 1828-1905, measured the speed of nerve impulses by means of photography. Published in 1890.

Nerve impulses, electric current of

JOSEPH ERLANGER, American physiologist, 1874-19??, with HERBERT S. GASSER, American physiologist, 1888-19??, studied and photographed the electric currents of nerve impulses, by combining electronic amplifiers and cathode-ray oscillographs. Recorded in 1924. Both shared the Nobel prize in 1944.

Nerve, injured, and its muscle; difference in potential

. . . See under *Potential difference.*

Nerve, intermedius, of Wrisberg

HEINRICH AUGUST WRISBERG, German anatomist, 1739-1808, described the pars intermedia of the facial nerve, now known as intermedius nerve, in 1777. Known also as *Wrisberg's pars intermedia.*

Nerve is exhausted by stimulation, belief that

JULIUS BERNSTEIN, Swiss physiologist, 1839-1917, propounded the theory that a nerve can be exhausted by continued stimulation. Recorded in 1877.

Nerve is not exhausted by stimulation, belief that

NIKOLAI IGOREVICH WEDENSKY, Russian physiologist, 1844-1918, demonstrated that a nerve cannot be exhausted by continued stimulation. Published in 1884.

Nerve, law of specific energies of

JOHANNES MÜLLER, German anatomist and physiologist, 1801-1858, propounded the law of specific energies of nerve or the law of specific irritability, which states that every sensory nerve gives rise to one form of sensation even if excited by stimuli other than the normal. Published in 1826. Known as *Müller's law.*

Nerve, long pedendal, eponymic description of

SAMUEL THOMAS SOEMMERRING, German anatomist, 1755-1830, described the long pudendal nerve. Recorded in 1790. Known as *Soemmerring's nerve.*

Nerve, make and break stimulation of

EDUARD FRIEDRICH WILHELM

PFLÜGER, German physiologist, 1829-1910, was first to formulate the laws concerning the behavior of nerves in response to make and break stimulation by galvanic current. Published in 1859.

Nerve, medial cutaneous, of arm

HEINRICH AUGUST WRISBERG, German anatomist, 1739-1808, described the medial cutaneous nerve of the arm, in 1777. Known as *Wrisberg's nerve.*

Nerve of pterygoid canal, early description of—1555

GUIDO GUIDI, Italian physician and anatomist, 1500-1569, described the nerve of the pterygoid canal, *circa* 1555. It was reported in his *De anatomia corporis humani,* published after his death, in 1611. Known as *Vidian nerve.*

Nerve of tooth, paste used to devitalize

. . . See under *Paste for devitalizing nerve of a tooth.*

Nerve, optic, vascular circle surrounding

ALBRECHT VON HALLER, Swiss physiologist and anatomist, 1708-1777, described a circle of arteries in the sclera, surrounding the entrance of the optic nerve. Known as *circle of Haller, circulus zinnii,* and *circulus arteriosus halleri.* Reported in 1756.

Nerve paralysis, experimental demonstration of

CLAUDE BERNARD, French physiologist, 1813-1878, discovered that nerves can be paralyzed experi-mentally by means of curare, a finding which enabled him to demonstrate the excitability of muscle. Reported in 1857.

Nerve plexus, submucous, of alimentary tract

GEORG MEISSNER, German anatomist and physiologist, 1829-1905, described a plexus of nerves in the submucous tissue of the alimentary canal, in 1853. Known as *Meissner's plexus.*

Nerve, severed, atrophy of

WILLIAM HOWSHIP DICKINSON, English physician, 1832-1913, proved that when a nerve is cut, as in case of a limb amputation, the proximal end eventually atrophies. Published in 1869.

Nerve, trigeminal, accurate description of

JOHANN FRIEDRICH MECKEL, German anatomist, 1714-1774, gave an accurate description of the trigeminal nerve, in 1748.

Nerve trunk, blocking of

. . . See under *Blocking of nerve trunk with local anesthesia.*

Nerve vibration in treatment of nervous disorders

JOSEPH M. GRANVILLE, English physician, 1833-1900, introduced a method for the treatment of nervous disorders by means of vibratory massage for the administration of which he invented a special device. Recorded in 1883.

Nerves and tendons, first clear distinction between

HEROPHILUS, Greek physician and anatomist in Egypt, 335-280 B. C., was the first to differentiate clearly between nerves and tendons. Exact date not available.

Nerves, motor and sensory, differentiation between

HEROPHILUS, Green physician and anatomist in Egypt, 335-280 B. C., was probably the first to differentiate between motor and sensory nerves. Exact date not available.

Nerves, tract of, in cervical region

HANS K. S. HELWEG, Danish psychiatrist, 1847-1901, described a crossed tract of fibers extending between the inferior olivary body of the medulla and the lower cervical or upper thoracic segments of the spinal cord. Reported in 1887. Known as *olivospinal tract* and *Helweg's bundle*.

Nervous impulse, velocity of, measurement of the

HERMANN L. F. VON HELMHOLTZ, German physiologist and physicist, 1821-1894, measured the velocity of nervous impulses by means of an instrument (pendulum-myograph) which he invented for the purpose of the experiment. Reported in 1850.

Nervous system, integrative action of

CHARLES SCOTT SHERRINGTON, English neurophysiologist, 1857-1952, introduced the term and the concept of "integrative action" with regard to the nervous system. Recorded in 1906.

Nessler's reagent

. . . See under *Ammonia, reagent for testing*.

Nettleship's disease

. . . See under *Urticaria pigmentosa, eponymic description of*.

Network of fibers in cytoplasm of cells

. . . See under *Golgi apparatus* .

Neubauer's artery

. . . See under *Artery, deep thyroid*.

Neubauer's ganglion

. . . See under *Ganglion formed by lower cervical and first thoracic ganglia*.

Neumann's disease

. . . See under *Pemphigus vegetans, early description of—1886*.

Neuralgias, classification of

HENRI VERGER, French physician, 1873-1930, devised a classification of the neuralgias, in 1904.

Neurasthenia, early description of

JEAN ANTOINE EUGÈNE BOUCHUT, French physician, 1818-1891, described neurasthenia in 1860.

Neurasthenia, first complete description of

GEORGE MILLER BEARD, American physician, 1839-1883, was the first to give a complete description of neurasthenia or nervous exhaustion, in April 1869. He wrote two more papers on the subject in 1879 and 1880. Known as *Beard's disease*.

Neurilemma, eponymic description of

THEODOR SCHWANN, German anatomist, 1810-1882, gave a clear description of the neurilemma, in 1839. Known as *sheath of Schwann*.

Neurilemma of medullated nerve fibers, demilunes of

... See under *Crescent-shaped cells beneath neurilemma.*

Neurinoma, introduction of term

JOSÉ VEROCAY, Uruguayan pathologist in Prague, 1876-1927, introduced the term *neurinoma,* to describe a type of fibroma derived from the endoneurium or the neurilemma. Recorded in 1910.

Neuritis fascians, early account of

... See under *Neuritis, interstitial.*

Neuritis, interstitial, early description of

HERMANN L. EICHHORST, Swiss physician, 1849-1921, described neuritis fascians, an interstitial neuritis, in 1873. Known as *Eichhorst's neuritis.*

Neuritis, peripheral, first description of

JOSEPH JULES DEJERINE, French neurologist, 1849-1917, was the first to describe peripheral neuritis resembling tabes dorsalis in which the tactile sense is normal but deep sensibility is diminished. Recorded in 1887. Known as *Dejerine's neurotabes.*

Neuroblast, introduction of term

WILHELM HIS, *père,* Swiss anatomist and embryologist, 1831-1904, is credited with introducing the term *neuroblast, circa* 1870.

Neuroblastoma, sympathetic, as distinct disease

JAMES HOMER WRIGHT, American pathologist, 1869-1928, described neuroblastoma sympatheticum as a separate clinical entity. Published in 1910.

Neurobuccal pouch

... See under *Buccal cavity, diverticulum of, in embryo.*

Neurocirculatory asthenia, early description of

... See under *Irritable heart.*

Neurodermatitis, eponymic description of

. . . See under *Lichen chronicus simplex.*

Neurofibroma, plexiform, first description of

PAUL VON BRUNS, German surgeon, 1846-1916, was the first to describe plexiform neurofibroma. Published in 1870.

Neurofibromas from sheath of Schwann or neurilemma

JOSÉ VEROCAY, Uruguayan pathologist in Prague, 1876-1927, demonstrated that neurofibromas are derived from the neurilemma. Published in 1910.

Neurofibromatosis, early description of

ROBERT WILLIAM SMITH, Scottish physician, 1807-1873, gave a good description of neurofibromatosis, later named von Recklinghausen's disease, in 1849.

Neurofibromatosis; von Recklinghausen's disease

FRIEDRICH DANIEL VON RECKLINGHAUSEN, German pathologist, 1833-1910, described a familial disease marked by developmental defects and the formation of multiple pedunculated soft tumors over the entire body, known as *neurofibro-matosis, multiple neuroma, neuro-matosis.* Recorded in 1882.

Neurogenic arthropathy, original description of

JEAN MARTIN CHARCOT, French neurologist, 1825-1893, described a condition of osteo-arthritis marked by joint enlargement due to trophic disturbances, in 1868. Known also as *Charcot's disease, Charcot's joints, tabetic arthro-pathy,* and *neuropathic arthritis.*

Neurogenic origin of heart beat in Limulus crab

ANTON JULIUS CARLSON, American physiologist, 1875-19??, discovered that section of the cardiac nerve in the Limulus crab causes the heart to stop beating, thus demonstrating the neurogenic origin of the heart beat in this animal. Recorded in 1912.

Neurogenic theory of action of heart, origin of

GIOVANNI ALFONSO BORELLI, Italian physiologist and physicist, 1608-1679, originated the neurogenic theory of the action of the heart. Published in 1680.

Neuroglia, discovery and naming of

RUDOLF LUDWIG KARL VIRCHOW, German pathologist, 1821-1902, recognized the nature of the supporting tissue of the central nervous system and named it *neuroglia.* Observed in 1846; recorded in 1854.

Neuroglia, silver tannin stain for

... See under *Silver tannin stain.*

Neuroma, first description of

WILLIAM WOOD, Scottish physician, 1774-1857, is credited with being the first to describe a neuroma, in 1828. There is a possibility that the condition was described earlier, in 1824, by DOMINIQUE JEAN LARREY, French army surgeon, 1766-1842.

Neuromyelitis optica, description of

EUGÈNE DEVIC, French physician, 1869-1930, described neuromyelitis optica, optic neuro-encephalomyel-opathy, an acute transverse myelitis marked by optic neuritis. Date not available. Known as *Devic's disease.*

Neuron doctrine, development of

HEINRICH WILHELM GOTTFRIED WALDEYER-HARTZ, German anatomist, 1836-1921, did extensive research in neurology which resulted in his proposal of the neuron theory or doctrine that the nervous system is composed of structural units called neurons and that there is no protoplasmic continuity between these units, the connection being through contact only. Published in 1891.

Neuron types, classification of—1899

ALEXANDER S. DOGIEL, Russian neurohistologist, 1852-1922, described and classified neuron types in spinal, sympathetic, intestinal, and other ganglia. Reported in 1899.

Neuropathic muscular atrophy, progressive, peroneal type of

JEAN MARTIN CHARCOT, French

neurologist, 1825-1893, with PIERRE MARIE (French neurologist, 1853-1940), described the peroneal form of progressive neuropathic muscular atrophy, in 1886. In the same year, HOWARD HENRY TOOTH, English physician, 1856-1925, described the same condition. The disease is thus known as the *Charcot-Marie-Tooth disease.*

Neuroses as compensation for social and physical inferiority, theory of

ALFRED ADLER, Austrian psychiatrist, 1870-1937, formulated the theory that neuroses are developed as compensations for physical and social inferiority. Published in English in 1917. First reported in 1907.

Neurosyphilis, treatment of, with induced malarial fever

. . . See under *Malarial fever in treatment of paralytic dementia.*

Neusser's granules

. . . See under *Leukocytes, basophilic granules of.*

Neutrophils, classification of, into five groups

JOSEPH ARNETH, German physician, 1873-19??, devised a formula which classified neutrophils into five groups, on the basis of the number of lobes. Recorded in 1904.

Neutrophils, classification of, into four groups

VICTOR SCHILLING, Austrian hematologist, 1883-19??, devised a modified Arneth's classification of neutrophils in which the cells are divided into four groups. Published in 1912. Known as *Schilling's hemogram.*

Newborn, hemorrhagic disease of

. . . See under *Hemorrhagic disease of newborn.*

Newborn, intracranial hemorrhage in, operation for

HARVEY W. CUSHING, Boston surgeon, 1869-1939, performed the first successful operation for intracranial hemorrhage in the newborn, in 1905.

Newborn, primary atrophy or marasmus of

. . . See under *Parrot's atrophy of the newborn.*

New tissue grows from preexisting cells

. . . See under *Growth of new tissue takes place by division of pre-existing cells.*

Newcomer's hemoglobinometer

. . . See under *Colorimeter with colored glass standards.*

Niacin, isolation of

CONRAD ARNOLD ELVEHJEM, American biochemist, 1901- , with R. J. MADDEN, F. N. STRONG, and D. W. WOOLLEY, isolated niacin or nicotinic acid. Reported in 1938.

Nicol's prism, invention of

WILLIAM NICOL, Scottish physicist, 1768-1851, prepared a polished prism of Iceland spar cut diagonally across the principal axis and held together by a transparent cement. A ray of light is split by the prism, so that one part is reflected while the other part passes through. Recorded in 1828.

Nicotine blocks passage of impulses through sympathetic ganglia, proof that

JOHN NEWPORT LANGLEY, English physiologist, 1852-1925, demonstrated that nicotine, applied to sympathetic ganglia, blocks the passage of impulses, *circa* 1889.

Nicotinic acid, isolation of

. . . See under *Niacin.*

Niemann-Pick disease; lipoid histiocytosis

ALBERT NIEMANN, German pediatrician, 1880-1921, was first to describe the disease of infants now known as *Niemann-Pick disease,* in 1914. It is marked by anemia, leukocytosis, enlargement of spleen and liver, and foamy appearance of the histiocytes. The disease was described more adequately by LUDWIG PICK, German pediatrician, 1868-1935, in a paper published in 1926.

Night blindness, congenital, in Japan

CHUTA OGUCHI, Japanese ophthalmologist, 1875-1945, described a type of congenital night blindness observed in Japan, in 1912. Known as *Oguchi's diseease.*

Nipple, circle of veins beneath areola of

ALBRECHT VON HALLER, Swiss physiologist and anatomist, 1708-1777, described a circle of veins beneath the areola of the nipple. Reported *circa* 1757. Known as *circulus venosus halleri.*

Nipple, Paget's disease of

JAMES PAGET, English surgeon, 1814-1899, described a cancerous disease of the nipple and areola of the breast. Published in 1874.

Nisbet's chancre

. . . See under *Chancre, lymphatic.*

Nissl granules or bodies

. . . See under *Nerve cells, Nissl bodies in.*

Nissl's degeneration

. . . See under *Nerve cell degeneration, etc.*

Nitrogen content of organic compounds, method for determining

JOHAN GUSTAV CHRISTOFFER KJELDAHL, Danish chemist, 1849-1900, devised a method for determining the amount of nitrogen in an organic compound. Published in 1883. Known as *Kjeldahl's method.*

Nitrogen, discovery of

DANIEL RUTHERFORD, Scottish physicist, 1749-1819, discovered nitrogen, in 1772.

Nitrogen fixation by bacteria

PIERRE E. M. BERTHELOT, French chemist, 1827-1907, investigated the action of bacteria in soils and demonstrated that bacteria growing in clay soils are capable of fixing nitrogen. Recorded in 1889.

Nitroglycerine for relief of angina pectoris, introduction of

WILLIAM MURRELL, English physician, 1853-1912, is credited with introducing nitroglycerine as a remedy for the relief of angina pectoris. Recorded in 1879.

Nitrous oxide as dental anesthetic, first use of

HORACE WELLS, American dentist, 1815-1848, is credited with being the first to use nitrous oxide successfully as a dental anesthetic, in 1844. When later demonstrations, including one at Harvard Medical School, failed, Wells committed suicide by cutting a vein in his arm and inhaling ether vapors at the same time.

Nitrous oxide, discovery of anesthetic properties of

HUMPHRY DAVY, English chemist and physicist, 1778-1829, was the first to discover the anesthetic properties of nitrous oxide and to suggest its use in surgery, in 1799. Reported in 1800.

Nitrous oxide-oxygen anesthesia in childbirth

FRANK WORTHINGTON LYNCH, American obstetrician, 1871-19??, introduced nitrous oxide-oxygen anesthesia in obstetrics. Recorded in 1915.

Nitrous oxide-oxygen-ether anesthesia, apparatus for administration

FREDERICK J. COTTON, American surgeon, 1869-1938, with W. M. BOOTHBY, devised an apparatus for the administration of nitrous oxide-oxygen-ether anesthesia. Reported in 1912.

Nobel prize, founding of

ALFRED BERNARD NOBEL, Swedish munitions manufacturer, 1833-1896, provided the funds for the distribution of prizes in several fields of human endeavor, in 1895. Nobel invented dynamite in 1866.

Nocardiosis, pure granulomatous, first description of

JOHN TINDAL CUTTINO, American pathologist, 1912- , with ANNE M. McCABE, described pure granulomatous nocardiosis, caused by *Nocardia intracellularis*. Published in 1949.

Nociceptor, introduction of term

CHARLES SCOTT SHERRINGTON, English neurophysiologist, 1857-1952, introduced the term *nociceptor*, to describe a receptor activated by pain or injury. Published in 1906.

Node of Keith and Flack

. . . See under *Sino-atrial node*.

Nodes on skull of syphilitic infants

JOSEPH PARROT, French physician, 1829-1883, described nodes on the outer table of the frontal and parietal bones of syphilitic children. Recorded in 1879. Known as *Parrot's nodes*.

Nodes, subcutaneous, in some cases of acute rheumatism

. . . See under *Rheumatism*.

Nodules in tendons and capsules of joints, in rheumatic conditions

PAUL CLAUDE H. MEYNET, French physician, 1831-1892, described nodular growths sometimes occurring in joint capsules and on tendon sheaths in cases of rheumatic disease, in 1864. Known as *Meynet's nodes* or *nodosities*.

Nodules on free edges of atrioventricular valves

GIUSEPPE ALBINI, Italian physiologist and anatomist, 1827-1911, described the remains of fetal structures sometimes seen on the free edges of the atrioventricular valves of infants in the form of gray, sago-grain nodules. First reported in 1867.

No-restraint method of treating insane, advocate of, in England

JOHN CONOLLY, Irish physician in England, 1794-1866, advocated, in 1839, the use of a humane, no-restraint method in handling the insane.

Norleucine, isolation of

EMIL ABDERHALDEN, Swiss pathologist and biochemist in Germany, 1877-1946, with A. WEIL, isolated norleucine, an amino acid found in the decomposition products of nervous tissue. Published in 1913.

North America, diseases of interior valley of

DANIEL DRAKE, American physician, 1785-1852, wrote a book on the principal diseases of the interior valley of North America. Published in 1850.

Nose, mucous membrane of; eponymic description

CONRAD VICTOR SCHNEIDER, German anatomist, 1614-1680, described the nasal mucous membrane, especially the lining of the respiratory portion. Recorded in 1660. Known as *Schneider's* or *Schneiderian membrane*.

Nose

. . . See also under *Nasal,* and under particular part of the nose.

Notch at upper border of tympanic sulcus

. . . See under *Tympanic sulcus, notch at upper border of.*

Notochord, discovery of

KARL ERNST VON BAER, German embryologist born in Estonia, 1792-1876, was the first to describe the chorda dorsalis or notochord. Recorded *circa* 1827.

Notochord, introduction of term

RICHARD OWEN, English physician, 1804-1892, is credited with the introduction of the term *notochord,* in 1848.

Novasurol, introduction of

. . . See under *Mercurial diuretic, first injection of.*

Novocaine, synthesis of

ALFRED EINHORN, German physician, 187?-19??, is credited with the synthesis of procaine or novocaine, in 1899.

Novy-MacNeal agar or medium

. . . See under *Trypanosomes, blood agar for cultivation of —* 1904.

Nuck's diverticulum

. . . See under *Round ligament, peritoneal diverticulum of.*

Nuclear fragments in erythrocytes; Howell's bodies

. . . See under *Red blood cells, nuclear particles in.*

Nuclear spindle in mitosis

OTTO BUTSCHLI, German zoologist, 1848-1920, described the spindle-shaped body observed in the nucleus in mitosis. Called *Butschli's nuclear spindle.* Exact date not available.

Nuclei arise by division of pre-existing nuclei

EDUARD ADOLF STRASBURGER,

German biologist, 1844-1912, propounded the doctrine that independent cell formations does not occur, as had been believed, but that new nuclei are formed by division of pre-existing nuclei. Published in 1880.

Nuclein, discovery of, in spermatozoa

FRIEDRICH MIESCHER, Swiss scientist, 1844-1893, is credited with discovering nuclein in spermatozoa. Recorded in 1874.

Nucleolus, introduction of term

GABRIEL GUSTAV VALENTIN, German physician, 1810-1883, is said to have introduced the term *nucleolus,* in 1836.

Nucleus beneath aqueduct of Sylvius

CARL FRIEDRICH OTTO WESTPHAL, German neurologist, 1833-1890, described a gray nucleus beneath the aqueduct of Sylvius giving rise to some of the fibers of the trochlear nerve. Recorded in 1887. The nucleus was described earlier, in 1885, by LUDWIG EDINGER, German neurologist. 1855-1918. Known as *Westphal's nucleus* and *Edinger's nucleus.*

Nucleus of cell, discovery of

ROBERT BROWN, Scottish botanist, 1773-1858, is credited with the discovery of the cell nucleus, in plants.

He was also the first to point out that the nucleus is a normal and important part of the cell. Recorded in 1831.

Nucleus of median and vestibular roots of auditory nerve

VLADIMIR MICHAILOVICH BECHTEREV, Russian neurologist, 1857-1927, described a nucleus of gray matter which gives origin to the fibers of the median and vestibular roots of the auditory nerve. Reported in 1892. Known as *Bechterev's nucleus.*

Nucleus of median root of auditory nerve

OTTO F. K. DEITERS, German anatomist, 1834-1863, described the lateral vestibular nucleus which gives origin to the median root of the auditory nerve. Recorded in 1865. Known as *Deiter's nucleus.*

Nyctalopia, first known description of

WILLIAM BRIGGS, English oculist, 1642-1704, gave the first recorded description of nyctalopia. Published in 1684.

Nystagmus in relation to semicircular canals

MARIE J. P. FLOURENS, French physiologist, 1794-1867, demonstrated the relation of the semicircular canals to nystagmus, in 1828.

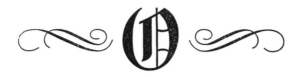

**Obelion, introduction of,
  as craniometric
  point**

PIERRE PAUL BROCA, French surgeon and anthropologist, 1824-1880, defined *obelion* as a craniometric point. Exact date not available.

**Objective, oil immersion,
  introduction of**

. . . See under *Oil immersion lens, introduction of.*

**Obstetric bag for dilating
  cervix uteri**

CAMILLE L. A. CHAMPETIER DE RIBES, French obstetrician, 1848-1915, devised an obstetric bag which he used to dilate the cervix uteri. Reported in 1888.

**Obstetric forceps, invention
  of first practical**

PETER CHAMBERLEN, English obstetrician, 1572-1626, is credited with the invention of the first practical obstetric forceps. It was kept by the Chamberlens as a family secret for nearly a century. The exact date of the invention is not available.

**Obstetric forceps with articu-
  lation allowing blades to
  move over each other**

CHRISTIAN C. G. KIELLAND, Norwegian obstetrician, 1871-1941, invented an obstetrical forceps with an articulation allowing the blades to move over each other; it has a marked cephalic curve but a slight pelvic curve. Report published in 1915. Called the *Kielland forceps.*

**Obstetric forceps with cephalic
  and pelvic curves,
  invention of**

ANDRE LEVRET, French obstetrician, 1703-1780, produced an improved obstetric forceps having cephalic and pelvic curves. Recorded in 1747. Known as *Levret's forceps.*

**Obstetrics, introduction of
  antisepsis in**

ÉTIENNE STÉPHANE TARNIER, French obstetrician, 1828-1897, is credited with introducing the methods of Lister in obstetrics. He was the first to use a solution of carbolic acid. Published in 1894.

**Occipital and preoccipital areas
  of cerebral cortex**

KORBINIAN BRODMANN, German neurologist, 1868-1918, described the occipital and preoccipital areas of the cerebral cortex. Recorded in 1908. Known as *Brodmann's areas.*

Occipital bone, ossification center which becomes basilar process of

THEODOR KERCKRING, German anatomist in Holland, 1640-1693, described an ossification center or small bone which becomes the basilar process of the occipital bone. Published in 1717. Known as *Kerckring's ossicle.*

Occipital convolution, posterior, of brain

ALEXANDER ECKER, German anatomist, 1816 - 1887, described the posterior occipital convolution of the brain, in 1869. Known as *Ecker's convolution.*

Occipitothalamic radiation

. . . See under *Optic radiation, description of.*

Occupational diseases, first important treatise on

BERNARDINO RAMAZZINI, Italian physician, 1633-1714, wrote the first adequate book on occupational diseases in which he dealt with pneumoconiosis, silicosis, lead poisoning, etc. Published in 1700.

Occupational diseases

. . . See also under name of particular disease, as *Chimney sweep's cancer.*

Ocular lens for oil immersion objective

. . . See under *Oil immersion lens, introduction of.*

Ocular muscles, motor anomalies of

. . . See under *Eye, motor anomalies,* etc.

Oculocardiac reflex, first description of

BERNARD ASCHNER, Austrian gynecologist, 1883 - 19??, discovered that pressure on the eyeballs causes a slowing of the beat of the heart. Reported in 1908. Known as *Aschner's phenomenon* or *reflex.*

Odontoid ligaments, lateral, eponymic description of

BURKHARD DAVID MAUCHART, German anatomist, 1696-1751, described the lateral odontoid ligaments, *circa* 1738. Known as *check ligaments, Mauchart's ligaments,* etc.

O'Dwyer tube

. . . See under *Intubation, laryngeal, in croup.*

Oedipus complex, introduction of concept of

SIGMUND FREUD, Austrian psychiatrist, 1856-1939, introduced the concept of an Oedipus complex, the erotic fixation of a son toward his mother. *Circa* 1896.

Oehl's layer

. . . See under *Stratum lucidum, eponymic description of.*

Oguchi's disease

. . . See under *Night blindness, congenital, in Japan.*

Ohara's disease

. . . See under *Tularemia, Japanese form of.*

Ohm's law of electric current

GEORG SIMON OHM, German physicist, 1787-1854, determined that the strength of an electric current is directly proportional to the electromotive force (voltage) and inversely proportional to the resistance of the circuit. This applies to direct current. Reported in 1827.

Oil immersion lens, introduction of

ERNST KARL ABBE, German physicist and mathematician, 1840-1905, developed and introduced the oil immersion lens, as well as a compensating ocular lens, in 1878. He reported it in a paper dated 1886.

Oil of chenopodium in ancylostomiasis

. . . See under *Hookworm disease, oil of chenopodium in.*

Ointment of benzoic and salicylic acids

ARTHUR WHITFIELD, English dermatologist, 1867-1947, devised an antiseptic ointment composed of benzoic and salicylic acids and petrolatum. Recorded in 1907. Known as *Whitfield's ointment.*

Ointment of calamine; Turner's cerate

DANIEL TURNER, English dermatologist, 1667-1740, produced a cerate or ointment containing calamine, *circa* 1700.

Ointment of yellow oxide of mercury, ophthalmic

ALEXANDER PAGENSTECHER, German ophthalmologist, 1828-1879, is credited with introducing an ointment of yellow mercuric oxide for use in the eye, about 1862. Known as *Pagenstecher's ointment.*

Olecranon, intratendinous bursa of; eponymic description

ALEXANDER MONROE, *primus,* 1697-1767, described the intraten-

dinous bursa of the olecranon, in 1726. Known as *Monroe's bursa.*

Olfactory bulb; tubercle of Morgagni

GIOVANNI BATTISTA MORGAGNI, Italian anatomist and pathologist, 1682-1771, is credited with describing the expanded portion of the olfactory nerve on the inferior surface of the anterior lobe of the cerebrum. Date not available. Known as *tubercle of Morgagni,* which also refers to the cuneiform cartilage of the larynx.

Olfactory mucous membrane, cells of

MAXIMILIAN J. S. SCHULTZE, German anatomist and histologist, 1825-1874, described the cells of the olfactory mucous membrane. Published in 1862. Known as *Schultze's cells.*

Olfactory nerves, function of

. . . See under *Cranial nerves, first pair, function of.*

Olfactory nerves, original description of

JOHN HUNTER, Scottish surgeon in England, 1728-1793, described the olfactory nerves in 1786.

Oligodendroglia, discovery and naming of

PIO DEL RIO HORTEGA, Spanish neurologist, 1882-1945, discovered and named the oligodendroglia, in 1921.

Olivospinal tract

. . . See under *Nerves, tract of, in cervical region.*

Ollier's disease

. . . See under *Dyschondroplasia, eponymic description of.*

Ollier's grafts

. . . See under *Skin grafts, intermediate thickness, introduction of.*

Ollier's layer

. . . See under *Periosteum, osteogenetic layer of.*

Omentopexy for relief of cirrhosis of liver

JAMES RUTHERFORD MORISON, English surgeon, 1853-1939, with DAVID DRUMMOND, introduced omentopexy to relieve ascites due to cirrhosis of the liver. Recorded in 1896. The same type of operation was devised independently by SAPE TALMA, Dutch surgeon, 1847-1918, in 1898. Known as *Morison-Talma operation.*

Oophoroma folliculare, first description of

FRITZ BRENNER, German physician, 1887-19??, was the first to describe a follicular ovarian tumor, oophoroma folliculare, in 1907. Known as *Brenner's tumor.*

Operating room, use of carbolic acid spray in

. . . See under *Carbolic acid spray in operating room.*

Operation for relief of esophageal stricture by use of a string

. . . See under *String operation, etc.*

Ophryospinal angle, eponymic description of

PAUL TOPINARD, French anthropologist, 1830-1911, described an angle formed at the anterior nasal spine by lines extending from the auricular point and the glabella. Published in 1876. Known as *Topinard's angle.*

Ophthalmia neonatorum, prophylaxis of, by use of silver nitrate solution

KARL S. F. CREDÉ, German gynecologist, 1819-1892, introduced the use of silver nitrate solution, instilled into the eyes of the newborn, as a method of prophylaxis for ophthalmia neonatorum. Reported in 1884.

Ophthalmology, first important textbook on, in the United States

GEORGE FRICK, American ophthalmologist, 1793-1870, is credited with the writing of the first complete textbook on ophthalmology, in 1823.

Ophthalmology, first printed book on

BENVENUTO GRASSI, Jerusalem physician in Italy, 12th century, wrote a classic work on ophthalmology which survived for more than four centuries. It was the first printed book on the subject. Published in 1474.

Ophthalmometer, invention of

LOUIS EMILE JAVAL, French ophthalmologist, 1839-1907, with H. SCHIOTZ, invented an ophthalmometer, in 1881.

Ophthalmoscope, early invention of

CHARLES BABBAGE, English mathematician, 1792-1871, is credited with the construction of a simple ophthalmoscope, in 1847.

Ophthalmoscope, first suggestion for the construction of

WILLIAM CUMMING, English physician, 1812-1886, observed the retinal reflex and the entrance of the optic nerve. As a result, he made the first suggestion for the construction of an instrument with which to examine the fundus of the eye. Recorded in 1846.

Ophthalmoscope in diseases of nervous system

JOHN HUGHLINGS JACKSON, English neurologist, 1835-1911, was the first to demonstrate the importance of ophthalmoscopy in the study of diseases of the nervous system. Recorded in 1864.

Ophthalmoscope, invention of first modern

HERMANN L. F. VON HELMHOLTZ, German physiologist and physicist, 1821-1894, is credited with the invention of the modern ophthalmoscope. Recorded in 1851.

Opisthion, introduction of, as craniometric point

PIERRE PAUL BROCA, French surgeon and anthropologist, 1824-1880, defined *opisthion* as a craniometric point. Exact date not available.

Opium addiction, treatment of, with medicine said to contain strychnine and gold chloride

. . . See under *Morphine addiction, treatment of,* etc.

Oppenheim's disease

. . . See under *Amyotonia congenita.*

Oppenheim-Urbach disease

. . . See under *Necrobiosis lipoidica diabeticorum.*

Oppilação is due to ancylostomiasis

. . . See under *Hypohemia intertropicalis.*

Opsonic index, introduction of term

ALMROTH EDWARD WRIGHT, English pathologist and bacteriologist, 1861-1947, introduced the term *opsonic index,* to indicate the relation between a normal serum and a particular serum with regard to phagocytic action. Recorded in 1904.

Opsonins in normal and immune serums

ALMROTH EDWARD WRIGHT, English pathologist and bacteriologist, 1861-1947, with STEWART RANKEN DOUGLAS, demonstrated the presence of opsonins in both normal and immune serums. Recorded in 1903.

Optic nerve, axial neuritis of

THEODOR LEBER, German ophthalmologist, 1840-1917, described a hereditary form of axial neuritis of the optic nerve. Recorded in 1871. Known as *Leber's optic atrophy* or *disease.*

Optic nerve, peripheral atrophy of

ERNST FUCHS, Austrian ophthalmologist, 1851-1930, described peripheral optic nerve atrophy, in 1885.

**Optic nerves, semi-
decussation of**

WILLIAM HYDE WOLLASTON, English physician and physicist, 1766-1828, is credited with suggesting the idea of semidecussation with regard to the optic nerves, in 1800.

**Optic neuro-encephalomyelo-
pathy**

... See under *Neuromyelitis optica*.

Optic papilla

... See under *Blind spot of retina*.

Optic radiation, description of

LOUIS PIERRE GRATIOLET, French anatomist and zoologist, 1815-1865, described the occipitothalamic radiation, a group of fibers from the lower visual centers which extend backward through the occipital portion of the internal capsule to the cortex of the occipital lobe. Published in 1856. Known as the *optic* or *occipitothalamic radiation, Gratiolet's optic radiation,* and *radiatio occipitothalamica.*

**Optic tract, fibers extending
from, to habenular ganglion**

LIVERI O. DARKSHEVICH, Russian neurologist, 1858-1925, described the nerve fibers which run from the optic tract to the habenular ganglion. Recorded in 1904.

**Optical activity in differentiating
chemical substances**

LOUIS PASTEUR, French scientist and bacteriologist, 1822-1895, is credited with discovering the use of polarization of light and optical activity as a means of differentiating chemical substances, *circa* 1847.

**Optical illusion in which a vertical
line seems to incline in a
direction opposite that of head**

HERMANN AUBERT, German physiologist, 1826-1892, was first to describe the optical illusion in which a vertical line seems to incline in a direction opposite from that in which the head inclines. Known as the Aubert phenomenon. Reported in 1865.

Optics, physiological, founder of

THOMAS YOUNG, English physician, 1773-1829, is regarded as the founder of physiological optics.

**Optochin, introduction of, in
treatment of pneumonia**

JULIUS MORGENROTH, German physician, 1871-1924, is credited with discovering the effectiveness of ethylhydrocupreine (optochin) in treating pneumococcal infections. Published in 1911.

Oral Surgery, Father of

JAMES E. GARRETSON, American dentist, 1828-1895, a pioneer in maxillary and oral surgery, is credited with being the Father of Oral Surgery.

**Orange Juice for scurvy,
early use of—1564**

BALDUINUS RONSSEUS, Dutch physician, 1525-1597, described the use of orange and lemon juice by Dutch sailors for the prevention and treatment of scurvy, in 1564.

**Orbicularis oculi, pars
lacrimalis of**

... See under *Tensor tarsi muscle*.

Orbital muscle of Müller

HEINRICH MÜLLER, German anatomist, 1820-1864, described the orbitalis muscle which bridges the inferior orbital fissure and, when contracted, tends to protrude the eye. Recorded in 1858.

Organ inferiority concept, first propounding of

ALFRED ADLER, Austrian psychiatrist, 1870-1937, was first to propound the theory of organ inferiority as it affects the mind. Report published in 1907.

Organ of Corti, outermost cells covering the

VIKTOR HENSEN, German pathologist, 1835-1924, discovered the outermost cells covering the organ of Corti. Reported in 1902. Known as *cells of Hensen.*

Organ of Jacobson, eponymic description of

. . . See under *Vomeronasal organ.*

Organ of Jacobson, eponymization of

GEORGES LEOPOLD C.F.D. CUVIER, French anatomist and naturalist, 1769-1832, is believed to have eponymized the vomeronasal organ as the *organ of Jacobson,* in 1811.

Organic compound, first synthesis of an

FRIEDRICH WÖHLER, German chemist, 1800-1882, was the first to synthesize an organic compound, urea, in 1828.

Organisms consist of cells, early recognition that

LORENZ OKEN, German naturalist and physiologist, 1779-1851, believed that organisms originate from and consist of cells. Published in 1805.

Organizers in embryonic development, introduction of concept of

HANS SPEMANN, German embryologist, 1869-1941, introduced the organizing-effect theory of embryonal development, stating that the interaction between the different regions of tissue results in structural development. Published in 1927 and 1931. Spemann received the Nobel prize in 1935.

Organs, excised, use of perfusion to keep alive

KARL FRIEDRICH W. LUDWIG, German physiologist, 1816-1895, is credited with introducing the idea of keeping organs and other excised parts alive by means or perfusion, in 1865.

Organs of taste

. . . See under *Papillae of tongue as organs of taste.*

Oriental sore, classic description of

JEAN LOUIS ALIBERT, French dermatologist, 1766-1837, gave a comprehensive description of oriental sore, in 1829.

Ornithology, first great atlas of

JOHN JAMES LAFOREST AUDUBON, American ornithologist, 1784-1851, prepared the first modern atlas of ornithology, *The Birds of America.* Published 1827-38. He also wrote, with WILLIAM MACGILLIVRAY, a five-volume text to accompany the atlas, titled *Ornithological Biography.* Published between 1831 and 1839.

Ornithology, first modern work on

WILLIAM TURNER, English physician and naturalist, 1510-1568, wrote the first modern ornithological work. Published in 1544.

Oroya fever, causative agent of

A. L. BARTON, Peruvian physician, 1874-19??, described the causative organism of Oroya fever, now known as *Bartonella bacilliformis,* in 1909.

Oroya fever

. . . See also under *Carrión's disease.*

Orthopedic hospital, founding of first

JEAN ANDRÉ VENEL, Swiss surgeon, 1740-1791, is credited with founding the first orthopedic hospital, at Orbe, Switzerland, in 1790.

Orthopedics, first book on

NICOLAS ANDRÉ, French physician, 1658-1742, is credited with the writing of the first book devoted entirely to orthopedics. It was published in 1741 under the title *L'orthopédie ou l'art de prévenir et de corriger dans les enfans, les difformités du corps.*

Orthopedics, origin of term

NICOLAS ANDRÉ, French physician, 1658-1742, coined the word *orthopedics,* or its French equivalent, in 1741.

Oscillating bed for vascular disease

. . . See under *Bed, seesawing, for cardiovascular,* etc.

Osgood-Schlatter disease

. . . See under *Tibial tuberosity, painful lesions of*—1903.

Osler-Vaquez disease

. . . See under *Polycythemia, splenomegalic.*

Osmosis, early observations on—1748

JEAN ANTOINE NOLLET, French physicist, 1700-1770, observed and described the double exchange of solutions, in 1748.

Osmosis, early observations on—1822

MICHELE FODERA, Italian physician, 1792-1848, studied the principles involved in osmosis. Reported in 1822.

Osmosis, first clear explanation of

RENÉ J. H. DUTROCHET, French physiologist, 1776-1847, gave the first satisfactory account of osmosis, in 1827.

Osmosis, introduction of term

THOMAS GRAHAM, Scottish chemist, 1805-1869, is credited with having introduced the term *osmosis* in 1854, on the basis of the words *endosmose* and *exosmose* introduced by Dutrochet in 1827.

Osmotic pressure, introduction of term

WILHEM F. P. PFEFFER, German scientist, 1845-1920, studied the forces of osmosis and introduced the term *osmotic pressure,* in 1877.

Ossicles, early description of

NICCOLO MASSA, Italian physician, 1499-1569, gave one of the earliest descriptions of the function of the ossicles. Published in 1536.

Ossification, hexosephosphoric esters in

. . . See under *Hexosephosphoric esters,* etc.

Osteitis, chronic sclerosing

CARL GARRE, Swiss surgeon, 1857-1928, described a form of chronic sclerosing osteitis or osteomyelitis, marked by small areas of necrosis but little suppuration, in 1893.

Osteitis deformans, eponymic description of

JAMES PAGET, English surgeon, 1814-1899, described a disease of bones marked by rarefaction, bowing of the long bones, and disfigurement of the flat bones. Recorded in 1877. Known as *Paget's disease*.

Osteitis deformans, introduction of term

VINCENZ CZERNY, German surgeon, 1842-1916, is credited with introducing the concept and term of *osteitis deformans*, in 1873. It was JAMES PAGET who gave the classic description of the disease.

Osteitis fibrosa and parathyroid glands

. . . See under *Parathyroid glands*, etc.

Osteitis fibrosa cystica, eponymic description of

FRIEDRICH DANIEL VON RECKLINGHAUSEN, German pathologist, 1833-1910, gave a full description of osteitis fibrosa cystica in 1891. Known, sometimes, as *Engel-Recklinghausen disease*. A preliminary report appeared in 1889.

Osteitis fibrosa cystica, first description of

GERHARD ENGEL, German physician, 1830-189?, gave the first recorded description of osteitis fibrosa cystica, in 1864.

Osteitis fibrosa disseminata

. . . See under *Precocious puberty in females*, etc.

Osteoarthritis, nodes on interphalangeal joints in

WILLIAM HEBERDEN, *père*, English physician, 1710-1801, described bony nodules appearing at the distal joints of the fingers in cases of osteoarthritis. Observed *circa* 1754; reported posthumously in 1802. Known as *Heberden's nodes*.

Osteochondritic epiphysial separation in congenital syphilis

FRIEDRICH RUDOLPH GEORG WEGNER, German pathologist, 1843-189?, described osteochondritic separation of the epiphyses in cases of congenital syphilis. Recorded in 1870. Known as *Wegner's disease*.

Osteochondritis deformans juvenilis, description of, in February, 1910

ARTHUR THORNTON LEGG, American orthopedic surgeon, 1874-1939, described osteochondritis deformans juvenilis, osteochondrosis of capitular epiphysis, in a report published February 17, 1910. The condition is known eponymically as *Legg-Calvé-Perthes disease*.

Osteochondritis deformans juvenilis, description of, in July, 1910

JACQUES CALVÉ, French surgeon, 1875-19??, described osteochondritis deformans juvenilis (osteochondrosis of capitular epiphysis) in a report published in July, 1910.

The condition is known as *Legg-Calvé-Perthes disease.*

Osteochondritis deformans juvenilis, description of, in October, 1910

GEORG CLEMENS PERTHES, German surgeon, 1869-1927, described osteochondritis deformans juvenilis (to which he referred as "arthritis deformans juvenilis") in a paper published in October, 1910. He published another report under the title "Osteochondritis deformans juvenilis" in June, 1913. The condition is known as *Legg-Calvé-Perthes disease.*

Osteochondritis dissecans, first description of

FRANZ KÖNIG, German surgeon, 1832-1910, was first to describe osteochondritis dissecans, a condition marked by splitting of joint cartilage, especially in the knee and shoulder joints. Published in 1888.

Osteochondritis dissecans, introduction of term

FRANZ KÖNIG, German surgeon, 1832-1910, was the first to use the term *osteochondritis dissecans;* he was also the first to describe the condition. Recorded in 1888.

Osteochondrosis of tuberosity of tibia

. . . See under *Tibial tuberosity, painful lesions of*—1903.

Osteoclasts, eponymic description of

CHARLES PHILIPPE ROBIN, French physician, 1821-1885, described osteoclasts, in a work on bone formation, in 1851. Known as *Robin's myeloplaxes.*

Osteodystrophia fibrosa; Albright's syndrome

. . . See under *Precocious puberty in females, pigmentation,* etc.

Osteogenesis imperfecta, eponymic description of

JOHANN GEORG C. F. M. LOBSTEIN, Alsatian pathologist, 1777-1835, described osteogenesis imperfecta (osteopsathyrosis), a condition in which the bones are subject to fractures because of abnormal brittleness, in 1833. Known as *Lobstein's disease.*

Osteomalacia due to vitamin D deficiency

JOHN PRESTON MAXWELL, English physician in China, 1871-19??, demonstrated that osteomalacia is caused by a deficiency of vitamin D. Recorded in 1930.

Osteomalacia, first description of

JEAN LOUIS PETIT, French surgeon, 1674-1750, is credited with giving the first description of osteomalacia, about 1705.

Osteomyelitis, chronic sclerosing

. . . See under *Osteitis, chronic sclerosing.*

Osteomyelitis, treatment of, by use of maggots

. . . See under *Maggot therapy,* etc.

Osteopathy, founder of

ANDREW TAYLOR STILL, American osteopathic physician, 1828-1917, founded osteopathy about 1875. The American School of Osteopathy was founded in Kirksville, Mo., in 1892.

Osteopetrosis; marmorization of bone

HEINRICH ERNST ALBERS-SCHÖN-

BERG, German surgeon, 1865-1921, described a condition in which there are bandlike areas of condensed bone near the epiphyseal lines of long bones and areas of condensation near the edges of small bones. Recorded in 1903. The disorder is known as *Albers-Schönberg disease, marble bone, ivory bone, marmorknochen,* etc.

Osteoplastic periostitis of metatarsal bones

JEAN EUGÈNE PAUZAT, French physician, 1851-1919, described osteoplastic periostitis of the metatarsal bones. Recorded in 1887. Known as *Pauzat's disease.*

Osteopsathyrosis, first description of

. . . See under *Osteogenesis imperfecta, eponymic description of.*

Otoliths, functions of

RUDOLPH MAGNUS, German physiologist in Holland, 1873-1927, studied the functions of the otoliths (otoconia) in the gelatinous film covering the maculae acusticae and demonstrated them to be comparable to those of the semicircular canals, published in 1926.

Otomycosis, early description of

ROBERT ROBERTOVICH WREDEN, Russian otologist to the Czars, 1837-1893, called attention to otomycosis in a treatise reporting six such cases. Published in 1867.

Otosclerosis, first successful treatment of, by fenestration

MAURICE LOUIS JOSEPH MARIE SOURDILLE, French otologist, 1896-, is said to have been the first to operate successfully for the restoration of hearing by fenestration in case of otosclerosis. Reported in 1937.

Otosclerosis, original description of

ADAM POLITZER, Austrian otologist, 1835-1920, described otosclerosis as a medical entity, in 1893, in a paper titled "On a peculiar affection of the labyrinthine capsule as a frequent cause of deafness."

Otosclerosis, use of fenestration in

. . . See under *Fenestration in treatment of partial deafness.* See also *Otosclerosis, first successful treatment of, by fenestration.*

Otoscope, invention of modern

ANTON FRIEDRICH VON TRÖLTSCH, German otologist, 1829-1890, is credited with devising the first modern otoscope, in 1860.

Otto's disease

. . . See under *Acetabulum, osteoarthitic protrusion of.*

Ovarian cystoma, drainage of, by tapping

ROBERT HOUSTOUN, English surgeon, 16??-1734, was the first to tap the cyst in a case of ovarian dropsy or cystoma. Recorded in 1726.

Ovarian disease, facial expression in

THOMAS SPENCER WELLS, English gynecologist, 1818-1897, described a peculiar anxious expression observed in patients with ovarian disease. Recorded in 1865. Known as *Wells's facies.*

Ovarian endometriomas, eponymic description of

JOHN ALBERTSON SAMPSON, American surgeon, 1873-1946, described ovarian endometriomas, in 1921. Known as *Sampson's implants, endometrial implants,* or *endometriosis.*

Ovarian hormone, carcinogenic effect of

ANTOINE MARCELLIN LACASSAGNE, French physician, 1884-19??, discovered that carcinoma of the breast can be produced in animals by estrone benzoate. Recorded in 1932.

Ovarian hormone in chronic mastitis

MAX CUTLER, American surgeon, 1899-   , was the first to prescribe ovarian hormone systematically in the treatment of chronic mastitis. Published in 1931.

Ovarian hormones, active principle of, preliminary report on

EDGAR ALLEN, American anatomist, 1892-1943, worked with E. A. DOISY (American biochemist and physiologist, 1893-   ) on the extraction of the active principle from ovarian hormones. Findings recorded in a preliminary report published in 1923.

Ovarian pregnancy, early description of

BENJAMIN JAN KOUWER, Dutch gynecologist, 1861-1933, is credited with giving the first description of an ovarian pregnancy. Recorded in 1897.

Ovariectomy, double, first successful

JOHN LIGHT ATLEE, American surgeon, 1799-1885, is credited with being the first to remove success-

fully both ovaries in a case of ovarian tumors. Published in 1843.

Ovariectomy, early successful

EPHRAIM McDOWELL, American surgeon, 1771-1830, performed one of several ovariectomies as early as 1809. Published in 1817. The operation, performed by abdominal section, is known as *McDowell's operation.*

Ovariotomy, early performance of

NATHAN SMITH, American surgeon, 1762-1829, performed the operation of ovariotomy on July 25, 1821. Recorded in 1822.

Ovariotomy, first attempted, in England

JOHN LIZARS, Scottish surgeon, *circa* 1785-1860, is credited with being the first to attempt ovariotomy in Great Britain. Recorded in 1825. Although the operation was unsuccessful, it stimulated further, more successful operations.

Ovariotomy for treatment of non-ovarian diseases

ROBERT BATTEY, American gynecologist, 1828-1895, devised an operation of ovariotomy for the treatment of non-ovarian diseases. Recorded in 1873. Battey's operation gained in importance later on because of the development of modern endocrinology.

Ovariotomy, introduction of term

CHARLES CLAY, English surgeon, 1801-1893, is credited with introducing the term *ovariotomy, circa* 1842. About four years later, and independently of Clay, JAMES YOUNG SIMPSON, Scottish obstetrician, 1811-1870, also introduced the term *ovariotomy.*

**Ovary, dermoid cysts of,
early description of**

MATTHEW BAILLIE, English physician, 1761-1823, described dermoid cysts of the ovary, in 1789.

**Ovary, line of insertion of
mesovarium in**

HEINRICH WILHELM GOTTFRIED WALDEYER-HARTZ, German anatomist, 1836-1921, described the line which forms the boundary of the insertion of the mesovarium in the ovary, at the hilus. Recorded in 1870. Known as *Waldeyer's line.*

Ovary, vascular layer of

HEINRICH WILHELM GOTTFRIED WALDEYER-HARTZ, German anatomist, 1836-1921, described the vascular layer of the ovary, in 1870.

**Ovary-stimulating hormone
of placenta**

. . . See under *Anterior pituitary-like factor,* etc.

**Oviducts, human, early
description of**

. . . See under *Uterine tubes.*

Ovum, germinal spot of

. . . See under *Germinal spot of animal egg.*

**Ovum, impregnated, passage
of, through uterine tube**

WILLIAM C. CRUIKSHANK, English surgeon, 1745-1800, demonstrated the passage of the impregnated ovum (in the rabbit) through the uterine tube into the uterus. Reported in 1797.

Ovum of mammals, discovery of

KARL ERNST VON BAER, German embryologist born in Estonia, 1792-1876, was the first to describe the mammalian ovum, in 1827. He demonstrated that the graafian follicles are not the eggs, as was believed before, but merely hold the "vesicles" which are the true eggs.

**Ovum of vertebrate animals is
single cell, proof that**

CARL GEGENBAUR, German anatomist, 1826-1903, is credited with being first to establish the fact that the ovum of a vertebrate animal is a single cell, in 1861.

**Ovum, small vesicle of
ovary containing the**

REGNIER DE GRAAF, Dutch anatomist, 1641-1673, studied the ovary and described the small vesicular sac of the ovarian cortex which contains the ovum. Work published in 1672. Known as *graafian follicle.* The term *graafian follicle* was suggested by ALBRECHT VON HALLER, Swiss anatomist, *circa* 1730.

Oxaluria, early description of

GOLDING BIRD, English physician, 1814-1854, described the condition marked by the presence of abnormal quantities of oxalic acid and oxalates in the urine. Known as *Bird's disease.* Reported in 1842.

**Oxophenarsine hydrochloride,
use of, in syphilis**

OTTO H. FOERSTER, American physician, 1876-19??, with R. L. MCINTOSH, L. M. WIEDER, H. R. FOERSTER, and G. A. COOPER, introduced the use of mapharsen, oxophenarsine hydrochloride, in the treatment of syphilis. Report dated Dec. 1935.

Oxygen, discovery and isolation of, by Priestley

JOSEPH PRIESTLEY, English chemist and clergyman, 1733-1804, isolated oxygen by igniting mercuric oxide. Recorded in 1774. Priestly called oxygen "dephlogisticated air."

Oxygen in combustion, function of

ANTOINE LAURENT LAVOISIER, French chemist, 1743-1794, discovered the function of oxygen in combustion, in 1776.

Oxygen, introduction of term

ANTOINE LAURENT LAVOISIER, French chemist, 1743-1794, is credited with the introduction of the name *oxygen,* previously called "dephlogisticated air" by its discoverer. *Circa* 1775.

Oxygen is used in recovery phase of muscular activity, demonstration that

ARCHIBALD V. HILL, English biophysicist, 1886-19??, demonstrated that oxygen is used in the recovery phase of muscular activity but not in the contracting phase. Reported, with W HARTREE, in 1920-1922. Received the Nobel prize in 1922.

Oxygen therapy, introduction of

JOHN SCOTT HALDANE, Scottish physiologist, 1860-1936, is credited with introducing modern oxygen therapy, in 1917.

Oxygen-nitrous oxide mixture, advocacy of

EDMUND ANDREWS, American physician, 1824-1904, suggested the use of an oxygen-nitrous oxide mixture. Recorded in 1868.

Oxyhemoglobin, introduction of term

ERNST F. I. HOPPE-SEYLER, German physiological chemist, 1825-1895, introduced the term *oxyhaemoglobin,* about 1862.

Oxyquinoline sulfate-scarlet red gauze for healing wounds and protecting grafts

ADALBERT G. BETTMAN, American physician, 1883-19??, devised a method for treating denuded areas and for protecting skin grafts by using gauze impregnated with scarlet red and oxyquinoline sulfate. Reported in 1931.

Ozena as clinical entity, recognition of

BERNHARD FRAENKEL, German physician, 1836-1911, recognized ozena as a clinical entity. Published in 1876.

Ozena, finding of bacillus in

BENJAMIN BENNO LOEWENBERG, German surgeon, 1836-19??, discovered a bacillus in the nasal secretion of a patient affected with ozena. Recorded in 1884. Other reports on the pathology and the organism were published later.

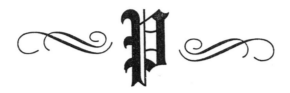

Pacchionian bodies, original description of

ANTONIO PACCHIONI, Italian anatomist, 1665-1726, described small arachnoid elevations which form clusters on the surface of the dura mater and produce depressions on the inner surface of the cranium. Pacchioni thought they were glands concerned with the production of lymph. Published in 1705.

Pacemaker of heart, designation of

THOMAS LEWIS, English physician, 1881-1945, designated the sino-auricular node as the pacemaker of the heart. Recorded in 1910.

Pacinian corpuscles, introduction of term

FRIEDRICH G. J. HENLE, German anatomist, 1809-1885, and RUDOLPH ALBERT VON KÖLLIKER (Swiss histologist, 1817-1905) are credited with introducing the term *Pacinian corpuscles,* in 1844.

Pacini's corpuscles; Pacinian corpuscles

FILIPPO PACINI, Italian anatomist, 1812-1883, described an end organ of the skin composed of a granular central bulb which encloses a terminal neurofibril. Recorded in 1840.

Known as *Vater-Pacini corpuscles,* after ABRAHAM VATER who is said to have described the corpuscle previously.

Pagenstecher's ointment

. . . See under *Ointment of yellow oxide of mercury, ophthalmic.*

Paget's disease of bone

. . . See under *Osteitis deformans.*

Paget's disease of nipple

. . . See under *Nipple, Paget's disease of.*

Pain and weather; relation between; early description of

SILAS WEIR MITCHELL, American neurologist, 1829-1914, described the relation of pain to weather as observed in a case of traumatic neuralgia. Published in 1877.

Pain, relief of, by infiltration of frontal lobes

. . . See under *Frontal lobes, infiltration of,* etc.

Painful heel, eponymic description of

EDUARD ALBERT, Austrian surgeon, 1841-1900, described the condition of painful heel. Recorded in 1893. Known as *achillodynia, Albert's disease,* and *Swediaur's disease.*

Pajot's hook

... See under *Hook for decapitating fetus in difficult labor.*

Palate, hard and soft, differentiation of

GABRIEL FALLOPIUS, Italian anatomist, 1523-1562, is credited with differentiating the hard palate from the soft palate, *circa* 1552. Previously both were known under the term *diaphragma oris.*

Palate, hard, small masses on each side of, in newborn

ALOIS EPSTEIN, German physician, 1849-1918, described small yellowish-white masses on each side of the raphe of the hard palate in newborn. Recorded in 1890. Known as *Epstein's pearls.*

Palatine nerve, anterior, point of emergence of

JEAN ANTOINE MEGLIN, French physician, 1756-1824, described the point of emergence of the anterior palatine nerve from the greater palatine foramen. Date not available. Known as *Meglin's point.*

Palatopharyngolaryngeal hemiplegia, eponymic description of

ANTONIO GARCIA TAPIA, Spanish physician, 1875-19??, described palatopharyngolaryngeal hemiplegia, also involving the sternocleidomastoid muscle and the tongue. Recorded in 1905. Known as *Tapia's syndrome.*

Paleocerebellum and neocerebellum, differentiation between

LUDWIG EDINGER, German neurologist, 1855-1918, was the first to distinguish between the paleocerebellum and the neocerebellum. Reported in 1885.

Paleocerebrum and neocerebrum, differentiation between

LUDWIG EDINGER, German neurologist, 1855-1918, was the first to distinguish between the paleocerebrum and the neocerebrum. Reported in 1885.

Palladium, discovery of

WILLIAM HYDE WOLLASTON, English physician and physicist, 1766-1828, discovered palladium in 1803. He named it *palladium* in allusion to the asteroid Pallas.

Palmaris brevis muscle, discovery of

GIOVANNI BATTISTA CANANO, Italian anatomist, 1515-1579, discovered the palmaris brevis muscle which tenses the palm of the hand. Exact date not available.

Palpebral fissure, widening of, in exophthalmic goiter

CARL STELLWAG VON CARION, Austrian ophthalmologist, 1823-1904, noted the widening of the palpebral fissure and the absence or infrequency of the winking movements in exophthalmic goiter. Recorded in 1869. Known as *Stellwag's sign.*

Palpitation, early use of quinine for

JEAN BAPTISTE SENAC, French physician, 1693-1770, was first to use quinine to control palpitation. Recorded in 1749.

Paludrine in treatment of malaria

... See under *Malaria, proguanil in treatment of.*

Pamaquine in treatment of malaria

. . . See under *Malaria, plasmoquine in treatment of.*

p-Aminobenzoic acid, recognition of

STEFAN ANSBACHER, German-American biochemist, 1905-   , is credited with recognizing *p*-aminobenzoic acid as a member of the vitamin B complex. Published in 1941.

Panaris, analgesic

. . . See under *Syringomyelia with atrophy and paralysis of hands and forearms.*

Panatrophy, local, first description of

WILLIAM RICHARD GOWERS, English neurologist, 1845-1915, was first to give a clear description of local panatrophy. Published in 1886.

Pancreas, accessory duct of

GIOVANNI DOMENICO SANTORINI, Italian anatomist, 1681-1739, described the accessory pancreatic duct. Published in 1724. Known as *Santorini's duct.*

Pancreas and duodenum, resection of, for carcinoma

. . . See under *Duodenopancreatectomy in treating carcinoma.*

Pancreas, excision of, causes thirst and polyuria

JOHANN CONRAD BRUNNER, Swiss anatomist, 1653-1727, experimenting with dogs, found that excision of the pancreas caused, in some cases, thirst and polyuria. Reported in 1683.

Pancreas, excretory duct of, in fowl; discovery of

MORITZ HOFFMANN, German anatomist, 1622-1698, is believed to have discovered the excretory duct of the pancreas in fowl, in 1642. It is also believed that this led to the discovery of the duct in man by WIRSUNG, in the same year.

Pancreas, excretory duct of, in man; discovery of

JOHANN GEORG WIRSUNG, German physician and anatomist, 159?-1643, discovered and described the pancreatic duct in man, in 1642. A copper-plate illustration accompanied the brief account. Wirsung described the duct again in 1643, in a letter written to JOHANNES RIOLAN, French anatomist.

Pancreas, glandular layer of cells which line acini of

CLAUDE BERNARD, French physiologist, 1813-1878, described the glandular layer of cells which line the acini of the pancreas. Reported in 1849.

Pancreas, insulin-producing cells of

. . . See under *Islands of Langerhans, discovery of.*

Pancreas, lesser; Winslow's pancreas

JACOBUS BENIGNUS WINSLOW, Danish anatomist in France, 1669-1760, described the lesser pancreas, the small portion of the gland lying dorsal of its head, in 1710.

Pancreas, secretory innervation of

IVAN PETROVICH PAVLOV, Russian physiologist, 1849-1936, is credited with discovering the innervation of the secretory mechanism of the pancreas, *circa* 1888.

Pancreatic islands, hydropic degeneration of

. . . See under *Islands of Langerhans,* etc.

Pancreatic juice, digestive action of, demonstration of

CLAUDE BERNARD, French physiologist, 1813-1878, demonstrated the digestive action of pancreatic juice. Reported in 1848.

Pancreatic necrosis, first description of

WILHELM BALSER, German physician, 1843-1898, was the first to describe pancreatic fat necrosis. Published in 1882.

Pancreatic proteolysis and acidity of medium

LUCIEN CORVISART, French physician, 1811-1882, demonstrated that pancreatic proteolysis can take place in acid, neutral, or alkaline media, at body temperature. Published between 1857 and 1863.

Panniculitis, nodular nonsuppurative—1925

FREDERICK P. WEBER, English physician, 1863-19??, described a disease characterized by the formation of painful nodules in the subcutaneous fatty tissue, known as *nodular nonsuppurative panniculitis* and as *Christian-Weber disease.* Reported in 1925.

Panniculitis, nodular nonsuppurative—1928

HENRY A. CHRISTIAN, American physician, 1876-1951, described

nodular nonsuppurative panniculitis, known as *Christian-Weber disease,* in 1928.

Panparnit in parkinsonism

. . . See under *Parkinsonism.*

Pansch's fissure

. . . See under *Fissure extending from central fissue to occipital lobe.*

Pantopaque in diagnosis of cerebral tumors, introduction of

THEODORE BEHN STEINHAUSEN, American radiologist, 1914-   , with C. E. DUNGAN, J. B. FURST, J. T. PLATI, S. W. SMITH, A. P. DARLING, and E. C. WOLCOTT, introduced pantopaque, ethyl iodophenylundecylate, as a contrast medium in the diagnosis of cerebral tumors. Published in 1944.

Pantopon in injectable form

HERMANN SAHLI, Swiss physician, 1856-1933, suggested the use of pantopon by injection. Recorded in 1909.

Pantothenic acid, isolation of

ROGER JOHN WILLIAMS, American biochemist, 1893-   , is credited with isolating pantothenic acid from the other components of the vitamin B complex, in 1936.

Papaverine in smooth muscle spasm

JAKOB PAL, Vienna physician, 1863-1936, suggested the use of papaverine for relief of spasm of smooth muscle. Recorded in 1914.

Papaverine, isolation of

GEORG MERCK, German chemist, 1815-1888, is credited with isolating papaverine, in 1848.

Papillae of tongue as organs of taste, recognition of

LORENZO BELLINI, Italian anatomist, 1643-1704, described the papillae of the tongue as the organs of taste. Reported in 1665.

Papin's digester

. . . See under *Pressure boiler for digesting organic matter.*

Pappataci fever, causative virus of

ROBERT DOERR, German bacteriologist, 1871-1952, with K. FRANZ and S. TAUSSIG, demonstrated that the causative organism of pappataci fever is a virus transmitted by the vector *Phlebotomus papatasii.* Recorded in 1909.

Pappataci fever, cultivation of virus of

HENRY EDWARD SHORTT, English physician, 1887-19??, with R. SANJIVA RAO and C. S. SWAMINATH, cultivated the virus of pappataci fever. Recorded in 1936.

Pappataci fever, first recorded description of

ALOIS PICK, Austrian physician, 1859-1918, is credited with giving the first description of pappataci fever. Published in 1886.

Pappataci fever, sandfly vector of

ROBERT DOERR, German bacteriologist, 1871-1952, demonstrated that the sandfly, *Phlebotomus,* is responsible for the transmission of pappataci fever. Published in 1908.

Para-aminosalicylic acid in tuberculosis

. . . See under *Tuberculosis, para-aminosalicylic acid in treatment of.*

Paracusia of Willis; psophacusia

THOMAS WILLIS, English physician and anatomist, 1621-1675, described a perversion of the sense of hearing in which the subject hears better in a noisy environment. Recorded in 1672.

Paradidymis, early description of

JOACHIM A. C. C. GIRALDES, Portuguese surgeon in Paris, 1808-1875, described the paradidymis, the body of closed tubes situated on the spermatic cord above the epididymis, in 1859. Known as *organ of Giraldes.*

Paraffin in microscopic technique, introduction of

THEODOR ALBRECHT EDWIN KLEBS, German bacteriologist, 1834-1913, introduced paraffin impregnation or embedding into microscopic technique. Recorded in 1869.

Paraldehyde, introduction of

VINCENZO CERVELLO, Italian physician, 1854-1919, is credited with introducing paraldehyde in medical usage, as a hypnotic. Recorded in 1884.

Paralysis, acute ascending spinal; Landry's paralysis

JEAN B. O. LANDRY, French physician, 1826-1865, described an acute ascending spinal paralysis, usually beginning in the muscles of the feet and gradually ascending to higher levels of the body. Recorded in 1859. Known as *Landry's paralysis.*

Paralysis agitans; Parkinson's disease

JAMES PARKINSON, English physician, 1755-1824, described a condition marked by "Involuntary tremulous motion with lessened muscular power, with a propensity to bend the trunk forward and to pass from a walking to a running pace, the senses and intellects being uninjured." Published in 1817. Also called *shaking palsy.*

Paralysis, congenital cerebral spastic; Little's disease
. . . See under *Cerebral spastic paralysis.*

Paralysis, general, early description of
THOMAS WILLIS, English physician, 1621-1675, gave the first clear description of general paralysis of the insane. Recorded in 1672. Known as *dementia paralytica, syphilitic meningoencephalitis,* etc.

Paralysis, progressive ascending
. . . See next entry.

Paralysis, unilateral ascending; eponymic description
CHARLES KARSNER MILLS, American neurologist, 1845-1931, was the first to describe unilateral progressive ascending paralysis. Published in 1900. Known as *Mills's disease.*

Paramoeba, discovery and naming of
CHARLES F. CRAIG, American pathologist, 1872-1950, described a genus of flagellate protozoans, two species of which (*hominis* and *migrans*) inhabit the intestine and cause dysentery-like symptoms. The genus is now called *Craigia.* Reported in 1906.

Paramyoclonus multiplex, original description of
NIKOLAUS FRIEDREICH, German neurologist, 1825-1882, described a disease marked by paroxysmal contractions of the muscles of the extremities (paramyoclonus multiplex), in 1881. Known as *Friedreich's disease.*

Paramyotonia congenita, original description of
ALBERT EULENBURG, German physician, 1840-1917, described paramyotonia congenita, a disease marked by spasm of certain muscles, as of neck and face, when they are called into use. Known as *Eulenburg's disease.* Date not available.

Parapsoriasis, introduction of term
LOUIS ANNE JEAN BROCQ, French dermatologist, 1856-1928, suggested the term *parapsoriasis,* to describe an exfoliative dermatitis not due to any known cause. Published in 1902.

Parasite, first demonstration of life cycle of
KARL THEODOR ERNST VON SIEBOLD, German zoologist and parasitologist, 1804-1885, studied sheep staggers and demonstrated for the first time the complete life cycle of a parasite. Reported in 1854.

Parasite
. . . See also under name of particular parasite.

Parasympathetic nervous system, introduction of term
JOHN NEWPORT LANGLEY, English physiologist, 1852-1925, introduced the term *parasympathetic nervous system,* for the craniosacral portion of the autonomic nervous system, in 1905.

Parasympathetic status, introduction of term

WILLIAM FERDINAND PETERSEN, American pathologist, 1887-19??, introduced the term *parasympathetic status, circa* 1923.

Parasyphilis, introduction of concept of

JEAN ALFRED FOURNIER, French syphilologist, 1832-1914, is credited with introducing the concept of parasyphilis, to describe a disease partly due to syphilis. Recorded in 1894.

Parathormone, isolation of

. . . See under *Parathyroid hormone*.

Parathyroid glands, active principle of, isolation of

ADOLPH M. HANSON, American physician, 1883-19??, is credited with isolating the active principle of the parathyroid glands. Reported in 1923.

Parathyroid glands and osteitis fibrosa

MAX ASKANAZY, German pathologist, 1865-1940, was the first to note the association of parathyroid tumors and decalcification, observed in a case of osteitis fibrosa cystica. Published in 1904.

Parathyroid glands and thyroid gland, functional independence of

GUSTAV MOUSSU, French physician, 1864-19??, demonstrated the independence, functionally, of the thyroid gland and the parathyroid glands. Published in 1897.

Parathyroid glands, first full account of

IVAR VICTOR SANDSTRÖM, Swedish anatomist, 1852-1889, was the first to give a full and systematic description of the parathyroid glands, in 1880.

Parathyroid glands, recognition of, as essential to life

MARCEL EUGÈNE E. GLEY, French physiologist, 1857-1930, described the parathyroid glands and demonstrated that they are essential for life, in 1891.

Parathyroid hormone in treatment of tetany

JAMES BERTRAM COLLIP, Canadian physician and biochemist, 1892- , is credited with being the first to use parathyroid hormone in the treatment of tetany. Published, with DOUGLAS BURROWS LEITCH, in 1925.

Parathyroid hormone, isolation of

JAMES BERTRAM COLLIP, Canadian physician and biochemist, 1892- , isolated the active principle of the parathyroid glands, in 1925.

Parathyroid tetany, first description of, in Germany

SALOMON LEVI STEINHEIM, German physician, 1789-1866, is credited with giving the first description of parathyroid tetany in Germany. Published in 1830.

Parathyroid tumors, excision of, in osteitis fibrosa

FELIX MANDL, Austrian surgeon, 1892- , was the first to treat successfully a case of osteitis fibrosa by excision of a parathyroid tumor. Published in 1925.

Paratyphoid fever, description and naming of

EMILE CHARLES ACHARD, French physician, 1860-1944, with RAOUL BENSAUDE (French physician, 1866-1938) gave a classic description of paratyphoid fever, gave it the name, and isolated *Bacillus paratyphosus B*, in 1896. The organism is now classified as *Salmonella paratyphi B*.

Paratyphoid fever

... See also under the names of the organisms involved.

Paravertebral triangle, eponymic description of

PIETRO GROCCO, Italian physician, 1856-1916, described a triangular region of dullness on the back on the side opposite to a pleural effusion. Published in 1902. Known as *Grocco's triangle*.

Parenchyma, introduction of term

ERASISTRATUS, Greek anatomist and physician, *circa* 300-250 B.C., is believed to have introduced the term *parenchyma*.

Paresthesia of lower limbs in young persons, without objective symptoms

OSKAR BERGER, German neurologist, 1844-1885, described a peculiar paresthesia affecting the lower extremities of young persons, usually accompanied by weaknes but presenting no objective symptoms. Reported in 1879. Known as *Berger's paresthesia*.

Parham-Martin band

... See under *Fracture, treatment of, with metal band*.

Parietal angle, eponymic description of

JEAN LOUIS ARMAND DE QUATREFAGES DE BRÉAU, French anthropologist and naturalist, 1810-1892, described the parietal angle. Published in 1872. Known as *Quatrefages' angle*.

Parietal cells

... See under *Acid cells of gastric mucosa*.

Parkinsonism, caramiphen in treatment of

ERNST GRÜNTHAL, Swiss physician, 19??- , introduced caramiphen or panparnit in the treatment of parkinsonism. Recorded in 1946.

Parkinsonism, diparcol in treatment of

JEAN SIGWALD, French physician, 19??- , with D. BOVET and G. DUMONT, introduced diparcol in the treatment of parkinsonism. Recorded in 1946.

Parkinsonism, encephalitis lethargica as cause of

... See under *Encephalitis lethargica*.

Parkinsonism, location of specific lesions in

CHARLES FOIX, French neurologist, 1882-1927, with his coworkers, located the site of the lesions in parkinsonism. Published in 1921.

Parkinsonism, profenamine in treatment of

JEAN SIGWALD, French physician,

19??-   , introduced profenamine hydrochloride in the treatment of parkinsonism. Also known as *lysivane* and *ethopropazine*. Published in 1949.

**Parkinsonism, trihexyphenidyl
in treatment of**

KENDALL BROOKS CORBIN, American physician, 1907-   , introduced the use of trihexyphenidyl in the treatment of parkinsonism. Recorded in 1949.

Parkinsonism

. . . See also under *Paralysis agitans*.

Park's aneurysm

. . . See under *Aneurysm in which arterial sac communicates with two veins*.

**Parotid gland duct, eponymic
description of**

NIELS STENSEN, Danish anatomist, 1638-1686, discovered the duct of the parotid gland in 1660. Published in 1662. Known as *Stensen's duct*.

Parotid gland, first excision of

PIERRE AUGUSTIN BÉCLARD, French anatomist, 1785-1825, is believed to have been the first to excise the parotid gland, in 1824.

**Parotitis and orchitis, first
modern account of**

ROBERT HAMILTON, English physician, 1721-1793, gave the first modern description of mumps followed by orchitis. Recorded in 1790.

**Parovarium, eponymic
description of**

. . . See under *Epoophoron*, etc.

**Paroxysmal tachycardia,
introduction of term**

LEON BOUVERET, French physician, 1850-1929, introduced the term *paroxysmal tachycardia*, in 1889.

Parrot's atrophy of the newborn

JOSEPH PARROT, French physician, 1829-1883, described a primary infantile atrophy or marasmus, in 1877.

Parrot's disease

. . . See under *Syphilitic pseudoparalysis in infants*.

Parrot's nodes

. . . See under *Nodes on skull of syphilitic infants*.

**Parthenogenesis, early
research in**

JACQUES LOEB, American biologist, 1859-1924, investigated the phenomena of parthenogenesis, successfully raising fatherless frogs to maturity. Report published in 1908.

**Pascal's law of transmission
of pressure in fluids**

BLAISE PASCAL, French scientist, 1623-1662, found that pressure applied anywhere to a body of confined fluid is transmitted equally in all directions. Enunciated in 1653.

**Paschen bodies in variola and
vaccinia—1886**

JOHN BROWN BUIST, Scottish physician, 1846-1915, was the first to note and demonstrate the inclusion bodies in the cells of tissues in cases of variola and vaccinia, later named *Paschen bodies*. Recorded in 1886.

**Paschen bodies in variola and
vaccinia—1906**

ENRIQUE PASCHEN, German bacteriologist, 1860-1936, gave a good description of the inclusion bodies in the cells of tissues in cases of variola and vaccinia. Published in 1906.

Passavant's bar, cushion, or ridge

. . . See under *Pharynx, Passavant's cushion of*.

Paste for devitalizing nerve of a tooth

WILLIAM ABBOT (also ABBOTTS), English physician, *circa* 1831-1900, was the originator of the first effective paste used to devitalize the nerves of teeth. It was composed of arsenic trioxide or arsenous acid, morphine, and creosote. Known as *Abbot's paste*. Exact date not available.

Pasteurella pestis, discovery of

. . . See under *Plague bacillus, discovery of*.

Pasteurella tularensis (Bacterium tularense), requirement of cystine for growth of

EDWARD FRANCIS, American physician and bacteriologist, 1872-19??, demonstrated that cystine is essential for the growth of *Pasteurella tularensis*, in 1923.

Patch test, early use of

JOSEF JADASSOHN, German dermatologist, 1863-1936, is credited with using the patch test as early as 1896.

Patella, epiphysitis of

SVEN JOHANSSON, Swedish surgeon, 1880-19??, described an epiphysitis involving an accessory cen-

ter of ossification at the apex of the patella. Recorded in 1922. The condition was reported a few months earlier, in December, 1921, by CHRISTIAN M. F. SINDING-LARSEN, Norwegian physician.

Patella, fracture of, special splint for

DAVID HAYES AGNEW, American surgeon, 1818-1892, invented a special splint for treating a fractured patella. He also devised a splint for fracture of the metacarpus. Reported in 1878.

Patella, pathologic fracture of cartilage of

KONRAD BUDINGER, Swiss physician in Austria, 1867-19??, described rupture (usually pathologic) of the cartilage of the patella, in 1906. The condition was also described by KARL LUDLOFF, in 1910, and by GEORGE ARTHUR LÄWEN, in 1925. Known as *Budinger-Ludloff-Läwen disease*.

Patellar tendon reflex, absence of, in tabes dorsalis

. . . See under *Knee jerk*.

Paternity, application of blood grouping in the jurisprudence of

. . . See under *Blood grouping in jurisprudence*, etc.

Paterson's bodies

. . . See under *Molluscum contagiosum, inclusion bodies in*.

Pathologic anatomy, founder of

GIOVANNI BATTISTA MORGAGNI, Italian anatomist and pathologist, 1682-1771, is considered the founder of the science of modern pathologic anatomy.

Pathological anatomy, atlas of, first complete

... See under *Atlas of pathological anatomy.*

Pathology, first American textbook on

WILLIAM EDMONDS HORNER, American anatomist and pathologist, 1793-1853, wrote what is believed to be the first American textbook on pathology. Published in 1829.

Pathology, first use of term, in modern sense

JEAN FRANÇOIS FERNEL, French physician, 1497-1558, is credited with being first to use the term *pathology,* in 1554.

Pathways in conduction in spinal cord, description of

CHARLES EDOUARD BROWN-SÉQUARD, British physiologist in France, 1817-1894, described the pathways of conduction in the spinal cord. Reported in 1863.

Paul's test

... See under *Smallpox, rabbit test for.*

Paul's tube

... See under *Glass drainage tube in intestinal operations.*

Pauzat's disease

... See under *Osteoplastic periostitis of metatarsal bones.*

Pavlov's pouch

... See under *Stomach pouch.*

Pavy's disease

... See under *Albuminuria, recurrent physiologic.*

Pawlik's folds

... See under *Vaginal folds bounding Pawlik's triangle.*

Pawlik's triangle

... See under *Triangle of vagina corresponding to trigonum vesicae.*

Payr's disease

... See under *Colon, kinking of, resulting in stasis.*

Pearson's Solution of Sodium Arsenate

... See under *Solution of sodium arsenate, Pearson's.*

Pecquet's cistern or reservoir

... See under *Receptaculum chyli.*

Pecquet's duct

... See under *Thoracic duct in dogs, discovery of.*

Pectinate ligament of iris, original description of

ALEXANDER FRIEDRICH HUECK, German-Estonian anatomist, 1802-1842, described the pectinate ligament of the iris, in 1826.

Pectinate ligament, spaces between the fibers of

FELICE FONTANA, Italian physiologist and naturalist, 1720-1805, described spaces between the fibers of the pectinate ligament which serve as passage between the sinus venosus and the anterior chamber of the eye. Published in 1765. Known as *Fontana's spaces* or *canal.*

Pectoralis major, furrow formed by

FRANCIS SIBSON, English anatomist, 1814-1876, described a furrow formed in some persons by the lower border of the pectoralis major muscle. Recorded in 1848. Known as *Sibson's furrow*.

Pectoriloquy, introduction of term

RENÉ T. H. LAENNEC, French physician, 1781-1826, is credited with introducing the term *pectoriloquy*, after his invention of the stethoscope and his study of auscultation. Published in 1819.

Pediatric clinic, first, in the United States

ABRAHAM JACOBI, American pediatrician, 1830-1919, is credited with founding the first pediatric clinic in the United States, in New York, in 1862.

Pediatrics, first book on, dealing with surgery

FELIX WÜRTZ, Swiss surgeon, 1518-1574, wrote the first book dealing with surgery of infants. Published in 1616.

Pediatrics, first book on, written by an Englishman

THOMAS PHAER, English pediatrician, 1510-1560, is credited with being the first Englishman to write a book devoted entirely to pediatrics. Published in 1545.

Pediatrics, first book on, written by a Frenchman

SIMON DE VALLAMBERT, French pediatrician, 1512-1576, is credited with producing the first work on pediatrics in French. Published in 1565.

Pediatrics, first printed book on

PAOLO BAGELLARDO, Italian physician, 14??-1494, is credited with producing the first printed book devoted entirely to pediatrics. Published in 1472.

Pediatrics, first textbook on, in America

WILLIAM POTTS DEWEES, American pediatrician, 1768-1841, is credited with writing the first textbook on pediatrics in America. Published in 1825.

Peking man

. . . See under *Sinanthropus pekinensis*.

Pel-Ebstein disease

. . . See under *Lymphadenoma with periodic attacks of pyrexia*.

Pellagra, early modern account of—1755

FRANÇOIS THIÉRRY, French physician, 1719-177?, described pellagra on the basis of patients under the care of GASPAR CASAL. Published in 1755. This is probably the earliest recorded description of pellagra.

Pellagra, early modern account of—1762

GASPAR CASAL, Spanish physician, 1679-1759, gave the earliest clear description of pellagra. Published posthumously in 1762. The substance of the book is said to have been written as early as 1735. Casal referred to pellagra as *mal de la rosa*. The pellagral lesions on the back of the neck are known as *Casal's collar* or *necklace*.

Pellagra, first hospital for, in Milan

A hospital for the treatment of pellagra was established in Milan, *circa* 1772, under the direction of

GAETANO STROMBIO. Strombio wrote a three-volume work on pellagra which appeared under the title *De Pellagra,* in 1786-1789.

Pellagra, introduction of term

FRANCESCO FRAPOLLI, Italian physician, 17??-177?, gave the first description of pellagra in Italy, in 1771. He also introduced the name pellagra (rough skin), in allusion to the outstanding lesion.

Pellagra without skin lesions, existence of

GAETANO STRAMBIO, Italian physician, 1752-1831, was the first to demonstrate that pellagra may occur without skin lesions. Recorded *circa* 1786.

Pellagra-preventive factor, discovery of

JOSEPH GOLDBERGER, American pathologist, 1874-1929, with G. A. WHEELER, R. D. LILLIE, and L. M. ROGERS, discovered the pellagra-preventive factor, *circa* 1926.

Pellegrini-Stieda disease

. . . See under *Knee, calcification of medial lateral ligament of.*

Pelves, early clinical classification of—1861

CARL C. T. LITZMANN, German gynecologist and obstetrician, 1815-1890, worked out a clinical classification of the female pelvis, in 1861.

Pelvic deformity, first record of

GIULIO CESARE ARANZI, Italian anatomist, 1530-1589, is said to have been the first to record a case involving pelvic deformity. Published in 1564.

Pelvic hematocele, classic description of

AUGUSTE NÉLATON, French surgeon, 1807-1873, gave a classic description of pelvic hematocele, in 1851.

Pelvic pain, control of, by cutting rami communicantes

MATHIEU JABOULAY, French surgeon, 1860-1913, cut the rami communicantes to relieve pelvic pain, in 1899.

Pelvimeter, invention of

JEAN LOUIS BAUDELOCQUE, French obstetrician, 1745-1810, invented the pelvimeter. Reported in 1781.

Pelviotomy, bilateral, for relief of dystocia

. . . See under *Dystocia, bilateral pelviotomy for relief of.*

Pelvis contracted in one of oblique diameters; Naegele's pelvis

FRANZ KARL NAEGELE, German obstetrician, 1778-1851, described a pelvis contracted in one of the oblique diameters with ankylosis of one sacroiliac synchondrosis, and imperfect development of the sacrum. Recorded in 1839.

Pelvis, deformed

. . . See under particular type of deformity, as *Kyphoscoliotic pelvis,* etc.

Pelvis, description of; including deformities

HENDRIK VAN DEVENTER, Dutch obstetrician, 1651-1724, gave an early account of the female pelvis and its deformities, *circa* 1701. This is considered the earliest accurate treatment of the subject.

Pelvis, external conjugate diameter of

JEAN LOUIS BAUDELOCQUE, French obstetrician, 1745-1810, described the external conjugate diameter of the pelvis, in 1781.

Pelvis, female, modern classification of

. . . See under *Female pelvis* and under *Pelves*.

Pelvis, instrument for measuring, internally

SAMUEL HANSON, American obstetrician, 1895-   , devised an instrument for making internal measurements of the pelvis through the vagina and rectum, in 1933. It is used mainly to determine the anteroposterior diameter and the biischial and interischial diameters.

Pelvis, osteomalacic, early report of

WILLIAM HUNTER, Scottish surgeon, 1718-1783, reported a case of osteomalacia of the female pelvis, in 1762. The condition is said to have been discovered by a country physician who brought it to the attention of Hunter.

Pelvis spinosa, first description of

HERMANN FRIEDRICH KILIAN, German gynecologist, 1800-1863, was the first to describe pelvis spinosa, a rachitic pelvis in which the crest of the pubis is unusually sharp. Published in 1854. Known as *Kilian's pelvis*.

Pelvis, spondylolisthetic, early description of

HERMANN FRIEDRICH KILIAN, German gynecologist, 1800-1863, de-scribed the spondylolisthetic pelvis, which he called "pelvis obtecta," a pelvis in which the fifth lumbar vertebra is displaced in front of the sacrum. Recorded in 1854. Known as *Kilian's pelvis*.

Pemphigus foliaceus, description of

PIERRE LOUIS A. CAZENAVE, French dermatologist, 1795-1877, gave an excellent description of pemphigus foliaceus, a form of pemphigus marked by flaccid, scabby bullae, in 1844.

Pemphigus vegetans, early description of

ISIDOR NEUMANN, Austrian dermatologist, 1832-1906, described pemphigus vegetans. Recorded in 1886. Known as *Neumann's disease*.

Penicillin, discovery of

SIR ALEXANDER FLEMING, Scottish bacteriologist, 1881-1955, discovered penicillin when he observed that cultures of Penicillium inhibited the growth of some bacteria, in 1928. Crude penicillin was introduced in 1929.

Penicillin, introduction of, in therapeutics

ERNST BORIS CHAIN, English biochemist, 1906-   , with H. W. FLOREY, A. D. GARDNER, N. G. HEATLY, M. A. JENNINGS, J. ORR-EWING, and A. G. SANDERS, introduced penicillin in therapeutics. The acceptance of penicillin was the result of their extensive work on the drug as a chemotherapeutic agent. Recorded in 1940.

Penicillium, bacteriostatic effect of

JOHN TYNDALL, English scientist,

1820-1893, discovered the selective growth-inhibiting effect of *Penicillium* on bacteria. Published in 1876.

Penis, erector mechanism of

CONRAD ECKHARD, German physiologist, 1822-1915, did important work on the mechanism of penile erection, experimenting with dogs. Recorded in 1863.

**Penis, fibrosis of corpora
    cavernosa of**

FRANÇOIS DE LA PEYRONIE, French surgeon, 1678-1747, described a disease of the penis marked by induration and fibrosis of the corpora cavernosa, *circa* 1702. Known as *Peyronie's disease, fibrous cavernitis, penis plasticus,* etc.

**Pentose nucleotides in
    normal blood**

HENRY JACKSON, American biochemist, 1892-   , demonstrated the presence of pentose nucleotides in normal blood. Published in 1924.

Pentosuria, first description of

ERNST LEOPOLD SALKOWSKI, German biochemist, 1844-1923, was the first to describe pentosuria. Published in 1895.

**Pentothal sodium, intro-
    duction of**

JOHN SILAS LUNDY, American physician, 1894-   , introduced the use of pentothal sodium. Published in 1935.

**Pepsin in gastric juice,
    discovery of**

THEODOR SCHWANN, German anatomist, 1810-1882, discovered pepsin in the gastric juice. Published in 1836.

**Peptic ulcer, vagotomy
    in treatment of**

LESTER REYNOLD DRAGSTEDT, American surgeon, 1893-   , with FREDERICK MITCHUM OWENS, introduced supra-diaphragmatic section of the vagus nerves in the treatment of duodenal ulcers. Published in 1943. The method was applied later, in 1944, to the treatment of gastric ulcers as well.

**Peptone and sodium chloride
    solution for indole formation**

. . . See under *Solution of peptone,* etc.

**Percussion of human body as a
    method of physical diag-
    nosis, invention of**

JOSEPH LEOPOLD AUENBRUGGER, Austrian physician, 1722-1809, introduced percussion of the chest as a method of physical diagnosis. Reported in 1761.

**Percussion sounds in diagnosis
    of pulmonary disease**

JOSEF SKODA, Austrian physician, 1805-1881, studied the percussion sounds characteristic of various pulmonary diseases and classified the sounds on the basis of their musical quality. The sound elicited above a line of pleural effusion is known as *Skodiac resonance.* Published in 1839.

**Percussor and pleximeter,
    introduction of**

PIERRE ADOLPHE PIORRY, French physician, 1794-1879, a pioneer in mediate percussion, invented a percussor and a pleximeter, in 1826. Reported in 1828.

Perez's bacillus

. . . See under *Coccobacillus foetidus ozaenae.*

Perfusion apparatus for keeping organs alive outside the body

ALEXIS CARREL, French surgeon, 1873-1944, with CHARLES LINDBERGH, devised a perfusion apparatus which permits organs to live outside the body. Called *Carrel-Lindbergh pump.* Exact date not available.

Perfusion to keep excised organs alive, introduction of

KARL FRIEDRICH W. LUDWIG, German physiologist, 1816-1895, is credited with introducing the idea of keeping excised organs and parts alive by perfusion or artificial circulation, in 1865.

Periarterial sympathectomy for relief of paresthesia and vasomotor disturbances

RENÉ LERICHE, French surgeon, 1870-19??, introduced periarterial sympathectomy for the relief of paresthesia and vasomotor disturbances. Published in 1916 and 1917. Known as *Leriche's operation.*

Periarteritis nodosa, eponymic description of

ADOLF KUSSMAUL, German physician, 1822-1902, with RUDOLF MAIER (German physician, 1824-1888), described periarteritis nodosa, an inflammatory disease of the coats of the medium-sized and small arteries. Published in 1866. Known as *Kussmaul's disease* and *Kussmaul-Maier disease.*

Pericardiectomy for adhesive pericarditis

FRANZ VOLHARD, German physician, 1872-1950, performed pericardiectomy for constrictive or adhesive pericarditis. Recorded in 1923. The procedure is also known as cardiolysis.

Pericardiectomy for relief of constrictive pericarditis

PAUL HALLOPEAU, French surgeon, 1876-1924, is credited with performing the first pericardiectomy for constrictive pericarditis. Published in 1921.

Pericardiocentesis, first performance of

FRANCISCO ROMERO, Spanish surgeon, 17??-18??, is credited with performing the first successful pericardiocentesis, *circa* 1808. Existing record dated 1814.

Pericarditis, chronic constrictive; first account

NORMAN CHEVERS, English physician, 1818-1886, gave the first accurate account of chronic constrictive pericarditis, in 1842.

Pericarditis, first description of

AVENZOAR, Arabian physician in Cordoba, circa 1091-1162, is believed to have been the first to describe pericarditis. Date not available.

Pericardium, adherent, retraction of intercostal tissue in

WILLIAM HENRY BROADBENT, English physician, 1835-1907, described a retraction of the intercostal tissue at the eleventh and twelfth ribs in cases of adherent pericardium. Published in 1895. Known as *Broadbent's sign.*

Perinaud's conjunctivitis

. . . See under *Conjunctivitis, infectious, caused by a leptothrix.*

Perineal fascia, superficial, deep layer of

. . . See under *Deep layer of superficial perineal fascia.*

Perineum, female, suture of ruptured

PHILIBERT JOSEPH ROUX, French surgeon, 1780-1854, sutured a ruptured female perineum, in 1832. Recorded in 1834.

Periodic law; Mendeleeff's law

DIMITRI IVANOVICH MENDELEEFF, Russian chemist, 1834-1907, discovered the periodic law of the elements in accordance with which the elements, when arranged in the sequence of the atomic weights, show a relationship in chemical properties. Recorded in 1869.

Periodic ophthalmoplegic migraine

. . . See under *Migraine, periodic, with paralysis of oculomotor muscles.*

Periosteum, fibers attaching, to bone

WILLIAM SHARPEY, English anatomist, 1802-1880, described connective tissue fibers which secure the periosteum to the bone. Recorded in *Quain's Anatomy,* in 1848. Known as *Sharpey's fibers.*

Periosteum, osteogenetic layer of

LÉOPOLD LOUIS X. E. OLLIER, French surgeon, 1830-1900, described the osteogenetic layer of the periosteum, in 1858. Known as *Ollier's layer.*

Peristalsis, early allusion to—1542

JEAN FRANÇOIS FERNEL, French physician, 1497-1558, made an early reference to peristalsis when he described the esophagus as contracting and pushing down the food. He stated that the same process is repeated in the intestine after the food is delivered by the stomach. Published in 1542.

Peritoneum, early description of

JAMES DOUGLAS, Scottish anatomist and obstetrician, 1675-1742, described the peritoneum. Recorded in 1730.

Peritoneum, process vaginalis of

. . . See under *Process vaginalis.*

Peritonitis complicating appendicitis

ALBERT JOHN OCHSNER, American surgeon, 1858-1925, called attention to the causes and methods of prevention of diffuse peritonitis which complicate appendicitis. Reported in 1901.

Peritonitis, first accurate description of

JOHANN GOTTLIEB WALTER, German physician, 1734-1818, gave the first clear description of peritonitis, in 1785.

Perkins' tractors

. . . See under *Tractors to draw out inflammation and allay pain.*

Pernicious anemia, dessicated stomach in treatment of

CYRUS CRESSEY STURGIS, American physician, 1891-   , with RAPHAEL ISAACS, discovered that the stomach contains an anti-pernicious anemia factor and advocated the use of desiccated stomach in treating the disease. Reported in 1929.

Pernicious anemia, etiologic relationship of achylia gastrica to

WILLIAM BOSWORTH CASTLE, American physician, 1897-   , demonstrated that pernicious anemia is due to the inability of the stomach to secrete an anti-pernicious-anemia factor. Reported in 1928.

Pernicious anemia, first description of

JAMES SCARFE COMBE, Scottish physician, 1796-1883, is credited with being the first to describe pernicious anemia. Report read May 1, 1822. Published in 1824.

Pernicious anemia, marrow changes in

WILLIAM PEPPER, American physician, 1843-1898, described bone marrow changes occurring in progressive pernicious anemia. Published in 1875.

Pernicious anemia of pregnancy

WALTER CHANNING, American physician, 1786-1876, was the first to describe pernicious anemia associated with pregnancy. Published in 1842.

Pernicious anemia, progressive, in pregnant women

EMILIO VALSUANI, Italian physician, 18??-189?, described progressive pernicious anemia occurring in pregnant or lactating women. Published in 1870. Known as *Valsuani's disease.*

Pernicious anemia, retinal hemorrhage in

ANTON BIERMER, German physician, 1827-1892, was the first to observe retinal hemorrhages in a case of pernicious anemia. Recorded in 1872.

Pernicious vomiting of pregnancy

. . . See under *Hyperemesis gravidarum.*

Peroneal artery, first successful ligation of

GEORGE JAMES GUTHRIE, English surgeon, 1785-1856, performed the first recorded successful ligation of the peroneal artery, of a German soldier wounded in the battle of Waterloo. Recorded in 1816.

Persecution mania, early description of

ERNEST CHARLES LASÈGUE, French physician, 1816-1883, gave an early description of persecution mania, in 1852. Known as *Lasègue's disease.*

Perspiration in maintenance of body temperature

CHARLES BLAGDEN, Enguish surgeon, 1748-1820, was the first to demonstrate the role of perspiration in the maintenance of constant body temperature. Recorded in 1775.

Pertik's diverticulum

. . . See under *Nasopharyngeal diverticulum.*

Pertussis, earliest reference to

AVICENNA, Persian physician and philosopher, 980-1037, gave an account of a disease which may have been pertussis, *circa* 1010.

Pertussis, early description of

THOMAS WILLIS, English physician and anatomist, 1621-1675, gave a clear description of pertussis. Published in 1675.

Pertussis, relation of Bordet-Gengou bacillus to

FRANKLIN BURR MALLORY, American pathologist, 1862-1941, with A. A. HOMER and F. F. HENDERSON, demonstrated the causal relation of the *Bordet-Gengou bacillus (Hemophilus pertussis)* to whooping cough. Recorded in 1913.

Pertussis

. . . See also under *Whooping cough.*

Pessary, "horseshoe," for retro-displacement of uterus

HUGH LENOX HODGE, American gynecologist, 1796-1873, designed a "horseshoe" type of pessary for correction of retrodisplacement of the uterus. Reported in 1866.

Pessary, single-stem type of, for prolapse

GEORGE GELLHORN, American gynecologist, 1870-1936, designed a single-stem, "plunger" type pessary for use in uterine prolapse, in 1908.

Petit's hernia

. . . See under *Hernia, lumbar, in Petit's triangle.*

Petit's triangle

. . . See under *Triangle, lumbar,* etc.

Petri dish, invention of

JULIUS PETRI, German bacteriologist, 1852-1921, devised a bacterial culture vessel consisting of two round rimmed plates, one serving as a cover for the other. Introduced in 1887. It is said that Petri's dish was a modification of a vessel used by KOCH.

Petrous bone, opening in, for petrosal branch of vidian nerve

GABRIEL FALLOPIUS, Italian anatomist, 1523-1562, described an opening in the petrous bone through which the petrosal branch of the vidian nerve passes. Published in 1561.

Peyer's patches

. . . See under *Lymph nodules in mucous membrane of small intestine.*

Peyronie's disease

. . . See under *Penis, fibrosis of corpora cavernosa of.*

Pfeifferella whitmori, isolation of

ALFRED WHITMORE, English surgeon in Indian Medical Service, 1876-1946, with C. S. KRISHNASWAMI, isolated the causative organisms of melioidosis, *circa* 1912. The name was introduced by STANTON and FLETCHER. The organism is now known as *Malleomyces pseudomallei.*

Pfeiffer's bacillus, discovery of

. . . See under *Influenza bacillus.*

pH, introduction of symbol

SØREN PETER LAURITZ SØRENSEN, Danish chemist, 1868-1939, introduced the symbol pH to indicate hydrogen ion concentration. Recorded in 1909. Known as *Sorensen's symbol.*

Phacoscope, invention of

HERMANN L. F. VON HELMHOLTZ, German physiologist and physicist, 1821-1894, is credited with inventing an early form of phacoscope, in 1851.

Phagocyte, introduction of term

ELIE METCHNIKOFF, Russian physiologist in France, 1845-1916, introduced the term *phagocyte* to describe a leukocyte having a scavenger function. Recorded in 1884.

Phagocytic index, devising of

JOSEPH ARNETH, German physician, 1873-19??, devised a phagocytic index based on the assumption that the neutrophils with three or more lobes have the greater phagocytic power. Reported in 1904.

Phagocytosis, introduction of theory of

ELIE METCHNIKOFF, Russian physiologist in France, 1845-1916, introduced the concept of scavenger cells (phagocytes) and the theory of phagocytosis. Reported in 1884.

Pharmacological Institute at Bonn, founding of

KARL BINZ, German pharmacologist and chemist, 1832-1912, founded the Pharmacological Institute at Bonn, in 1869.

Pharmacopeia, early German

VALERIUS CORDUS, German physician and pharmacologist, 1515-1544, compiled the earliest form of pharmacopeia, in the modern sense. Published in 1535.

Pharmacopeia, first German

ORTOLFF VON BAYRLANT, Würzburg physician, 15th century, compiled the first German pharmacopeia, which was also a textbook of medicine. Published in 1477.

Pharyngeal bursa, chronic inflammation of

GUSTAV LUDWIG TORNWALDT, German physician, 1843-1910, described pharyngeal bursitis associated with cyst formation, suppuration, and nasopharyngeal stenosis. Published in 1885. Known as *Tornwaldt's bursitis*. The condition was described earlier, in 1874, by HERMANN WENDT, German physician, 1838-1875.

Pharyngeal tonsil, eponymic description of

EMIL ZUKERKANDL, Austrian anatomist, 1849-1910, described the pharyngeal or nasal tonsil, *circa* 1882. Known as *Zukerkandl's tubercle*.

Pharyngotomy, first, in England

EDWARD COCK, English surgeon, 1805-1892, is credited with performing the first pharyngotomy in England. Recorded in 1856.

Pharynx and larynx, miliary tuberculosis of; early description

EMILE ISAMBERT, French physician, 1827-1876, an authority on laryngeal tuberculosis, described miliary tuberculosis of the larynx and pharynx, in 1871. Known as *Isambert's disease*.

Pharynx, lateral recess of

JOHANN CHRISTIAN ROSENMÜLLER, German anatomist, 1771-1826, described the lateral pharyngeal recess, in 1808. Known as *fossa of Rosenmüller*.

Pharynx, Morgagni's sinus of

. . . See under *Sinus of Morgagni, pharyngeal*.

Pharynx, Passavant's cushion of

GUSTAV PASSAVANT, German surgeon, 1815-1893, described a bulge on the posterior pharyngeal wall produced by the contraction of the superior and middle constrictor muscles of the pharynx in the act of deglutition. Published in 1862. Known as *Passavant's bar, cushion,* or *ridge.*

Phase-contrast microscope, invention of

FRITZ ZERNICKE, Dutch physicist, 1888-19??, invented the phase-contrast microscope which alters the phase relationship of the light passing through the object and the light passing around the object. Received the Nobel prize in physics, in 1953.

Phenindione (phenylindanedione), introduction of

JEAN PIERRE SOULIER, French physician, 19??-   , with JEAN GUEGUEN, introduced phenindione as an anticoagulant. Published in 1947.

Phenolsulfonphthalein as purgative

. . . See under *Phthaleins as purgatives.*

Phenolsulfonphthalein excretion by kidney

JOHN JACOB ABEL, Baltimore pharmacologist and physiologist, 1857-1938, in cooperation with L. G. ROWNTREE, American internist, 1883-   , discovered that phenolsulfonphthalein is excreted by the kidney. Reported in 1909. The discovery led to the use of the material in kidney function tests.

Phenolsulfonphthalein test for kidney function

JOHN T. GERAGHTY, American ur-

ologist, 1876-1924, with LEONARD G. ROWNTREE (American internist, 1883-   ), devised and introduced the phenolsulfonphthalein test for kidney function, in 1910.

Phenoltetrachlorphthalein in liver function tests

JOHN JACOB ABEL, American pharmacologist and physiologist, 1857-1938, was instrumental in the wide acceptance of phenoltetrachlorphthalein as a testing agent for liver function. Recorded in 1909.

Phenylindanedione, introduction of

. . . See under *Phenindione.*

Pheochromocytoma, first description of

FELIX FRÄNKEL, German pathologist, 1829-1897, was the first to describe pheochromocytoma, a chromaffin cell tumor containing epinephrine. Published in 1886.

Phlebograph, invention of

JAMES MACKENZIE, Scottish cardiologist in England, 1853-1925, devised a phlebograph, an instrument with which he recorded the pulsation of veins, in 1892. He also made simultaneous tracings, especially of the radial artery and jugular vein. The phlebograph is considered the forerunner of the modern polygraph .

Phlebotomus fever

. . . See under *Pappataci fever.*

Phlegmasia alba dolens, early description of

CHARLES WHITE, English surgeon, 1728-1813, was probably the first to give a clinical description of phlegmasia alba dolens. Published in 1784.

Phlogiston theory, introduction of

GEORG ERNST STAHL, German physiologist and chemist, 1660-1734, with JOHANN BECHER, developed the phlogiston theory of combustion. It stated that all inflammable materials contain the combustible substance phlogiston which is identical in all matter but merely varies in amount. Proposed in 1697.

Phlogiston theory, rejection of

ANTOINE LAURENT LAVOISIER, French chemist, 1743-1794, demonstrated the true nature of combustion and exploded the phlogiston theory of Stahl, *circa* 1775.

Photelometer of Sheard-Sanford

. . . See under *Colorimeter, photoelectric, introduction of.*

Photometer to measure light of electric arc

ROBERT W. BUNSON, German chemist, 1811-1899, invented a photometer with which to measure the light of an electric arc, which he was investigating, in 1844.

Photosynthesis, early recognition of

JAN INGENHOUSZ, Dutch physician and naturalist, 1730-1799, discovered that green plants absorb carbon dioxide in the presence of light but not in darkness, and that they give off oxygen in the process. He also differentiated between this process of photosynthesis and the respiration of plants whereby carbon dioxide is given off constantly. Recorded in 1779.

Phototherapy, Father of

NIELS R. FINSEN, Danish physician, 1860-1904, is regarded as the Father of Modern Phototherapy.

Phrenicotomy in treatment of pulmonary tuberculosis

ERNST FERDINAND SAUERBRUCH, German surgeon, 1875-1951, introduced phrenicotomy in the treatment of pulmonary tuberculosis. Published in 1913.

Phrenicotomy in treatment of pulmonary tuberculosis, suggestion for

CARL ADOLPH ERNST STUERTZ, German physician, 1870-19??, suggested phrenicotomy for the treatment of pulmonary tuberculosis or basal lung disease of other types. Recorded in 1911.

Phrenicotomy, phrenic exeresis in

WILLY FELIX, German surgeon, 1880-19??, developed phrenic exeresis as a method of phrenicotomy, in 1922.

Phrenicotomy, phrenic resection in

OTTO GOETZE, German surgeon, 1890-19??, developed phrenic resection as a method of phrenicotomy, in 1922.

Phrenology, founder of

FRANZ J. GALL, German anatomist, 1758-1828, is considered the founder of phrenology.

Phthaleins as purgatives, study of

JOHN JACOB ABEL, Baltimore phar-

macologist and physiologist, 1857-
1938, in cooperation with L. G.
ROWNTREE, American internist,
1883-19??, studied the action of the
phthaleins and their derivatives
with regard to their function as purgatives. Recorded in 1909. Abel
and Rowntree also studied the excretion of phthaleins and discovered that phenolsulfonphthalein is
eliminated by the kidney.

Phthaleins in kidney
function tests

. . . See under *Phenolsulfonphthalein excretion by kidney.*

Physiognomy, founder
of—1586

GIOVANNI BATTISTA DELLA PORTA,
Italian physician, 1536-1605, studied the relation of moral character
and aesthetic qualities to facial features; he is regarded as the founder
of physiognomy. His work was
published in 1586.

Physiological chemistry labora-
tory, first, in United
States

RUSSELL HENRY CHITTENDEN,
American physiological chemist,
1856-1943, is believed to have
founded the first laboratory for
physiological chemistry in the United States.

Physiology as a branch of
science, establish-
ment of

ALBRECHT VON HALLER, Swiss
physiologist and antomist, 1708-
1777, is credited with elevating
physiology to the level of a special
branch of science. His work *Ele-
menta Physiologiae Corporis Humani,* published between 1757 and

1766, was an important influence in
this direction.

Physiology, Father of

ERASISTRATUS, Greek anatomist
and physician, *circa* 300-250 B.C.,
is considered the *Father of Physiology.*

Physiology, first European
textbook of

RENÉ DESCARTES, French scientist
and philosopher, 1596-1650, wrote
a textbook of physiology which is
believed to have been the first one
in Europe. It was published posthumously in 1661, and is referred
to as *Tractatus de homine.*

Physiology, first journal of

JOHANN CHRISTIAN REIL, Dutch
physiologist, 1759-1813, founded
the *Archiv für die Physiologie,* the
first journal of physiology.

Physiology, first use of
term, in modern sense

JEAN FRANÇOIS FERNEL, French
physician, 1497-1558, is credited
wtih being first to use the term
physiology, in 1552.

Physostigmine in myas-
thenia gravis

. . . See under *Myasthenia gravis.*

Physostigmine in treatment
of glaucoma, introduc-
tion of

LUDWIG LAQUEUR, German opthalmologist, 1839-1909, introduced
the use of physostigmine as a mio-
tic in treating glaucoma. Published
in 1876.

Physostigmine, original
work on—1863

THOMAS RICHARD FRASER, British

pharmacologist, 1841-1920, did valuable and original work on physostigmine. Reported in 1863.

Pill of iron, quinine, strychnine, and arsenic

WILLIAM AITKEN, Scottish physician, 1825-1892, compounded a pill containing reduced iron, quinine sulfate, strychnine, and arsenic trioxide. Known as *Aitken's pill*, and used as a hematinic. Date not available.

Pills of ferrous carbonate, introduction of

PIERRE BLAUD, French physician, 1774-1858, was successful in compounding pills of ferrous carbonate. He reported it in 1832. Known as chalybeate pills and as *Blaud's pills*.

Pills of ferrous iodide, introduction of

STEPHAN BLANKAART, Dutch physician, 1650-1702, was the first to prepare pills of ferrous iodide. Exact date not available.

Pilocarpine action on heart

JOHN NEWPORT LANGLEY, English physiologist, 1852-1925, studied the action of pilocarpine on the heart. Recorded in 1875.

Piltdown skull, description of

ARTHUR KEITH, Scottish anthropologist and anatomist, 1866-1955, described the Piltdown skull (*Eoanthropus*) which was discovered by Charles Dawson in 1911-12. Published in 1913-14.

Pinhole method to illustrate refraction

CHRISTOPH SCHEINER, German physicist, 1575-1650, devised a simple method to demonstrate refraction by means of a card provided with a pinhole. Recorded in 1619. Known as *Scheiner's test*.

Pink disease

. . . See under *Erythredema polyneuropathy*.

Pinkeye, causative organism of

JOHN ELMER WEEKS, American ophthalmologist, 1853-1949, discovered that the organism responsible for Egyptian ophthalmia, discovered by ROBERT KOCH in 1883, is also the cause of pinkeye. Recorded in 1886. Known as *Koch-Weeks bacillus*.

Pinkus' disease

. . . See under *Lichen nitidus*.

Pirquet test

. . . See under *Tuberculin test by application to abrasion of skin*.

Pithecanthropus erectus, Java man, discovery of

MARIE E. F. T. DUBOIS, Dutch anatomist and paleontologist, 1858-1941, discovered the prehistoric Java man, *Pithecanthropus erectus*, in 1891. The bones were found in Java, hence the name.

Pituitary, anterior, adrenocorticotropic factor of

JAMES BERTRAM COLLIP, Canadian physician and biochemist, 1892- , with E. M. ANDERSON and D. L. THOMSON, isolated an impure extract of the anterior pituitary containing an adrenocorticotropic principle. Published in 1933.

Pituitary, anterior, and activity of gonads

PHILIP EDWARD SMITH, American

physiologist, 1884-19??, with EARL
THERON ENGLE, produced precocious sexual maturity in mice by implantation of anterior pituitary tissue, thus demonstrating the effect
of the gland upon the gonads. Published in 1927.

Pituitary, anterior, and sugar metabolism

BERNARDO ALBERTO HOUSSAY, Argentinian physiologist, 1887-19??,
with ALFREDO BIASOTTI, demonstrated the effect of the anterior
pituitary on sugar metabolism. He
showed that hypophysectomy resulted in almost complete disap-
pearance of diabetes caused by de-
pancreatization. Published in 1930.

Pituitary, anterior, diabeto- genic hormone of

BERNARDO ALBERTO HOUSSAY, Argentinian physiologist, 1887-19??,
was the first to observe the diabetogenic action of extracts of the anterior pituitary. Published in 1930.

Pituitary, anterior, diabeto- genic hormone of

FRANK GEORGE YOUNG, English
physician, 1908-   , produced experimental diabetes in animals by
injections of anterior pituitary extracts. Reported in 1937.

Pituitary basophilism, original description of

. . . See under *Basophilism, pituitary,* etc.

Pituitary, differentiation of lobes of

NICHOLAS PAULESCO, Rumanian
surgeon, 186?-19??, found that the
anterior lobe of the pituitary gland
was essential to life while the posterior lobe was expendable. Recorded in 1908.

Pituitary enlargement in rela- tion to acromegaly

. . . See under *Acromegaly, enlargement of pituitary in relation to.*

Pituitary extract of posterior lobe is exytocic

HENRY H. DALE, English physiologist, 1875-19??, demonstrated that
the most important action of an extract of the posterior lobe of the
pituitary gland is oxytocic in nature. Recorded in 1909.

Pituitary growth hormone

. . . See under *Growth hormone.*

Pituitary obesity, early description of—1823

PIERRE FRANÇOIS OLIVE RAYER,
French dermatologist, 1793-1867,
described pituitary obesity, in 1823.

Pituitary tumor associated with amenorrhea

ANTON DE HAEN, French physician, 1704-1776, wrote about amenorrhea associated with a pituitary
tumor. Published in 1759.

Pituitary tumor in acromegaly contains chromophil cells

CARL BENDA, German physician,
1857-1933, demonstrated that pituitary tumors in acromegaly contain
chromophil cells. Published in
1900.

Pituitary tumor in acromegaly, first successful operation on

HERMANN SCHLOFFER, Austrian
surgeon, 1868-1937, is credited
with being the first to operate successfully for pituitary tumor in acromegaly, in man. Recorded in
1906.

Pituitary with relation to reproduction

SAMUEL JAMES CROWE, Baltimore physician, 1883-19??, with H. W. CUSHING and J. HOMANS, gave the first demonstration of the relationship between the pituitary gland and the reproductive system. Recorded in 1910.

Pituitrin, oxytocic action of

HENRY HALLETT DALE, English physiologist, 1875-19??, demonstrated the oxytocic effect of pituitrin. Published in 1909.

Pityriasis nigra

. . . See under *Tinea nigra*.

Pityriasis rosea as clinical entity, early recognition of—1834

CAMILLE MELCHIOR GIBERT, French dermatologist, 1797-1866, is credited with being first to establish pityriasis rosea as a clinical entity, in 1834. Known as *Gibert's disease*.

Pityriasis rubra, early description of

FERDINAND VON HEBRA, Austrian dermatologist, 1816-1880, gave an early description of pityriasis rubra, in 1857. Known as *Hebra's pityriasis, tinea cruris*, etc.

Pityriasis rubra pilaris, early description of

MARIE G. A. DEVERGIE, French dermatologist, 1798-1879, described pityriasis rubra pilaris, a chronic skin disease marked by small follicular papules which are grouped in patches and by scattered pinkish scaling patches. Published in 1856. Known as *Devergie's disease* and *lichen ruber acuminatus*.

Pityriasis versicolor, causative organism of

CARL FERDINAND EICHSTEDT, German dermatologist, 1816-1892, discovered *Malassezia furfur*, the causative agent of pityriasis versicolor. Reported in 1846. Known also as *Malassezia tropica* and *Microsporon furfur*.

Placenta, detailed description of, with illustrations

FABRICIUS AB AQUAPENDENTE, Italian anatomist and surgeon, 1537-1619, gave what is probably the first detailed description of the placenta, accompanied by illustrations. *Circa* 1600.

Placenta, early description of—1552

BARTOLOMMEO EUSTACHIUS, Italian anatomist, 1524-1574, described the placenta in 1552, but the work was not published in his lifetime. It appeared in 1714.

Placenta, external expression of, early suggestion for —1767

JOHN HARVIE, English obstetrician, *floruit* uncertain, suggested the external manual expression of the placenta "without violence." Reported in 1767, nearly 90 years before Credé proposed his manual expression, in 1854.

Placenta, introduction of term

GABRIEL FALLOPIUS, Italian anatomist, 1523-1562, is credited with the introduction of the term *placenta*. He referred to the structure as *placenta uterina*, literally "uterine cake," in his work published in 1561.

Placenta, method of expressing; by Credé

KARL S. F. CREDÉ, German gynecologist, 1819-1892, described a method for manual expression of the placenta by grasping the uterus through the abdominal wall, kneading it, and pressing downward. First reported in 1854; a more accurate description was published in 1860. Known as *Credé's method*.

Placenta previa, management of; early description

FRANÇOIS MAURICEAU, French obstetrician, 1637-1709, was probably the first to describe the management of placenta previa. Published in 1668.

Placenta previa, puncture of amnotic sac in

. . . See under *Amniotic sac, puncture of, to check hemorrhage*.

Plácido's disk

. . . See under *Keratoscope, invention of*.

Plague and typhus, differentiation between

WILLIAM BOGHURST, English apothecary, 1631-1685, was probably the first to differentiate between plague and typhus, in 1666. Published in 1894.

Plague bacilli, transmission of, by rats

ALEXANDER RENNIE, English physician, 1859-1940, held to the theory that the plague bacilli are transmitted by rats. Recorded in 1894.

Plague bacillus, discovery of—1894

SHIBASABURO KITASATO, Japanese bacteriologist, 1852-1931, discovered the plague bacillus *(Pasteurella pestis)*. Reported in 1894. In the same year, the organism was discovered independently by ALEXANDRE E. J. YERSIN, French bacteriologist, 1863-1943.

Plague vaccine, successful inoculation of animals with

ALEXANDRE EMIL JEAN YERSIN, French bacteriologist, 1863-1943, with L. C. A. CALMETTE and A. BORREL, successfully inoculated animals with anti-plague vaccine. Recorded in 1895.

Plague vaccine, successful production of—1906

WALDEMAR MORDECAI WOLFF HAFFKINE, Russian bacteriologist, 1860-1930, developed an anti-bubonic plague vaccine composed of a six-week-old culture of *Pasteurella pestis*, killed by heat and treated with phenol. Recorded in 1906.

Plane of foramen magnum extended through basion and opithion

LOUIS J. M. DAUBENTON, French physician and naturalist, 1716-1799, described a hypothetical plane formed by the extension of the plane of the foramen magnum through the basion and opisthion points, *circa* 1751. Known as *Daubenton's plane*.

Plane passing through nasion and basion perpendicular to median plane of cranium

. . . See under *Craniometric plane passing through nasion and basion*.

Planes used as landmarks in topography of abdomen and thorax

CHRISTOPHER ADDISON, English anatomist, 1869-1951, described several planes, lines, and points used as landmarks in the topography of the thorax and abdomen. Some of these were described in a paper published in 1899. (See also under name of particular plane.)

Planigraphy, first description of

. . . See under *Tomography*.

Plant cells, early recognition of

MARCELLO MALPIGHI, Italian anatomist, 1628-1694, observed the existence of cells in plants. Recorded in a two-part work published in 1675-1679.

Plants and animals, binomial classification of

. . . See under *Binomial nomenclature*, etc.

Plasma cell mastitis, first description of

FRANK EARL ADAIR, American surgeon, 1887-19??, was the first to describe plasma cell mastitis, marked by lesions simulating carcinoma. Published in 1933.

Plasma, derivation of, by method of plasmapheresis

. . . See under *Plasmapheresis*.

Plasma, method of dehydrating

. . . See under *Sera, method of dehydrating*.

Plasmapheresis, method of

JOHN JACOB ABEL, Baltimore pharmacologist and physiologist, 1857-1938, devised a method of plasma removal known as plasmapheresis. It was reported in 1914. In this procedure, blood is removed from a subject and the plasma separated by centrifugation. The cells are then suspended in a suitable medium, as citrate-saline, and reinjected into the donor. The plasma is thus obtained without loss of erythrocytes.

Plasmodium cynomolgi, pre-erythrocytic stage of

HENRY EDWARD SHORTT, English parasitologist, 1887-19??, with P. C. C. GARNHAM and B. MALAMOS, demonstrated the pre-erythrocytic phase of *Plasmodium cynomolgi*, in the monkey. Recorded in 1948.

Plasmodium falciparum, life cycle of

ETTORE MARCHIAFAVA, Italian pathologist, 1847-1935, studied and determined the life cycle of *Plasmodium falciparum*, the causative agent of estivo-autumnal malaria. Published in 1892.

Plasmodium falciparum, pre-erythrocytic forms of

HENRY EDWARD SHORTT, English parasitologist, 1887-19??, with P. C. C. GARNHAM and B. MALAMOS, demonstrated the pre-erythrocytic forms of *Plasmodium falciparum*. Recorded in 1949.

Plasmodium vivax, pre-erythrocytic forms of

HENRY EDWARD SHORTT, English parasitologist, 1887-19??, with P. C. C. GARNHAM and B. MALAMOS, demonstrated the pre-erythrocytic forms of *Plasmodium vivax*. Recorded in 1948.

**Plasmoquine in treatment
of malaria**

. . . See under *Malaria, plasmoquine in treatment of.*

**Plaster-of-paris bandage,
introduction of**

ANTHONIUS MATHIJSEN, Nether-
land surgeon, 1805-1878, introduced the use of plaster-of-paris
bandages, in 1852.

**Plaster-of-paris bandage,
use of, in treating spinal
column disorders**

LEWIS ALBERT SAYRE, American
surgeon, 1820-1900, is credited
with being first to use plaster-of-
paris bandages, in form of a jacket,
in the treatment of spinal column
diseases, such as Pott's disease,
scoliosis, etc. Recorded in 1877.

Plastic surgery, Father of

CARL FERDINAND VON GRAEFE,
German surgeon, 1787-1840, is
considered the Father of Modern
Plastic Surgery.

Plastic surgery

. . . See also under name of part
involved, as *Cleft palate.*

**Platyspondylisis, first
description of**

PIERRE NAU, French physician,
18??-19??, was the first to describe
platyspondylisis (platyspondylia),
in 1904.

Plaut's angina

. . . See under *Vincent's infection or
angina.*

**Pleasure-pain principle,
introduction of**

SIGMUND FREUD, Austrian psychiatrist, 1856-1939, introduced the

concept of the pleasure-pain principle. *Circa* 1888.

Pleural effusion, dullness in

PIETRO GROCCO, Italian physician,
1856-1916, described a triangle of
dullness in the paravertebral region
on the opposite side of a pleural
effusion. Recorded in 1902. Known
as *Grocco's triangle.*

**Pleuritic exudate, sign of
resorption of**

CALVIN ELLIS, American physician,
1826-1883, described a curved line
of dullness which marks the limits
of the exudate in pleuritic effusions.
Reported in 1874. Known as *Ellis's
curve.*

Pleximeter, introduction of

. . . See under *Percussor and pleximeter.*

**Plica lacrimalis, eponymic
description of**

. . . See under *Lacrimal fold, eponymic description of.*

Plotz's bacillus

. . . See under *Typhus-like fever,
bacillus found in.*

**Plugs found in sputum in cases
of bronchiectasis, bron-
chitis, abscess, etc.**

FRANZ DITTRICH, German physician, 1815-1859, described masses
of varying whitish or yellowish
color found in the sputum of patients affected with pulmonary abscess, bronchiectasis, bronchitis,
etc. Reported in 1850. Known as
Dittrich's plugs.

Plummer-Vinson syndrome

. . . See under *Dysphagia with
glossitis and anemia.*

Pneumococcus, discovery of

LOUIS PASTEUR, French scientist and bacteriologist, 1822-1895, is credited with the definite discovery of the pneumococcus. Recorded in 1881.

Pneumococcus, early description of

JOSEPH PARROT, French physician, 1829-1883, gave what is possibly the earliest adequate description of the pneumococcus. Recorded in 1881.

Pneumococcus in mouth of healthy subject

GEORGE MILLER STERNBERG, American bacteriologist, 1838-1915, discovered the presence of pneumococci in the saliva of healthy subjects. He produced septicemia in rabbits by the injection of human saliva. Recorded in 1881.

Pneumococcus, rapid typing method for

ALBERT BRUCE SABIN, American bacteriologist, 1906-   , devised a rapid "stained slide" test for typing of pneumococci. Reported in 1929. Known as *Sabin's rapid method.*

Pneumococcus, typing of, based on capsular swelling

FRED NEUFELD, German bacteriologist, 1861-1945, devised a method of typing pneumococci on the basis of capsular swelling. Published in 1902.

Pneumoencephalography, introduction of

. . . See under *Ventriculography.*

Pneumonectomy, first successful

. . . See under *Lung, total removal of.*

Pneumonectomy for malignancy in a tuberculous patient

HOWARD LILIENTHAL, American surgeon, 1861-1946, performed pneumonectomy in a tuberculous patient for sarcoma of the lung. Reported in 1933.

Pneumonia, atypical, caused by virus

HOBART ANSTETH REINMANN, American physician, 1897-   , described an atypical form of pneumonia "probably caused by a filtrable virus." Published in 1938.

Pneumonia, causal relation of *Diplococcus pneumoniae* to

ALBERT FRAENKEL, German physician, 1848-1916, definitely proved that the *Diplococcus pneumoniae* is the causal agent of lobar pneumonia, in 1884.

Pneumonia, earliest references to

HIPPOCRATES, Greek physician, *circa* 460-377 B. C., recognized and described pneumonia. Exact date not available.

Pneumonia, early description of—2nd century

ARETAEUS THE CAPPADOCIAN, Greek physician in Rome, *circa* 81-138 A. D., gave an early account of pneumonia in his treatise on the causes and symptoms of acute and chronic diseases. Exact date not available.

Pneumonia, Friedländer type of, isolation of causative agent

CARL FRIEDLÄNDER, German pathologist, 1847-1887, is credited with isolating *Klebsiella pneumoniae,* the causative agent of Friedländer pneumonia, in 1883.

Pneumonia, lipoid, first description of

GEORGE FRANKLIN LAUGHLEN, American pathologist, 1888-19??, described pneumonia following nasopharyngeal injection of oil. Published in 1925.

Pneumonia, lobar, diplococci in

GEORGE MILLER STERNBERG, American bacteriologist, 1838-1915, and LOUIS PASTEUR, French scientist and bacteriologist, 1822-1895, working independently, discovered small diplococci in the sputum of patients ill with lobar pneumonia. Recorded in 1881.

Pneumonia, lobar, first classic description of

RENÉ T. H. LAENNEC, French physician, 1781-1826, gave the first classic description of the pathologic changes and physical signs in lobar pneumonia. Reported in 1819.

Pneumonia, pneumococcal, skin test for

THOMAS FRANCIS, JR., American pathologist, 1900-   , developed a skin test to determine the presence of antibody in pneumococcal pneumonia. Known as the *Francis test. Circa* 1932.

Pneumonolysis by use of galvanocautery

HANS CHRISTIAN JACOBAEUS, Swedish surgeon, 1879-1937, devised a method of pneumonolysis in which he used galvanocautery to divide pleural adhesions. Reported in 1915.

Pneumopericardium, first clear description of

ISIDORE BRICHETEAU, French physician, 1789-1861, gave the first clear description of pneumopericardium, in 1844.

Pneumoperitoneum in treatment of tuberculosis

. . . See under *Tuberculosis.*

Pneumotaxic center, eponymic description of

THOMAS WILLIAM LUMSDEN, English physician, 1894-   , described a center in the upper part of the pons which rhythmically inhibits inspiration thus allowing expiration to begin. Published in 1923. Known as *Lumsden's center.*

Pneumothorax, artificial, early suggestion of

JAMES CARSON, English physician, 1772-1843, suggested the induction of artificial pneumothorax in treating pulmonary tuberculosis, in 1821.

Pneumothorax, artificial, early use of, in tuberculosis

CARLO FORLANINI, Italian physician, 1847-1918, suggested the use of artificial pneumothorax in treating tuberculosis as early as 1882, but did not apply it clinically until 1888. Reported in 1894.

Pneumothorax, use of nitrogen in

LUDOLPH BRAUER, German physician, 1865-1951, used nitrogen in the production of artificial pneumothorax for the treatment of tuberculosis. Published in 1906.

Podalic version, combined, introduction of

JOHN BRAXTON HICKS, English gynecologist, 1823-1897, introduced combined podalic version. Recorded in 1864.

Point at which palatine nerve emerges from palatine foramen

JEAN ANTOINE MEGLIN, French physician, 1756-1824, described the point of emergence of the anterior palatine nerve from the greater palatine foramen. Known as *Meglin's point*. Date not available.

Poirier's line

. . . See under *Nasolambdoid line*.

Poiseuille's law regarding flow in capillary tubes

JEAN LÉONARD MARIE POISEUILLE, French physiologist, 1799-1869, pronounced a law which states that the speed with which a liquid flows in capillary tubes is proportional to the square of the diameter. Published in 1840.

Poisons, effect of, on frog's heart

JOHANN ERNST OSWALD SCHMIE-DEBERG, German pharmacologist, 1838-1921, was first to investigate the effects of poisons on the heart of the frog. Reported in 1870.

Poisons

. . . See also under name of particular poison, as *Arsenic, Lead, Snake venom*, etc.

Poitou colic

. . . See under *Lead colic, early recognition as definite syndrome*.

Polarized light affected by magnetic field

MICHAEL FARADAY, English chemist and physicist, 1791-1867, dis-covered the influence of a magnetic field on polarized light, in 1845.

Polioencephalomyelitis; Strümpell's disease

ERNST ADOLF GUSTAV GOTTFRIED STRÜMPELL, German physician, 1853-1925, described a form of acute encephalitis of infants. Recorded in 1885.

Poliomyelitis, deformities resulting from, early description of

JACOB VON HEINE, German orthopedist, 1800-1879, is credited with being the first to describe the various deformities caused by poliomyelitis. Reported in 1840. Poliomyelitis is sometimes referred to as *Heine-Medin disease*.

Poliomyelitis, epidemic nature of, first observation on

KARL OSKAR MEDIN, Swedish physician, 1847-1927, was first to call attention to the epidemic character of acute anterior poliomyelitis, in 1890.

Poliomyelitis, gamma globulin in prophylaxis of

WILLIAM MCDOWELL HAMMON, American physician, 1904- , with L. I. CORIELL, J. STOKES, P. F. WEHRLE, and C. R. KLIMT, was the first to try gamma globulin in the prophylaxis of poliomyelitis. Recorded in 1952.

Poliomyelitis, infantile, atrophy of anterior horns in

JEAN MARTIN CHARCOT, French neurologist, 1825-1893, was the first to demonstrate the atrophy of the anterior horns of the spinal cord in infantile poliomyelitis. Recorded in 1870, with ALEX JOFFROY. The possibility of such atrophy was suggested earlier by JACOB VON HEINE and by GUILLAUME B. A. DU-CHENNE.

Poliomyelitis, infantile, first clear clinical account of

JOHN BADHAM, English physician, 1764-1842, gave the first adequate clinical account of infantile poliomyelitis, in a report of four cases. Published in 1835.

Poliomyelitis, infantile, first recorded description of

MICHAEL UNDERWOOD, English pediatrician, 1737-1820, gave the first recorded description of infantile poliomyelitis, under the title of "Debility of the lower extremities." Recorded in 1789.

Poliomyelitis, infectiousness of

OTTO IVAR WICKMAN, German physician, 1872-1914, was the first to confirm that poliomyelitis is an infectious disease. Published in 1907.

Poliomyelitis, Kenny treatment of

. . . See under *Kenny treatment of poliomyelitis.*

Poliomyelitis, transmission of, from man to monkeys —1909

KARL LANDSTEINER, American pathologist, 1868-1943, transmitted poliomyelitis from man to monkeys, by injection of an emulsion of spinal cord derived from a patient. Reported in 1909.

Poliomyelitis, transmission of, to monkeys—1909

SIMON FLEXNER, American path-ologist and bacteriologist, 1863-1946, with PAUL A. LEWIS, transmitted poliomyelitis to monkeys using cultures of a filtrable virus, in 1909.

Poliomyelitis vaccine, early form of

JOHN ALBERT KOLMER, American pathologist, 1886-19??, with ANNA M. RULE, developed an early crude form of poliomyelitis vaccine which he used on monkeys. Recorded in 1934.

Poliomyelitis vaccine, introduction of

JONAS EDWARD SALK, American bacteriologist, 1914-   , developed a poliomyelitis vaccine composed of three types of virus treated with formaldehyde. Widely accepted in 1954. Known as *Salk's vaccine.*

Poliomyelitis virus will grow in cultures of different tissues, discovery that

JOHN F. ENDERS, American bacteriologist, 1897-   , with FREDERICK C. ROBBINS (American pediatrician, 1916-   ) and THOMAS H. WELLER (American physician, 1915-   ), demonstrated that the poliomyelitis virus will grow in cultures of different tissues. All three shared the Nobel prize in 1954.

Politzer bag

. . . See under *Middle ear, bag for inflating.*

Pollen is cause of hay fever, early proof that—1831

JOHN ELLIOTSON, English surgeon, 1786-1868, "ascertained" that pollen is the cause of hay fever. Recorded in 1831.

Pollen is cause of hay fever, early proof that—1873

CHARLES HARRISON BLACKLEY, English homeopath, 1820-1900, demonstrated that pollen can cause asthma, catarrh, and skin reactions in sensitive subjects. Recorded in 1873.

Pollen, reproduction of plants by means of

ROBERT BROWN, Scottish botanist, 1773-1858, was the first to discover the part played by pollen in the reproduction of plants. Observed in 1827; reported in 1828.

Polyarthritis in children; Still's disease

GEORGE FREDERIC STILL, English pediatrician, 1868-1941, described a form of chronic joint disease, "chronic articular rheumatism," in children. Recorded in 1897.

Polycythemia hypertonica, original description of

FELIX GAISBÖCK, Austrian physician, 1868-19??, described a condition marked by polycythemia, hypertension, hypertrophy of the heart, etc., but without enlargement of the spleen. Reported in 1905. Known as *Gaisböck's disease.*

Polycythemia, phenylhydrazine hydrochloride in

HANS EPPINGER, Austrian physician, 1879-1946, with KARL KLOSS, introduced phenylhydrazine hydrochloride in the treatment of polycythemia. Published in 1918.

Polycythemia, splenomegalic; Osler's disease

WILLIAM OSLER, Canadian-English physician, 1849-1919, described polycythemia with cyanosis and enlarged spleen. Recorded in 1903. Known also as *Osler-Vaquez disease.*

Polycythemia, splenomegalic; Vaquez's disease

LOUIS HENRI VAQUEZ, French physician, 1860-1936, described polycythemia with cyanosis and splenomegaly. Recorded in 1892. Known also as *Osler-Vaquez disease.*

Polygraph, early form of

JAMES MACKENZIE, Scottish cardiologist in England, 1853-1925, is credited with producing the forerunner of the modern polygraph, in 1892. It was a phlebograph with which Mackenzie obtained tracings of veins and simultaneous tracings of the radial artery and jugular vein. Later, in 1902, Mackenzie described an improved form with which he made simultaneous recordings of the pulse, blood pressure, apex beat, etc.

Polyhedral cells of cochlear duct, description of

FRIEDRICH M. CLAUDIUS, German anatomist, 1822-1869, gave a lucid description of the polyhedral cells of the cochlear duct. Recorded in 1852.

Polymorphism, discovery of phenomenon of

ERNST EILHARD MITSCHERLICH, German chemist, 1794-1863, discovered and described polymorphism, in 1844.

Polymyxin, discovery of

. . . See under *Aerosporin.*

Polyposis of colon, first description of

HUBERT VON LUSCHKA, German anatomist, 1820-1875, is credited with giving the first clear description of polyposis of the colon, in 1861.

Polyserositis; mediastinoperi- carditis

. . . See under *Liver, pseudocir- rhosis of, with pericarditis.*

Polyuria caused by excision of pancreas

. . . See under *Pancreas, excision of,* etc.

Pompholyx, original de- scription of

WILLIAM TILBURY FOX, English dermatologist, 1836-1879, gave the original description of pompholyx or dyshidrosis, in 1873.

Poncet's disease

. . . See under *Tuberculous arth- ritis, multiple,* etc.

Ponfick's shadow

. . . See under *Achromacyte, early description of.*

Popliteal bursitis, classic description of

. . . See under *Cyst formed by her- niation of synovial membrane of a joint.*

Population increases faster than food supply, theory that

THOMAS ROBERT MALTHUS, Eng- lish political economist, 1766-1834, proposed a theory that the normal increase in population is more rapid than the increase in food supply, unless the growth of population is slowed by war and disease. He, therefore, advocated sexual conti- nence as a means of keeping the population in line with the food supply. First report published in 1798. The doctrine is known as *Malthusianism.*

Porokeratosis, early de- scription of—1875

ISIDOR NEUMANN, Austrian derma- tologist, 1832-1906, described por- okeratosis under the name derma- titis circumscripta herpetiformis, in 1875.

Porokeratosis, eponymic de- scription of

VITTORIO MIBELLI, Italian derma- tologist, 1860-1910, described a disease of the skin marked by hy- pertrophy of the stratum corneum, followed by progressive atrophy. Recorded in 1893. Known as *Mi- belli's disease No. 2* and as *poro- keratosis excentrica.*

Porro's operation

. . . See under *Caesarean section with hysterectomy and adnexec- tomy.*

Portal vein and vena cava, communication between

NIKOLAI VLADIMIROVICH ECK, Rus- sian physiologist, 1847-19??, pro- duced an artificial communication between the portal vein and the vena cava, for the study of liver diseases and the relation of the liver to metabolism. Published in 1877. Known as *Eck's fistula.*

Portal veins, accessory, eponymic descrip- tion of

MARIE PHILIBERT CONSTANT SAP-

PEY, French anatomist, 1810-1896, described the accessory portal veins. Recorded in 1859. Known as *Sappey's veins*.

Portes' operation

... See under *Caesarean section, Portes' classic method of.*

Posada-Wernicke disease

... See under *Coccidioidomycosis.*

Position, operative, for gallbladder surgery

JOHN W. ELLIOT, American surgeon, 1852-1925, devised a position for gallbladder surgery in which the patient's lower chest is elevated by placing a support under the small of the back. Published in 1895.

Positive and negative charges of electricity, early concept of—1753

BENJAMIN FRANKLIN, American statesman and scientist, 1706-1790, promulgated the theory that electricity is of two kinds, positive and negative, in 1753.

Posterior elastic lamina of cornea, early description of—1729

BENEDICT DUDDELL, English ophthalmologist, 1690-1752, is believed to have described the posterior elastic lamina of the cornea as early as 1729. Known as *Duddell's membrane.*

Posterior elastic lamina of cornea, early description of—1758

JEAN DESCEMET, French surgeon, 1732-1810, described the thin membrane between the substantia pro-

pria and the endothelial layer of the cornea (lamina elastica posterior), in 1758. Known as *Descemet's membrane.*

Posterior ligament of knee joint, eponymic description of

MARC JEAN BOURGERY, French anatomist, 1797-1869, described the posterior ligament of the knee, ligamentum popliteum obliquum. Exact date not available. Known as *Bourgery's ligament.*

Posterior root fibers divide into ascending and descending branches

FRIDTJOF NANSEN, Norwegian explorer and scientist, 1861-1930, was the first to demonstrate that the posterior root fibers of the spinal cord divide into ascending and descending branches, upon entering the substance of the cord. Recorded in 1886.

Posterior scleral protuberance, early description of

FRIEDRICH AUGUST VON AMMON, Dresden ophthalmologist, 1799-1861, described the posterior scleral protuberance and the pyriform scleral fissure present in early fetal life. Reported in 1838.

Posterior vertex presentation, conversion of

... See under *Scanzoni maneuver.*

Postganglionic, introduction of term

JOHN NEWPORT LANGLEY, English physiologist, 1852-1925, is credited with introducing the term *postganglionic, circa* 1894.

Postmortem warts

. . . See under *Dissecting-room warts.*

Posture, classic study of

RUDOLF MAGNUS, German physiologist in Holland, 1873-1927, did original work in the study of posture and postural mechanisms. His book, titled *Körperstellung,* was published in 1924.

Potassium and sodium tartrate; Rochelle salt

PIERRE SEIGNETTE, French apothecary, 1660-1719, is credited with introducing potassium and sodium tartrate as a laxative, in 1682. The name is derived from the city of Rochelle, where Seignette lived.

Potassium chloride in myasthenia gravis

LOUIS PHILIPPE EUGENE LAURENT, English physician, 1895- , with WILLIAM WERNER WALTHER, introduced the use of potassium chloride in the treatment of myasthenia gravis. Published in 1935.

Potassium iodide in treatment of epilepsy

WILLIAM O'CONNOR, English physician, 18??-1880, is believed to have been the first to use potassium iodide in the treatment of epilepsy. Recorded in 1857.

Potassium iodide in treatment of syphilis

WILLIAM WALLACE, Irish physician, 1791-1837, is credited with introducing potassium iodide in the treatment of syphilis. Recorded in 1833.

Potential difference between injured nerve and its muscle

CARLO MATTEUCCI, Italian scientist, 1811-1868, demonstrated that there is a difference in electric potential between an injured nerve and its muscle. Recorded in 1838.

Pott's disease, tuberculous origin of

JACQUES M. DELPECH, French orthopedist, 1777-1832, demonstrated the tuberculous origin of Pott's disease, in 1816.

Pott's fracture of the fibula

PERCIVALL POTT, English surgeon, 1714-1788, described a typical fracture of the lower end of the fibula, sometimes associated with injury to the medial malleolus and the lower tibial articulation. Recorded in 1765. Known as *Pott's fracture.*

Pouch of Douglas

. . . See under *Rectouterine pouch.*

Poulet's disease

. . . See under *Rheumatic osteoperiostitis.*

Powder of opium and ipecac, compounding of

THOMAS DOVER, English physician, 1660-1742, who believed in sweating as a therapeutic measure, invented a powder of opium and ipecac, which he described in his book *The Ancient Physician's Legacy to his Country,* in 1733.

Prausnitz-Küstner reaction

. . . See under *Hypersensitiveness, local, production of.*

Precancerous dermatosis, first description of

JOHN TEMPLETON BOWEN, American dermatologist, 1857-1941, was the first to describe precancerous dermatosis, in 1912. Known as *Bowen's disease* and *Bowen's epithelioma.*

Precentral area of cerebral cortex, eponymic description of

ALFRED WALTER CAMPBELL, Australian neurologist and psychiatrist, 1868-1937, described the precentral area of the cerebral cortex concerned with integration and transmission of motor impulses in response to sensory stimulation. Recorded in 1905. Known as *psychomotor area* and *Campbell's area.*

Precipitins in medicolegal tests for human blood

PAUL THEODORE UHLENHUTH, German bacteriologist, 1870-19??, is credited with being the first to use precipitins in medicolegal identification of human blood. Reported in 1901.

Precocious puberty in females, pigmentation, and osteitis fibrosa disseminata

FULLER ALBRIGHT, American physician, 1900-   , described a syndrome characterized by osteitis fibrosa disseminata, areas of pigmentation (often segmental), and endocrine dysfunction, with precocious puberty in females. Report of five cases published in 1937. Known as the *Albright syndrome* and as the *Albright-McCune-Sternberg syndrome.*

Preganglionic fibers originate in central nervous system, proof that

WALTER H. GASKELL, English physiologist and anatomist, 1847-1914, established that the preganglionic neurons originate in the central nervous system. Reported in 1886.

Preganglionic, introduction of term

JOHN NEWPORT LANGLEY, English physiologist, 1852-1925, is credited with introducing the term *preganglionic, circa* 1894.

Pregnancy, abdominal, first successful operation for

JOHN KING, American surgeon, 1776-184?, performed the first successful operation for abdominal pregnancy, in 1817.

Pregnancy, interstitial, first description of

WILHELM JOSEPH SCHMITT, Austrian obstetrician, 1760-1827, was the first to describe interstitial pregnancy, i.e., gestation in that part of the uterine tube which is within the wall of the uterus. Recorded in 1801.

Pregnancy sign consisting of bluish coloration of vaginal mucosa —1838

JEAN MARIE JACQUEMIER, French obstetrician, 1806-1879, described a bluish spot on the vaginal mucosa, below the urethral opening, appearing during the early weeks of pregnancy. Reported in 1838. Known as *Jacquemier's sign.*

Pregnancy sign consisting of bluish coloration of vaginal mucosa —1887

JAMES READ CHADWICK, American gynecologist, 1844-1905, described a bluish coloration of the vaginal mucosa occurring from about the 6th to the 12th week of pregnancy. Reported in 1887. Known as *Chadwick's sign.*

Pregnancy test based on presence of protective ferment in body

. . . See under *Serum reaction based on,* etc.

Pregnancy test by injection of urine into immature female mice

SELMAR ASCHHEIM, German physician, 1878-19??, with BERNHARDT ZONDEK, German physician, 1891-19??, developed a test for pregnancy in which the subject's urine is injected subcutaneously in immature female mice. A positive reaction is marked by congestion and hemorrhages of the ovaries in the mice. Recorded in 1928. Known as *Aschheim-Zondek test.*

Pregnancy test by injection of urine into rabbits

MAURICE H. FRIEDMAN, American physiologist, 1903-   , developed a modification of the Aschheim-Zondek test for pregnancy in which the urine of a pregnant woman is injected into female rabbits. Pregnancy is indicated by the formation of corpora lutea and corpora haemorrhagica. Reported, with M. E. LAPHAM, in 1931.

Pregnancy test with subject's citrated blood

ZACHARIAS TAYLOR BERCOVITZ, American physician, 1895-   , invented a test for pregnancy in which a few drops of the subject's prepared blood are instilled in the eye; if the pupil reacts by contraction or dilatation, the test is positive. Known as the *Bercovitz test.* Reported in 1930.

Pregnancy, *Xenopus* toad test for

CHARLES WILLIAM BELLERBY, English physician, 19??-   , introduced the *Xenopus* toad test for the diagnosis of pregnancy. This followed by four years the discovery that the toad responds by ovulation to the injection of gonadotropic hormone. Recorded in 1934.

Pregnanediol, isolation of

GUY FREDERIC MARRIAN, English biochemist, 1904-   , isolated pregnanediol, a degeneration product of progesterone. Published in 1929.

Preiser's disease

. . . See under *Navicular, carpal, osteoporosis of.*

Preisz-Nocard bacillus

. . . See under *Pseudotuberculosis in cattle, sheep, etc., causative agent of.*

Preperitoneal space

. . . See under *Prevesical space of Retzius.*

Presenile dementia associated with cerebral sclerosis

ALOIS ALZHEIMER, German neurologist, 1864-1915, described a presenile condition marked by symptoms of progressive mental weakness and associated with cortical cerebral sclerosis. Reported in 1907. Known as *Alzheimer's disease*.

Pressometer, Jarcho's

. . . See under *Instrument for measuring pressure during injection of radiopaque material into uterus*.

Pressor substance of adrenal gland

EDWARD ALBERT SHARPEY-SCHAFER, English physician, 1850-1935, with GEORGE OLIVER, demonstrated the presence of a pressor substance in the adrenal medulla. First reported in 1894. It was later named epinephrine by JOHN JACOB ABEL.

Pressure boiler for digesting organic matter

DENIS PAPIN, French physicist, 1647-1714, devised an apparatus for boiling and digesting organic matter under pressure, hence at a temperature higher than the boiling point of water. Recorded in 1682. Known as *Papin's digester*.

Pressure on eyeballs causes slowing of heart

. . . See under *Oculocardiac reflex*.

Prevesical space of Retzius

ANDERS ADOLF RETZIUS, Swedish anatomist, 1796-1860, described a space between the bladder and the symphysis pubis. Published in 1849. Known as *space of Retzius* and *preperitoneal space*. Sometimes also called *cave of Retzius*.

Price-Jones method for measuring red blood cells

. . . See under *Red blood cells, method for measuring*.

Pringle's disease or adenoma

. . . See under *Sebaceous adenoma*.

Probe for detecting bullets and other metal objects in the body

HOWARD LILIENTHAL, American surgeon, 1861-1946, devised a probe for detecting bullets and other metal objects in the body by means of an elementary electric circuit. Reported in 1901. Known as *Lilienthal's probe*.

Probe for dilating lacrimal duct in case of stenosis

DOMINIQUE ANEL, French surgeon, *circa* 1679-1730, invented a probe which he used in treatment of stenosis of the lacrimal duct. Reported in 1713.

Probe for locating lead bullets

AUGUSTE NÉLATON, French surgeon, 1807-1873, invented a probe tipped with porcelain for locating lead bullets, which stained the tip when touched. Recorded in 1837. Known as *Nélaton's probe*. The device was used in locating a bullet in Garibaldi's leg.

Procaine, first clinical use of

HEINRICH FRIEDRICH WILHELM BRAUN, German surgeon, 1862-1934, is credited with introducing procaine in clinical use. Recorded in 1905.

Procaine penicillin G (duracillin), introduction of

WALLACE EDGAR HERRELL, American scientist, 1909-   , with D. R. NICHOLS and F. R. HEILMAN, produced procaine penicillin G or duracillin. Recorded in 1947.

Procaine, synthesis of —1899

ALFRED EINHORN, German chemist, 185?-19??, is credited with the synthesis of procaine or novocaine. Recorded in 1899.

Procerus muscle, early description of

. . . See under *Pyramidalis nasi muscle.*

Process vaginalis of peritoneum, first description of

PIETER CAMPER, Dutch anatomist, 1722-1789, is believed to have been the first to describe the process vaginalis of the peritoneum, also known as the processus vaginalis testis, *circa* 1775.

Proctoclysis, continuous; Murphy drip

JOHN BENJAMIN MURPHY, American surgeon, 1857-1916, introduced the method of continuous proctoclysis, used in infections of the peritoneum, in which salt solution is administered per rectum drop by drop, with the patient in Fowler's position. Recorded in 1908-9.

Prodigiosus toxin in treatment of sarcoma

. . . See under *Sarcoma, use of erysipelas toxin in treatment of.*

Proetz's treatment

. . . See under *Sinuses, paranasal, displacement irrigation of.*

Profenamine in treatment of parkinsonism

. . . See under *Parkinsonism.*

Progeria, a form of infantilism, eponymic description of

HASTINGS GILFORD, English physician, 1861-1941, described progeria, a form of infantilism marked by smallness of stature, absence of pubic and facial hair, wrinkling of skin, and general appearance of old age. Reported in 1904. Known as *Hutchinson-Gilford disease.*

Progeria, first recorded case of

JONATHAN HUTCHINSON, English surgeon, 1828-1913, was the first to describe a case of progeria in a boy. Published in 1886.

Progeria, introduction of term

HASTINGS GILFORD, English physician, 1861-1941, is credited with introducing the term *progeria,* in connection with a case reported by him in 1904.

Progesterone, crystalline, in Germany

ADOLPH FRIEDRICH JOHANN BUTENANDT, German chemist, 1903-   , succeeded in obtaining crystalline progesterone. Recorded in 1934.

Progesterone, discovery and crystallization of

WILLARD MYRON ALLEN, American physician, 1904-   , with GEORGE WASHINGTON CORNER, American anatomist, 1889-   , discovered progesterone, the corpus luteum hormone, in 1929. He also proved that progesterone is necessary for the preservation of early pregnancy. In 1934, with OSKAR

WINTERSTEINER, he produced crystalline progesterone.

Progressive ascending paralysis or hemiplegia

CHARLES KARSNER MILLS, American neurologist, 1845-1931, described a case of unilateral progressive ascending paralysis, in 1900. Known as *Mills's disease.*

Progressive descending paralysis

. . . See under *Descending paralysis, progressive unilateral.*

Progressive hypertrophic interstitial neuropathy

JOSEPH JULES DEJERINE, French neurologist, 1849-1917, with JULES SOTTAS (French neurologist, 1866-1943), gave the first descripton of progressive hypertrophic interstitial neuropathy, in 1893. Known as *Dejerine-Sottas disease.*

Progressive lenticular degeneration, eponymic description of

SAMUEL ALEXANDER KINNIER WILSON, American neurologist in England, 1877-1937, gave a classic description of progressive familial lenticular degeneration, in 1912. The condition was described earlier, in 1861, by FRIEDRICH THEODOR FRERICHS. Known as *Kinnier Wilson's disease.*

Progressive lenticular degeneration, original description of

FRIEDRICH T. VON FRERICHS, German pathologist, 1819-1885, gave the first description of progressive lenticular degeneration, a disease marked by bilateral degeneration of the corpus striatum, cirrhosis of the liver, etc., in 1861.

Progressive muscular atrophy, early description of

WILLIAM JOHN LITTLE, English surgeon, 1810-1894, described progressive muscular atrophy, in a paper titled *On the nature and treatment of the deformities of the human frame.* Published in 1853.

Progressive muscular atrophy; Hoffmann's atrophy

JOHANN HOFFMANN, German neurologist, 1857-1919, described hereditary familial spinal muscular atrophy affecting the legs, feet, forearms, and hands. Reported *circa* 1889. Known as *Hoffmann's atrophy, Hoffmann-Werding syndrome,* etc.

Progressive muscular atrophy, spinal cord lesions in

JULES BERNARD LUYS, French neurologist, 1828-1897, described the degeneration of the anterior horn cells associated with progressive muscular atrophy, in 1860.

Progressive neuropathic muscular atrophy of peroneal type

. . . See under *Neuropathic muscular atrophy,* etc.

Progressive ophthalmoplegia, early description of

FRIEDRICH W. E. A. VON GRAEFE, German ophthalmologist, 1828-1870, described progressive ophthalmoplegia, a creeping paralysis affecting first one eye muscle and then another, in 1868.

Progressive pigmentary dermatosis

JAY FRANK SCHAMBERG, American

dermatologist, 1870-1934, described progressive pigmentary dermatosis, in 1901. Known as *Schamberg's disease.*

Progressive spastic paraplegia in children with hereditary syphilis

ANTONIN BERNARD JEAN MARFAN, French pediatrician, 1858-1942, described progressive spastic paraplegia in children with hereditary syphilis, in 1892. Known as *Marfan's disease.*

Progressive spinal muscular atrophy, description of, in 1849

GUILLAUME BENJAMIN AMAND DUCHENNE, French neurologist, 1806-1875, was the first to describe progressive spinal muscular atrophy, in 1849. The disease is known also as *Duchenne-Aran muscular atrophy, Cruveilhier's disease,* and as myelopathic muscular atrophy.

Progressive spinal muscular atrophy, description of, in 1850

FRANÇOIS AMILCAR ARAN, French physician, 1817-1861, described progressive spinal muscular atrophy in 1850, after the condition was described by G. B. A. DUCHENNE in 1849. The condition is known as myelopathic muscular atrophy, *Duchenne-Aran muscular atrophy,* and as *Cruveilhier's disease.*

Proguanil in treatment of malaria
. . . See under *Malaria.*

Prolan A and prolan B, discovery of

BERNARD ZONDEK, German gynecologist in Israel, 1891-19??, with

SELMER ASCHHEIM, discovered prolan A and B in human pregnancy urine, in 1927.

Promin in treatment of leprosy
. . . See under *Leprosy.*

Pronephros, introduction of term

EDWIN RAY LANKESTER, English zoologist, 1847-1930, is credited with introducing the term *pronephros, circa* 1885.

Prontosil, introduction of

GERHARD DOMAGK, German pharmacologist, 1895- , introduced prontosil, the first of the sulfonamides, as a therapeutic agent against hemolytic streptococci, in 1935.

Prophase, introduction of term
. . . See under *Mitosis, three stages of.*

Proprioceptor and *proprioception,* introduction of terms

CHARLES SCOTT SHERRINGTON, English neurophysiologist, 1857-1952, introduced the terms *proprioceptor* and *proprioception,* in 1906. He wrote, "the deep receptors may be termed proprioceptors, and the deep field a field of proprioception."

Prostate, cancer of, stilbestrol in treatment of

CHARLES HUGGINS, American surgeon, 1901- , with CLARENCE VERNARD HODGES, used stilbestrol in the treatment of metastatic carcinoma of the prostate. Recorded in 1941.

Prostate, carcinoma of; first record

GEORGE LANGSTAFF, American surgeon, 1780-1846, was the first to describe carcinoma of the prostate. Published in 1817.

Prostate, carcinoma of, radical operation for

HUGH HAMPTON YOUNG, Baltimore urologist, 1870-1945, introduced the radical operation for carcinoma of the prostate. Recorded in 1905.

Prostate, hypertrophy and carcinoma of; distinction between

JOHN ADAMS, English surgeon, 1806-1877, is credited with being the first to distinguish between benign hypertrophy and carcinoma of the prostate. Published in 1851.

Prostate, introduction of term

HEROPHILUS, Greek physician and anatomist in Egypt, 335-280 B.C., is credited with the introduction of the term *prostate,* in allusion to the gland's position before the bladder. It is derived from the Greek *pro* (before) and *histanai* (to set). Exact date not available.

Prostate, sarcoma of; first recorded case

RICHARD ANTHONY STAFFORD, American physician, 1801-1866, was the first to describe a case of sarcoma of the prostate in a child of five. Recorded in 1839.

Prostate, subsidiary lobe of

EVERARD HOME, English surgeon, 1756-1832, described a subsidiary lobe of the prostate. Published in 1811. Known as *Home's lobe* or *gland, subtrigonal gland,* and *third lobe of prostate.*

Prostatectomy, conservative perineal

HUGH HAMPTON YOUNG, Baltimore urologist, 1870-1945, introduced the method of conservative perineal prostatectomy. Recorded in 1903.

Prostatectomy, dilatable bag for controlling hemorrhage in

. . . See under *Prostatectomy, suprapubic.*

Prostatectomy, median perineal, introduction of

FRANCIS SEDGWICK WATSON, American urologist, 1853-1942, was the first to perform median perineal prostatectomy. Recorded in 1905.

Prostatectomy, perineal; first in France

JOAQUIN ALBARRAN Y DOMINGUEZ, Cuban surgeon and urologist in France, 1860-1912, is credited with being the first to perform perineal prostatectomy in France. Published in 1909.

Prostatectomy, punch operation

HUGH HAMPTON YOUNG, Baltimore urologist, 1870-1945, introduced the so-called punch operation for the removal of small prostatic bars, etc. Recorded in 1913.

Prostatectomy, retropubic, introduction of

TERENCE JOHN MILLIN, English urologist, 19??-   , introduced the method of retropubic prostatectomy. Recorded in 1945.

Prostatectomy, suprapubic, bag for controlling hemorrhage following

JAMES EMMONS BRIGGS, American

surgeon, 1869-1942, devised a distensible bag for the control of hemorrhage following suprapubic prostatectomy. Introduced in 1905. Published in 1906.

Prostatectomy, suprapubic, early performance of—1895

EUGENE FULLER, American surgeon, 1858-1930, was probably the first to perform suprapubic prostatectomy, in 1895.

Prostatectomy, suprapubic, early performance of—1900

PETER J. FREYER, English surgeon, 1851-1921, performed and described suprapubic prostatectomy, in 1900.

Prostatic fluid, crystals in

. . . See under *Crystals in prostatic fluid.*

Prostatic obstruction, galvanocautery in

. . . See under *Galvanocautery.*

Prostigmine, use of, in myasthenia gravis

LAZAR REMEN, Westphalian physician, 1907-   , introduced the use of prostigmine in the treatment of myasthenia gravis. Recorded in 1932.

Protamine insulin, introduction of

. . . See under *Insulin, protamine, etc.*

Protamine zinc insulin, introduction of

ROBERT BEWS KERR, Canadian scientist, 1908-   , with C. H. BEST, W. R. CAMPBELL, and A. A. FLETCHER, suggested the combination of insulin with zinc to slow down the rate of absorption. To this combination protamine was added later to form protamine zinc insulin. Recorded in 1936.

Protective mimicry of animals, early explanation of

HENRY WALTER BATES, English naturalist, 1825-1892, described and explained the protective mimicry of animals whereby they are able to evade their enemies. Published in 1862.

Protective mimicry, warning colors in

JOHANN FRIEDRICH THEODOR MÜLLER, German naturalist, 1821-1897, described the warning coloration of certain animals whereby they warn their would-be enemies. Published in 1878.

Protein, fat, and carbohydrate breakdown in body

MAX JOSEF VON PETTENKOFER, German chemist and hygienist, 1818-1901, with CARL VON VOIT, made the first determination of the amounts of protein, fat, and carboyhdrate broken down in the body. Published in 1862.

***Protein*, introduction of term**

GERARDUS JOHANN MULDER, Dutch chemist, 1802-1880, working with organic material obtained a complex substance which he believed to be the basic constituent of all organized bodies and hence named it *protein*, from the Greek *protos*, first. Recorded in 1838.

Protein molecule is composed of monoamino and diamino acids

EDMUND DRECHSEL, German chemist, 1843-1897, demonstrated

that the protein molecule contains both monoamino and diamino acids. Published in 1891.

Protein precipitation by neutral salts

PETER LUDVIG PANUM, Danish physiologist, 1820-1885, precipitated protein by use of neutral salts. Published in 1852.

Protein reaction using glacial acetic and sulfuric acids

ALBERT ADAMKIEWICZ, Polish pathologist, 1850-1921, described a color reaction for albumin in which sulfuric and glacial acetic acids are used. Reported in 1875. Known as the *Adamkiewicz test.*

Protein, reagent for detection of

AUGUST NICOLAS EUGÈNE MILLON, French chemist, 1812-1867, was one of the first to discover a reagent for the detection of proteins. Recorded in 1849.

Proteins, structure of, basic research in

. . . See under *Immunochemistry and structure of proteins.*

Proteus vulgaris, isolation of

GUSTAV HAUSER, German bacteriologist, 1856-1935, was the first to isolate *Proteus vulgaris.* Recorded in 1885.

Protoplasm, fundamental units of

. . . See under *Fundamental units of protoplasm.*

Protoplasm, introduction of term

JOHANNES EVANGELISTA VON PURKINJE, Bohemian physiologist, 1787-1869, introduced the term *protoplasm,* in 1839, to describe the embryonic ground substance. Recorded by JOSEPH ROSENTHAL, one of Purkinje's students, in 1839.

Protoplasm is identical in all living cells

MAXIMILIAN J. S. SCHULTZE, German anatomist and histologist, 1825 - 1874, demonstrated that the protoplasm of all living cells is almost identical. Published in 1863.

Protozoa, microscopic, first observation of

ANTONJ VAN LEEUWENHOEK, Dutch naturalist, 1632-1723, is believed to have been the first to see microscopic protozoa, in 1675.

Prowazek's bodies; Prowazek-Halberstaedter bodies

. . . See under *Trachoma, cytoplasmic inclusion bodies in.*

Prurigo mitis, original description of

ROBERT WILLAN, English dermatologist, 1757-1812, gave the first description of prurigo mitis, now defined as a mild form of prurigo, under the name *ichthyosis cornea,* circa 1796.

Prurigo nodularis, eponymic description of

JAMES NEVIN HYDE, American dermatologist, 1840-1910, gave a full description of prurigo nodularis, in 1909. Known as *Hyde's disease.*

Prurigo nodularis, first description of

WILLIAM AUGUSTUS HARDAWAY, American physician, 1850 - 1923, was the first to describe prurigo nodularis, later named *Hyde's disease.* Recorded in 1879.

Prurigo, summer

. . . See under *Summer prurigo.*

**Pruritus ani, treatment of,
by division of nerves**

CHARLES BENT BALL, Irish surgeon, 1851-1916, devised an operation for the relief of pruritus ani by cutting the nerve fibers which supply the area involved. Reported in 1887.

Prussak's fibers

. . . See under *Tympanic membrane, Prussak's fibers of.*

Prussak's space or pouch

. . . See under *Middle ear, space in attic of.*

**Pseudohemophilia, hereditary;
hemorrhagic diathesis**

EVERARD ALGERNON WILLEBRAND, German physician in Finland, 1892-   , described a hereditary form of pseudohemophilia marked by prolonged bleeding time but a normal coagulation time and normal number of platelets. It occurs in both males and females. First recorded in 1926. Known as *Willebrand's disease.*

**Pseudohypertrophic muscular
dystrophy, early description of—1865**

WILHELM GRIESINGER, German neurologist, 1817 - 1868, described pseudohypertrophic muscular dystrophy, a condition in which the muscles of the shoulder girdle and sometimes also of the pelvic girdle undergo dystrophy, beginning with hypertrophy and ending in atrophy. Reported in 1865. Known as *Duchenne-Griesinger disease;* also as *Erb's paralysis* or *dystrophy.*

**Pseudohypertrophic muscular
dystrophy, early description of—1868**

GUILLAUME B. A. DUCHENNE, French neurologist, 1806-1875, described progressive muscular dystrophy with pseudohypertrophy, in 1868.

**Pseudohypertrophic muscular
dystrophy, early description of—1884**

WILHELM H. ERB, German neurologist, 1840-1921, described progressive muscular dystrophy with pseudohypertrophy, in 1884.

Pseudoleukemia, naming of

JULIUS FRIEDRICH COHNHEIM, German pathologist, 1839 - 1884, described and named pseudoleukemia, in 1865.

**Pseudomonas pyocyanea
(Pseudomonas aeruginosa), isolation of**

CARLE GESSARD, French physician, 1850-1917, is credited with the isolation of *Pseudomonas aeruginosa.* Recorded in 1882.

**Pseudosclerosis of Westphal-
Strumpell**

CARL FRIEDRICH OTTO WESTPHAL, German neurologist, 1833 - 1890, described pseudosclerosis, a condition marked by rigidity, tremor, optic atrophy, etc. Published in 1883. The condition was also described by ADOLF GUSTAV GOTTFRIED VON STRUMPELL (German neurologist, 1853-1925), in 1898.

**Pseudotuberculosis in cattle,
sheep, etc., causative
agent of**

EDMOND ISIDORE ÉTIENNE NOCARD,

French veterinarian, 1850 - 1903, described an organism causing pseudotuberculosis in sheep, cattle, and horses. Recorded in 1885. Known as *Corynebacterium pseudotuberculosis,* also as *Preisz-Nocard bacillus.* (Hugo von Preisz, Hungarian bacteriologist, 1860-1940.)

Psittacosis, causative agent of, is filtrable

SAMUEL PHILLIPS BEDSON, English bacteriologist, 1886-19??, with GEORGE TRENCH WESTERN and SAMUEL LEVY SIMPSON, determined that the causative agent of psittacosis is filtrable. Recorded in 1930.

Psittacosis, first description of, in man

JACOB RITTER, Swiss physician, 18??-1896, is credited with giving the first description of psittacosis in man, in 1879.

Psittacosis in man, diagnosis of, by injection

THOMAS MILTON RIVERS, New York physician, 1888 - 19??, with GEORGE PACKER BERRY (1898-), devised a method for the diagnosis of psittacosis in man by the injection of sputum in white mice. Published in 1935.

Psophacusia, original description of

... See under *Paracusia of Willis.*

Psoriasis as separate skin disease, establishment of

ROBERT WILLAN, English dermatologist, 1757-1812, is credited with recognizing psoriasis as a skin dis-

ease entity separate from other diseases, *circa* 1796. Published in 1808.

Psoriasis, bleeding points in

HEINRICH AUSPITZ, Austrian physician, 1835 - 1886, described the bleeding points produced by the removal of the scales in psoriasis. Recorded in 1870.

Psoriasis buccalis; leukoplakia buccalis

ANTOINE P. E. BAZIN, French dermatologist, 1807 - 1878, gave an account of psoriasis buccalis, in 1861.

Psychasthenia, eponymic description of

PIERRE MARIE FELIX JANET, French psychiatrist, 1859 - 1947, gave a good clinical picture of psychasthenia, in 1903. Known as *Janet's disease.*

Psychiatry, first American book on

BENJAMIN RUSH, American physician, 1745-1813, wrote a book on psychiatry which is considered the first book on the subject in the United States. Published in 1812.

Psychiatry, first journal of

JOHANN CHRISTIAN REIL, Dutch physiologist, 1759-1813, is credited with being instrumental in founding the first journal of psychiatry, titled *Magazin für psychische Heilkunde,* in 1805.

Psychiatry, "open door" school of

PHILIPPE PINEL, French alienist, 1745-1826, advocated the abolition of forcible restraint in treating the insane, and the introduction of the "open door" methods in psychiatry. Published in 1801.

Psychical process, reaction time involved in
. . . See under *Reaction time.*

Psychoanalysis, introduction of
SIGMUND FREUD, Austrian psychiatrist, 1856 - 1939, introduced the first concept and method of psychoanalysis, *circa* 1895. He called the approach "free association."

Psychobiology, development of concept and introduction of term of
ADOLF MEYER, Swiss - American psychiatrist, 1866-1950, developed the concept of psychobiology and introduced the term, in the United States, in 1915.

Psychogalvanic reflex, eponymic description of
IVAN ROMANOVICH TARCHANOFF, Russian physiologist, 1848 - 1909, discovered the psychogalvanic reflex, a decrease in the electrical resistance of the body resulting from emotional excitation. Recorded in 1890. Known as *Tarchanoff's phenomenon.*

Psychology, experimental, founder of
WILHELM MAX WUNDT, German physiologist, 1832-1920, is regarded as the founder of experimental psychology. His classic work was published in 1873-4.

Psychomotor area of cortex
. . . See under *Precentral area of cerebral cortex.*

Psychophysics, founder of
GUSTAV THEODOR FECHNER, Ger-man physicist and psychologist, 1801-1887, is regarded as one of the founders of psychophysics.

Psychotherapy, substitution of, for hypnotic suggestion
AMBROISE AUGUSTE LIÉBEAULT, French physician, 1823 - 1904, is credited with introducing psychotherapy which he used instead of hypnotic suggestion. Recorded in 1889.

Pterygoid canal, early description of
GUIDO GUIDI, Italian physician and anatomist, 1500-1569, described the pterygoid canal, which provides passage for the vidian artery and nerve, *circa* 1555. Recorded after his death, in 1611. Known as *Vidian canal.*

Ptyalin, isolation of—1845
LOUIS MIALHE, French physician, 1807-1886, is credited with being first to isolate the salivary enzyme ptyalin, in 1845.

Pubic ligament, inferior, early description of
JULIUS CAESAR ARANTIUS, Italian physician, 1530-1589, described the inferior pubic ligament, in 1571.

Public health, early advocacy of
JOHANN PETER FRANK, German physician, 1745-1821, advocated public control of health problems as early as 1766.

Public health, first comprehensive treatise on
JOHANN PETER FRANK, German physician, 1745-1821, wrote the first comprehensive treatise on public health. It appeared in six volumes between 1779 and 1817.

Pudendal, introduction of term

FRANÇOIS MAURICEAU, French obstetrician, 1637-1709, is credited with introducing the term *pudendal* into the vocabulary of obstetrics. Recorded in 1668.

Puerperal fever, contagious nature of; early recognition—1772

JOHN LEAKE, English physician, 1729-1792, recognized the contagious nature of puerperal fever. Recorded in 1772.

Puerperal fever, contagious nature of; early recognition—1795

ALEXANDER GORDON, Scottish obstetrician, 1752-1799, formulated a theory expounding the contagiousness of puerperal fever. Published in 1795. Gordon suggested the disinfection of the clothes of the attending physician and of the midwife.

Puerperal fever, contagious nature of; early recognition — 1842-3

OLIVER WENDELL HOLMES, American physician and author, 1804-1894, recognized the contagiousness of puerperal fever and was the first to definitely establish the fact. Published 1842-3.

Puerperal fever, contagious nature of; early recognition — 1847

IGNAZ PHILIPP SEMMELWEIS, Hungarian obstetrician, 1818-1865, recognized the contagiousness of puerperal fever and attributed its spread to contamination by the hands of physicians and other attendants, *circa* 1840. He advocated antisepsis in childbirth cases. Recorded in 1847.

Puerperal fever, cultivation of streptococcus of

LOUIS PASTEUR, French bacteriologist and scientist, 1822-1895, cultivated the streptococcus from a case of puerperal fever. Published in 1879.

Puerperal fever, early modern work on

CHARLES WHITE, English surgeon, 1728-1813, is credited with being the first since Hippocrates to contribute substantially to the understanding and treatment of puerperal fever. Published in 1773.

Puerperal fever, first recorded reference to

HIPPOCRATES, Greek physician, 460-375 B. C., left the earliest known description of puerperal fever. Exact date not available.

Puerperal fever, introduction of term

EDWARD STROTHER, English physician, 1675-1737, is credited with introducing the term *puerperal fever,* in 1716.

Puerperal fever, septicemic nature of; first recognition

IGNAZ PHILIPP SEMMELWEIS, Hungarian obstetrician, 1818-1865, was the first to recognize that puerperal fever is a septicemia. Recorded in 1847.

Puerperal fever, vaginal secretions in relation to

ALBERT SIEGMUND GUSTAV DÖDERLEIN, German obstetrician, 1860-1941, studied the vaginal secretions and their role in the initiation of puerperal fever. Recorded in 1892.

Puerperal septicemia, bacterial origin of
. . . See under *Septicemia, puerperal*, etc.

Puerperal septicemia, contagiousness of—1843
OLIVER WENDELL HOLMES, American physician, 1804-1894, recognized the contagiousness of puerperal fever or septicemia. Reported in 1843.

Puerperal septicemia, contagiousness of—1847
IGNAZ PHILIPP SEMMELWEIS, Hungarian obstetrician, 1818-1865, recognized the contagiousness and the septicemic nature of puerperal fever. Reported in 1847. He also attributed the spread of puerperal septicemia to contamination by the hands of physicians and midwives.

Puerperal septicemia
. . . See also under *Puerperal fever*.

Pulmonary arteries, terminal, aneurysm of
. . . See under *Aneurysm of terminal pulmonary arteries*.

Pulmonary arteries, tubercles in semilunar valves of
. . . See under *Corpora arantii*.

Pulmonary artery, dilatation of
CHARLES LAUBRY, French physician, 1872-1941, with D. ROUTIER and R. HEIM DE BALSAC, described idiopathic dilatation of the pulmonary artery. Published in 1940.

Pulmonary artery, sclerosis of, with cyanosis, dyspnea, etc.
ABEL AYERZA, Argentinian physician, 1861-1918, described a condition marked by sclerosis of the pulmonary artery, chronic cyanosis, dyspnea, bronchitis, etc. Reported in 1901. Known as *Ayerza's disease* or *syndrome*.

Pulmonary artery stenosis or atresia, operation for relief of
ALFRED BLALOCK, Baltimore surgeon, 1899-   , devised an operation for the relief of congenital pulmonary artery obstruction by creating an artificial ductus arteriosus. In this operation an anastomosis is made between a pulmonary artery and an artery arising from the aortic arch. Reported in association with HELEN B. TAUSSIG, in 1945. Known as the *Blalock-Taussig operation*.

Pulmonary aspergillosis, first description of
RUDOLF LUDWIG KARL VIRCHOW, German pathologist, 1821-1902, is credited with being first to describe pulmonary aspergillosis, in 1856.

Pulmonary circulation, discovery of
MICHAEL SERVETUS, Spanish physician and theologian, 1511-1553, is probably the earliest observer to give an adequate description of the lungs. His concepts were published in 1546. Some thirteen years later, MATTEO R. COLOMBO, Italian anatomist, *circa* 1516-1559, gave a very good description of the pulmonary circulation. Some medical historians believe that Colombo merely repeated the observations of Servetus, a belief which this author does not uphold.

Pulmonary diastolic murmur, eponymic description of

GRAHAM STEELL, English physician, 1851-1942, described a diastolic murmur heard in pulmonary valve insufficiency. Recorded in 1888. Known as *Graham Steell murmur*.

Pulmonary embolectomy, first attempted operation of

FRIEDRICH TRENDELENBURG, German surgeon, 1844-1924, made the first attempt to excise a pulmonary embolus, without success, in 1908.

Pulmonary embolectomy, first successful performance of

MARTIN KIRSCHNER, German surgeon, 1879-1942, performed the first successful pulmonary embolectomy in accordance with a procedure suggested by FRIEDRICH TRENDELENBURG. Recorded in 1924.

Pulmonary fat embolism, classic description of

ALDRED SCOTT WARTHIN, American physician, 1867-1931, gave a classic description of traumatic lipemia and fatty embolism of the lung. Recorded in 1913.

Pulmonary fat embolism, first description of

FRIEDRICH ALBERT ZENKER, German pathologist, 1825-1898, is believed to have been the first to give an account of pulmonary fat embolism. Recorded in 1862.

Pulmonary tuberculosis, removal of apex in

THEODORE TUFFIER, French surgeon, 1857-1929, effected cure of pulmonary tuberculosis by excising the apex of the lung. Published in 1897.

Pulmonary tuberculosis

. . . See also under *Tuberculosis*.

Pulmonary valve insufficiency, murmur of

GRAHAM STEELL, English physician, 1851-1942, described a diastolic murmur heard in pulmonary valve insufficiency. Recorded in 1888. Known as *Graham Steell murmur*.

Pulmonary

. . . See also under *Lung*, and under name of particular part involved.

Pulse, bigeminal, first clear description of

LUDWIG TRAUBE, German physician, 1818-1876, is credited with being first to give a clear description of a bigeminal pulse. Published in 1872.

Pulse clock, first description of

SANTORIUS SANCTORIUS, Italian physician, 1561-1636, devised a pulsilograph or pulse clock for the purpose of determining the pulse rate. Recorded in 1626.

Pulse count, introduction of—1707

JOHN FLOYER, English physician, 1649-1734, was probably the first to make a study of the pulse count. He invented a special watch, which indicated an interval of a minute and its divisions, for use in his pulse studies. Reported in 1707.

Pulse, instrument for registering the

. . . See under *Sphygmograph*, etc.

Pulse, mid-diastolic wave in
ALEXANDER GEORGE GIBSON, English physician, 1875-1950, was the first to describe a mid-diastolic wave in the jugular pulse, observed when the pulse is slow. Recorded in 1907. Known as the *b*-wave.

Pulse smaller during expiration
FRANZ RIEGEL, German physician, 1843-1904, demonstrated that the volume of the pulse appears smaller during expiration. Recorded in 1883.

Pulse, temporary slowing of, on bending forward or in process of sitting down
SIEGMUND ERBEN, Austrian physician, 1863-19??, observed that the pulse is temporarily slowed on bending forward and while one is in process of sitting down, due to stimulation of the vagus. Described in 1912.

Pulse watch, invention of
... See under *Pulse count.*

Pulse wave, velocity of; early determination
ERNST HEINRICH WEBER, German physician, 1795-1878, with EDUARD FRIEDRICH WILHELM WEBER, German physiologist, 1806-1871, determined the velocity of the pulse wave, in 1825.

Pupil, artificial, first recorded construction of
WILLIAM CHESELDEN, English surgeon, 1688-1752, was the first to construct an artificial pupil in a patient whose normal pupil had been obliterated by inflammation, *circa* 1725.

Pupil, artificial, iridencleisis for
... See under *Iridencleisis.*

Pupil, change in shape of, after death
LOUIS HENRI ANTONIN RIPAULT, French physician, 1807-1856, demonstrated that pressure upon the eye after death causes the pupil to change shape permanently. In the living subject the pupil regains its normal shape. Recorded in 1841. Known as *Ripault's sign.*

Pupil, dilatation of, in response to psychic stimuli
OSWALD C. E. BUMKE, German neurologist, 1877-1950, discovered the peculiar dilatation of the pupil in response to certain psychic stimuli, a phenomenon not operative in dementia praecox. Recorded in 1904. Known as *Bumke's pupil.*

Pupil, dilating mechanism of
JOSEPH LISTER, English surgeon, 1827-1912, is credited with giving the first clear description of the dilating mechanism of the pupil, in 1853.

Pupil, illumination of, by light placed in mouth
HERMANN DAVIDSOHN, German physician, 1842-1911, devised a method for illuminating the pupils by placing a light in the mouth. Fluid or other matter in the maxillary sinus causes a reduction in the illumination on the affected side. Introduced *circa* 1880. Known as *Davidsohn's sign.*

Pupil, irregular contraction of, in tabes dorsalis
WILLIAM RICHARD GOWERS, English neurologist, 1845-1915, described an irregular contraction of the pupil, in response to light, observed in tabes dorsalis. Reported in 1895. Known as *Gowers' sign.*

Pupil, irregularity of, in early tabes dorsalis

EMIL BERGER, Austrian ophthalmologist, 1855-1926, described an irregularity of the pupil, usually elliptical, as a sign of early tabes dorsalis. Reported in 1889.

Pupil, three sets of images seen in

JOHANNES EVANGELISTA VON PURKINJE, Bohemian physiologist, 1787-1869, described the appearance of three pairs of images of a single object, reflected from the anterior and posterior surfaces of the lens and from the cornea, seen when looking into the pupil. Recorded in 1823. The phenomenon was described also, about the same time, by LOUIS JOSEPH SANSON, French physician, 1790-1841. Known as *Purkinje-Sanson images.*

Pupil which reacts to accommodation but not to light

. . . See under *Argyll Robertson pupil.*

Pupillary contraction in response to light

ROBERT WHYTT, Scottish physician, 1714-1766, was the first to demonstrate that the contraction of the pupils in response to light is a reflex action. Published in 1751. Known as *Whytt's reflex.*

Pupillary contraction without accommodation or convergence

OTTO HAAB, Swiss ophthalmologist, 1850-1931, described pupillary contraction when the subject directs his attention to a bright object already in the field of vision, without using accommodation or convergence. Reported in 1891. Known as *Haab's reflex* and *cerebral cortex reflex.*

Pupillary membrane of fetus

EBERHARD JACOB VON WACHENDORF, Dutch anatomist, 1703-1758, described a thin membrane filling in the pupil in the fetus up to the sixth or seventh month, in 1754. Known as *Wachendorf's membrane.*

Pupillary reaction in diagnosis of pregnancy

. . . See under *Pregnancy test with subject's citrated blood.*

Purkinje's cells or corpuscles

. . . See under *Cerebellum, branching neurons in cortex of.*

Purkinje's fibers or network

. . . See under *Heart, beaded muscular fibers in subendocardial layer of.*

Purkinje's images

. . . See under *Retina, images on, produced by blood vessels.*

Purkinje's vesicle

. . . See under *Embryo, germinal vesicle of.*

Purkinje-Sanson images

. . . See under *Pupil, three sets of images seen in.*

Purpura, abdominal, eponymic description of

EDUARD HENOCH, German pediatrician, 1820-1910, described a nonthrombopenic form of purpura marked by abdominal symptoms, first described by ROBERT WILLAN in 1796. Recorded in 1868. Known as *Henoch's purpura.*

Purpura, abdominal, first description of

ROBERT WILLAN, English dermatologist, 1757-1812, was the first to describe a nonthrombopenic form of purpura marked by abdominal symptoms, as diarrhea, vomiting, etc. Recorded in 1796. Known also as *purpura nervosa* and *Henoch's purpura*.

Purpura annularis telangiectodes, eponymic description of

DOMENICO MAJOCCHI, Italian dermatologist, 1849-1929, described a skin disease marked by an eruption on the lower extremities which is at first telangiectatic, then purpuric and atrophic. Published in 1896. Known as *Majocchi's disease* and *purpura annularis telangiectodes*.

Purpura as a medical entity, first description of

AMATUS LUSITANUS, (JOÃO RODRIGUEZ DE CASTELLO BRANCO), Spanish physician, 1511-1568, was the first to describe a case of purpura, not associated with fever, as a medical entity. Recorded in 1556.

Purpura, experimental production of

FRANÇOIS MAGENDIE, French physiologist, 1783-1855, produced purpura experimentally, in 1833.

Purpura fulminans, original description of

EDUARD HENOCH, German pediatrician, 1820-1910, described a type of purpura characterized by rapid exacerbation and severe prostration, often terminating fatally in twenty-four hours. Reported in 1874.

Purpura hemorrhagica, early description of—1735

RUDOLPH AUGUST BEHRENS, German physician, 16??-1747, described purpura hemorrhagica under the name of *morbus maculosus haemorrhagicus*, in 1735.

Purpura hemorrhagica or haemorrhagica

. . . See also under *Thrombopenic purpura*.

Purpura nervosa

. . . See under *Purpura, nonthrombopenic, marked by acute intestinal symptoms*.

Purpura, nonthrombopenic, marked by acute intestinal symptoms

EDUARD HENOCH, German pediatrician, 1820-1910, described a nonthrombopenic form of purpura characterized by gastrointestinal symptoms, hematuria, renal colic, etc. Reported in 1868. Known as *Henoch's purpura*. Also called *purpura nervosa*.

Purpura, nonthrombopenic, of Schönlein

JOHANN LUCAS SCHÖNLEIN, German physician, 1793-1864, described a form of nonthrombocytopenic purpura often associated with pains in the joints. Published in 1837. Known as *Schönlein's purpura*.

Purtscher's disease

. . . See under *Retina, traumatic angiopathy of*.

Pus, composition of; early observation

JULIUS FRIEDRICH COHNHEIM,

German pathologist, 1839-1884, demonstrated that pus is composed chiefly of leukocytes which have passed through the walls of the capillaries. Recorded in 1867.

Putnam-Dana syndrome

. . . See under *Spinal cord, subacute combined degeneration of,* etc.

Putrefaction, chemical products of

PETER LUDVIG PANUM, Danish physiologist, 1820-1885, is credited with being first to study the chemical products of putrefaction. The results influenced the concept of putrid intoxication. Published in 1856.

Putrefaction, founder of theory of

THEODOR SCHWANN, German anatomist, 1810-1882, is regarded as the founder of the theory of putrefaction and fermentation. He demonstrated that putrefaction is produced by living cells. Recorded in 1837.

Pyelography, introduction of

FRIEDRICH VOELCKER, German surgeon, 1872-19??, is credited with introducing pyelography. Recorded in 1905.

Pyemia, introduction of term

PIERRE ADOLPHE PIORRY, French physician, 1794-1879, introduced the term *pyemia,* about 1828.

Pygmies are not a retrograde or degenerate type

JEAN LOUIS ARMAND DE QUATREFAGES DE BRÉAU, French anthropologist and naturalist, 1810-1892, established that pygmies are not, as it was believed, a degenerate or retrograde type of Negro but are descendants of ancient races. Published in 1887.

Pyknic body build, description of

ERNST KRETSCHMER, German psychiatrist, 1888-19??, described the short, thick, and stocky build known as the pyknic type. Published in 1927.

Pylorectomy, first recorded, for carcinoma

JULES ÉMILE PÉAN, French surgeon, 1830-1898, is credited with performing the first recorded pylorectomy, on April 9, 1879.

Pyloric muscle, hypertrophy of, early description

JEAN CRUVEILHIER, French pathologist, 1791-1874, gave an early description of pyloric stenosis due to hypertrophy of the pyloric muscle. Reported in 1829-1835.

Pyloric sphincter, description of

HERMANN D. STIEVE, German anatomist, 1886-19??, described the pyloric sphincter. Recorded in 1919.

Pyloric stenosis, congenital hypertrophic, first record of

PATRICK BLAIR, English surgeon, 166?-1728, gave the first account of congenital hypertrophic pyloric stenosis, based on the dissection of a child. Published in 1717.

Pyloric stenosis, congenital hypertrophic, first record of, in America

HEZEKIAH BEARDSLEY, American physician, 1748-1790, is credited with describing the first case of congenital hypertrophic pyloric stenosis recorded in America. Published in 1788.

Pyloric stenosis, congenital, Ramstedt's operation for

CONRAD RAMSTEDT, German surgeon, 1867-19??, devised an operation for the relief of congenital pyloric stenosis by cutting through the serosa and muscular layer of the pylorus down to the mucous membrane. Recorded in 1912. Known as *Ramstedt's operation* and *Frédet-Ramstedt operation*. PIERRE FRÉDET, French surgeon, 1870-19??, described the operation in 1908.

Pyloric stenosis due to hypertrophy of pyloric muscle

. . . See under *Pyloric muscle, hypertrophy of*, etc.

Pyloroplasty, first recorded operation of

PIETRO LORETA, Italian surgeon, 1831-1889, is credited with performing the first successful operation of pyloroplasty. Recorded in 1882.

Pylorus, resection of— Billroth I

CHRISTIAN ALBERT THEODOR BILLROTH, Austrian surgeon, 1829-1894, devised an operation for the resection of the pylorus in which the duodenal stump is united by anastomosis with the greater curvature of the stomach. Reported in 1881. Called *Billroth I operation*.

Pylorus, resection of— Billroth II

CHRISTIAN ALBERT THEODOR BILL-ROTH, Austrian surgeon, 1829-1894, devised an operation for the excision of the pylorus in which the stomach and the duodenum are closed and union of the stomach and intestine is effected by gastroenterostomy. Known as *Billroth II operation*. Reported in 1885.

Pyodermatitis vegetans or pyodermite végétante

FRANÇOIS HENRI HALLOPEAU, French dermatologist, 1842-1919, described dermatitis vegetans, pyodermatitis vegetans, or pyodermite végétante, in 1889.

Pyorrhea alveolaris, early description of—1594

JACQUES GUILLEMEAU, French physician, 1550-1613, gave a good description of pyorrhea alveolaris. Recorded in 1594.

Pyorrhea alveolaris, early description of—1746

PIERRE FAUCHARD, French dentist, 1678-1761, described pyorrhea alveolaris or alvelodental periostitis, in 1746. Known as *Fauchard's disease*.

Pyorrhea alveolaris, early description of—1876

JOHN M. RIGGS, American dentist, 1810-1885, described pyorrhea alveolaris and suggested a method of treatment, in 1876. Known as *Riggs's disease*.

Pyorrhea alveolaris, scraping in treatment of

JOHN M. RIGGS, American dentist, 1810-1885, introduced the method of scraping for the treatment of pyorrhea alveolaris. Recorded in 1876.

Pyramidal cells, giant, of
cerebral cortex
... See under *Giant pyramidal
cells,* etc.

Pyramidal cells, solitary, in
cerebral cortex
... See under *Meynert's cells.*

Pyramidal tract,
introduction of term
PAUL EMIL FLECHSIG, German
neurologist, 1847-1929, is credited
with the introduction of the term
pyramidal tract, about 1876.

Pyramidalis nasi muscle,
early description of
GABRIEL FALLOPIUS, Italian anatomist, 1523-1562, described the
procerus or pyramidalis nasi muscle, one of the muscles of facial expression. Recorded in 1561.

Pyramidon, introduction of
... See under *Aminopyrine.*

Pyriform scleral fissure of
early fetal life
FRIEDRICH AUGUST VON AMMON,
Dresden ophthalmologist, 1799-
1861, described the pyriform scleral
fissure of early fetal life, the posterior scleral protuberance, and the
cilia on the inner surface of the
ciliary body, in 1838-1847.

Pyrogens in distilled water,
discovery of
FLORENCE BARBARA SEIBERT,
American chemist, 1897-   , discovered thermostable products of
bacteria in distilled water capable
of producing fever when injected.
Published in 1923. Known as *distilled water pyrogens.*

Pyrosoma bigeminum
... See under *Texas cattle fever,*
etc.

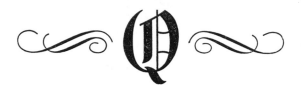

"Q" fever and primary atypical pneumonia

MICHAEL GEORGE PARKE STOKER, English physician, 19??- , showed a relationship between primary atypical pneumonia and "Q" fever. He also brought forward evidence of the existence of "Q" fever in England. Published in 1949.

"Q" fever, description of

EDWARD HOLBROOK DERRICK, Australian physician, 19??- , gave the first description of "Q" fever, "a new fever entity" caused by *Coxiella burnetii*, first noted in Australia. Recorded in 1937. Known also as *Queensland fever* and *quadrilateral fever*.

"Q" fever, discovery of causative agent of

FRANK MACFARLANE BURNET, Australian physician, 1899- , with MAVIS FREEMAN, discovered *Coxiella burnetii*, the causative organism of "Q" fever. Recorded in 1937.

"Q" fever, isolation of causative agent of, in United States

HERALD R. COX, American bacteriologist, 1907- , was the first to isolate *Coxiella burnetii*, the causa-tive agent of "Q" fever, in the United States, *circa* 1937.

Quadrilateral fever

. . . See under *"Q" fever, description of*.

Quain's fatty degeneration

. . . See under *Heart, fatty or fibrous degeneration of*.

Quarantine, introduction of

GILBERT BLANE, English physician, 1749-1834, formulated the principles which formed the basis of the *Quarantine Act* of Great Britain. Introduced in 1799.

Quartan malarial parasite, differentiation of, from tertian

. . . See under *Malarial parasite, differentiation of*, etc.

Quatrefages' angle

. . . See under *Parietal angle*.

Queckenstedt's sign or test

. . . See under *Subarachnoid space, patency of, in spine*.

Queensland fever

. . . See under *"Q" fever, description of*.

Quervain's disease

. . . See under *Tenosynovitis of muscles of thumb*.

Queyrat's erythroplasia, eponymic description of

AUGUSTE QUEYRAT, French physician, 1872-19??, described a precancerous dermatosis now known as erythroplasia of Queyrat. Recorded in 1911.

Quinacrine hydrochloride in treatment of malaria

... See under *Malaria, atabrine in treatment of.*

Quincke's edema or disease

... See under *Angioneurotic edema, eponymic description of.*

Quincke's pulse

... See under *Fingernails, alternate flushing and blanching of.*

Quincke's sign

... See under *Fingernails, alternate flushing and blanching of.*

Quinidine in auricular fibrillation

... See under *Auricular fibrillation.*

Quinine in auricular fibrillation

KAREL FREDERIK WENCKEBACH, Dutch physician, 1864-1940, is credited with being the first to recognize and demonstrate the value of quinine in cardiac arrhythmia, as in auricular fibrillation. Recorded in 1914.

Quinine, isolation of

JOSEPH B. CAVENTOU, French pharmacologist, 1795-1877, with PIERRE J. PELLETIER, French chemist, 1788-1842, isolated the alkaloid quinine, in 1820.

Quinine, local anesthetic action of

HENRY THIBAULT, American physician, 1879-19??, discovered the local anesthetic property of quinine when given by injection. Recorded in 1907.

Quinine urea anesthesia in treatment of anal fissure

RAOUL BENSAUDE, French physician, 1866-1938, was first to use quinine urea anesthesia in the treatment of anal fissure. Date not available.

Quinquaud's disease

... See under *Folliculitis decalvans, eponymic description of.*

Quinsy, early mention of

ARETAEUS THE CAPPADOCIAN, Greek physician in Rome, *circa* 81-138 A. D., described quinsy or angina. Exact date not available.

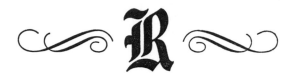

Rabies, first protective treatment against

Louis Pasteur, French scientist and bacteriologist, 1822-1895, administered the first protective treatment for rabies in man on July 6, 1885.

Rabies, inclusion bodies diagnostic of

Adelchi Negri, Italian physician and pathologist, 1876-1912, described small round or oval inclusion bodies occurring in the protoplasm and often in the processes of nerve cells, especially of the hippocampus, of animals dying of rabies. Recorded in 1903. Known as *Negri bodies*.

Rabies, infectiousness of; early demonstration

Georg Gottfried Zinke, German physician, 1771-1849, transmitted rabies from an affected dog to a healthy dog by injection of saliva, thus demonstrating the infectiousness of the disease. Recorded in 1804.

Rabies virus in blood, demonstration of

Louis Pasteur, French scientist and bacteriologist, 1822-1895, with C. Chamberland and P. P. E. Roux, demonstrated the presence of rabies virus in the blood of a rabid animal. Published in 1884.

Rabies

. . . See also under *Hydrophobia*.

Race classification on basis of cranial index

Anders Adolf Retzius, Swedish anatomist, 1796-1860, introduced a method for classifying races on the basis of the cephalic or cranial index. Recorded in 1842.

Racemic acid, preparation of

Louis Pasteur, French scientist and bacteriologist, 1822-1895, is credited with discovering racemic acid. Recorded in 1853.

Radiatio occipitothalamica

. . . See under *Optic radiation, description of*.

Radioactive isotopes in leukemia

John Hundale Lawrence, American physician, 1904-   , with K. G. Scott and L. W. Tuttle, used radioactive phosphorus in the study of leukemia. Recorded in 1939.

Radioactive tracer compounds in fat metabolism

Rudolf Schoenheimer, American biochemist, 1898-1941, introduced the use of radioactive tracer compounds in the study of amino acid and fat metabolism, in the 1930s.

Radioactivity of uranium, discovery of

ANTOINE HENRI BECQUEREL, French physicist, 1852-1908, discovered the phenomenon of radioactivity in uranium, in 1896.

Radium, beta rays of, are effective in destroying cells

ROBERT ABBE, American surgeon, 1851-1928, demonstrated that the beta rays of radium, not the gamma rays, are effective in cell destruction. Published in 1914.

Radium, discovery of

PIERRE CURIE, French chemist, 1859-1906, with MARIE SKLODOW-SKA CURIE (Polish-French chemist, 1867-1934), discovered and isolated radium from pitchblende, in 1898. The Curies and A. H. BEC-QUEREL received the Nobel prize in 1903. Mme. Curie received the Nobel prize again in 1911.

Radium, occupational injuries caused by—1916

THOMAS ORDWAY, American physician, 1877-19??, gave an early description of occupational injuries caused by radium. Published in 1916.

Radius, distortion of lower end of

... See under *Wrist, deformity of, caused by distortion of radius.*

Radius, dorsal tubercle of

JOSEPH LISTER, English surgeon, 1827-1912, described the dorsal tubercle of the radius, in 1865. Known as *Lister's tubercle.*

Radius, fracture of, with "silver-fork" deformity

ABRAHAM COLLES, Irish surgeon, 1773-1843, described a fracture at the distal end of the radius marked by a characteristic "silver-fork" deformity. Recorded in 1814. Known as *Colles' fracture.*

Radon tube, small, invention of

GIOACCHINO FAILLA, American radiological physicist, 1891- , developed a small radon tube, known as gold radon seed, in 1924.

Railway spine or brain; Erichsen's disease

JOHN ERIC ERICHSEN, English surgeon, 1818-1896, described a condition occasionally following train accidents which may assume the form of traumatic neurasthenia or hysteria. Reported in 1866. Known as *railway spine, railway brain, railway neurosis,* and *Erichsen's disease.*

Rales, sonorous and *sibilant,* introduction of terms

RENÉ T. H. LAENNEC, French physician, 1781-1826, is credited with introducing the terms *sonorous rales* and *sibilant rales,* after his invention of the stethoscope and his study of auscultation. Published in 1819.

Rami communicantes, cutting of, for relief of pelvic pain

... See under *Pelvic pain, control of,* etc.

Ramon's flocculation test

... See under *Diphtheria toxin and antitoxin, determination of potency of.*

Ramsden ocular

. . . See under *Microscope ocular made of two planoconvex lenses.*

Ramstedt's operation

. . . See under *Pyloric stenosis, congenital,* etc.

Raphe of corpus callosum, description of

FRANÇOIS CHAUSSIER, French physician, 1746-1828, described the median raphe of the corpus callosum, *circa* 1807.

Rasmussen's aneurysm

. . . See under *Aneurysm of terminal pulmonary arteries.*

Rat-bite fever, causative organism of

HENRY VANDYKE CARTER, English physician in India, 1831-1897, discovered the organism *Spirillum minus* in the rat. Recorded in 1887. At this time the relationship of the *Spirillum minus* to rat-bite fever was not fully appreciated.

Rat-bite fever, discovery of causative agent of —1916

KENZO FUTAKI, Japanese physician, 1873-19??, with his colleagues (F. TAKAKI, T. TANIGUCHI, and S. OSUMI), discovered the causative agent of rat-bite fever to be *Spirillum minus.* Reported in 1916.

Rat-bite fever, first medical record of

WHITMAN WILCOX, American physician, 18??-1877, reported "violent symptoms from the bite of a rat." Published in 1840.

Rat-bite fever, salvarsan in treatment of

SAHACHIRO HATA, Japanese physician, 1873-1938, was the first to use salvarsan in the treatment of rat-bite fever, in Japan. Recorded in 1912.

Rat-bite fever, *Streptobacillus moniliformis* in

ANDRÉ LEMIERRE, French physician, 1875-19??, with J. REILLY, A. LAPORTE, and M. MORIN, isolated *Streptobacillus moniliformis* from a patient with rat-bite fever. Published in 1937.

Rat-growth unit of vitamin A

HENRY CLAPP SHERMAN, American chemist, 1875-19??, with HAZEL E. MUNSELL, introduced the rat-growth unit of vitamin A, which is the daily amount necessary to maintain a weekly gain of 3 Gm. in test rats depleted of vitamin A. Known as *Sherman-Munsell unit.* Exact date not available.

Rathke's pouch

. . . See under *Buccal cavity, diverticulum of, in embryo.*

Rauber's layer

. . . See under *Blastoderm, external layer of.*

Rayer's disease

. . . See under *Xanthoma, eponymic description of.*

Raynaud's disease or syndrome

. . . See under *Vascular spasm in extremities, especially in digits.*

Ray's mania

. . . See under *Moral insanity or mania, eponymic description of.*

Rays pass from object to eye, not vice versa

ALHAZEN, Arabian mathematician, physicist, and optician, *circa* 965-1039, propounded the belief that the rays of light concerned with vision travel from the object to the eye, and not from the eye to the object, as some observers held at the time. Exact date not available.

Reaction time of mental process, early measurement of —1868

FRANS C. DONDERS, Dutch physician, 1818-1889, was probably the first to measure the reaction time involved in a mental process, in 1868.

Receptaculum chyli, eponymic description of

JEAN PECQUET, French anatomist, 1622-1674, who discovered the thoracic duct in the dog, described the receptaculum chyli, the dilated lower portion of the thoracic duct. Recorded in 1651. Known as *Pecquet's cistern* or *reservoir*.

Reciprocal innervation, early study of

CHARLES SCOTT SHERRINGTON, English neurophysiologist, 1857-1952, is credited with being first to study the mechanism and phenomena of reciprocal innervation. Recorded in 1893.

Recklinghausen's disease

. . . See under *Neurofibromatosis*.

Reclus' disease

. . . See under *Ligneous phlegmon*.

Reclus' disease of breast

. . . See under *Breasts, painless cystic enlargement of*.

Rectal columns; columns of Morgagni

GIOVANNI BATTISTA MORGAGNI, Italian anatomist and pathologist, 1682-1771, described vertical folds of mucous membrane in the upper part of the anal canal, or in the rectum. Published in 1719. Known as *columns of Morgagni*.

Rectal sinuses of Morgagni

. . . See under *Sinuses of Morgagni, rectal*.

Rectal valves, eponymic description of

JOHN HOUSTON, Irish physician, 1802-1845, described the transverse folds of the rectal wall which form the rectal valves, in 1830. Known as *Houston's valves*.

Rectouterine pouch; rectouterine excavation; pouch of Douglas

JAMES DOUGLAS, Scottish anatomist and obstetrician, 1675-1742, described the recess or pouch formed by a fold of peritoneum extending down between the rectum and the uterus. Known also as *cul-de-sac of Douglas*. *Circa* 1730.

Rectovesical fascia, early description of

CHARLES PIERRE DENONVILLIERS, French surgeon, 1808-1872, gave an early description of the rectovesical fascia situated between the rectum and the prostate. Reported in 1836.

Rectum, excision of, for cancer

RICHARD VON VOLKMANN, German surgeon, 1830-1889, is said to have been the first to excise the rectum for cancer. Recorded in 1878.

**Rectum, sacral method
of excision of**

PAUL KRASKE, German surgeon, 1851-1930, devised the sacral method of excision of the rectum in case of carcinoma. Recorded in 1887.

**Rectus oculi inferior, lateralis,
medialis, superior;
origin of**

... See under *Eye muscles originate from margin of optic canal.*

**Red blood cells carry oxygen,
discovery that**

JUSTUS VON LIEBIG, German chemist, 1803-1873, is believed to have been first to suggest that the red blood cells are oxygen carriers, in 1851.

**Red blood cells, earliest
observation of**

JAN SWAMMERDAM, Dutch physician and naturalist, 1637-1680, is credited with being first to discover and describe the red blood cells, in 1658.

**Red blood cells, early accurate
account of**

ANTONJ VAN LEEUWENHOEK, Dutch naturalist, 1632-1723, is credited with giving the first adequate description of the red blood cells, in 1674.

**Red blood cells, granules
in, in malaria**

WILHELM AUGUST PAUL SCHÜFFNER, German pathologist, 1867-1949, described small round granules appearing in the red blood cells of malarial patients at the time the parasites develop. Known as *Schüffner's dots* or *granules.* Recorded in 1904.

**Red blood cells, method for
measuring**

CECIL PRICE-JONES, English hematologist, 1863-1943, developed a method for direct measurement of red blood cells and for the recording of the results in the form of a graph expressing distribution in a stained specimen. Recorded in 1910. Known as *Price-Jones method.*

**Red blood cells, nuclear
particles in**

WILLIAM HENRY HOWELL, American physiologist, 1860-1945, described certain small round or oval bodies seen in some erythrocytes. They are believed to be nuclear fragments. Reported in 1890. Known as *Howell's bodies, nuclear particles, nuclear fragments,* etc.

Red blood cells, stroma of

ALEXANDER ROLLET, Austrian physiologist, 1834-1903, described the stroma of erythrocytes which supports the hemoglobin, in 1882. Known as *Rollet's stroma.*

**Red Cross, originator
of idea of a**

JOHN PRINGLE, Scottish physician, 1707-1782, is credited with originating the idea of a Red Cross. He is also called the founder of modern military medicine. His book on the diseases of the army appeared in 1752.

Red flap; jockey-strap itch

... See under *Tinea cruris, fungous origin of.*

Red nucleus, function of

CONSTANTIN VON MONAKOW, Russian neurologist in Switzerland, 1853-1930, described the function of the red nucleus. Recorded in 1909.

Red-staining nuclear substance of cells

LEOPOLD AUERBACH, German anatomist, 1828-1897, was first to describe the nuclear substance of cells having an affinity for red dyes. He called the substance *erythrophil*. Date not available.

Reflex action, introduction of concept of

MARSHALL HALL, English physiologist, 1790-1857, introduced the concept of and the term *reflex action*. Published in 1833.

Reflex, first use of term

JOHANN AUGUST UNZER, German physiologist, 1747-1809, was probably the first to use the word *reflex* with reference to motor reactions. Published in 1771.

Reflexes and volitional action, distinction between

MARSHALL HALL, English physiologist, 1790-1857, demonstrated the difference between unconscious reflexes and volitional acts, in a study on the reflex function of the medulla oblongata and the spinal cord. Published in 1833.

Refraction, early study of

ALHAZEN, Arabian mathematician, physicist, and optician, *circa* 965-1039, noted and studied the phenomena of refraction, about 1005.

Refraction, fundamental work on

ALLVAR GULLSTRAND, Swedish ophthalmologist, 1862-1930, did basic research on the dioptrics of the eye. He received the Nobel prize in 1911.

Refraction, small errors in, may cause nervous disturbances, observation that

GEORGE MILBRY GOULD, American ophthalmologist and lexicographer, 1848-1922, wrote on the psychologic influence of errors of refraction, demonstrating that even very small abnormalities may cause marked nervous irritation. Reported in 1888.

Rehfuss method

. . . See under *Fractional test meal examination*.

Reichert's cartilage

. . . See under *Cartilage of hyoid arch of embryo*.

Reichmann's disease

. . . See under *Gastrosuccorrhea*.

Reid's base line at level of base of skull

ROBERT WILLIAM REID, Scottish anatomist, 1851-1939, described an imaginary line extending from the infra-orbital ridge through the external auditory meatus to the midline of the occiput. Published in 1884.

Reisseisen's muscles

. . . See under *Bronchial tubes, muscular fibers of*.

Reissner's canal

. . . See under COCHLEA, *membranous canal of*.

Reissner's fiber

. . . See under *Spinal cord, fiber in central canal of*.

Reissner's membrane

. . . See under *Membrane, vestibular, of cochlea.*

Reiter's syndrome, eponymic description of

HANS REITER, German physician, 1881-19??, described a disease marked by urethritis, conjunctivitis, polyarthritis, etc. Recorded in 1916.

Reiter's syndrome, pre-eponymic description of

NOËL FIESSINGER, French physician, 1876-19??, with EDGAR LEROY, described the condition which was later given the name of *Reiter's syndrome.* Published in 1916.

Rejuvenation by means of testicular transplants

SERGEI VORONOFF, Russian physiologist, 1866-1951, experimented with rejuvenation by means of testicular transplants. First reported in 1919. Published in 1923. Known as *Voronoff's operation.*

Rejuvenation operation

. . . See under *Impotence, treatment of, by occlusion of vas deferens.*

Relapsing fever, African tick variety of

PHILIP HEDGELAND ROSS, English physician, 1876-1929, with A. D. MILNE, discovered the organism responsible for the African variety of relapsing fever. Recorded in 1904.

Relapsing fever, American, discovery of spirochete in a case of

THOMAS FLOURNOY, American physician, 1877-19??, with

CHARLES NORRIS and A. M. PAPPENHEIMER, discovered a spirochete in a case of American relapsing fever. Reported in 1906.

Relapsing fever, Asiatic, original description of

HENRY VANDYKE CARTER, English physician in India, 1831-1897, described the Asiatic form of relapsing fever, which he was able to reproduce in monkeys. Published in 1882.

Relapsing fever, causative agent of

JOSEPH EVERETT DUTTON, English physician, 1874-1905, with JOHN L. TODD (English physician, 1876-1949), demonstrated that the cause of relapsing fever in monkeys is the organism now called *Spirillum duttoni* or *Borrelia duttonii.* Reported in 1905.

Relapsing fever, causative agent of

OTTO H. F. OBERMEIER, German physician, 1843-1873, discovered *Borrelia recurrentis (Spirochaeta obermeieri)* in the blood of patients stricken with relapsing fever, during the German epidemic of 1872. Recorded in 1873.

Relapsing fever, contagious nature of

PIERRE MARIE SILLIAU, French physician, 18??-189?, demonstrated the contagious nature of relapsing fever and gave a good description of the epidemic at Réunion. Published in 1869.

Relapsing fever, demonstration of communicability of

OSIP OSIPOVICH MOCZUTKOWSKY

(MOSCHUTKOWSKY), Russian physician, 1845-1903, demonstrated the communicability of relapsing fever by inoculating healthy subjects with the blood of relapsing fever patients. He also proved the pathogenic significance of the spirochete. Published in 1879.

Relapsing fever, early reference to

DAVID LIVINGSTONE, Scottish explorer and physician in Africa, 1813-1873, described "a peculiar relapsing fever" which often followed the bite of a tick, in 1857.

Relapsing fever, first definite reference to

JOHN RUTTY, Dublin physician, 1697-1775, made the first definite reference to relapsing fever when he observed it in 1741, in association with typhus fever, in Dublin.

Relapsing fever, introduction of term

DAVID CRAIGIE, Scottish physician, 1793-1866, is credited with introducing the name *relapsing fever,* in his description of the Edinburgh epidemic of 1843. Published in 1843.

Relapsing fever, large spirillum in

OTTO H. F. OBERMEIER, German physician, 1843-1873, observed the presence of a large spirillum in the blood of a patient suspected of having relapsing fever. Recorded in 1868.

Relapsing fever, reproduction of, in monkeys

HENRY VANDYKE CARTER, English physician in India, 1831-1897, studied relapsing fever and reproduced it in monkeys, in 1882.

Relapsing fever, transmission of, by body louse — 1907

FREDERICK PERCIVAL MACKIE, English physician, 1875-1944, demonstrated that relapsing fever is transmitted by *Pediculus corporis.* Published in 1907.

Relapsing fever, transmission of, by body louse — 1913

CHARLES JULES HENRI NICOLLE, French bacteriologist, 1866-1936, with L. BLAIZOT and E. CONSEIL, demonstrated that relapsing fever can be transmitted by the body louse *Pediculus corporis.* Recorded in 1913.

Relapsing spastic spinal paralysis, early description of

MAX FRIEDMANN, German neurologist, 1858-1925, described "recurring, apparently luetic, so-called spastic spinal paralysis in youth," known as relapsing infantile spastic spinal paralysis, in 1892.

Remak's band

. . . See under *Axis-cylinder, eponymic description of.*

Remak's fibers

. . . See under *Nerve fibers, peripheral nonmedullated.*

Remak's ganglion or ganglia

. . . See under *Heart, intrinsic ganglia of.*

Renal calculi, composition of

. . . See under *Urinary calculi.*

Renal corpuscle

. . . See under *Kidney, corpuscle of,* etc.

Renal decortication, first performance of, in chronic nephritis

GEORGE MICHAEL EDEBOHLS, American surgeon, 1853-1908, was the first to perform renal decortication for the relief of chronic nephritis. Reported in "The cure of chronic Bright's disease by operation," in 1901.

Renal dropsy, first description of

GULIELMUS DE SALICETO, Italian surgeon, *circa* 1200-1277, described dropsy caused by contracted kidneys. Published in 1476.

Renal epistaxis, early description of—1866

WILLIAM W. GULL, English physician, 1816-1890, described a disease, usually of middle age, marked by renal hemorrhage, but having no demonstrable lesion. Reported in 1866. Known also as *renal hemophilia, essential renal hematuria,* and *angioneurotic hematuria.*

Renal excretory ducts, discovery of

LORENZO BELLINI, Italian anatomist, 1643-1704, discovered the renal excretory ducts. Reported in 1662.

Renal fascia, description of

DIMITRU GEROTA, Rumanian surgeon, 1867-1939, described the renal or perirenal fascia in 1895. Known as *Gerota's fascia.*

Renal function, coefficient for estimating, based on urea index

... See under *Coefficient for estimating renal function.*

Renal function, secretion theory of

RUDOLF P. H. HEIDENHAIN, German physiologist, 1834-1897, formulated the so-called secretion theory of renal function. First reported in 1874.

Renal glomerulus, capsule surrounding

... See under *Capsule surrounding renal glomerulus.*

Renal hemophilia

... See under *Renal epistaxis, early description of.*

Renal pyramid

... See under *Kidney, pyramid of; eponymic description.*

Renal tubules, rodlike cells in

RUDOLF P. H. HEIDENHAIN, German physiologist, 1834-1897, described columnar or rodlike cells in the renal tubules, in 1861. Known as *Heidenhain's rods.*

Rendu-Osler-Weber disease

... See under *Telangiectasis, hereditary hemorrhagic.*

Rendu's tremor

... See under *Tremor, hysterical and volitional.*

Renon-Delille syndrome

... See under *Dyspituitarism marked by tachycardia,* etc.

Reproduction of plants by means of pollen

... See under *Pollen, reproduction of plants by means of.*

Resectoscope operating in a water medium

MAXIMILIAN STERN, American surgeon, 1877-19??, devised a resectoscope, a cystoscopic instrument using a cutting current which is capable of operating in a water medium. Recorded in 1926.

Resorcinol, introduction of, in dermatology

PAUL GERSON UNNA, German dermatologist, 1850-1929, introduced the use of resorcinol in treating skin disorders. Recorded in 1886.

Respiration, center of

... See under *Center of respiration.*

Respiration, diaphragmatic type of, in tuberculosis; advocacy of

SIGARD ADOLPHUS KNOPF, American physician, 1857-1940, advocated the training of patients with apical tuberculosis to breathe chiefly by means of the diaphragm, in order to reduce motion in the affected area. Known as *Knopf's treatment.* Introduced about 1900.

Respiration, inhibitory center of

... See under *Pneumotaxic center, eponymic description of.*

Respiration, irregularity of, Cheyne-Stokes type

JOHN CHEYNE, Scottish physician, 1777-1836, was the first to describe an irregularity of breathing now known as Cheyne-Stokes respiration, in 1818. The condition was described later, in 1854, by WILLIAM STOKES, Irish physician, 1804-1878.

Respiration is regulated by carbon dioxide content of blood, proof that

JOHN SCOTT HALDANE, Scottish physiologist, 1860-1936, demonstrated that respiration is regulated by the concentration of carbon dioxide in the blood stream. Reported in 1914.

Respiration like combustion involves liberation of heat, carbon dioxide, and water

ANTOINE LAURENT LAVOISIER, French chemist, 1743-1794, with PIERRE SIMON DE LAPLACE (French astronomer and physicist, 1749-1827), showed that respiration is a form of combustion accompanied by liberation of heat, carbon dioxide, and water. Published in 1784.

Respiration, role of vagus nerve in

HENRY HEAD, English neurologist, 1861-1940, described the action of the vagus in respiration. Reported in 1889.

Respiatory center, location of, early allusion to—1789

LAZARO SPALLANZANI, Italian physiologist, 1729-1799, was possibly the earliest observer to locate, in a general way, the respiratory center, in 1789. The report was published posthumously in 1803.

Respiratory center, location of, in medulla oblongata —1812

JULIEN J. C. LEGALLOIS, French physician, 1770-1814, is credited with having located the center of respiration in the medulla oblongata, in 1812.

Respiratory center, location of, in medulla oblongata —1837

MARIE J. P. FLOURENS, French physiologist, 1794-1867, located the respiratory center in the medulla oblongata with more accuracy than the previous investigators. He placed it at the "posterior end of the rhombic groove." The observation was made *circa* 1837, but the report appeared in 1842.

Respiratory ferment, function of

OTTO HEINRICH WARBURG, German biochemist, 1883-19??, did fundamental research in the field of cellular respiration, discovered respiratory enzymes, and described the nature and function of cytochrome oxidase. Published in 1926 and 1929.

Respiratory gases, apparatus for analyzing

JOHN SCOTT HALDANE, Scottish physiologist, 1860-1936, invented an apparatus for the analysis of respiratory gases. Reported in 1892.

Respiratory movements, mechanism of, early recognition

GEORG ERHARD HAMBERGER, German physician, 1697-1755, studied the mechanism of respiration and demonstrated that the internal intercostal muscles aid in expiration while the external intercostal muscles are inspiratory in function. *Circa* 1740.

Respiratory muscles

. . . See under *Respiratory movements.*

Respiratory quotient, first determination of

HENRI VICTOR REGNAULT, French scientist, 1810-1878, with JULES REISET, made the first determination of the respiratory quotient. Published in 1849.

Rest as part of treatment in surgical disorders

JOHN HILTON, English surgeon, 1804-1878, advocated complete rest in surgical disorders. Reported in 1863.

Reticulocytes, early description of

VICTOR CLARENCE VAUGHAN, American pathologist, 1851-1929, described reticulocytes, in 1903.

Reticuloendothelial cytomycosis

. . . See under *Histoplasmosis.*

***Reticuloendothelial system,* introduction of term**

KARL ALBERT LUDWIG ASCHOFF, German pathologist, 1866-1942, introduced the term *reticuloendothelial system,* in 1924.

Reticuloendotheliosis, nonlipid

. . . See under *Letterer-Siwe disease, eponymic description of.*

Retina, angiomatosis of; eponymic description

EUGEN VON HIPPEL, German ophthalmologist, 1867-1939, described a disease of the retinal vessels marked by the formation of multiple angiomas. Reported in 1895. Known as *angiomatosis retinae, von Hippel's disease,* and *Lindau-von Hippel disease.*

Retina, central artery of; eponymic description

JOHANN GOTTFRIED ZINN, German anatomist, 1727-1759, described the central artery of the retina.

Published in 1755. Known as *Zinn's central artery*.

Retina, detachment of, ignipuncture in treatment of

JULES GONIN, Swiss ophthalmologist, 1870-1935, introduced a method of treating detachment of the retina by means of ignipuncture of the retinal fissure through an incision in the sclera. Reported in 1927.

Retina, detachment of

. . . See also under *Retinal detachment*.

Retina, images on, produced by blood vessels

JOHANNES EVANGELISTA VON PURKINJE, Bohemian physiologist, 1787-1869, described images formed on the retina by the shadows of the blood vessels. Recorded in 1823. Known as *Purkinje's images*.

***Retina*, introduction of term**

HEROPHILUS, Greek physician and anatomist in Egypt, 335-280 B. C., is credited with introducing the name *retina, circa* 295 B. C. It is based on the Latin *rete*, a net.

Retina, nerve endings in

MAXIMILIAN J. S. SCHULTZE, German anatomist and histologist, 1825-1874, wrote a classic monograph on the nerve endings in the retina. Published in 1866.

Retina, traumatic angiopathy of

OTMAR PURTSCHER, German ophthalmologist, 1852-1927, described traumatic angiopathy of the retina associated with lymphorrhagia. Recorded in 1912. Known as *Purt-*

scher's disease, liporrhagia retinalis, etc.

Retina, traumatic edema of

RUDOLF BERLIN, German ophthalmologist, 1833-1897, described traumatic edema of the retina (commotio retinae) in a paper published in 1873.

Retina, vertebrate, classic account of

SANTIAGO RAMÓN Y CAJAL, Spanish neurologist, 1852-1934, gave a classic description of the retina of vertebrates. Published in 1894.

Retinal action currents, demonstration of

ALARIK FRITHIOF HOLMGREN, Swedish physiologist, 1831-1897, demonstrated the existence of retinal action currents, in 1865. Reported in 1870.

Retinal changes in chronic nephritis

WILLIAM RICHARD GOWERS, English neurologist, 1845-1915, described certain retinal changes observed in patients with chronic nephritis. Recorded in 1876.

Retinal detachment, diathermy in treatment of

SVEN LARSSON, Danish ophthalmologist, 189?-   , introduced superficial diathermy in the treatment of retinal detachment. Recorded in 1930.

Retinal detachment, diathermy in treatment of

KARL SAFÁR, German ophthalmologist, 1899-   , introduced multiple electrode diathermy in the treatment of retinal detachment. Recorded in 1932.

Retinal hemorrhage in pernicious anemia

. . . See under *Pernicious anemia,* etc.

Retinal hemorrhages and tumor of the brain

LUDWIG TÜRCK, Austrian neurologist, 1810-1868, called attention to the relationship between retinal hemorrhage and tumor of the brain. Recorded in 1853.

Retinal rods, early description of

. . . See under *Rods of retina.*

Retinitis exudativa, first description of

GEORGE COATS, English ophthalmologist, 1876-1915, described exudative retinopathy or retinitis exudativa, in 1908. Known as *Coats's disease.*

Retinitis pigmentosa, familial; eponymic description

JOHN ZACHARIAS LAURENCE, English physician, 1830-1874, described four cases of retinitis pigmentosa occurring in the same family and associated with developmental defects, as hypogenitalism, mental deficiency, etc. Recorded in 1866. Known as *Laurence-Moon-Biedl syndrome.*

Retinochoroiditis juxtapapillaris, eponymic description of

EDMUND ZEUTHEN JENSEN, Danish ophthalmologist, 1861-1950, described retinochoroiditis juxtapapillaris, a condition distinguished by a small inflammatory spot on the fundus of the eye, close to the optic papilla. It is found usually in young healthy individuals. Reported in 1908. Known as *Jensen's disease.*

Retinoscopy, introduction of

FERDINAND L. J. CUIGNET, French ophthalmologist, 1823-18??, introduced the method or retinoscopy, in 1873. Known as *Cuignet's test.*

Retrolental fibroplasia, original description of

THEODORE LASATER TERRY, American ophthalmologist, 1899-1946, was the first to describe retrolental fibroplasia. Published in 1942. Known as *Terry's syndrome.*

Retroperitoneal veins

. . . See under *Veins extending from mesentery to vena cava.*

Retrosternal pain in angina pectoris, description of

JEAN B. T. BAUMÈS, French physician, 1756-1828, described the retrosternal pain of angina pectoris. Known as *Baumès' sign.* Date not available.

Retzius' lines; lines of Retzius

. . . See under *Tooth enamel, concentric lines in.*

Retzius' space

. . . See under *Prevesical space of Retzius.*

Retzius' veins

. . . See under *Veins extending from mesentery to vena cava.*

Reverdin's needle

. . . See under *Aneurysm needle with eye near point.*

Rh factor, discovery of—1940

KARL LANDSTEINER, American pathologist, 1868-1943, with ALEXANDER S. WIENER, discovered the Rh factor, in 1940.

Rh factor, discovery of—1941

PHILIP LEVINE, American pathologist, 1900-   , with L. BURNHAM, E. M. KATZIN, and P. VOGEL, discovered the Rh factor. Reported with reference to a case of erythroblastosis fetalis due to blood incompatibility between the mother and the child, in 1941. The Rh factor was discovered independently of Levine and his associates by PAUL MOUREAU, in occupied Belgium, also in 1941.

Rheoscopic frog effect, original description of

CARLO MATTEUCCI, Italian scientist, 1811-1868, demonstrated that when a nerve of a muscle-nerve preparation is brought in contact with a contracting muscle, the muscle of the nerve-muscle preparation follows with a contraction, thus illustrating the passage of an electric current. Published in 1843.

Rheumatic endocarditis, early description of

DAVID DUNDAS, English physician, 17??-1841, described nine cases of a "peculiar disease of the heart," now known to have been rheumatic endocarditis. Recorded in 1809.

Rheumatic fever and endocarditis

JEAN BAPTISTE BOUILLAUD, French physician, 1796-1881, described the frequent incidence of endocarditis in cases of rheumatic fever. Recorded in 1840.

Rheumatic fever, cortisone in treatment of

PHILIP S. HENCH, American physician, 1896-   , with C. H. SLOCUMB, A. R. BARNES, H. L. SMITH, H. F. POLLEY, and E. C. KENDALL, introduced cortisone in the treatment of rheumatic fever. Recorded in 1949.

Rheumatic fever

. . . See also under *Rheumatism, acute.*

Rheumatic osteoperiostitis, eponymic description of

ALFRED POULET, French physician, 1848-1888, described osteoperiostitis associated with rheumatic disease, *circa* 1876. Known as *Poulet's disease.*

Rheumatism, acute, streptococci in

FREDERICK JOHN POYNTON, English physician, 1869-1943, with ALEXANDER PAINE, concluded, after extensive study, that a streptococcus was the cause of acute rheumatism. Published in 1913.

Rheumatism, acute, throat infection and

BERNARD SCHLESINGER, American physician, 1896-   , studied the relationship of throat infection to acute rheumatism in children and demonstrated that the hemolytic streptococcus was the causative agent. Recorded in 1930.

Rheumatism, cardiac complications of

WILLIAM CHARLES WELLS, American physician, 1757-1817, described cardiac complications of rheumatism. Recorded in 1812.

Rheumatism, introduction of term

GUILLAUME DE BAILLOU, French physician, 1538-1616, is believed to have been the first to use the word *rheumatism* in the modern sense. Recorded in 1642.

Rheumatism, salicylates in treatment of

THOMAS JOHN MACLAGAN, Scottish physician, 1838-1903, introduced the use of salicylates in the treatment of rheumatism. Recorded in 1876.

Rheumatism, subcutaneous nodes in acute

LOUIS H. F. FÉRÉOL, French physician, 1825-1891, described subcutaneous nodosities occurring about the joints in some cases of acute articular rheumatism. Known as *Féréol's nodes* or *nodosities*. Recorded in 1859.

Rheumatoid arthritis, cortisone in treatment of

PHILIP S. HENCH, American physician, 1896- , with E. C. KENDALL, C. H. SLOCUMB, and H. F. POLLEY, introduced cortisone and ACTH in the treatment of rheumatoid arthritis. Published in 1949.

Rhinoplasty, introduction of

CARL FERDINAND VON GRAEFE, German surgeon, 1787-1840, introduced the first satisfactory technique of rhinoplasty. Published in 1818.

Rhinoplasty, pioneer work in

GASPARE TAGLIACOZZI, Italian surgeon, 1546-1599, developed a method for performing rhinoplasty by the use of a pedicle flap taken from the arm. He reported his work in 1587 and 1597.

Rhinoscleroma, organism found in

ANTON R. VON FRISCH, Austrian surgeon and bacteriologist, 1849-1917, described the organism *Klebsiella rhinoscleromatis,* found in rhinoscleroma. Published in 1874.

Rhodesian skull, description of

GRAFTON ELLIOT SMITH, English neuroanatomist, 1871-1937, described the so-called Rhodesian skull found at Broken Hill, Rhodesia, in 1921. Published in 1922.

Rhodium, discovery of

WILLIAM HYDE WOLLASTON, English physician and physicist, 1766-1828, is credited with the discovery of rhodium, in 1803. The name is an allusion to the rose-red color of some of the rhodium salts.

Rhodopsin, discovery of, in retinal rods

. . . See under *Visual purple.*

Rib cartilages, nonsuppurative swelling of

ALEXANDER TIETZE, German surgeon, 1864-1927, described a nonsuppurative but painful swelling of the rib cartilages. Published in 1921. Known as *Tietze's disease.*

Riboflavin, chemical structure of

PHILIPP ELLINGER, German biochemist, 1888-19??, with WALTER KOSCHARA, established the chemical formula of riboflavin. Published in 1934.

Riboflavin deficiency, early description of

WILLIAM HENRY SEBRELL, American physician, 1901- , with ROY

EDWIN BUTLER, described aribo-flavinosis, in 1938.

Ribs, cervical, classification of

WENZEL LEOPOLD GRUBER, Bohemian anatomist in Russia, 1814-1890, developed a classification of cervical ribs. Reported in 1869.

Rice diet in hypertension

. . . See under *Hypertension*.

Richter's hernia

. . . See under *Hernia in which only part of intestinal lumen is involved*.

Rickets, classic description of—1650

FRANCIS GLISSON, English physician, 1597-1677, gave a classic description of rickets, under the name of *rachitis*, in 1650. Known as *Glisson's disease*.

Rickets, cod liver oil in treatment of

. . . See under *Cod liver oil in rickets*, etc.

Rickets combined with scurvy, first description of

JULIUS OTTO LUDWIG MOELLER, German physician, 1819-1887, was the first to describe acute rickets associated with scurvy. Recorded in 1859.

Rickets, differentiation of, from scurvy

WALTER BUTLER CHEADLE, English pediatrician, 1836-1910, investigated rickets and scurvy, and presented a clear differentiation between the two, in 1878.

Rickets, distention of abdomen in early

RICHARD CLEMENT LUCAS, English surgeon, 1846-1915, is credited with being first to describe the abdominal distention observed in most cases of early rickets. Recorded in 1887. Known as the *Lucas sign*.

Rickets, early description of —1582

BARTHOLOMAEUS REUSNER, Swiss physician, 16th century, gave a brief description of rickets, under the name of *tabes infantum*, in 1582.

Rickets, early description of —1645

DANIEL WHISTLER, English physician, 1619-1684, gave the first description of rickets as a clinical entity, in his graduation thesis. Published in 1645.

Rickets is a deficiency disease, experimental proof that

EDWARD MELLANBY, English physiologist, 1884-19??, was the first to demonstrate that rickets is a deficiency disease. Published in 1918.

Rickets, use of ultraviolet rays in

. . . See under *Ultraviolet rays in treatment of rickets*.

Rickettsia prowazeki, isolation of

. . . See under *Typhus, causative agent of; first isolation*.

Rickettsia quintana or *pediculi*, isolation of

HANS WILLI TÖPFER, German physician, 1876-19??, isolated *Ricksettsia pediculi* or *quintana* from lice taken from patients affected with trench fever. Recorded in 1916.

Rickettsia rickettsii

. . . See under *Rocky Mountain spotted fever, naming of causative agent of.*

Rickettsiae, yolk-sac method for cultivating

HERALD R. COX, American bacteriologist, 1907-   , developed the so-called yolk-sac method for cultivating rickettsiae in high concentrations. Exact date not available.

Ridley's sinus

. . . See under *Sinus, circular, eponymic description of.*

Riedel's disease or struma

. . . See under *Thyroiditis, chronic or ligneous.*

Riedel's lobe

. . . See under *Liver, tongue-shaped lobe of.*

Rieder's cell

. . . See under *Leukocyte with divided nucleus in acute leukemia.*

Riesman's eyeball sign in diabetic coma

. . . See under *Diabetic coma, softness of eyeball in.*

Riesman's eyeball sign in exophthalmic goiter

. . . See under *Exophthalmic goiter, eye bruit in.*

Riesman's myocardosis

. . . See under *Heart, noninflammatory fibrotic disease of.*

Rieux's hernia

. . . See under *Hernia, retrocecal, first description of.*

Rift Valley fever, first description of

ROBERT DAUBNEY, English physician, 1891-   , with JOHN RICHARD HUDSON, gave the first description of enzootic hepatitis or Rift Valley fever, a virus disease of sheep, cattle, and man, in Kenya. Published in 1931.

Right-handed persons, dominance of left cortical hemisphere in

HUGO CARL LIEPMANN, German neurologist, 1863-1925, is credited with discovering that in right-handed persons there is a dominance of the left cortical hemisphere, in 1904.

Rigor mortis, Nysten's law of

PIERRE HUBERT NYSTEN, French pediatrician, 1774-1817, described the course of rigor mortis in the following order: the muscles of mastication; the muscles of the face and neck; the muscles of the arms and upper trunk; the muscles of the lower trunk, thighs, legs, and feet. Introduced *circa* 1812.

Ring compounds from chain compounds, method for making

OTTO DIELS, German chemist, 1876-19??, in cooperation with KURT ALDER, German chemist, 1907-   , developed a practical and inexpensive method for making ring compounds from chain compounds (as butadiene) by forcing them to combine with maleic anhydride. Both shared the Nobel prize in 1950.

Ring of adenoid tissue formed by tonsils etc.

HEINRICH WILHELM GOTTFRIED

WALDEYER-HARTZ, German anatomist, 1836-1921, described a ring of lymphatic tissue formed by the faucial, lingual, and pharyngeal tonsils. Published in 1884. Known as *Waldeyer's tonsillar ring.*

Ringer's solution, introduction of

SIDNEY RINGER, English physiologist, 1834-1910, compounded a solution of sodium, potassium and calcium chlorides in recently boiled water. Recorded in 1880. There are several variants of the formula.

Ringlike bodies in erythrocytes in some forms of anemia

RICHARD CLARKE CABOT, American physician, 1868-1939, discovered the loops or ringlike bodies seen in stained erythrocytes in some cases of anemia. Reported in 1903. Known as *Cabot's ring bodies.*

Ringworm, treatment of, by x-rays

RAYMOND JACQUES ADRIEN SABOURAUD, French dermatologist, 1864-1938, suggested the use of x-rays in the treatment of ringworm. Recorded in 1904.

Ripault's sign of death

. . . See under *Pupil, change in shape of, after death.*

Ritter's disease

. . . See under *Dermatitis exfoliativa of newborn.*

Ritter-Valli law

. . . See under *Nerve, cut, loss of irritability of.*

Rivalta's test for exudate

. . . See under *Exudate and transudate, differentiation between.*

Rivinian ducts

. . . See under *Glands, sublingual, smaller ducts of.*

Rivinus' gland

. . . See under *Gland, sublingual, eponymic description of.*

Rivinus' notch

. . . See under *Tympanic sulcus, notch at upper border of.*

Robin spaces

. . . See under *Artery, spaces in external coat of.*

Robin's myeloplaxes

. . . See under *Osteoclasts, eponymic description of.*

Robinson's circle

. . . See under *Arterial circle of Robinson.*

Robinson's disease

. . . See under *Hidrocystoma, eponymic description of.*

Rochelle salt

. . . See under *Potassium and sodium tartrate.*

Rocky Mountain spotted fever, causative organism of

HOWARD TAYLOR RICKETTS, American pathologist, 1871-1910, described the causative organism of Rocky Mountain spotted fever, which he observed in blood smears. Recorded in 1909.

Rocky Mountain spotted fever, differentiation of, from typhus

HOWARD TAYLOR RICKETTS, American pathologist, 1871-1910, with RUSSELL MORSE WILDER (American physician, 1885-19??), differentiated between typhus and Rocky Mountain spotted fever. Recorded in 1910.

Rocky Mountain spotted fever, development of vaccine for

ROSCOE ROY SPENCER, American physician, 1888-19??, with RALPH ROBINSON PARKER, American entomologist, 1888-1949, developed a prophylactic vaccine for Rocky Mountain spotted fever, consisting mainly of the phenolized and emulsified organs of infected ticks. *Circa* 1917.

Rocky Mountain spotted fever, early description of

JOHN F. ANDERSON, American physician, 1873-19??, described a "new disease, spotted fever of the Rocky Mountains," in 1903. He also described the tick responsible for the transmission of the disease, now called *Dermacentor andersoni.*

Rocky Mountain spotted fever, first description of

EDWARD ERNEST MAXEY, American physician, 1867-1934, is credited with giving the first description of Rocky Mountain spotted fever, to which he referred as "the spotted fever of Idaho." Recorded in 1899.

Rocky Mountain spotted fever, naming of causative agent of

SIMEON BURT WOLBACH, American pathologist, 1880-1954, named the causative organism of Rocky Mountain spotted fever *Dermacentroxenus rickettsi,* in 1919. The organism is now better known as *Rickettsia rickettsii.*

Rocky Mountain spotted fever, tick responsible for transmitting

JOHN F. ANDERSON, American physician, 1873-19??, described the reddish-brown tick responsible for the transmission of Rocky Mountain spotted fever, in 1903. Known as *Dermacentor andersoni.*

Rocky Mountain spotted fever, tick responsible for transmitting

HOWARD TAYLOR RICKETTS, American pathologist, 1871-1910, further demonstrated that the wood tick *Dermacentor andersoni* is the vector of Rocky Mountain spotted fever. Recorded in 1906. Ricketts died of typhus a few years later.

Rodent ulcer, eponymic description of

EDMUND KROMPECHER, Hungarian pathologist, 1870-1926, described rodent ulcer or basal cell carcinoma, in 1900. Called *Krompecher's tumor.*

Rodent ulcer of eyelid, eponymic description of

ARTHUR JACOB, Irish ophthalmologist, 1790-1874, reported "observations respecting an ulcer of peculiar character which attacks the eyelids and other parts of the face." Published in 1827. Known as *Jacob's ulcer.*

Rods and cones, layer of; eponymic description

ARTHUR JACOB, Irish ophthalmologist, 1790-1874, described the layer of rods and cones in the retina, in 1819. Known as *Jacob's membrane.*

Rods of Corti, eponymic description of

ALFONSO CORTI, Italian anatomist,

1822-1888, described rodlike bodies arranged in a double row so as to form a spiral tunnel, the tunnel of Corti, a part of the cochlea. Recorded in 1851.

Rods of retina, early description of—1674

ANTONJ VAN LEEUWENHOEK, Dutch naturalist, 1632-1723, described the retinal rods, which he observed with his crude microscope, in 1674.

Roentgen cinematography, development of direct

CESARE GIANTURCO, American radiologist, 1905- , with W. C. ALVAREZ, developed a method of direct roentgen cinematography, producing a roentgen ray motion picture of the stomach, in 1932.

Roentgen rays, discovery of

WILHELM KONRAD ROENTGEN, German physicist, 1845-1923, observed that an active Crookes tube affected a fluorescent screen at a distance of about two yards. He called the unknown rays "x-rays." Observed on October 8, 1895; recorded in January 1896. Roentgen received the Nobel prize in 1901.

Roentgen rays in treatment of cancer, first successful use of

TAGE ANTON ULTIMUS SJÖGREN, Swedish surgeon, 1859-1939, is credited with being the first to use x-rays successfully in the treatment of cancer, in June 1899.

Roentgen rays, intensifying screen for

MICHAEL IDVORSKY PUPIN, American engineer, 1858-19??, introduced an intensifying screen in the early x-ray technique. Recorded in 1896.

Roentgen rays

. . . See also under *X-ray* and *X-rays.*

Roentgenokymograph, invention of

. . . See under *X-ray kymography.*

Roger's disease

. . . See under *Ventricles, communication between, abnormal.*

Rokitansky's disease

. . . See under *Liver, acute yellow atrophy of.*

Rolando's area

. . . See under *Motor area of cerebral cortex.*

Rolando's fibers

. . . See under *Medulla oblongata, external arcuate fibers of.*

Rolando's gelatinous substance

. . . See under *Spinal cord, substance covering posterior horn of.*

Rolando's tubercle

. . . See under *Tuberculum cinereum.*

Rollet's cells

. . . See under *Acid cells of gastric mucosa.*

Rollet's disease

. . . See under *Chancre, mixed form of.*

Rollet's stroma

. . . See under *Red blood cells, stroma of.*

Rollier's method

. . . See under *Sunlight in treatment of extrapulmonary tuberculosis.*

Romanovsky stain
... See under *Eosin-methylene blue stain.*

Romberg's disease
... See under *Facial hemiatrophy, eponymic description of.*

Romberg's sign in tabes dorsalis
... See under *Tabes dorsalis.*

Room, allergen-free
... See under *Allergen-proof room.*

Rorschach test
... See under *Ink blot intelligence test.*

Rosenmüller's fossa
... See under *Pharynx, lateral recess of.*

Rosenmüller's gland
... See under *Lacrimal gland, palpebral portion of.*

Rosenmüller's organ or body
... See under *Epoophoron, eponymic description of.*

Rosenmüller's valve
... See under *Lacrimal fold, eponymic description of.*

Rosenthal's canal
... See under *Cochlea, spiral canal of.*

Rosenthal's vein
... See under *Vein, basal cerebral, etc.*

Roseola infantilis (infantum), original description of
JOHN ZAHORSKY, American pediatrician, 1871-19??, described roseola infantilis as a disease entity, in 1910. Known also as *exanthema subitum, parascarlatina, Dukes' disease,* etc.

Rossbach's disease
... See under *Hyperchlorhydria, eponymic description of.*

Ross's bodies in syphilis
EDWARD HALFORD ROSS, English pathologist, 1875-1928, described "spherical copper-colored" bodies found in the tissue fluids and in the blood of patients with syphilis, about 1905. Known as *Lymphocytozoon pallidum.*

Rostan's asthma
... See under *Cardiac asthma, eponymic description of.*

Round ligament, peritoneal diverticulum of
ANTON NUCK, Dutch anatomist, 1650-1692, described a diverticulum or sac of peritoneum which accompanies the round ligament of the uterus in its passage through the inguinal canal. Published in 1691. Known as *canal of Nuck* and *Nuck's diverticulum.*

Round ligaments, shortening of, for correction of retroversion of uterus
... See under *Uterus, operation for retroversion of,* etc.

Rous sarcoma
... See under *Cancer, transmission of, by cell-free filtrate.*

Royal Orthopaedic Hospital, in London, founder of
WILLIAM JOHN LITTLE, English surgeon, 1810-1894, is credited with founding the Royal Orthopaedic Hospital in London, in 1838.

Rubber bag for dilating cervix of uterus
ROBERT BARNES, English obstetri-

cian, 1817-1907, devised a series of graduated dilatable rubber bags for inducing labor by dilating the cervix. Reported in 1858. Known as *Barnes's bags*.

Rubber bag

. . . See also under *Bag, rubber,* etc.

Rubber gloves in surgery, early advocacy of

THOMAS WATSON, English physician, 1792-1882, is credited with suggesting the use of rubber gloves in surgical procedures. Recorded in 1843.

Rubber gloves in surgery, introduction of

WILLIAM S. HALSTED, American surgeon, 1852-1922, is credited with introducing the use of rubber gloves in surgery, at the Johns Hopkins Hospital. Reported in 1894.

Rubber tube drains, introduction of

EDOUARD P. M. CHASSAIGNAC, French surgeon, 1804-1879, introduced the use of rubber tube drains, a procedure which revolutionized surgical drainage technique. Recorded in 1859.

Rubella during pregnancy, effect of, on infant

NORMAN MCALISTER GREGG, Australian physician, 189?- , described congenital cataract in an infant following German measles in the mother during pregnancy. Recorded in 1941.

Rubella, introduction of term

HENRY RICHARD LOBB VEALE, Scottish physician, 1832-1908, introduced the term *rubella* as another name for German measles, in 1866.

Rubella, transmission of, to monkeys

KARL HABEL, American epidemiologist, 1908- , successfully transmitted rubella to *Macacus mulatta* monkeys. Published in 1942.

Rubeola scarlatinosa, first description of

NILS FEODOROVICH FILATOV, Russian pediatrician, 1846-1902, described a form of German measles with a scarlatiniform rash, which he named *rubeola scarlatinosa*. Recorded in 1887. The same or a similar condition was described by CLEMENT DUKES (English physician, 1845-1925) in 1900. He called it the "fourth disease." There is no universal agreement about the existence of this disease as a clinical entity. Known as *Filatov-Dukes disease*.

Rubidium, discovery of

ROBERT W. BUNSEN, German chemist, 1811-1899, in collaboration with G. R. KIRCHHOFF, German physicist, 1824-1887, discovered the element rubidium, in 1860. The name is derived from the Latin *rubidus,* red, in allusion to the two red lines of its spectrum.

Rubin test for tubal patency

. . . See under *Uterine tubes, inflation patency test for.*

Rubner's law of growth quotient

. . . See under *Growth quotient, law of constant.*

Rubrospinal tract;
    Monakow's tract

CONSTANTIN VON MONAKOW, Russian neurologist in Switzerland, 1853-1930, described the rubrospinal tract, a bundle of nerve fibers descending from the red nucleus through the lateral column of the spinal cord to the sacral region. Recorded in 1909. Known as *Monakow's bundle, fibers, tract;* also as *fasciculus intermediolateralis* and *prepyramidal tract.*

Ruffini's corpuscle or end organ

ANGELO RUFFINI, Italian anatomist, 1864-1929, described specialized nerve endings in the skin and subcutaneous tissue of the fingers, composed of a terminal branching enclosed within a sheath. Published in 1893.

Rummo's disease

. . . See under *Heart, downward displacement of.*

Rumpel-Leede sign or
    phenomenon

. . . See under *Scarlet fever, petechial constriction test for.*

Rust's disease

. . . See under *Tuberculous spondylitis of neck.*

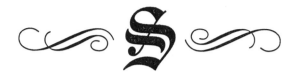

Sabin's rapid method for typing pneumococci

ALBERT BRUCE SABIN, American bacteriologist, 1906-   , devised a rapid "stained slide" method for typing of pneumococci. Reported in 1929.

Saccharin, introduction of

CONSTANTIN FAHLBERG, German chemist, 1851-192?, is credited with being first to prepare saccharin, *circa* 1878. Recorded in 1879. In the United States, saccharin was first prepared by IRA REMSEN, American chemist, 1846-1927, in 1879.

Sacro-iliac ligament, lower bundle of posterior

MARIE F. X. BICHAT, French anatomist and physiologist, 1771-1802, gave the first description of the lower bundle of the posterior sacro-iliac ligament. Reported in his text in 1801.

Saddle nose, eponymic description of

EMANUEL ZAUFAL, Austrian rhinologist and otologist, 1833-1910, described the condition known as saddle nose, and pointed out that if associated with alopecia it may be considered pathognomonic of congenital syphilis. Recorded *circa* 1875. Known as *Zaufal's sign.*

Saemisch's ulcer

. . . See under *Cornea, serpiginous ulcer of.*

Saenger's operation

. . . See under *Caesarean section, Saenger's operation of.*

Safe period in sexual intercourse

KYUSAKU OGINO, Japanese gynecologist, 1891-   , introduced the concept of a "safe period" in sexual intercourse. Published in 1930.

Sakel's method

. . . See under *Schizophrenia, insulin shock treatment of.*

Salicin, isolation of

RAFFAELE PIRIA, Italian chemist, 1815-1865, is credited with isolating salicin, in 1839.

Saline infusions and low temperature in treatment of shock

FREDERICK MADISON ALLEN, American physician, 1879-19??, introduced the method of treating shock by using saline infusions and reduced temperature, in 1939.

Saliva, digestive action of

LAZARO SPALLANZANI, Italian physiologist, 1729-1799, discovered the digestive action of saliva. Recorded in 1780.

Salivary glands, innervation of
CARL FRIEDRICH WILHELM LUDWIG, German physiologist, 1816-1895, gave the first clear description of the nerves of the salivary glands. Recorded in 1851.

Salk's vaccine
. . . See under *Poliomyelitis vaccine.*

Salmonella aertrycke (Salmonella typhimurium), discovery of, in patients
HERBERT EDWARD DURHAM, English bacteriologist, 1866-1945, discovered *Salmonella typhimurium* in patients affected with food posioning. Recorded in 1898.

Salmonella cholerae-suis, discovery of
. . . See under *Swine plague,* etc.

Salmonella enteritidis, description of
AUGUST GÄRTNER, German bacteriologist, 1848-1934, described a widely distributed parasite which causes epidemic diarrheal disease in rodents and gastroenteritis in man. Recorded in 1888. Known as *Gärtner's bacillus* and *Salmonella enteritidis.* The organism is a frequent cause of food poisioning.

Salmonella foetida
. . . See under *Coccobacillus foetidus ozaenae.*

Salmonella paratyphi C, description of
ERICH A. HUBENER, German bacteriologist, 1870-19??, with PAUL T. UHLENHUTH (German bacter-

iologist, 1870-19??), was first to describe *Salmonella paratyphi C,* in 1908.

Salmonella typhimurium, isolation of—1892
FREDRICH AUGUST JOHANNES LOEFFLER, German bacteriologist, 1852-1915, isolated *Salmonella typhimurium.* Recorded in 1892.

Salmonella typhimurium, isolation of—1900
JEAN DANYSZ, Polish pathologist in France, 1860-1928, isolated *Salmonella typhimurium,* the causative agent of mouse typhoid and of food poisoning in man, in 1900.

Salpinography, first use of
WILLIAM HOLLENBACK CARY, American gynecologist, 1883-19??, was the first to apply salpingography, in 1914. He used the procedure to determine the patency of the tubes, utilizing collargol as a contrast medium.

Salpinx, introduction of term, in reference to oviduct
GABRIEL FALLOPIUS, Italian anatomist, 1523-1562, was the first to popularize the comparison of the uterine tube to a trumpet, and thus call it *salpinx,* the Greek term for trumpet. Introduced *circa* 1553.

Salt, iodized, for prevention of goiter
. . . See under *Iodized salt.*

Salt-free diet in treatment of hypertension
FREDERICK MADISON ALLEN, American physician, 1879-19??, introduced salt and water restriction in the treatment of hypertension. Reported in 1920.

Salvarsan, discovery of

... See under *Arsphenamine.*

Sampson's implants

... See under *Ovarian endometriomas.*

Sanarelli's bacillus

... See under *Bacillus icteroides.*

Sand filter for air bacteria

JULIUS PETRI, German bacteriologist, 1852-1921, invented a sand filter to separate bacteria from the air. Recorded in 1888.

Sanders' bed

... See under *Bed, seesawing, for cardiovascular,* etc.

Sanocrysin, introduction of

... See under *Tuberculosis, sanocrysin in treatment of.*

Santorini's cartilages

... See under *Larynx, corniculate cartilages of.*

Santorini's duct

... See under *Pancreas, accessory duct of.*

Sappey's veins

... See under *Portal veins, accessory,* etc.

Sarcina ventriculi, discovery of

JOHN GOODSIR, Scottish physician, 1814-1867, discovered and described *Sarcina ventriculi,* an organism found in the stomach of animals and man. Recorded in 1842.

Sarcoidosis, early description of, in 1889

ERNEST BESNIER, French dermatologist, 1831-1909, described lupus pernio, later classified as sarcoidosis, in 1889.

Sarcoidosis, early description of, in 1899

CAESAR P. M. BOECK, Norwegian pathologist, 1845-1917, described sarcoidosis or lupus pernio, in 1899.

Sarcolemma, early recognition of

ANTONJ VAN LEEUWENHOEK, Dutch naturalist, 1632-1723, is credited with recognizing the sarcolemma as early as 1675.

Sarcoma, multiple idiopathic hemorrhagic, eponymic description of

MORITZ KAPOSI, Hungarian dermatologist, 1837-1902, described multiple bluish nodules of the skin marked by hemorrhages and a tendency toward malignancy, in 1872. Known as multiple idiopathic hemorrhagic sarcoma or *Kaposi's sarcoma.*

Sarcoma of liver and adrenals, congenital

WILLIAM PEPPER, American physician, 1874-1947, described congenital sarcoma of the liver and adrenals, in 1901. Known as *Pepper type of adrenal mediastinal tumor.*

Sarcoma, transplantation of—1902

CARL OLUF JENSEN, Copenhagen veterinary surgeon and pathologist, 1864-1934, proved that carcinoma and sarcoma can be transplanted, and retransplanted, in mice and rats. Published in 1902.

Sarcoma, use of erysipelas toxin in treatment of

WILLIAM B. COLEY, American

surgeon, 1862-1936, tried the method of using erysipelas and prodigiosus toxins in the treatment of sarcoma. Reported ten cases in 1893.

Sarcoptes scabiei, demonstration of

SIMON FRANÇOIS RENUCCI, French physician, 179?-185?, demonstrated the *Sarcoptes scabiei,* the itch mite which produces scabies in man. Recorded in 1835.

Sarcoptes scabiei, first description of

GIOVANNI COSIMO BONOMO, Italian physician, 16??-1697, gave the first good description of the itch mite *Sarcoptes scabiei,* in 1687.

Saw, wire, for cutting bone

. . . See under *Wire saw.*

Scabies, parasitic nature of

JOHANN ERNST WICHMANN, German physician, 1740-1802, demonstrated the parasitic cause of scabies. Recorded in 1786.

Scabies, relation of itch mite to

AVENZOAR, Arabian physician in Cordoba, *circa* 1091-1162, noted that the causative agent of scabies is the itch mite *Sarcoptes scabiei.* Exact date not available.

Scabies

. . . See also under *Sarcoptes scabiei.*

Scale for measuring size of urethral sounds and catheters

JOSEPH FRANÇOIS BENOIT CHARRIÈRE, French surgeon and instrument maker, 1803-1876, devised a scale for measuring the size of catheters and urethral sounds in which consecutive numbers differ by 1/3 mm. in diameter, *circa* 1850.

Scalene tubercle on upper surface of first rib

JACQUES LISFRANC DE SAINT MARTIN, French surgeon, 1790-1847, described the scalene tubercle on the upper surface of the first rib receiving the insertion of the scalenus anterior muscle. Published in 1815. Called *Lisfranc's tubercle.*

Scalenotomy for relief of symptoms due to cervical rib

ALFRED WASHINGTON ADSON, American surgeon, 1887-1951, developed the method of scalenotomy for the relief of symptoms due to cervical rib. Reported in 1927.

Scanzoni maneuver, introduction of

FRIEDRICH WILHELM SCANZONI, German obstetrician, 1821-1891, developed a procedure for changing a posterior vertex presentation into an anterior presentation. Published in 1849.

Scaphoid, carpal, osteoporosis of

. . . See under *Navicular, carpal, osteoporosis of.*

Scapula, congenitally high, eponymic description of

OTTO GERHARD KARL SPRENGEL, German surgeon, 1852-1915, gave a classic description of the condition marked by congenital abnormal elevation of the scapula. Recorded in 1891. Known as *Sprengel's deformity.*

**Scapula, congenitally high,
first description of**

MORITZ MICHAEL EULENBURG, German physician, 1811-1877, was first to describe a congenital abnormal elevation of the scapula, in 1863.

**Scapula, first excision of,
in England**

ROBERT LISTON, Scottish surgeon in England, 1794-1847, is credited with being the first in England to remove a scapula, *circa* 1834.

**Scar hypertrophy resembling
keloid**

CAESAR HENRY HAWKINS, English surgeon, 1798-1884, described cicatricial hypertrophy resembling keloid tissue, in 1833.

Scarlatina, introduction of term

. . . See under *Scarlet fever.*

**Scarlet fever antitoxin,
development of**

GEORGE F. DICK, American physician, 1881-19??, with his wife GLADYS R. H. DICK, developed an effective scarlet fever antitoxin. Reported April 19, 1924.

**Scarlet fever, differentiation
of, from measles**

THOMAS SYDENHAM, English physician, 1624-1689, described scarlet fever and differentiated it from measles. Recorded in 1675.

**Scarlet fever, early good
description of**

DANIEL SENNERT, German physician, 1572-1637, accurately described scarlet fever in 1619.

**Scarlet fever immunization
with scarlatinal toxin**

GEORGE F. DICK, American physi-

cian, 1881-19??, with his wife GLADYS R. H. DICK, developed a substance, obtained from cultures of scarlet fever streptococci, for the use in immunizing against scarlet fever. Reported Feb. 16, 1924.

**Scarlet fever in New England,
first report of**

WILLIAM DOUGLASS, American physician, 1691-1752, was the first to record cases of scarlet fever in New England, under the name of *angina ulcusculosa.* Recorded in 1736.

**Scarlet fever, introduc-
tion of term**

THOMAS SYDENHAM, English physician, 1624-1689, is credited with introducing the term *scarlet fever,* in 1676. The name *scarlatina,* previously spelled *scarlattina,* was also introduced by Sydenham at the same time.

**Scarlet fever, petechial con-
striction test for**

THEODOR RUMPEL, German physician, 1862-1923, discovered that in a patient with scarlet fever constriction of the arm produces petechiae. Recorded in 1909. The phenomenon was also described by CARL STOCKBRIDGE LEEDE, in 1911. Known as *Rumpel-Leede sign* or *phenomenon.*

**Scarlet fever serum obtained
by immunization of horses**

ALPHONSE RAYMOND DOCHEZ, American physician, 1882-19??, prepared a specific antiscarlatinal serum by the immunization of horses to the scarlet fever organism. Reported, with LILLIAN SHERMAN, February 16, 1924.

Scarlet fever, skin test for susceptibility to

GEORGE F. DICK, American physician, 1881-19??, with his wife GLADYS R. H. DICK, devised a skin test for determining susceptibility to scarlet fever, in 1924.

Scarlet fever, streptococcal origin of

EDWARD EMANUEL KLEIN, English physician, 1844-1925, was probably the first to suggest that scarlet fever is caused by a streptococcus. Recorded in 1887.

Scarlet fever toxin, isolation of

GEORGE F. DICK, American physician, 1881-19??, with his wife GLADYS R. H. DICK, isolated the erythrogenic toxin of the streptococci causing scarlet fever, *circa* 1924.

Scarpa's fascia

. . . See under *Fascia of abdomen, deep layer of superficial.*

Scarpa's foramen

. . . See under *Foramen for palatine nerve.*

Scarpa's ganglion

. . . See under *Ganglion of vestibular nerve.*

Scarpa's hernia

. . . See under *Hernia, sliding or slipping.*

Scarpa's triangle

. . . See under *Femoral triangle, eponymic description of.*

Schachowa's spiral tubule

. . . See under *Uriniferous tubule,* etc.

Schamberg's disease

. . . See under *Progressive pigmentary dermatosis.*

Scheiner's test

. . . See under *Pinhole method to illustrate refraction.*

Schenck's disease

. . . See under *Sporotrichosis, first description of.*

Scheuermann's disease

. . . See under *Vertebrae, necrosis of epiphyses of.*

Schilder's disease

. . . See under *Encephalitis periaxialis diffusa,* etc.

Schiller's test for carcinoma of uterine cervix

. . . See under *Carcinoma of uterine cervix,* etc.

Schistosomiasis, cause of

. . . See under *Bilharziasis, discovery of cause of.*

Schistosomiasis, intestinal; Manson's schistosomiasis

PATRICK MANSON, Scottish parasitologist, 1844-1922, described a condition marked by inflammation of the liver and intestines and caused by *Schistosoma mansoni.* Published in 1898.

Schizomycetes, key for identification of

DAVID HENDRICKS BERGEY, American bacteriologist, 1860-1937, prepared a systematic arrangement for the identification of the class of microorganisms known as the *Schizomycetes,* about 1923.

Schizophrenia, insulin shock treatment of

MANFRED SAKEL, American psychiatrist, 1900- , introduced the use of insulin shock in the treatment of mental disorders, especially schizophrenia, in 1929. Recorded in 1934. Known as *Sakel's method.*

Schizophrenia, introduction of concept of

PAUL EUGEN BLEULER, Swiss psychiatrist, 1857-1939, introduced the concept of schizophrenia, *circa* 1911.

Schizophrenia, introduction of term

PAUL EUGEN BLEULER, Swiss psychiatrist, 1857-1939, introduced the term *schizophrenia, circa* 1911.

Schizophrenia, treatment of, with metrazol

LAZLO DE MEDUNA, Budapest psychiatrist, 1896- , introduced the camphor-metrazol convulsion treatment of schizophrenia, in 1934. Recorded in 1935.

Schlemm's canal

. . . See under *Canal of Schlemm, eponymic description of.*

Schmidt television phenomenon

JAKOB EDWARD SCHMIDT, American physician and lexicographer, 1905- , observed that if the line of vision is moved across an operating oscilloscope or television receiver screen in a horizontal direction at the rate of about 8 feet per second, vertical figures or lines seem to incline or tilt momentarily in the direction in which the eyes are moving. First observed in 1948; reported in 1958. Known as *Schmidt phenomenon* or *effect.*

Schmorl's nodule or nodules

. . . See under *Vertebra, Schmorl's nodule of.*

Schneider's membrane

. . . See under *Nose, mucous membrane of.*

Schönlein's disease or purpura

. . . See under *Purpura, nonthrombopenic.*

School children, regular inspection of; early advocacy

RUDOLPH LUDWIG KARL VIRCHOW, German pathologist, 1821-1902, was instrumental in the establishment of regular inspection of school children and in the improvement of school hygiene in Germany. Recorded in 1869.

Schridde's disease

. . . See under *Dropsy, congenital generalized.*

Schüffner's dots or granules

. . . See under *Red blood cells, granules in, in malaria.*

Schultze's cells

See under *Olfactory mucous membrane, cells of.*

Schultz's disease

. . . See under *Agranulocytosis, first description of.*

Schwann, sheath of

. . . See under *Neurilemma, eponymic description of.*

Sciatica caused by injury to intervertebral disk

JOEL ERNEST GOLDTHWAIT, American physician, 1866-19??, suggested that intervertebral disk injury may be the cause of "sciatica," "lumbago," "paraplegia," etc. Reported in 1911.

Sciatica, early description of

DOMENICO COTUGNO, Italian anatomist, 1736-1822, described sciatica in 1764. Known as *Cotugno's disease*.

Sciatica, intervertebral disk herniation in

WILLIAM JASON MIXTER, American physician, 1880-19??, with JOSEPH SEATON BARR, demonstrated the role played by intervertebral disk herniation in the causation of "sciatica." Published in 1934.

Sciatica, introduction of term

DOMENICO COTUGNO, Italian anatomist, 1736-1822, is believed to have coined the word *sciatica,* a term he first used in 1764.

Sciatica, Lasègue's sign in

ERNST CHARLES LASÈGUE, French physician, 1816-1883, demonstrated that elevation of the extended lower extremity causes pain along the sciatic nerve, in sciatica. Recorded by J. J. FORST, LASÈGUE's pupil, in 1881.

Sciatica, nervous, original description of

DOMENICO COTUGNO, Italian anatomist, 1736-1822, was the first to describe two types of sciatica, the nervous and the arthritic. Recorded in 1764.

Sciatica with atrophy of muscles of leg; Landouzy's sciatica

LOUIS T. J. LANDOUZY, French physician, 1845-1917, described a form of sciatica complicated by atrophy of the muscles of the affected leg. Published in 1875. Known as *Landouzy's sciatica*.

Scissors for craniotomy in difficult labor

CLAUDE P. H. BLOT, French obstetrician, 1822-1888, invented a kind of scissors for performing craniotomy in cases of difficult labor. Known as *Blot's scissors*. Exact date not available.

Scleredema adultorum; Buschke's scleredema

ABRAHAM BUSCHKE, German physician, 1868-1943, described a condition marked by hardening of the subcutaneous tissue, often beginning on the head, and terminating after several weeks or months. *Circa* 1900.

Sclerema neonatorum, first description of

MICHAEL UNDERWOOD, English pediatrician, 1737-1820, was the first to describe sclerema neonatorum, a disease of infancy marked by hardening and tightening of the skin, depression of respiration and pulse, etc. Published in 1784. Known as *Underwood's disease*.

Scleroderma, differentiation of, from ichthyosis, etc.

CARLO CRUSIO, Italian physician, 1628-170?, was the first to differentiate between scleroderma and several of the diseases with which it had been confused, as leprosy, ichthyosis, etc. Recorded in the form of an abstract in 1754.

Scleroderma, diffuse, description of

PAUL KLEMPERER, American phy-

sician, 1887-19??, with A. D. POL-
LACK and G. BAEHR, described diffuse scleroderma and incorporated
it into a larger group known as diffuse collagen disease. Published in
1942.

Scleroderma, introduction of term

W. GINTRAC (also Gintrack),
English physician, 1817-1862, is
credited with introducing the term
scleroderma, in 1847.

Scleroderma neonatorum, first description of

. . . See under *Sclerema neonatorum.*

Scoliosis, treatment of, by plaster jackets and bandages

EDVILLE GERHARDT ABBOTT,
American surgeon, 1871-1938,
devised a treatment for scoliosis
consisting of the application of a
series of plaster jackets and bandages, the aim being to achieve grad-
ual overcorrection. Reports published in 1911 and 1912. The treatment is known as *Abbott's method*
or *treatment.*

Scoliotic pelvis, early description of

CARL C. T. LITZMANN, German
gynecologist and obstetrician,
1815-1890, described the scoliotic
pelvis (one with a small oblique
diameter), in 1853.

Scoliotic pelvis

. . . See also under *Pelvis.*

Scurvy, advocacy of vegetables and fruit for

JOHN HUXHAM, English physician,
1692-1768, advocated the inclusion
of vegetables, fruit, and fruit juices
in the diet of sailors for the prevention of scurvy. Recorded in
1766.

Scurvy, classic description of—1753

JAMES LIND, Scottish physician,
1716-1794, presented a classic description of scurvy, in 1753.

Scurvy, early description of—1250

JEAN DE JOINVILLE, French chronic-
ler, 122?-1317, was the first to record a description of scurvy, *circa*
1250.

Scurvy, early description of—1614

DANIEL SENNERT, German physician, 1572-1637, gave a good description of scurvy in 1614.

Scurvy in guinea pigs, experimental production of

AXEL HOLST, German physician,
1861-1931, demonstrated the experimental production of scurvy in
guinea pigs, thus pointing to the
use of these animals in the evaluation of antiscorbutic foods and
preparations. First published in
1907.

Scurvy, infantile, classic description of

THOMAS BARLOW, English physician, 1845-1945, gave a classic description of infantile scurvy, including an account of the pathological
changes involved, in 1883. A less
thorough account was presented by
Barlow in 1881. The disease is
known eponymically as *Barlow's
disease* and as *Moeller-Barlow disease.*

Scurvy, infantile, differentiation of, from rickets

WALTER BUTLER CHEADLE, English pediatrician, 1836-1910, investigated infantile scurvy and rickets, and gave a clear differentiation between the two. Reported in 1878.

Scurvy, infantile, early description of

JULIUS OTTO LUDWIG MOELLER, German physician, 1819-1887, presented a good description of infantile scurvy, in 1859. Infantile scurvy is known as *Moeller-Barlow disaese* and *Barlow's disease*.

Scurvy, introduction of lemon juice for prevention of, in British navy

. . . See under *Lemon juice for seamen*, etc.

Seaweed, use of, in goiter

. . . See under *Goiter, use of Seaweed in*.

Sebaceous adenoma, eponymic description of

JOHN JAMES PRINGLE, English dermatologist, 1855-1922, described sebaceous adenoma, in 1890. Known as *Pringle's disease* or *adenoma*.

Seborrheic eczema of Unna

PAUL GERSON UNNA, German dermatologist, 1850-1929, described seborrheic eczema, in 1887. Known as *Unna's disease*.

Secretin, crystalline, first preparation of

GUNNAR ÅGREN, Swedish pharmacologist, 1907-   , was the first to prepare crystalline secretin. Recorded in 1934.

Secretin, discovery of

WILLIAM MADDOCK BAYLISS, English physician and physiologist, 1860-1924, working with ERNEST HENRY STARLING (English physiologist, 1866-1927) discovered secretin in the duodenal secretions. Reported in 1902.

Secretion theory of renal function

. . . See under *Renal function, secretion theory of*.

Sedimentation of erythrocytes, early observation of

HERMANN NASSE, German physician,1807-1892, observed sedimentation of erythrocytes in certain diseases, in 1836.

Sedimentation rate, Wintrobe's method for determining

MAXWELL MYER WINTROBE, American internist and hematologist, 1901-   , with J. WALTER LANDSBERG, introduced a standardized technique for the erythrocyte sedimentation test. Published in 1935. An earlier paper appeared in 1933.

Segmentation cavity of blastoderm, discovery of

KARL ERNST VON BAER, German embryologist born in Estonia, 1792-1876, described the segmentation cavity of the blastoderm, in 1827.

Segmentation of mammalian ovum, first description of

EDOUARD VAN BENEDEN, Belgian embryologist, 1846-1910, gave the first complete description of the segmentation of mammalian ova. Reported in 1875.

Seidlitz mineral springs in Bohemia, medical appreciation of

FRIEDRICH HOFFMANN, German physician, 1660-1742, is credited with being first to describe the medicinal virtues of the Seidlitz mineral springs, in Bohemia, in 1724.

Seidlitz powder, introduction of

FRIEDRICH HOFFMANN, German physician, 1660-1742, discovered that the water of the Seidlitz spring near Prague contained medicinal mineral salts. These were proved to be chiefly magnesium sulfate. The present Seidlitz Powder does not contain magnesium sulfate, but is composed of potassium and sodium tartrate, sodium bicarbonate, and tartaric acid, the latter being wrapped separately. It was introduced about 1815.

Selenic acid, discovery of

ERNST EILHARD MITSCHERLICH, German chemist, 1794-1863, is credited with discovering selenic acid, in 1827.

Selenium, discovery of

JÖNS JAKOB BERZELIUS, Swedish chemist, 1779-1848, discovered the element selenium in 1817. It was named selenium on the basis of the Greek term *selene,* the moon.

Semicircular canals, early description of

GABRIEL FALLOPIUS, Italian anatomist, 1523-1562, described the semicircular canals of the ear. Recorded in 1561.

Semilunar bone, chronic osteitis of

ROBERT KIENBÖCK, Austrian physician, 1871-1953, described a slowly progressive osteitis involving the semilunar bone. Recorded in 1910. Known as *Kienböck's disease.*

Semilunar ganglion, excision of, for trigeminal neuralgia —1884

JAMES EWING MEARS, American surgeon, 1838-1919, was the first to suggest excision of the semilunar ganglion in treatment of trigeminal neuralgia. Recorded in 1884.

Semilunar ganglion, excision of, for trigeminal neuralgia —1890

WILLIAM ROSE, English surgeon, 1847-1910, excised the semilunar ganglion for the relief of trigeminal neuralgia. Recorded in 1890. The patient survived for more than two years.

Semilunar ganglion, excision of, for trigeminal neuralgia —1900

HARVEY WILLIAMS CUSHING, American neurosurgeon, 1869-1939, devised an operation for the excision of the semilunar ganglion in trigeminal neuralgia. Recorded in 1900. The route of approach is below the middle meningeal artery. Known as Cushing's operation No. 1.

Semilunar valves of aorta and pulmonary arteries, tubercles in

. . . See under *Corpora arantii.*

Seminiferous tubules, sustentacular cells of

ENRICO SERTOLI, Italian histologist, 1842-1910, described elongated cells in the seminiferous tubules of the testes which support the spermatids until they mature to become spermatozoa. Recorded in 1865. Known as *Sertoli's cells*.

Sensational-type personality, introduction of concept of

CARL GUSTAV JUNG, Swiss psychiatrist, 1875-19??, introduced the concept of a sensational-type personality, the fourth of his four types of personality; it is the type in which actions and attitudes are determined by sensation, rather than by feeling or reflective thinking. Presented *circa* 1908.

Sensorium commune, introduction of concept of

GEORG PROCHASKA, Czechoslovakian physiologist, 1749-1820, is credited with introducing the concept of a sensorium commune, the part of the cortex which coordinates all the impressions passing to the individual nerve centers. Recorded in 1784.

Sensory aphasia, eponymic description of

CARL WERNICKE, German psychiatrist, 1848-1905, described sensory aphasia, a condition marked by inability to understand spoken, written, or tactile speech symbols, due to central lesion. Published in 1874. Known as *Wernicke's aphasia*.

Sensory innervation of striated muscle

. . . See under *Striated muscle*, etc.

Septal deviation, early mention of

JULES HIPPOLYTE CLOQUET, French physician, 1787-1840, described deviation of the nasal septum. Published in 1821.

Septal deviation

. . . See also under *Nasal septum*.

Septicemia, causation of, by suppurative phlebitis

JOHN HUNTER, Scottish surgeon in England, 1728-1793, demonstrated that septicemia may be caused by suppurative phlebitis, in 1774.

Septicemia, classic description of

RUDOLPH L. K. VIRCHOW, German pathologist, 1821-1902, gave a classic description of septicemia in 1856. He pointed out that infected emboli were the cause of metastatic abscesses.

Septicemia, cryptogenetic, first description of

WILHELM OLIVIER LEUBE, German physician, 1842-1912, described a form of septicemia which occurs without an apparent local infection, in 1878.

Septicemia, introduction of term

PIERRE ADOLPHE PIORRY, French physician, 1794-1879, introduced the term *septicemia*, in 1837.

Septicemia, puerperal, bacterial origin of

LOUIS PASTEUR, French scientist and bacteriologist, 1822-1895, proved the bacterial origin of puerperal septicemia by cultivating the streptococci obtained in cases of pureperal sepsis. Reported in 1879.

Septicemia, puerperal

. . . See also under *Puerperal septicemia*.

Sera, method of dehydrating

EARL W. FLOSDORF, American bacteriologist, 1904- , with STUART MUDD, developed a method for dehydrating plasma, sera, etc., by vacuum desiccation in the frozen state. Reported in 1935. The method is called *lyophilization*.

Serous surface approximation in intestinal surgery, introduction of principle of

ANTOINE LEMBERT, French surgeon, 1802 - 1851, introduced an approximating suture which assures the union of serous surface with serous surface in suturing intestine. This laid the foundation for modern intestinal and gastric surgery. Published in 1826. Known as *Lembert's suture*.

Serpiginous angioma, eponymic description of

JONATHAN HUTCHINSON, English surgeon, 1828-1913, described angioma serpiginosum, a skin disorder marked by the appearance of small vascular points arranged in ring-shaped figures. Reported in 1892. Known also as *Hutchinson's disease* and as *infective angioma*.

Serres' glands in infants

ANTOINE E. R. A. SERRES, French physician, 1786 - 1868, described pearly epithelial masses found occasionally on the gums of infants. Published in 1817. Known as *gingival glands*.

Sertoli's cells

. . . See under *Seminiferous tubules, sustentacular cells of*.

Serum for treatment of snakebite

. . . See under *Snakebite serum*.

Serum potency destroyed by heat

. . . See under *Bactericidal power of immune serum*.

Serum proteins, significance of

ERNEST HENRY STARLING, English physiologist, 1866-1927, is credited with discovering the functions of serum proteins. Recorded in 1896.

Serum reaction based on presence of protective ferment in body

EMIL ABDERHALDEN, Swiss physiologist and pathologist working in Germany, 1877-1950, devised a reaction or test based on the principle that when a foreign protein is introduced into the blood, the body reacts by elaborating a protective ferment which causes the disintegration of the foreign protein. The reaction was first applied to the test for pregnancy, and reported in 1912. It is known as the *Abderhalden* or the *Abderhalden-Fauser reaction*.

Serum sickness, early description of—1905

CLEMENS PETER PIRQUET VON CESENATICO, Austrian pediatrician, 1874 - 1929, with BELA SCHICK (Austrian pediatrician, 1877-19??), made a study of serum sickness and evaluated its importance to medicine. Recorded in 1905.

Seton in treatment of ununited fractures

PHILIP SYNG PHYSICK, American surgeon, 1768-1837, introduced the use of a seton in the treatment of ununited fractures. Recorded in 1822.

Seton, introduction of use of

ROGER OF PALERMO, Italian surgeon, *circa* 1140-1210, is credited with introducing the use of the seton. Recorded in 1170.

Sever's disease
. . . See under *Calcaneus, epiphysitis of.*

Sewage oxidation, catalytic effect of cesium on
JAKOB EDWARD SCHMIDT, American physician and lexicographer, 1905-   , investigating the problem of catalysis in sewage oxidation, discovered that the addition of minute quantities of cesium, or certain other elements related to cesium, greatly accelerated the rate of oxidation. Recorded in 1934.

Sewage purification by bacterial action
WILLIAM JOSEPH DIBDIN, English engineer, 1850 - 1925, introduced the use of bacteria in the purification of sewage. Recorded in 1897.

Sewer system for Berlin, Germany
RUDOLF LUDWIG KARL VIRCHOW, German pathologist, 1821 - 1902, suggested the construction of a pipe sewer system for Berlin. Recorded in 1868. The plan was carried out in 1884 by JAMES HOBRECHT.

Sex chromosomes
. . . See under *Chromosomes, accessory.*

Sham feeding, introduction of method of
IVAN PETROVICH PAVLOV, Russian physiologist, 1849-1936, developed the method of "sham feeding," *circa* 1889.

Sharpey's fibers, eponymic description of
. . . See under *Periosteum, fibers attaching, to bone.*

Sheath of Henle
. . . See under *Nerve fibers, connective tissue between.*

Shepherd's fracture
. . . See under *Talus, fracture of; eponymic description.*

Sherman-Munsell unit
. . . See under *Rat-growth unit of vitamin A.*

Shigella alkalescens, first description of
FREDERICK WILLIAM ANDREWES, English pathologist, 1859 - 1932, described the *Shigella alkalescens,* sometimes the cause of diarrheal disease in man. Recorded in 1918.

Shigella sonnei, eponymic description of
CARL SONNE, Danish bacteriologist, 1882-1948, described a strain of the Shigella group of organisms, one of the commonest causes of bacillary dysentery in temperate climates. First recorded in 1914. Also known as *Sonne's bacillus.*

Shock, constriction of peripheral vessels in
JOHN DAVID MALCOLM, English surgeon, 1852 - 1921, is credited with being first to demonstrate that shock is associated with constriction of peripheral vessels. Published in 1893.

Shock is due to exhaustion of vasomotor center
GEORGE WASHINGTON CRILE,

American surgeon, 1864-1943, introduced the theory that shock is the result of exhaustion of the vasomotor center. Recorded in 1901.

Shock, treatment of, with saline infusions and reduced temperature

. . . See under *Saline infusions.*

Shoulder dislocation, sign of

LOUIS A. DUGAS, American surgeon, 1806-1884, described a practical test for dislocation of the shoulder. In dislocation, if the hand of the affected side is placed on the opposite shoulder, the elbow on the affected side cannot be made to touch the side of the chest. Recorded in 1857.

Shrapnell's membrane

. . . See under *Tympanic membrane, flaccid portion of.*

Sibson's fascia or aponeurosis

FRANCIS SIBSON, English anatomist, 1814-1876, described an expansion of fascia covering and strengthening the dome of the pleura. Recorded between 1855 and 1869.

Sibson's furrow

. . . See under *Pectoralis major, furrow formed by.*

Sicklemia

. . . See under *Anemia, sickle-cell, first clear description of.*

Side-chain theory of immunity, introduction of

PAUL EHRLICH, German bacteriologist and pathologist, 1854-1915, propounded a theory which holds that the protoplasm is composed of very complex organic molecules consisting of a stable central group and less stable lateral or side-chain groups, the latter taking part in immunological transformations. Reported in 1885. Known as *Ehrlich's side-chain theory.*

Siemens' syndrome

. . . See under *Congenital ectodermal dysplasia.*

Sigault's operation

. . . See under *Symphysiotomy, first successful.*

Sign language for deaf-mutes, invention of

GIOVANNI BONIFACIO, Italian physician, 1574-16??, devised a sign language for deaf-mutes, in 1616.

Silkworm disease, parasitic nature of

AGOSTINO BASSI, Italian physician, 1773 - 1856, showed that muscardine, a disease of silkworms, is caused by a fungus now known as *Botrytis bassiana.* Reported in 1835.

Silkworm, metamorphosis of; early description

MARCELLO MALPIGHI, Italian anatomist, 1628 - 1694, described the structure and life history of the silkworm *Bombyx mori.* Recorded in 1669.

Silver, colloidal, first use of

CARL C. B. CREDÉ, German surgeon, 1847-1929, is credited with introduction of colloidal silver in surgery, about 1897.

Silver nitrate for staining nerve cells, introduction of

CAMILLO GOLGI, Italian histologist, 1844-1926, is credited with introducing the silver nitrate stain for nerve cells, *circa* 1894.

Silver nitrate solution for eyes of newborn

. . . See under *Ophthalmia neonatorum, prophylaxis of,* etc.

Silver tannin stain for neuroglia

NICOLAS ACHUCARRO, Spanish histologist, 1881 - 1918, devised the silver-tannin stain for impregnating connective tissue, especially neuroglia. Published in 1911. Method is known as *Achucarro's stain.*

Silver wire sutures, introduction of

JAMES MARION SIMS, American surgeon, 1813-1883, introduced the use of silver wire as suture material, in 1858.

Silver-fork fracture of radius

. . . See under *Radius, fracture of,* etc.

Simian society, first clear description of

SOLLY ZUCKERMAN, English zoologist, 1904- , was the first to give a clear description of the simian society, in a work titled "The social life of monkeys and apes." Published in 1932.

Simmonds' disease, eponymic description of

. . . See under *Hypophysial cachexia.*

Simmonds' disease, pre-eponymic description of

L. K. GLINSKI, Polish physician, 18??-19??, described the condition later to be known as Simmonds' disease, in 1913.

Simonart's bands

. . . See under *Amniotic bands of fetus.*

Sims' position

. . . See under *Lithotomy position,* etc.

Sims' speculum

. . . See under *Vaginal speculum, duckbill, introduction of.*

Sinanthropus pekinensis, description of skull of

GRAFTON ELLIOT SMITH, English neuroanatomist, 1871-1937, described the skull of the "Peking man," *Sinanthropus pekinensis,* discovered by W. C. PEI on December 2, 1929. Published in 1931. Pei's brief account appeared in 1929.

Sino-atrial node, discovery of

MARTIN W. FLACK, English physiologist, 1882-1931, with ARTHUR KEITH (Scottish anatomist and anthropologist, 1866 - 1955), discovered the sino-atrial node. Reported in 1907. Known as *node of Keith and Flack.*

Sinus, circular, eponymic description of

HUMPHREY RIDLEY, English physician and anatomist, 1653 - 1708, described a venous sinus around the pituitary. Recorded in 1695. Known as *Ridley's sinus.*

Sinus, maxillary, eponymic description of

NATHANIEL HIGHMORE, English physician and anatomist, 1613-1685, described the maxillary sinus in 1651. Known as *antrum of Highmore.*

Sinus of external jugular vein

. . . See under *External jugular vein.*

Sinus of Morgagni, pharyngeal

GIOVANNI BATTISTA MORGAGNI, Italian anatomist and pathologist, 1682-1771, described a space in the nasopharynx between the upper border of the superior constrictor muscle and the base of the skull, covered by the fascia pharyngo-basilaris. Recorded *circa* 1717.

Sinus of Valsalva

. . . See under *Aortic sinus, eponymic description of.*

Sinus, venous, of sclera, eponymic description of

ERNEST ALEXANDRE LAUTH, Alsatian anatomist and physiologist, 1803-1837, described the venous sinus of the sclera, a circular canal near the junction of the sclera with the cornea, which gives rise to the anterior ciliary veins. Published in 1829. The structure was also described by FRIEDRICH S. SCHLEMM (German anatomist, 1795-1858) in 1830. Known as *Lauth's canal* and as *Schlemm's canal.*

Sinuses, confluence of; torcular Herophili

HEROPHILUS, Greek physician and anatomist in Egypt, 335-280 B.C., described the confluens sinuum, the confluence of the superior sagittal, straight, occipital, and transverse sinuses of the dura mater. Exact date not available.

Sinuses of Morgagni, rectal

GIOVANNI BATTISTA MORGAGNI, Italian anatomist and pathologist, 1682 - 1771, described the spaces between the vertical folds of the rectum, i.e., between the columns of Morgagni. Recorded between 1717 and 1719.

Sinuses, paranasal, displacement irrigation of

ARTHUR WALTER PROETZ, American otolaryngologist, 1888 - 19??, introduced a method for treating infected nasal sinuses by irrigation under negative pressure. Recorded in 1926. Known as *Proetz's treatment.*

Siphon drainage in empyema

GOTTHARD BULAU, German physician, 1835-1900, is believed to have been the first to use siphon drainage in treating empyema. Known as *Bulau drainage.* Date not available.

Sippy treatment of peptic ulcer

BERTRAM WELTON SIPPY, American physician, 1866-1924, devised a diet for the treatment of peptic ulcer consisting of a milk-cream mixture supplemented by antacid powders. Published in 1915. Known as *Sippy diet.*

Skein test for color vision

. . . See under *Wool skein test for color vision.*

Skeletal traction, pin for

FRITZ STEINMANN, Swiss surgeon, 1872-1932, invented a surgical pin or nail for insertion into the distal fragment of a fractured bone in order to provide a hold for skeletal traction. Published in 1907. Known as *Steinmann's pin* or *nail.*

Skin diseases, early classification of

JEAN LOUIS ALIBERT, French dermatologist, 1766-1837, considered by some as the founder of the modern school of dermatology in France, classified skin diseases, particularly in his *Monographie des dermatoses*, published in 1832.

Skin diseases, early classification of

FERDINAND VON HEBRA, Austrian dermatologist, 1816-1880, attempted to classify skin diseases on the basis of pathologic anatomy. Recorded in 1845.

Skin diseases, parasitic cause of many

FERDINAND VON HEBRA, Austrian dermatologist, 1816-1880, demonstrated that many skin disorders are caused by parasites, *circa* 1850.

Skin diseases

. . . See also under name of particular disease.

Skin grafts, early successful transplantation of

GIUSEPPE BARONIO, Italian surgeon, 1759 - 1811, performed successful transplantation of skin grafts in animals. Recorded in 1804.

Skin grafts, early successful transplantation of, in man

JACQUES LOUIS REVERDIN, Swiss surgeon, 1842-1908, was the first to use free skin transplants, as opposed to the pedunculated flaps used previously. Recorded in 1869.

Skin grafts, intermediate thickness, introduction of

LÉOPOLD LOUIS X. E. OLLIER, French surgeon, 1830 - 1900, was the first to describe intermediate thickness skin grafts. Published in 1872. Known as *Ollier's grafts*.

Skin, hyperelasticity of, with joint involvement and pseudotumors

EDVARD L. EHLERS, German dermatologist, 1863-1937, reported a syndrome characterized by hyperelasticity and fragility of the skin, overextensibility of joints, and formation of pseudotumors. Reported in 1901. The condition was reported in 1908 by HENRI A. DANLOS. Known as *Ehlers - Danlos syndrome*.

Skin, idiopathic localized atrophy of

ROBERT WILLIAM TAYLOR, American dermatologist, 1842-1908, gave the first description of idiopathic localized atrophy of the skin, in 1875. The same disorder was described later, in 1902, by HERXHEIMER and HARTMANN under the name of *acrodermatitis chronica atrophicans*. Known as *Taylor's disease*.

Skin, lines of tension of

CARL VON LANGER, Austrian anatomist, 1819 - 1887, discovered and mapped the lines of normal tension in the skin. These lines also indicate the direction along which the skin stretches least; the skin stretches most in a direction perpendicular to these lines. Reported in 1861. Known as *Langer's lines* and *Langer's fissure lines*.

Skodaic resonance in pleural effusion

JOSEF SKODA, Austrian physician, 1805 - 1881, described a resonant sound elicited by percussion above a pleural effusion. Published in 1839.

Skull sutures, small bones in

OLE WORM, Danish anatomist, 1588-1654, described small, adventitious bones in the suture lines of the skull. Date not available. Known as *Wormian bones;* so named by Worm's nephew, THOMAS BARTHOLIN, in 1656.

Skull, vertebrate theory of origin of

RICHARD OWEN, English physician, 1804 - 1892, proposed the vertebrate theory of the origin of the skull. Reported in 1848.

Sleeping sickness, African, causative agent of

DAVID BRUCE, British pathologist and bacteriologist, 1855-1931, and JOSEPH EVERETT DUTTON (English physician, 1874-1905) discovered the trypanosome causing African sleeping sickness. Reported in 1902.

Sleeping sickness, African, spinal fluid in

ALDO CASTELLANI, Italian pathologist, 1878-19??, discovered the organism *Trypanosoma gambiense* in the spinal fluid of patients affected with African sleeping sickness. Recorded in 1903.

Sleeping sickness, African, vector in

DAVID BRUCE, British pathologist and bacteriologist, 1855-1931, demonstrated (with NABARRO) that the vector involved in African sleeping sickness is the tsetse fly. Reported in 1903.

Sleeping sickness

. . . See also under *Encephalitis,* *epidemic,* and *Trypanosomiasis, African.*

Slit lamp used in examining the eye, invention of

ALLVAR GULLSTRAND, Swedish ophthalmologist, 1862 - 1930, invented an illuminating instrument having a slitlike opening which allows a flat beam of light to be projected into the eye, *circa* 1902. Known as *Gullstrand's slit lamp.*

Slow-drip method of blood transfusion

. . . See under *Blood transfusion by slow-drip method.*

Sluder's neuralgia

. . . See under *Sphenopalatine ganglion neuralgia.*

Small doses of drugs, effect of

HORATIO CHARLES WOOD, Philadelphia physician, 1841-1920, was the first to investigate the effect of drugs in small doses. Published in 1874.

Small intestine, internal strangulation of

JOHN HILTON, English surgeon, 1804 - 1878, with GOLDING BIRD, English physician, 1814-1854, performed the first recorded operation for the relief of internal strangulation of the small intestine, in 1847. No anesthesia was used, and the patient died nine hours after the operation.

Small intestine

. . . See also under *Intestinal, Intestine,* and under the name of the particular part of the intestine.

Smallpox, coagulation necrosis in formation of lesions of

CARL WEIGERT, German pathologist and histologist, 1845-1904, explained the formation of smallpox lesions by pointing out the necrotizing effect of the virus upon the skin. This resulted in the introduction of the term "coagulation necrosis" for the process involved. Recorded in 1874-75.

Smallpox, early description of

ABŪ BAKR MUHAMMED IBN ZAKARIYĀ AL-RĀZI, better known as RHAZES, Arabian physician, 850-923, gave the first medical description of smallpox, *circa* 910.

Smallpox, inclusion bodies in lesions of

GIUSEPPE GUARNIERI, Italian pathologist, 1856-1918, described certain inclusion bodies found in the cells of tissues affected with vaccinia and smallpox. Reported in 1894. Known as *Guarnieri's bodies*.

Smallpox inoculation, American method of

ADAM THOMSON, American physician, 17?? - 1767, is credited with introducing the "American" method of inoculation against smallpox. Recorded in 1750.

Smallpox occurs only once in same subject, observation that

AVERROES, Arabian physician in Cordoba, 1126-1198, is believed to have been first to note that smallpox occurs only once in the same subject. Date not available.

Smallpox, Paschen bodies in

. . . See under *Paschen bodies.*

Smallpox, rabbit test for diagnosis of

GUSTAV PAUL, German bacteriologist, 1859-1935, devised a test for the diagnosis of smallpox in which matter from a suspected pustule is rubbed into the eye of a rabbit; if epitheliosis develops, the test is positive. Recorded in 1915. Known as *Paul's test.*

Smallpox vaccination, cowpox matter in

EDWARD JENNER, English physician, 1749-1823, introduced the use of cowpox lymph matter in vaccinating against smallpox. Previously the matter used in the process was taken from human cases of smallpox. First vaccination performed on May 14, 1796. Recorded in 1798.

Smallpox vaccination, early performance of—1701

JAMES PYLARINO (Giacomo Pylarini), Italian physician, 1659-1715, inoculated 3 Constantinople children with smallpox virus, in 1701. Recorded in 1715. Pylarino is considered by some as the first immunologist.

Smallpox vaccination, first, in America

ZABDIEL BOYLSTON, American physician, 1679 - 1766, is believed to have been the first in America to inoculate patients against smallpox, in 1721.

Smallpox vaccination, first, in Philadelphia

JOHN REDMAN COXE, American physician, 1773-1864, was the first to inoculate against smallpox in Philadelphia, *circa* 1802.

Smallpox vaccination, first, in United States

BENJAMIN WATERHOUSE, American physician, 1754-1846, is credited with being the first to perform vaccination against smallpox by the Jennerian method in the United States, in July 1800.

Smallpox vaccination

. . . See also under *Variolation.*

Smooth muscle cells, isolation of

RUDOLPH ALBERT VON KÖLLIKER, Swiss anatomist and histologist, 1817-1905, is credited with being first to isolate smooth muscle cells. Published in 1848.

Smooth muscle, differentiation of, from striped

. . . See under *Muscle, smooth and striped,* etc.

Smooth muscle in wall of arterioles

. . . See under *Arterioles, smooth muscle in.*

Snake venom is protein, demonstration that

SILAS WEIR MITCHELL, American neurologist, 1829 - 1914, with EDWARD TYSON REICHERT, demonstrated that snake venom is protein in nature. Recorded in 1886.

Snakebite serum, development of—1897

LEON C. A. CALMETTE, French bacteriologist, 1863 - 1933, developed a serum for the treatment of snakebite. Reported in 1897. Known as *Calmette's serum.*

Snakes, venomous, first substantial work on

FRANCESCO REDI, Italian naturalist, 1626-1697, wrote the first substantial treatise on poisoning by snakes. He demonstrated that the venom is not effective unless injected. Published in 1664.

Snakes, venomous, of India, description of

JOSEPH FAYRER, English surgeon, 1824-1907, described the venomous snakes of India in a paper published in 1872.

Snapping hip disorder; Perrin-Ferraton disease

MAURICE PERRIN, French surgeon, 1826-1889, described the condition of snapping hip, caused by the movement of a band of fascia lata over the greater trochanter of the femur, *circa* 1866. The same condition was described later, in 1905, by LOUIS FERRATON, French orthopedic surgeon, 1860-1932.

Snare for removing polyps from nose and throat

WILLIAM CHAPMAN JARVIS, American laryngologist, 1855-1895, invented a snare used to remove polyps from the nose and throat. Reported in 1882. Known as *Jarvis's snare.*

Snellen test types or chart

HERMANN SNELLEN, Dutch ophthalmologist, 1834-1908, devised a set of type of varying sizes for testing the acuteness of central vision. Recorded in 1862.

Sodium amytal, introduction of

IRVINE HEINLY PAGE, American physician, 1901-   , introduced sodium amytal as an anesthetic. Recorded in 1923.

Sodium amytal, introduction of, by intravenous injection

LEON GROTIUS ZEFRAS, American physician, 1897-   , with J. T. C. McCALLUM, H. A. SHONLE, E. E. SWANSON, J. B. SCOTT, and G. H. A. CLOWES, studied the induction of anesthesia in man by intravenous injection of sodium isoamyl-ethyl-barbituric acid. Published in 1929.

Sodium citrate, anticoagulant effect of

ALBERT HUSTIN, Belgian physician, 1882 - 19??, discovered the anticoagulant effect of sodium citrate upon blood and advocated its use in transfusions. Recorded in 1914.

Sodium iodide in uretero-pyelography

EARL DORLAND OSBORNE, American urologist, 1895-   , with C. G. SUTHERLAND, A. J. SCHOLL, and L. G. ROWNTREE, introduced the use of sodium iodide in ureteropyelography. Published in 1923.

Sodium salicylate in treating varicose veins

. . . See under *Varicose veins*.

Sodium sulfate, introduction of

JOHANN RUDOLF GLAUBER, German chemist, 1604-1670, prepared sodium sulfate and introduced it as a cathartic, in 1656. Known as *Glauber's salt*.

Soemmerring's ganglion

. . . See under *Substantia nigra, eponymic description of*.

Soemmerring's ligament

. . . See under *Lacrimal gland, suspensory ligament of*.

Soemmerring's spot

. . . See under *Macula lutea, early description of*.

Soft palate, paralysis of, in diphtheria

JOHN HUXHAM, English physician, 1692-1768, was the first to describe paralysis of the soft palate in a case of diphtheria which he, incidentally, mistook for scarlet fever. Recorded in 1757.

Soft palate, plastic operation for

. . . See under *Staphylorrhaphy*.

Soft palate, recurrent paralysis of; eponymic description

GEORG AVELLIS, German laryngologist, 1864-1916, described a syndrome involving recurrent paralysis of the soft palate, ipsilateral involvement of the vocal cord, etc. Published in 1891. Known as *Avellis's syndrome*.

Soldier's heart, early description of

. . . See under *Irritable heart*.

Solution disinfectant, for hand and abdomen sterilization

ELLICE McDONALD, American surgeon, 1876-19??, introduced a solution of orthophenylphenate, sodium oleate, acetone, and alcohol, for use in sterilizing the skin of the abdomen and the hands. Recorded in 1915. Known as *McDonald's solution*.

Solution, disinfectant, for hand sterilization

FRANCIS B. HARRINGTON, American surgeon, 1854-1914, compounded a hand disinfecting solution composed of mercuric chloride, hydrochloric acid, alcohol, and water. Reported in 1904. Known as *Harrington's solution*.

Solution of aluminum acetate; Burow's solution

KARL AUGUST BUROW, German surgeon, 1809 - 1874, devised an astringent and antiseptic solution known as *Solution of Aluminum Acetate* or *Burow's solution*. It was originally compounded from alum and lead acetate. Reported in 1857.

Solution of arsenic and mercuric iodides

MICHAEL D. DONOVAN, Irish physician and pharmacist, 1809-1876, invented a solution of arsenic and mercuric iodides. Reported in November 1839. Used in skin diseases and, formerly, as a tonic. Known as *Donovan's solution*.

Solution of chlorinated soda and sodium bicarbonate, compounding and application of

ALEXIS CARREL, French surgeon, 1873-1944, and HENRY D. DAKIN (English chemist in the United States, 1880 - 1952) developed a solution of chlorinated soda and sodium bicarbonate for use in irrigating wounds. Reported in 1915.

Solution of chlorinated soda, Labarraque's

ANTOINE G. LABARRAQUE, French chemist and apothecary, 1777-1850, compounded a solution of chlorinated soda, for use as a disinfectant. Recorded in 1825. Known as *Labarraque's solution* and as *sodium hypochlorite solution*.

Solution of Iodine, Strong; Lugol's Solution

JEAN GUILLAUME AUGUSTE LUGOL, French physician, 1786-1851, produced a solution of iodine, later known as *Liquor Iodi Fortis, Strong Solution of Iodine, Compound Solution of Iodine*, and *Lugol's Solution*, in 1829. The solution was designed by Lugol for use in tuberculous conditions.

Solution of peptone and sodium chloride for indole formation

EDWARD K. DUNHAM, American pathologist, 1860-1922, invented a solution consisting of 1% peptone and 0.5% sodium chloride in distilled water. It is used as a culture medium for bacteria to determine the formation of indole, as in the case of the spirillum of cholera. Reported *circa* 1887.

Solution of potassium arsenite, introduction of

THOMAS FOWLER, English physician, 1736-1801, introduced the use of solution of potassium arsenite in the treatment of "agues, remitting fevers, and periodic headaches," in 1786. Known as *Fowler's solution*.

Solution of sodium arsenate, Pearson's

GEORGE PEARSON, English physician, 1751-1828, introduced a solution of sodium arsenate which is one-tenth the strength of Solution of Sodium Arsenate, in 1774. Known as *Pearson's Solution of Sodium Arsenate*.

Solution of sodium hypochlorite

. . . See under *Solution of chlorinated soda*.

Sonne's bacillus

. . . See under *Shigella sonnei, etc.*

Sound, surgical, invention of

ERASISTRATUS, Greek anatomist and physician, *circa* 300-250 B.C., is believed to have invented the surgical sound. Date not available.

Sound transmission through cranial bones in diagnosis of ear diseases

AUGUST LUCAE, German otologist, 1835-1911, is credited with being the first to evaluate the transmission of sounds through the cranial bones as an aid in the diagnosis of ear diseases. Recorded in 1870.

Sound, uterine, in diagnosis of retrodisplacement

JAMES YOUNG SIMPSON, Scottish obstetrician, 1811-1870, introduced a uterine sound for the diagnosis of retrodisplacement of the uterus. Recorded in 1843.

Soxhlet apparatus

. . . See under *Apparatus for extracting fatty material.*

Space under perineal fascia

ABRAHAM COLLES, Irish surgeon, 1773 - 1843, described the space under the perineal fascia which contains the ischiocavernosus, the transverse perineal muscle, and other structures. Recorded in 1811. Known as *Colles' space.*

Spastic pseudosclerosis, eponymic description of

ALFONS M. JAKOB, German psychiatrist, 1884 - 1931, described a type of pseudosclerosis characterized by partial degeneration of the pyramidal system and sometimes also of the extrapyramidal system, occurring usually in middle age. Jakob called it spastic pseudosclero-

sis. Report published in 1921. Known also as *Jakob's disease* and *Jakob-Creutzfeldt disease.*

Specific dynamic action of foodstuffs, introduction of concept of

MAX RUBNER, German physiologist, 1854 - 1932, introduced the concept of and the term "specific dynamic action of foodstuffs." Published in 1902.

Specific heat, definition of

JOSEPH BLACK, Scottish chemist, 1728-1799, defined the concept of "specific heat." Reported in 1754.

Spectroscope in analysis of blood

KARL VIERORDT, German physiologist, 1818 - 1884, is credited with having been the first to use the spectroscope in the analysis of oxyhemoglobin, bile, and urine. Recorded in 1876.

Spectroscope, invention of

The early spectroscopes consisted merely of a prism, and as such were known for a long time. The first advanced form of spectroscope, with a diffraction grating, was invented by JOSEPH FRAUENHOFER, German physicist, 1787 - 1826, in 1814. He identified 576 lines of the spectrum; these are known as *Frauenhofer's lines.*

Spectroscopy, **introduction of term**

ARTHUR SCHUSTER, English physicist, 1836-1902, is credited with the introduction of the term *spectroscopy*, to designate a specific branch of physical science, in 1882.

Spectrum analysis, development of methods of

ROBERT W. BUNSEN, German chemist, 1811-1899, is credited with developing methods of spectrum analysis, in 1859.

Speculum for ear, with illumination

PHILIPP BOZZINI, Austrian surgeon, 1773-1809, devised an aural speculum provided with mirror reflectors and illumination. Recorded in 1807.

Speech center in anterior cerebral lobes, placing of

JEAN BAPTISTE BOUILLAUD, French physician, 1796-1881, pointed out that the speech center is located in the anterior cerebral lobes. Reported in 1825.

Speech center in third left frontal convolution

PIERRE PAUL BROCA, French surgeon and anthropologist, 1824-1880, localized the speech center in the third left frontal convolution. Reported in 1861.

Speech, physiology of, classic treatise on

FRANS C. DONDERS, Dutch physician, 1818-1889, wrote a classic report on the physiology of speech, in 1870.

Speech, voluntary abstaining from, as seen in psychoses

ADOLF KUSSMAUL, German physician, 1822-1902, described a form of voluntary mutism occasionally seen in the insane. Published in 1877. Known as *Kussmaul's aphasia*.

Speed of nerve impulses

... See under *Nerve impulse.*

Spee's curve

... See under *Line extended along buccal cusps of teeth.*

Spengler's fragments in tuberculous sputum

CARL SPENGLER, Swiss physician, 1861-1937, described small round bodies occurring in the sputum of tuberculous patients, in 1900.

Spermatozoa, early description of—1674

ANTONJ VAN LEEUWENHOEK Dutch naturalist, 1632-1723, is credited with being first to describe spermatozoa which, according to legend, were actually discovered by one of his students. Published in 1677.

Spermatozoa, function of, in fertilization

RUDOLPH ALBERT VON KÖLLIKER, Swiss anatomist and histologist, 1817-1905, described the function of spermatozoa in the process of fertilization. Published in 1841.

Spermatozoa, origin of, in testicular cells

RUDOLPH ALBERT VON KÖLLIKER, Swiss anatomist and histologist, 1817-1905, established that spermatozoa originate in the cells of the testicle. Published in 1841.

Spermatozoon, cytoplasm and nucleus of

FRANZ SCHWEIGGER-SEIDEL, German physiologist, 1834-1871, demonstrated that a spermatozoon contains a nucleus and cytoplasm. Published in 1865.

Spermatozoon enters ovum and union of pronuclei occurs, demonstration that

WILHELM A. O. HERTWIG, German embryologist, 1849-1922, demonstrated that in the process of fertilization the spermatozoon enters the ovum and the male and female pronuclei unite. Published in 1875.

Spermin crystals in prostatic fluid

. . . See under *Crystals in prostatic fluid.*

Spermin, isolation of, from testis

ALEXANDER VASILYEVICH VON POEHL, Russian chemist, 1850-1898, is credited with being first to isolate spermin from the testis. Published in 1891.

Sphenoid, lesser wings of; eponymic description

GIOVAN FILIPPO INGRASSIA, Italian physician and anatomist, 1510-1580, described the lesser wings of the sphenoid bone, *circa* 1568. Published in 1603. Known as *Ingrassia's wings.*

Sphenoid sinuses, first description of

BERENGARIUS OF CAPRI, Italian anatomist, 1480-1550, is believed to have been the first to describe the sphenoid sinuses, in 1521.

Sphenomandibular ligament, spine for attachment of

JOHANN BAPTIST SPIX, German anatomist, 1781-1826, described a spine at the edge of the mandibular foramen to which the sphenomandibular ligament is attached, *circa* 1810. Known as *Spix's spine.*

Sphenopalatine ganglion, eponymic description of

JOHANN FRIEDRICH MECKEL, German anatomist, 1714-1774, described the sphenopalatine gan-

glion, composed of the facial, sympathetic, and other nerves, located in the sphenomaxillary fossa. Published in 1748. Known as *Meckel's ganglion.*

Sphenopalatine ganglion neuralgia, eponymic description of

GREENFIELD SLUDER, American laryngologist, 1865-1928, gave the first description of sphenopalatine ganglion neuralgia, in 1910. Known as *Sluder's neuralgia.*

Sphenoparietal sinus, description and naming of

GILBERT BRESCHET, French anatomist, 1784-1845, described and named the sphenoparietal sinus, *circa* 1827.

Sphygmograph, earliest form of—1854

KARL VIERORDT, German physiologist, 1818-1884, devised a sphygmograph with which he traced the human pulse. He also used the instrument to estimate blood pressure, by measuring the force necessary to obliterate the pulse. Recorded in 1854.

Sphygmograph, early form of—1860

ÉTIENNE JULES MAREY, French physiologist, 1830-1904, invented a sphygmograph in 1860. This instrument was variously modified later, and served as the basis of the modern sphygmograph. Marey's chief contribution was the reduction of inertia by means of light drums, styluses, and levers.

Sphygmomanometer, air-type, portable

PIERRE CARL EDOUARD POTAIN,

French physician, 1825-1901, invented a portable air sphygmomanometer, in 1889.

Sphygmomanometer, early form of

SAMUEL SIEGRIED VON BASCH, German physician, 1837-1905, invented an early form of sphygmomanometer and was a pioneer in the science of recording blood pressure. Recorded in 1876.

Sphygmomanometer, first simple clinical

SCIPIONE RIVA-ROCCI, Italian physician, 1863-1943, is credited with inventing the first practical clinical sphygmomanometer. Recorded in 1896.

Sphygmomanometer with pressure gauge

HAROLD LESLIE BARNARD, English physiologist, 1868-1908, with LEONARD ERSKINE, English physician, 1866-19??, devised a sphygmomanometer provided with a pressure gauge. Recorded in 1897.

Spinal anesthesia, continuous, introduction of

WILLIAM THOMAS LEMMON, American physician, 1896-   , introduced continuous spinal anesthesia, in 1940.

Spinal anesthesia with cocaine, introduction of

AUGUST K. G. BIER, German surgeon, 1861-1949, introduced the use of cocaine in spinal anesthesia. Reported in 1899.

Spinal anesthesia

. . . See also under *Anesthesia.*

Spinal arthropathy, neurotic, first description of

JOHN KEARSLEY MITCHELL, Philadelphia physician, 1798-1858, is believed to have been first to describe neurotic spinal arthropathy, in 1831.

Spinal braces, introduction of

LORENZ (LAURENTIUS) HEISTER, German surgeon and anatomist, 1683-1758, is credited with introducing the use of spinal braces, *circa* 1710.

Spinal column and pharynx, space between

PHILIPP JAKOB W. HENKE, German anatomist, 1834-1896, described the potential space, filled with connective tissue, between the spinal column and the pharynx and esophagus, in 1878. Known as *Henke's space.*

Spinal cord, central canal of

JEAN FRANÇOIS FERNEL, French physician, 1497-1558, described the central canal of the spinal cord, in 1542.

Spinal cord, disease of posterior columns of

EDWARD STANLEY, English surgeon, 1793-1862, is said to have been first to describe disease of the posterior columns of the spinal cord. Recorded in 1840.

Spinal cord, fiber in central canal of

ERNST REISSNER, Riga anatomist, 1824-1878, described the free fiber in the central canal of the spinal cord. Published in 1864. Known as *Reissner's fiber.*

Spinal cord, length of fibers of

EDWARD FLATAU, Polish neurologist, 1869-1932, made the observation that the longer the fibers of the spinal cord the nearer they are to the periphery. Reported in 1894.

Spinal cord, pathways of conduction in

... See under *Pathways of conduction in spinal cord*.

Spinal cord, posterior root fibers of, divide on entering cord

... See under *Posterior root fibers divide*.

Spinal cord, regeneration of

LAZARO SPALLANZANI, Italian physiologist, 1729-1799, was the first to propound the doctrine of regeneration of the spinal cord. Published in 1768.

Spinal cord, subacute combined degeneration of, in relation to pernicious anemia—1884

OTTO LEICHTENSTERN, German physician, 1845-1900, is credited with giving the first description of subacute combined degeneration of the spinal cord, under the name of "progressive pernicious anemia in tabetics." Published in 1884.

Spinal cord, subacute combined degeneration of, in relation to pernicious anemia—1891

JAMES JACKSON PUTNAM, American neurologist, 1846-1918, described dorsolateral sclerosis such as occurs in pernicious anemia. Reported in 1891. In the same year, CHARLES LOOMIS DANA, American neurologist, 1852-1935, also wrote on subacute combined degeneration of the spinal cord. The condition is known as *Putnam-Dana syndrome*.

Spinal cord, subacute combined degeneration of, in relation to pernicious anemia—1900

JAMES S. R. RUSSELL, English physician, 1863-1939, with F. E. BATTEN and JAMES S. COLLIER, gave a description of subacute combined degeneration of the spinal cord in its relation to pernicious anemia. Reported in 1900.

Spinal cord, substance covering posterior horn of

LUIGI ROLANDO, Italian anatomist, 1773-1831, described a gelatinous substance which forms a sheath around the posterior horn of the spinal cord and forms a lining of the central canal. Known as *Rolando's gelatinous substance* and *substantia gelatinosa*. Recorded in 1809.

Spinal cord, tract of ascending anterolateral fibers of

WILLIAM RICHARD GOWERS, English neurologist, 1845-1915, described a bundle of nerve fibers in the anterior and lateral funiculus of the spinal cord composed of several smaller tracts. Reported in 1880 or 1879. Known as *Gowers' tract* or *column* and *fasciculus ventrolateralis superficialis*.

Spinal cord, transverse lesion of, causes loss of reflexes

HENRY CHARLTON BASTIAN, English neurologist, 1837-1915, promulgated the law that in case of transverse lesion of the spinal cord above the lumbar enlargement, the tendon reflexes in the lower extremities are completely lost. Reported in 1890. Known as the *Bastian-Bruns law*.

Spinal cord tumor, successful removal of

WILLIAM RICHARD GOWERS, English neurologist, 1845-1915, with V. A. H. HORSLEY, is credited with being the first to remove successfully a tumor of the spinal cord, in 1888.

Spinal fluid, isolation of meningococci from —1896

OTTO J. L. HEUBNER, German pediatrician, 1843-1926, is credited with isolating meningococci from cerebrospinal fluid, in 1896.

Spinal ganglia, early description of—1899

ALEXANDER S. DOGIEL, Russian neurohistologist, 1852-1922, described the spinal ganglia in man and other mammals, in 1899.

Spinal nerve roots, distribution of

CHARLES SCOTT SHERRINGTON, English neurophysiologist, 1857-1952, studied the distribution of the ventral and dorsal spinal nerve roots and demonstrated that every posterior spinal nerve root supplies a definite area of the skin. Published in 1892.

Spinal nerves, anterior roots of, are motor

. . . See under *Motor function of anterior roots.*

Spinal nerves, early description of

THOMAS WILLIS, English physician and anatomist, 1621-1675, de-scribed the spinal nerves. Published posthumously in 1684.

Spinal puncture, diagnostic value of

PAUL FÜRBRINGER, German physician, 1849-1930, showed that the method of spinal puncture has diagnostic value. Recorded in 1895.

Spinal puncture

. . . See also under *Lumbar puncture.*

Spinal reflexes, cerebral inhibition of

IVAN MICHAILOVICH SETCHENOV, Russian neurologist, 1829-1905, is credited with discovering that the cerebrum is capable of inhibiting spinal reflexes. Published in 1863.

Spindle-shaped figure in mitosis

. . . See under *Nuclear spindle in mitosis.*

Spine on outer edge of external pterygoid plate

FILIPPO CIVININI, Italian anatomist, 1805-1844, described a small process or eminence on the outer edge of the external pterygoid plate, giving attachment to the pterygospinous ligament. Recorded in 1830. Known as *Civinini's spine.*

Spinocerebellar tracts, ventral and dorsal

LUDWIG EDINGER, German neurologist, 1855-1918, was the first to give a description of the ventral and dorsal spinocerebellar tracts. Recorded in 1885.

Spiral canal of cochlea

. . . See under *Cochlea, spiral canal of.*

Spiral mucous bodies in gastric secretion in hyper-chlorhydria

VALERY JAWORSKI, Polish physician, 1849-1925, described spiral mucous bodies or corpuscles found in the gastric secretion of patients with marked hyperchlorhydria, in 1887. Known as *Jaworski's corpuscles*.

Spirals of mucin threads in sputum of asthmatics

HEINRICH CURSCHMANN, German physician, 1846-1910, described coiled or spiral mucinous threads found occasionally in the small pellets expectorated by asthmatic patients. Reported in 1882. Known as *Curschmann's spirals*.

Spirillium, introduction of term

OTTO FRIEDRICH MÜLLER, Danish bacteriologist, 1730-1784, introduced the term *spirillum,* about 1773.

Spirillum minus as cause of rat-bite fever

HENRY VANDYKE CARTER, English physician in India, 1831-1897, was the first to describe *Spirillum minus* as the cause of rat-bite fever. Recorded in 1887.

Spirit of Ether, Compound

. . . See under *Compound Spirit of Ether.*

Spirit of Ether; Hoffmann's drops

FRIEDRICH HOFFMANN, German physician, 1660-1742, is credited with the original compounding of Spirit of Ether. Recorded *circa* 1729.

Spirochaeta pallida, discovery of

. . . See under *Syphilis, causative agent of.*

Spirochaeta refringens in pure culture

HIDEYO NOGUCHI, Japanese bacteriologist in America, 1876-1928, cultivated the *Spirochaeta refringens* in pure culture, in 1912.

Spirometer, early invention of

JOHN HUTCHINSON, English physician, 1811-1861, invented an early form of spirometer for measuring the air taken in and breathed out by the lungs. Reported in 1846.

Spiroptera carcinoma, discovery of

JOHANNES FIBIGER, Danish bacteriologist, 1867-1926, described the *Spiroptera* carcinoma, discovered in the stomach of rats infested by the nematode *Spiroptera.* First report in 1913.

Spix's spine

. . . See under *Sphenomandibular ligament, spine for attachment of.*

Spleen, corpuscle of; eponymic description

MARCELLO MALPIGHI, Italian anatomist, 1628-1694, described lymph nodules of the spleen associated with central arteries. Recorded in 1666. Each such lymph nodule is known as a *splenic corpuscle* or *malpighian corpuscle* of the spleen.

Spleen, first extirpation of

CARL FRIEDRICH QUITTENBAUM, German surgeon, 1793-1852, is credited with being first to perform a splenectomy and thus establish it as a surgical possibility. Performed in 1829; recorded in 1836.

Spleen, floating, anchorage of

BERNHARD BARDENHEUER, German surgeon, 1839-1913, devised an operation for fixing a floating spleen by making a pocket in the parietal peritoneum. Published in 1895.

Spleen is not essential to life, proof that

GIUSEPPE ZAMBECCARI, Italian surgeon, 1655-1728, experimenting with animals demonstrated that the spleen is not essential to life. Recorded in 1680.

Splenic anemia of infants, early description of—1866

WILHELM GRIESINGER, German neurologist, 1817-1868, is credited with being first to describe infantile splenic anemia, a condition marked by anemia, enlargement of the spleen, etc., in 1866. Known also as *infantile splenomegaly, infantile pseudoleukemic anemia,* and as *von Jaksch's anemia* or *disease.*

Splenic anemia of infants, early description of—1889

RUDOLF VON JAKSCH, Austrian physician in Czechoslovakia, 1855-1947, described infantile anemia in children, in 1889. Known as *von Jaksch's anemia* or *disease, infantile pseudoleukemic anemia,* etc.

Splenic corpuscle

. . . See under *Spleen, corpuscle of,* etc.

Splenization in lobar pneumonia, early description of

LOUIS JOSEPH DESNOS, French physician, 1828-1893, described the splenization stage of lobar pneumonia. Exact date not available. Known as *splenopneumonia, Desnos' pneumonia,* and as *Grancher's pneumonia.*

Splenization in lobar pneumonia, early description of—1883

JACQUES JOSEPH GRANCHER, French physician, 1843-1907, described the splenization of the lung in lobar pneumonia, in 1883. Known as *Grancher's pneumonia, Desnos' pneumonia,* and as *splenopneumonia.*

Splenomegaly, early description of—1892

MAURICE GEORGES DEBOVE, French physician, 1845-1920, described essential splenomegaly, a condition marked by enlargement of the spleen and progressive anemia. Reported in 1892.

Splenomegaly of undetermined origin

GUIDO BANTI, Italian physician, 1852-1925, gave the first description of splenomegaly accompanied by anemia, cirrhosis of the liver, leukopenia, etc. Reported in 1882. Known as *Banti's disease.*

Splitting of chromosomes in act of reproduction

THEODOR BOVERI, German zoologist, 1862-1915, was the first to point out that the splitting of chromosomes is a part of the mechanism of reproduction. Reported in 1888.

Spondylitis deformans; ankylosing spondylitis—1884

ERNST A. G. G. STRÜMPELL, German physician, 1853-1925, described ankylosing spondylitis in 1897, but made reference to it earlier, in 1884. Known as *Strümpell-Marie disease.*

Spondylitis deformans; ankylosing spondylitis—1892

VLADIMIR MICHAILOVICH BECHTEREV, Russian neurologist, 1857-1927, described ankylosing spondylitis in 1892. Known as *Bechterev's disease.*

Spondylitis deformans; ankylosing spondylitis—1898

PIERRE MARIE, French neurologist, 1853-1940, described ankylosing spondylitis in 1898. Known as *Marie-Strümpell arthritis* and *Strümpell-Marie disease.*

Spondylolisthesis, first description of and introduction of term

CARL VON ROKITANSKY, Austrian pathologist, 1804-1878, was the first to describe spondylolisthesis. Recorded in 1839. He also introduced the term *spondylolisthesis.*

Sponge, burnt, in treatment of goiter

BRADFORD WILMER, English physician, 1739-1796, introduced the use of burnt sponge in the treatment of goiter. Recorded in 1779. Known as the "Coventry treatment," in allusion to the place where it was first used.

Spongioblast, introduction of term

WILHELM HIS, *père,* Swiss anatomist and embryologist, 1831-1904, is credited with introducing the term *spongioblast, circa* 1880.

Spontaneous generation, disproval of

LOUIS PASTEUR, French scientist and bacteriologist, 1822-1895, studied fermentation in 1857 and was able to disprove, in 1861, the prevalent theory of spontaneous generation.

Spore formation by bacteria, discovery of

FERDINAND J. COHN, German bacteriologist, 1828-1898, made the discovery that bacteria are able to form spores. *Circa* 1872.

Sporotrichosis, earliest description of—1898

BENJAMIN ROBINSON SCHENCK, American surgeon, 1842-1920, described a disease marked by the formation of ulcerating nodules in the skin, lymph nodes, subcutaneous tissue, etc. It is caused by *Sporotrichum schenckii* or *beurmanni.* Recorded in 1898. Known as *Schenck's disease.*

Sporotrichosis, early description of—1906

CHARLES LUCIEN DE BEURMANN, French dermatologist, 1851-1923, with HENRI GOUGEROT, described sporotrichosis, a chronic infection characterized by the formation of nodular lesions which have a tendency to break down and form ulcers. It is caused by *Sporotrichum schenckii.* Reported in 1906. Known as *de Beurmann-Gougerot disease.* Published in 1912.

Spreading factor; hyaluronidase; Duran-Reynals' factor

FRANCISCO DURAN-REYNALS, French-American physician, 1899-, demonstrated that the injection of extracts of normal rabbit testicle into the skin along with vaccine virus greatly facilitates the spread of the infection. The phenomenon is due to the presence of an enzyme (hyaluronidase) which aids the hydrolysis of the cement substance of the tissues involved. Reported in 1928.

Sprengel's deformity

... See under *Scapula, congenitally high,* etc.

Sprue, nontropical, eponymic description of

THORVALD EINAR HESS THAYSEN, Danish physician, 1883-1936, described nontropical sprue or idiopathic steatorrhea, in 1929. The condition was described earlier, in 1888, by SAMUEL JONES GEE, English physician, 1839-1911. Known as *Gee-Thaysen disease.*

Sprue, tropical, early description of

WILLIAM HILLARY, English physician, 170?-1763, described sprue of the Island of Barbados. Recorded in 1759.

Sprue, tropical, effectiveness of liver extract in

WILLIAM BOSWORTH CASTLE, American physician, 1897-　　, proved the effectiveness of injectable liver extract in the treatment of tropical sprue. Reported *circa* 1930.

Stähli's pigment line

... See under *Cornea, brown line of degeneration in.*

Stain for use on protozoan parasites

GUSTAV GIEMSA, German chemist, 1867-1948, devised many stains, the best known being the one composed of azure II-eosin, azure II, methanol, etc., and used to stain protozoan parasites, as the *Leishmania, trypanosomes,* etc. Introduced *circa* 1903.

Stain

... See also under name of particular stain, as *Methylene blue.*

Staining of bacteria, first experiments in—1871

CARL WEIGART, German pathologist and histologist, 1845-1904, was the first to stain bacteria successfully, *circa* 1871.

Staining of bacteria, first experiments in—1878

WILHELM FRIEDRICH VON GLEICHEN, German naturalist, 1717-1783, is credited with being the first to stain bacteria, with indigo and carmine. Recorded in 1778.

Stannic chloride, discovery of

ANDREAS LIBAVIUS (LIBAU), German chemist, 1546-1616, is credited with discovering stannic chloride which he prepared in 1605 by distilling tin with mercuric chloride. He called it *Spiritus argenti vivi sublimati.* It was named after him, *Spiritus fumans Libavii.* In the early World War, stannic chloride was used as an irritating smoke screen.

Stapes, early description of —1557

GIOVAN FILIPPO INGRASSIA, Italian physician and anatomist, 1510-1580, gave the first accurate description of the stapes, *circa* 1557. Published in 1603.

Staphylococcus pyogenes aureus, discovery of

ALEXANDER OGSTON, Scottish surgeon and bacteriologist, 1844-1929, is credited with the discovery of the *Staphylococcus pyogenes aureus,* about 1881.

Staphylococcus pyogenes, classification of

ANTON JULIUS FRIEDRICH ROSENBACH, German physician and bacteriologist, 1842-1923, divided the *Staphylococcus pyogenes* into the *albus* and *aureus.* Recorded in 1884.

Staphylorrhaphy, first recorded, in America

JOHN COLLINS WARREN, American surgeon, 1778-1856, introduced staphylorrhaphy in the United States. Recorded in 1828.

Staphylorrhaphy, first recorded, in France

PHILIBERT JOSEPH ROUX, French surgeon, 1780-1854, is credited with performing the first staphylorrhaphy in France, in 1819.

Starvation treatment in diabetes mellitus

FREDERICK MADISON ALLEN, American physician, 1879-19??, introduced a dietary treatment for diabetes mellitus, consisting of certain days of fasting followed by a restricted diet. Recorded in 1914.

Static electricity, use of, in treating nervous disorders

WILLIAM W. GULL, English physician, 1816-1890, investigated the use of static electricity in the treatment of nervous disorders, in 1849.

Static electricity, use of, in treatment of spasmodic disorders

THOMAS ADDISON, English physician, 1793-1860, is believed to have been the first to use static electricity in treating spasmodic diseases, in 1837.

Statistics, introduction of, in medicine

PIERRE C. A. LOUIS, French physician, 1787-1872, is credited with the introduction of statistical methods in the study and reporting of disease. Recorded in 1825.

Statistics

... See also under *Medical statistics.*

Status lymphaticus, original description of

RICHARD BRIGHT, English physician, 1789-1858, made original observations on the condition status lymphaticus. Recorded in 1838.

Status marmoratus

... See under *Corpus striatum syndrome.*

Steam sterilization in surgery, introduction of

ERNST VON BERGMANN, German surgeon born in Latvia, 1836-1907, introduced steam sterilization in surgery. Recorded in 1886.

Steinach's operation or method

... See under *Impotence, treatment of, by occlusion of vas deferens.*

Steinmann's pin or nail

... See under *Skeletal traction, pin for.*

Stellwag's sign

. . . See under *Winking, absence or infrequency of, in goiter.*

Stenosis of lacrimal duct, treatment of, by dilatation

. . . See under *Lacrimal duct, stenosis of,* etc.

Stensen's duct

. . . See under *Parotid gland duct, eponymic description of.*

Stereoroentgenometer, invention of

CLAYTON RICHARDSON JOHNSON, American radiologist, 1896-   , invented a stereoroentgenometer for measuring the solid dimensions of an object and for localizing points from stereoscopic roentgenograms. Recorded in 1927.

Sternum, angle formed by body and manubrium of

PIERRE CHARLES ALEXANDRE LOUIS, French physician, 1787-1872, described the angle formed by the body and the manubrium of the sternum. Published in 1825. Known as *Louis's angle.*

Stethoscope, invention of

RENÉ T. H. LAENNEC, French physician, 1781-1826, invented the stethoscope in 1816. In his first experiment, Laennec used a paper notebook rolled to form a tube through which he heard the heart sounds much clearer than through the immediate application of the ear to the chest. Reported in 1818; published in 1819.

Stethoscope, use of, in measuring systolic and diastolic blood pressure

BRUNO FELLNER, German physician, 18??-1926, is credited with being first to suggest the use of the stethoscope in the measurement of systolic and diastolic blood pressure. Published in 1907.

Stevens-Johnson syndrome in children, eponymic description of

ALBERT MASON STEVENS, American pediatrician, 1884-19??, with F. C. JOHNSON, described a condition in children marked by fever, generalized eruption, purulent conjunctivitis, etc. Published in 1922.

Stevens-Johnson syndrome in children, pre-eponymic description of

ROBERT RENDU, French pediatrician, 1886-19??, was the first to describe the condition later called the Stevens-Johnson syndrome. Published in 1916. See under *Stevens-Johnson syndrome in children,* above.

Sticker's disease

. . . See under *Erythema infectiosum.*

Stieda's fracture

. . . See under *Femur, fracture of internal condyle of.*

Stieda's process

. . . See under *Talus, posterior process of.*

Stilbestrol, discovery of

EDWARD CHARLES DODDS, English chemist, 1899-19??, with L. GOLDBERG, W. LAWSON, and R. ROBINSON, discovered stilbestrol. Recorded in 1938.

Stiller's disease

. . . See under *Asthenic body type,* etc.

Stilling's bundle

. . . See under *Medulla oblongata, solitary fasciculus of.*

Still's disease

. . . See under *Polyarthritis in children.*

Stomach contractions as cause of hunger pains

. . . See under *Hunger pains are caused by cramplike contractions.*

Stomach, desiccated, in treatment of pernicious anemia

. . . See under *Pernicious anemia,* etc.

Stomach exploration by means of a light passed down the esophagus

. . . See under *Gastrodiaphany, introduction of.*

Stomach, first excision of

CARL SCHLATTER, Swiss surgeon, 1864-1934, is credited with the performance of the first successful gastrectomy. Recorded in 1897.

Stomach, first roentgenographic outline of, in guinea pig

WOLF BECHER, German physician, 1862-1906, was the first to show the outline of the stomach in the guinea pig by means of x-rays and a lead contrast medium. Reported in 1896.

Stomach movements recorded by means of a balloon

. . . See under *Balloon, use of, in recording stomach movements.*

Stomach, oblique muscle fibers of

HYACINTHE GAVARD, French anatomist, 1753-1802, was the first to describe the oblique muscle fibers of the stomach wall, *circa* 1792. Known as *Gavard's muscle.*

Stomach pouch; Pavlov's pouch

IVAN PETROVICH PAVLOV, Russian physiologist, 1849-1936, developed a method for isolating a portion of the stomach from the rest of the organ without severing the nerve supply. By means of this "stomach pouch," which had an external opening on the abdominal wall, Pavlov studied the mechanism of gastric secretion. Recorded in 1897.

Stomach, primary atrophy of

SAMUEL FENWICK, English physician, 1821-1902, described primary atrophy of the stomach, in 1880. Known as *Fenwick's disease.*

Stomach suspension by plication of ligaments

. . . See under *Gastroptosis, operation for,* etc.

Stomach tube, early invention of—1140

AVENZOAR, Arabian physician in Cordoba, *circa* 1091-1162, is credited with the invention of a primitive form of stomach tube, *circa* 1140.

Stomach tube, early invention of—1810

GUILLAUME DUPUYTREN, French surgeon, 1777-1835, invented an early form of stomach tube. Reported in 1810.

Stomach tube, first use of, in gastric lavage

PHILIP SYNG PHYSICK, American surgeon, 1768-1837, was the first to use a stomach tube in a case of poisoning, in the United States, in 1805. Published in 1812. ALEXANDER MONRO *secundus,* Scottish physician, 1733-1817, had devised a similar apparatus in 1767.

Stomach tube, flexible rubber

CARL A. EWALD, German physician, 1845-1915, is believed to have introduced a flexible rubber tube for aspirating the contents of the stomach, in 1875.

Stovaine, introduction of

. . . See under *Amylocaine, introduction of.*

Stovarsol in treatment of amebiasis

. . . See under *Amebiasis,* etc.

Strabismus, correction of, by myotomy

JOHANN F. DIEFFENBACH, German surgeon, 1792-1847, was the first to use myotomy in the successful treatment of stabismus. Reported in 1839 and 1842.

Strabismus, operation for—1857

FREIDRICH W. E. A. VON GRAEFE, German ophthalmologist, 1828-1870, devised an operation for the treatment of strabismus, in 1857.

Stratum granulosum of skin

PAUL GERSON UNNA, German dermatologist, 1850-1929, described the stratum granulosum of the skin, in 1876.

Stratum lucidum, eponymic description of

EUSEBIO OEHL, Italian anatomist, 1827-1903, gave a clear description of the structure of the skin, especially of the stratum lucidum, in 1857. The stratum lucidum is known as *Oehl's layer.*

Straus's reaction

. . . See under *Glanders, diagnostic reaction for.*

Strawberry gallbladder, original description of

WILLIAM CARPENTER MACCARTY, American pathologist, 1880-19??, described a condition of the gallbladder marked by hyperplasia of the lining folds in which are embedded cholesterin-fat granules. The mass formed has a strawberry-like appearance and may fill the entire gallbladder. Published in 1910.

Streptococcus erysipelatis (*Streptococcus pyogenes*), discovery of

FRIEDRICH FEHLEISEN, German physician, 1854-1924, is credited with the discovery of *Streptococcus pyogenes,* formerly known as *Streptococcus erysipelatis.* Recorded in 1882.

Streptococcus pyogenes, isolation of

ANTON JULIUS FRIEDRICH ROSENBACH, German physician and bacteriologist, 1842-1923, is credited with isolating *Streptococcus pyogenes.* Recorded in 1884.

Streptococcus viridans in bacterial endocarditis

. . . See under *Bacterial endocarditis, isolation of causative agent of.*

Streptomycin, discovery of

SELMAN ABRAHAM WAKSMAN, American microbiologist, 1888- , discovered streptomycin, in

1944. Received the Nobel prize in 1952.

Streptothrix madurae, isolation of

JEAN HYACINTHE VINCENT, French bacteriologist, 1862-1950, isolated the organism *Streptothrix madurae*, in 1894.

Streptothrix muris ratti, isolation of, in rat-bite fever

HUGO SCHOTTMÜLLER, German physician and bacteriologist, 1867-1936, isolated *Streptothrix muris ratti* from patients bitten by rats and demonstrated it to be the cause of rat-bite fever. Recorded in 1914.

Stress, adaptation syndrome to

. . . See under *Adaptation syndrome to stress.*

Stretch reflex, discovery of

CHARLES SCOTT SHERRINGTON, English neurophysiologist, 1857-1952, described the stretch reflex, the reflex contraction of a muscle which has been subjected to passive stretching. Recorded in 1927.

Striated muscle, differentiation of, from smooth

. . . See under *Muscle, smooth and striped,* etc.

Striated muscle, early description of

WILLIAM BOWMAN, English ophthalmologist and anatomist, 1816-1892, described striated muscle, in 1840.

Striated muscle fiber, dark line in center of light band of

WILLIAM M. DOBIE, English anatomist, 1828-1915, described a dark line (actually a membrane) in the center of a light band of a striated muscle fiber. It serves to limit the sarcomere. Reported in 1849. Known as *Dobie's line, Krause's membrane, Amici's disk,* etc.

Striated muscle, sensory innervation of

CHARLES SCOTT SHERRINGTON, English neurophysiologist, 1857-1952, demonstrated the sensory innervation of striated muscle, in 1894.

Stricture of

. . . See under name of part or structure involved.

String operation for relief of esophageal stricture

ROBERT ABBE, American surgeon, 1851-1928, developed the string method treatment for esophageal stricture, reported in 1893, in which a string is passed through the stricture by way of a gastric fistula and the mouth. By pulling the string up and down, the lumen of the stricture is enlarged, so that a bougie may be passed.

Stromuhr, invention of

. . . See under *Blood flow, instrument for measuring velocity of.*

Strong Solution of Iodine

. . . See under *Solution of Iodine, Strong;* etc.

Strophanthus, introduction of, as a medicinal substance

THOMAS RICHARD FRASER, British pharmacologist, 1841-1920, is credited with introducing strophanthus (*Strophanthus kombe* and *Strophanthus hispidus*), a digitalis-like substance, as a medicine, in 1892. Previously strophanthus was known as an arrow poison.

Strümpell's disease

. . . See under *Polioencephalomyelitis*.

Strychnine, discovery of

JOSEPH B. CAVENTOU, French pharmacologist, 1795-1877, with PIERRE J. PELLETIER, French chemist, 1788-1842, isolated the alkaloid strychnine, in 1819.

Subacute bacterial endocarditis, early description of

GEORGE HILARO BARLOW, English physician, 1806-1866, with GEORGE OWEN REES (English physician, 1813-1889), reported a case of subacute bacterial endocarditis, in 1843.

Subacute bacterial endocarditis, palmar and plantar hemorrhagic spots in

THEODORE CALDWELL JANEWAY, American physician, 1872-1917, is credited with describing the hemorrhagic spots or nodes on the soles and palms observed in cases of subacute bacterial endocarditis. Date not available. Known as *Janeway's nodes* or *spots*.

Subacute bacterial endocarditis, renal lesions in

GEORGE BAEHR, American physician, 1887-19??, demonstrated the renal lesions associated with subacute bacterial endocarditis. Published in 1912.

Subacute bacterial endocarditis, *Streptococcus endocarditidis* in

EMANUEL LIBMAN, American cardiologist, 1872-1946, with HERBERT LOUIS CELLER, demonstrated that *Streptococcus endocarditidis* is the most common organism found in cases of subacute bacterial endocarditis. Published in 1910.

Subacute combined degeneration of spinal cord

. . . See under *Spinal cord*.

Subarachnoid space, patency of, in spine

HANS HEINRICH GEORG QUECKENSTEDT, German neurologist, 1876-1918, devised a maneuver to test the patency of the spinal subarachnoid space by compressing the veins in the neck. Published in 1916. Known as *Queckenstedt's sign* or *test*.

Subcallosal gyrus, eponymic description of

EMIL ZUCKERKANDL, Austrian anatomist, 1849-1910, described the gray substance covering the under surface of the rostrum of the corpus callosum, *circa* 1895. Known as gyrus subcallosus or *Zuckerkandl's convolution*.

Subclavian artery, early ligation of—1813

ABRAHAM COLLES, Irish surgeon, 1773-1843, ligated the subclavian artery in 1811 and 1813.

Subclavian artery, early ligation of—1819

GUILLAUME DUPUYTREN, French surgeon, 1777-1835, performed a ligation of the subclavian artery in 1819.

Subconscious and unconscious minds, early work on

RUDOLPH HERMANN LOTZE, German physician, 1817-1881, was an early investigator of the subconscious and unconscious minds. Recorded in 1852.

Sublingual duct, longer and larger, discovery of

CASPAR BARTHOLIN, Danish anatomist, 1655-1738, discovered the longer and larger of the sublingual ducts. Reported in 1685. Known as *duct of Bartholin*.

Sublingual granuloma of infancy

FRANCESCO FEDE, Italian pediatrician, 1832-1913, described a sublingual granuloma occurring in infants during dentition, resulting from abrasion of the frenum linguae by the lower central incisors. Reported in 1890. The same condition was described by ANTONIO RIGA, Italian physician, nineteenth century. Known as *Fede's disease* and *Fede-Riga disease*.

Submaxillary gland duct, eponymic description of

THOMAS WHARTON, English anatomist, 1610-1673, discovered the duct of the submaxillary gland. Recorded in 1656. Known as *Wharton's duct*.

Submaxillary glands, innervation of

KARL FRIEDRICH W. LUDWIG, German physiologist, 1816-1895, studied and demonstrated the innervation of the submaxillary glands. Published in 1851.

Submucous nerve plexus of alimentary tract

. . . See under *Nerve plexus, submucous*, etc.

Subsartorial canal

. . . See under *Canal of Hunter*.

Substantia nigra, eponymic description of

SAMUEL THOMAS SOEMMERRING, German anatomist, 1755-1830, described a region of gray matter dorsal of the basis pedunculi. Recorded in 1798. Known as *Soemmerring's ganglion*.

Subthalamic nucleus, eponymic description of

JULES BERNARD LUYS, French neurologist, 1828-1897, described a nucleus in the hypothalamus, forming a part of the descending pathway from the corpus striatum. Recorded in 1865. Known as *Luys' nucleus, body of Luys, nucleus hypothalamicus*, etc.

Subthalamic region, first clear description of

AUGUSTE HENRI FOREL, Swiss neurologist, 1848-1931, gave the first clear description of the subthalamic region, including the fibers running from the nucleus ruber to the thalamus. Recorded in 1872 and 1877. Known as *campus Foreli*.

Subtrigonal gland

. . . See under *Prostate, subsidiary lobe of*.

Subtrochanteric osteotomy of femur for ankylosis of hip joint

FREDERICK JAMES GANT, English surgeon, 1825-1905, introduced subtrochanteric osteotomy of the femur for ankylosis of the hip joint. Known as *Gant's operation*. Recorded *circa* 1865.

Succinylcholine chloride, clinical use of

H. BRÜCKE, Austrian physician, 19??- , with K. H. GINZEL, H. KLUPP, F. PFAFFENSCHLAGER, and G. WERNER, reported clinical use of succinylcholine chloride, in 1951.

Succinylcholine chloride, introduction of

DANIEL BOVET, French pharmacologist, 19??- , with F. BOVET-NITTI, S. GUARINO, V. G. LONGO, and M. MAROTTA, introduced succinylcholine chloride, a strong inhibitor of neuromuscular transmission. Published in 1949.

Sudeck's atrophy

... See under *Bone atrophy following injury.*

Sudoriparous glands; sweat glands; description of

HERMANN BOERHAAVE, Dutch physician, 1668-1738, was the first to give a good description of the sweat glands or sudoriparous glands. Reported in 1693. Known as *Boerhaave's glands.*

Sudoriparous glands

... See also under *Sweat glands.*

Sugar in diabetic urine is glucose, proof that

MICHEL E. CHEVREUL, French chemist, 1786-1889, investigated the sugar in diabetic urine and proved it to be glucose. Reported in 1815.

Sugar, test solution for; Fehling's solution

... See under *Fehling's solution.*

Suggestion as means of treatment, introduction of

FRANZ ANTON MESMER, German physician, 1734-1815, who popularized the concept of animal magnetism in 1779, may be said to have laid the foundation for the development of suggestion therapy.

Sulcus, hypothalamic; sulcus of Monro

ALEXANDER MONRO, *secundus,* Scottish anatomist, 1733-1817, described the shallow curved sulcus on the wall of the third ventricle of the brain. Published in 1783. Known as *sulcus of Monro.*

Sulfadiazine, clinical application of

MAXWELL FINLAND, American physician, 1902- , with E. STRAUSS and O. L. PETERSON, introduced sulfadiazine into therapeutics. Reported in 1941.

Sulfaguanidine in treatment of bacillary dysentery in children, introduction of

ELI KENNERLY MARSHALL, JR., Baltimore pharmacologist, 1889-19??, with ANDREW C. BRATTON, L. B. EDWARDS, and E. L. WALKER, introduced the use of sulfaguanidine in the treatment of bacillary dysentery in children. Published in 1941.

Sulfaguanidine in treatment of intestinal infections, introduction of

ELI KENNERLY MARSHALL, JR., Baltimore pharmacologist, 1889-19??, with ANDREW C. BRATTON, H. J. WHITE, and J. T. LITCHFIELD, introduced the use of sulfaguanidine in the treatment of intestinal infections. Recorded in 1940.

Sulfamerazine, synthesis of

RICHARD OWEN ROBLIN, American

chemist, 1907-   , with J. H. WILLIAMS, P. S. WINNEK, and J. P. ENGLISH, synthesized sulfamerazine. Recorded in 1940.

Sulfanilamide, first American report on

PERRIN H. LONG, Baltimore physician, 1899-   , is credited with making the first American report on the therapeutic value of sulfanilamide. Published in 1937.

Sulfanilamide, first preparation of

PAUL GELMO, Vienna chemist, 1879-19??, was the first to prepare sulfanilamide, in 1908.

Sulfanilamide in treatment of wounds

NATHAN KENNETH JENSEN, American surgeon, 1910-   , with L. W. JOHNSRUD and M. C. NELSON, used local implantation of sulfanilamide in the treatment of compound fractures. Recorded in 1939.

Sulfapyridine in treatment of pneumonia

GLADYS MARY EVANS, English physician, 19??-   , with WILFRID FLETCHER GAISFORD, introduced sulfapyridine in the treatment of pneumonia. Reported in 1938.

Sulfapyridine in treatment of pneumonia

LIONEL ERNEST HOWARD WHITBY, English pathologist, 1895-   , demonstrated the effectiveness of sulfapyridine in the treatment of pneumonia. Published in 1938.

Sulfasuxidine, clinical application of

EDGAR JACOB POTH, American phy-

sician, 1899-   , with FRANK LOUIS KNOTTS, introduced the use of sulfasuxidine in treatment of gastrointestinal infections. Recorded in 1941.

Sulfathiazole, clinical application of

OTTO GSELL, German physician, 1895-   , is credited with the clinical application of sulfathiazole. Published in 1940.

Sulfhemoglobinemia in United States

T. W. CLARKE, American pediatrician, 1878-19??, is credited with having presented the earliest record of a case of sulfhemoglobinemia in the United States. Published in 1909.

Sulfonal, introduction of

EUGEN BAUMANN, German physician and biochemist, 1846-1896, is credited with introducing sulfonal, in 1886. Also known as sulfonmethane.

Sulfonal, introduction of, in therapeutics

ALFRED KAST, German physician, 1856-1903, is credited with introducing sulfonal in therapeutics. Published in 1888.

Sulfonethylmethane, introduction of

. . . See under *Trional, introduction of.*

Sulfonmethane, introduction of

. . . See under *Sulfonal, introduction of.*

Sulfuric acid, discovery of

VALERIUS CORDUS, German physician and pharmacologist, 1515-1544, is believed to be the discoverer of sulfuric acid, in 1540.

Sulphetrone, introduction of

GLADWIN ALBERT HURST BUTTLE, American biochemist, 1899-   , with T. DEWING, G. E. FOSTER, W. H. GRAY, S. SMITH, and D. STEPHENSON, described sulphetrone, proposed for the treatment of tuberculosis. Published in 1938.

Sulphonal, introduction of

. . . See under *Sulfonal, introduction of.*

Summer prurigo, eponymic description of

JONATHAN HUTCHINSON, English surgeon, 1828-1913, described summer prurigo, a condition marked by intense itching and the development of deep-seated papules, in 1878. Known also as *prurigo aestivalis* and as *Hutchinson's prurigo.*

Sunlight, bactericidal action of

ARTHUR H. DOWNES, English physician, 1851-1938, described the bactericidal action of sunlight and the effect of sunlight on other organisms. Published in 1877.

Sunlight in treatment of extra-pulmonary tuberculosis

AUGUSTE ROLLIER, Swiss physician, 1874-19??, reintroduced the use of sunlight and insolation in the treatment of surgical tuberculosis. Published in 1913. Known as *Rollier's method.*

Sunlight, therapeutic value of

. . . See under *Actinic rays.*

Superficial fascia, superficial layer of, over lower portion of abdomen

PIETER CAMPER, Dutch anatomist, 1722-1789, described the superficial layer of the superficial fascia over the lower part of the abdomen, known as *fascia of Camper.* Recorded *circa* 1770.

Supraclavicular node; signal node

ÉMILE TROISIER, French physician, 1844-1919, described the enlargement of the left supraclavicular lymph node occasionally associated with abdominal tumors. Recorded in 1886. Known as *Virchow-Troisier node* or *gland.*

Suprameatal spine, original description of

FRIEDRICH G. J. HENLE, German anatomist, 1809-1885, described a pointed bony process extending from the temporal bone above and behind the auditory meatus, *circa* 1838. Known as *Henle's spine.*

Suprameatal triangle, eponymic description of

WILLIAM MACEWEN, Scottish surgeon, 1848-1924, described a surgical triangle lying between the lower posterior edge of the root of the zygoma and the superior posterior edge of the external auditory meatus, in 1893. Known as *Macewen's triangle* and *suprameatal triangle.*

Suprapubic cystotomy, first record of

PIERRE FRANCO, French surgeon, 1500-1561, is believed to have performed the first recorded suprapubic cystotomy, in 1556.

**Suprapubic lithotomy,
introduction of**

PIERRE FRANCO, French surgeon,
1500-1561, introduced the method
of suprapubic lithotomy, in 1556.

**Suprarenal capsule, action
of extracts of**

GEORGE OLIVER, English physician, 1841-1915, with E. A. SCHA-
FER, studied the physiologic action
of extracts of the suprarenal capsules and noted the pressor effect.
Recorded in 1894.

**Suprarenal glands, first
description of**

BARTOLOMMEO EUSTACHIUS, Italian anatomist, 1524-1574, is believed to have given the first description of the adrenal glands, in
1564.

**Suramin in treatment of
trypanosomiasis**

. . . See under *Trypanosomiasis*.

Surgery, antiseptic, founder of

JOSEPH LISTER, English surgeon,
1827-1912, is considered the
founder of antiseptic surgery. Early
work published in 1867.

**Surgery, first text on, in
the United States**

JOHN S. DORSEY, American surgeon, 1783-1818, wrote what is
probably the first surgical work in
the United States. Published in
1813.

Surgery, German, Father of

WILHELM FABRY (FABRICIUS HIL-
DANUS), German surgeon, 1560-
1634, is regarded as the Father of
German Surgery.

**Surgical anatomy, first
known treatise on**

GULIELMUS DE SALICETO, Italian
surgeon, 1201-1277, wrote the first
known work on surgical anatomy,
circa 1275.

**Surgical drainage, rubber
tubes in**

. . . See under *Rubber tube drains,*
etc.

**Surgical dressings with
carbolic acid**

. . . See under *Carbolic acid,* etc.

Surgical mask, introduction of

WILLIAM HUNTER, English physician, 1861-1937, is credited with
introducing the use of a gauze surgical mask in the operating room,
in 1900.

**Surgical operations with aid
of hypnotism, early
reports of—1843**

JOHN ELLIOTSON, English surgeon,
1786-1868, reported "numerous
cases of surgical operations without
pain in the mesmeric state," in 1843.
He also noted the antagonism and
remarked upon "the opposition of
many members of the Royal Medical and Chirurgical Society and
others to the reception of the ines-
timable blessings of mesmerism."

**Surgical refrigeration in treat-
ment of traumatized limbs**

FREDERICK MADISON ALLEN,
American physician, 1879-19??, introduced surgical refrigeration in
the treatment of traumatized and
potentially infected limbs. Reported
in 1937.

Surra, trypanosomes in; discovery of

GRIFFITH EVANS, English veterinarian in India, 1835-1935, discovered parasites (*Trypanosoma evansi*) in the blood of horses affected with surra, a disease of horses and other domestic animals in India, China, etc. Published in 1881.

Suspension laryngoscopy, introduction of

GUSTAV KILLIAN, German laryngologist and rhinologist, 1860-1921, introduced suspension laryngoscopy. Recorded in 1912.

Suspensory ligament of eye; suspensory ligament of Lockwood

CHARLES BARRETT LOCKWOOD, English surgeon, 1856-1914, described a thickened area of the orbital fascia between the sheaths of the inferior rectus and the inferior oblique muscles and Tenon's capsule. Published in 1885. Known also as *Lockwood's ligament*.

Suspensory ligament of lens

JOHANN GOTTFRIED ZINN, German anatomist, 1727-1759, described a fibrous ring part of which forms the suspensory ligament of the crystalline lens. Recorded in 1755. Known as *zonule of Zinn, ciliary zonule*, and *zone of Zinn*.

Suspensory ligament of ovary; Clado's band

SPIRO CLADO, French gynecologist, 1856-1905, described the suspensory ligament of the ovary which, covered with peritoneum, is known as *Clado's band*. Recorded *circa* 1892.

Suspensory muscle of duodenum

WENZEL TREITZ, Austrian physician and anatomist, 1819-1872, described muscle fibers sometimes occurring in the suspensory ligament of the duodenum, extending from the right crus of the diaphragm to the duodenojejunal junction. Published in 1857. Known as *Treitz's muscle*.

Sustentacular cells of seminiferous tubules

. . . See under *Seminiferous tubules*.

Sweat glands, early description of—1833

JOHANNES EVANGELISTA VON PURKINJE, Bohemian physiologist, 1787-1869, described the sweat glands and their ducts. Recorded in 1833.

Sweat glands

. . . See also under *Sudoriparous glands*.

Sweating sickness, first English account of

JOHN CAIUS, English physician, 1510-1573, wrote the first English book on the sweating sickness, *"A boke, or conseill against the disease commonly called the sweate, or sweatyng sicknesse."* Published in 1552.

Sweating sickness; miliary fever

EURICIUS CORDUS, German physician and botanist, 1486-1535, gave an early account of an acute infectious disease characterized by fever, sweating, and skin lesions; known as *miliary fever* and *sweating sickness*. Reported in 1529.

Swine plague, discovery of causative organism of

DANIEL ELMER SALMON, American pathologist, 1850-1914, and THEOBALD SMITH (American pathologist, 1859-1934) discovered the causative organism of swine plague, now known as *Salmonella cholerae-suis,* in 1886.

Sycosis barbae, classic description of

JEAN LOUIS ALIBERT, French dermatologist, 1766-1837, gave an account of sycosis barbae in 1825. The condition is also known as *Alibert's mentagra.*

Sycosis barbae, ectothrix causing, description of

DAVID GRUBY, French dermatologist, 1810-1898, is credited with giving the first description of the trichophyton *ectothrix,* the causative agent of sycosis barbae, in 1842.

Sycosis vulgaris, classic description of

JEAN LOUIS ALIBERT, French dermatologist, 1766-1837, gave a classic description of sycosis vulgaris, in 1825.

Sydenham's chorea

. . . See under *Chorea minor.*

Syme's amputation

. . . See under *Ankle joint, Syme's amputation at.*

Sympathectomy, cervical, for exophthalmic goiter

. . . See under *Exophthalmic goiter.*

Sympathectomy for relief of hypertension, introduction of

MATHIEU JABOULAY, French surgeon, 1860-1913, is credited with introducing sympathectomy as treatment for vascular hypertension. Published in 1900.

Sympathetic nervous system, first published figure of

GUIDO GUIDI, Italian physician and anatomist, 1500-1569, wrote a book on anatomy, published posthumously in 1611, which contains the first known published figure of the sympathetic nervous system.

Sympathetic nervous system, introduction of term

JOHN NEWPORT LANGLEY, English physiologist, 1852-1925, introduced the term *sympathetic nervous system,* for the thoracolumbar portion of the autonomic nervous system, in 1905.

Sympathetic ophthalmia, early description of

FRIEDRICH W. E. A. VON GRAEFE, German ophthalmologist, 1828-1870, described sympathetic ophthalmia, in 1866.

Sympathetic ophthalmia, first description of, as a distinct disease

WILLIAM MACKENZIE, Scottish ophthalmologist, 1791-1868, was the first to describe sympathetic ophthalmia as a distinct disease or entity. Recorded in 1830.

Sympathetic outflow and lateral horn cells

CHARLES SCOTT SHERRINGTON, English neurophysiologist, 1857-1952, was first to associate the lateral horn cells with the outflow of sympathetic fibers. Recorded in 1892.

Sympathetic ramisection in treatment of spastic paralysis

NORMAN DAWSON ROYLE, Australian surgeon, 18??-1944, introduced sympathetic ramisection in the treatment of spastic paralysis. Published in 1924.

Sympathetic status, introduction of term

WILLIAM FERDINAND PETERSEN, American pathologist, 1887-19??, introduced the term *sympathetic status, circa* 1923.

Sympathin, discovery and naming of

WALTER BRADFORD CANNON, American physiologist, 1871-1945, demonstrated that the peripheral sympathetic nerve endings are activated by a substance resembling epinephrine, which he named *sympathin*. Reported in 1931.

Symphysiotomy, early advocacy of

PIETER CAMPER, Dutch anatomist, 1722-1789, is said to have advocated symphysiotomy in cases of difficult labor. Date not available.

Symphysiotomy, first successful

JEAN RENÉ SIGAULT, French surgeon, 1740-180?, performed the first successful pubic symphysiotomy. Recorded in 1777. Known as *Sigault's operation*.

Symphysiotomy, popularization of, in Germany

EDUARD CASPAR JACOB VON SIEBOLD, German obstetrician, 1801-1861, is credited with popularizing pubic symphysiotomy for relief of difficult labor, in Germany.

Synapse, introduction of term

CHARLES SCOTT SHERRINGTON, English neurophysiologist, 1857-1952, introduced the term *synapse,* in 1897. It is said that the word was suggested to him by a "Euripidean scholar" named VERRALL.

Syndactylism, operation for correction of

DAVID HAYES AGNEW, American surgeon, 1818-1892, devised a method for the operative correction of webbed fingers. Described in 1883.

Synovectomy, early description of

ALFRED MIGNON, French surgeon, 1854-19??, described synovectomy involving the knee joint. Published in 1899.

Synovial membranes, folds or pads on

CLOPTON HAVERS, English physician and anatomist, 1653-1702, described folds or pads on the surface of synovial membranes, having a secretory or pressure adjusting function, in 1691. Known as *Haversian glands.*

Synovitis, chronic, eponymic description of

BENJAMIN COLLINS BRODIE, English surgeon, 1783-1862, described chronic synovitis associated with pulpy degeneration of the affected structures. Published in 1813 and 1818.

Synovitis, symmetrical, of knee joint, in prenatal syphilis

HENRY HUGH CLUTTON, English surgeon, 1850-1909, is credited with what may be the first description of symmetrical synovitis of the knee joint, associated with congenital syphilis. Published in 1886.

Syphilide, introduction of term

JEAN L. M. ALIBERT, French dermatologist, 1766-1837, described the cutaneous lesion of syphilis and named it *syphilide,* in 1832.

Syphilis and gonorrhea, differentiation between

BENJAMIN BELL, Scottish physician, 1749-1806, is said to have been the first to differentiate between syphilis and gonorrhea. Recorded in 1793.

Syphilis as cause of aneurysm, early suggestion of

AMBROISE PARÉ, French surgeon, 1510-1590, suggested that some forms of aneurysm are caused by syphilis. Recorded in 1575.

Syphilis as cause of aortic aneurysm

SAMUEL WILKS, English physician, 1824-1911, was instrumental in the acceptance of syphilis as a cause of aortic aneurysm. He accomplished this through his work on visceral syphilis. Published in 1863.

Syphilis, bismarsen in treatment of

JOHN HINCHMAN STOKES, American physician, 1885-19??, with STANLEY OWEN CHAMBERS, introduced bismarsen into the treatment of syphilis. Recorded in 1927. Bismarsen was synthesized in 1924 by G. W. RAIZISS.

Syphilis, bismuth in treatment of

FELIX BALZER, French physician, 1849-1929, was the first to use bis-

muth in the treatment of syphilis. Recorded in 1889.

Syphilis, calomel ointment as prophylactic against

ELIE METCHNIKOFF, Russian physiologist in France, 1845-1916, with PIERRE P. E. ROUX, introduced ointment of mild mercurous chloride as a prophylactic against syphilis, in 1903.

Syphilis, causative agent of

FRITZ RICHARD SCHAUDINN, German bacteriologist, 1871-1906, with P. E. HOFFMANN, discovered *Spirochaeta pallida* or *Treponema pallidum,* the causative agent of syphilis, in 1904. Recorded in 1905.

Syphilis, complement fixation test for

AUGUST VON WASSERMANN, German bacteriologist, 1866-1925, with ALBERT NEISSER and CARL BRUCK, developed a specific blood test for the diagnosis of syphilis. Recorded May 10, 1906. Known as the *Wassermann test.* In the same year, LASZLO DETRE, Hungarian pathologist, 1875-1939, developed an almost identical test independently of Wassermann.

Syphilis, dark field in examination for

KARL LANDSTEINER, American pathologist, 1868-1943, with VIKTOR MUCHA (Austrian pathologist, 1877-19??), introduced the dark field method for the detection of the *Treponema pallidum.* Published in 1906.

Syphilis, demonstration of inoculability of

JULIUS BETTINGER, German physician, 1802-1887, demonstrated the inoculability of syphilis. The report of the experiment was published without title and anonymously in 1856.

Syphilis, division of, into three stages

PHILIPPE RICORD, French urologist and dermatologist, 1800-1889, was the first to divide syphilis into three stages, now known as the primary, secondary, and tertiary stages. Published in 1838.

Syphilis, first description of

RODRIGO R. DIAZ DE ISLA, Spanish surgeon, 1462-1542, is believed to have been the first to describe syphilis, which he recognized in members of Columbus's crew, in 1493.

Syphilis, first mention of, in English literature

THOMAS GALE, English surgeon, 1507-1586, is credited with introducing the word *syphilis* into the English language. He used it in his "Certaine Works of Chirurgerie," published in 1563.

Syphilis, heart involvement in

GIOVANNI MARIA LANCISI, Italian physician, 1654-1720, is credited with being the first to describe syphilitic heart disease. Published in 1728.

Syphilis in children, first recorded reference to

SIMON DE VALLAMBERT, French pediatrician, 1512-1576, was the first to record a reference to syphilis in children. Published in 1565.

Syphilis, introduction of term

GIROLAMO FRACASTORO, Italian pathologist, 1483-1553, gave syphilis its name in a poem titled *Syphilis Sive Morbus Gallicus*, published in 1530. The poem recognized the venereal cause of the disease and included most of the knowledge of the time regarding it.

Syphilis, Kolmer's modification of Wassermann's test for

JOHN ALBERT KOLMER, American pathologist, 1886-19??, developed a modification of the Wassermann test for syphilis. Published in 1922. Known as *Kolmer's test*.

Syphilis, microscopic flocculation test for

LOUIS YOLANDO MAZZINI, American serologist, 1894-   , developed a rapid, microscopic flocculation test for syphilis. Recorded in 1939. Known as the *Mazzini test*.

Syphilis, mixed primary lesions of

JOSEPH GRÜNPECK, German physician, 1473-1532, is said to have been the first to describe mixed primary lesions and multiple primary lesions of syphilis. Extant record dated 1496.

Syphilis, neurological manifestations of, early observations on

NICCOLO MASSA, Italian physician, 1499-1569, described the neurological effects of syphilis. Published in 1532.

Syphilis, penicillin in treatment of

JOHN FRIEND MAHONEY, American physician, 1889-19??, with R. C. ARNOLD and A. HARRIS, introduced the use of penicillin in the treatment of early syphilis. Recorded in 1943.

Syphilis, quantitative precipitation test for

REUBEN LEON KAHN, American bacteriologist, 1887-19??, developed a quantitative precipitation test for syphilis. Recorded in 1922. Known as the *Kahn test*.

Syphilis, transmission of, to apes

THEODOR ALBRECHT EDWIN KLEBS, German bacteriologist, 1834-1913, experimented with the transmission of syphilis to animals and succeeded in producing the disease in apes. Reported in 1878.

Syphilis, treatment of, by injection of mercuric chloride

GUIDO BACCELLI, Italian physician, 1832-1916, introduced the use of mercuric chloride by injection in the treatment of syphilis. Reported in 1893.

Syphilis, visceral lesions of

NICOLAUS LEONICENUS, Italian physician, 1428-1524, recognized the fact that syphilis may produce visceral lesions. He also recognized and described a case of syphilitic hemiplegia. Recorded in 1497.

Syphilitic aortitis, early description of—1885

KARL G. P. DOEHLE, German pathologist, 1855-1928, described a form of aortitis now known to be due to syphilis. Recorded in 1885. Called *Doehle-Heller aortitis*.

Syphilitic aortitis, early description of—1899

ARNOLD HELLER, German pathologist, 1840-1913, described aortitis and aortic aneurysm, and established the role of syphilis in the causation of these conditions. Reported in 1899. Known as *Doehle-Heller aortitis*.

Syphilitic aortitis, *Treponema pallidum* in

KARL REUTER, German physician, 1860-19??, was the first to find *Treponema pallidum* in the wall of a syphilitic aorta. Recorded in 1906.

Syphilitic bursitis, eponymic description of

ARISTIDE AUGUSTE STANISLAUS VERNEUIL, French surgeon and anatomist, 1823-1895, described syphilitic disease of the bursae, *circa* 1860. Known as *Verneuil's bursitis* or *disease*.

Syphilitic endarteritis of cerebral vessels, early description of—1868

THOMAS CLIFFORD ALLBUTT, English physician, 1836-1925, reported a case of cerebral disease in a syphilitic patient and called attention to the endarteritis of the cerebral vessels. Published in 1868.

Syphilitic endarteritis of cerebral vessels, early description of—1874

OTTO J. L. HEUBNER, German pediatrician, 1843-1926, gave an accurate description of inflammation of the intima of cerebral vessels due to syphilis. Published in 1874. Called *Heubner's disease*.

Syphilitic hemiplegia, early description of—1497

NICOLAUS LEONICENUS, Italian physician, 1428-1524, gave a good description of syphilitic hemiplegia, in 1497.

Syphilitic infants, nodes on skull of

. . . See under *Nodes on skull of syphilitic infants.*

Syphilitic meningoencephalitis

. . . See under *Paralysis, general,* etc.

Syphilitic pseudoparalysis in infants

JOSEPH PARROT, French physician, 1829-1883, described syphilitic pseudoparalysis in infants due to epiphyseal separation. Published in 1871. Known as *Parrot's disease.*

Syphilitic sailors of Columbus, treatment of

RODRIGO R. DIAZ DE ISLA, Spanish physician, 1462-1542, is credited with treating the syphilitic sailors of Columbus on their return from America. Published in 1542.

Syphilitic spastic spinal paralysis

WILHELM H. ERB, German neurologist, 1840-1921, described a syphilitic form of spastic spinal paralysis, in 1875. Called *Erb's paralysis* and *Erb-Charcot disease.*

Syphilitic symptoms, exacerbation of, after administration of antisyphilitic drugs

KARL HERXHEIMER, German dermatologist, 1861-1944, described the phenomenon of exacerbation in the syphilitic lesions and symptoms sometimes following the administration of antisyphilitic drugs. Reported in 1902. Known as *Herxheimer's reaction* and *Jarisch-Herxheimer reaction.*

Syringe for treatment of lacrimal passages

DOMINIQUE ANEL, French surgeon, *circa* 1679-1730, devised a delicate syringe which he used in treating diseases of the lacrimal passages. Reported in 1713.

Syringe, metal, invention of

. . . See under *Hypodermic syringe,* etc.

Syringomyelia, early description of

WILLIAM WITHEY GULL, English physician, 1816-1890, described syringomyelia in a report titled "Case of progressive atrophy of the muscles of the hands: enlargement of the ventricle of the cord in the cervical region, with atrophy of the gray matter." Published in 1862.

Syringomyelia, first adequate account of

JACOB AUGUSTUS LOCKHART CLARKE, English physician, 1817-1880, with JOHN HUGHLINGS JACKSON, gave the first complete description of syringomyelia. Published in 1867.

Syringomyelia, traumatic, eponymic description of

ROBERT KIENBÖCK, Austrian physician, 1871-1953, described traumatic cavity formation in the spinal cord. Published in 1902. Known as *Kienböck's disease* of the spinal cord.

Syringomyelia with atrophy and paralysis of hands and forearms

AUGUSTIN MARIE MORVAN, French

physician, 1819-1897, described a type of syringomyelia marked by atrophy, analgesic paralysis, and painless ulceration affecting the forearms and hands. Published in 1883. Known as *Morvan's disease* and *analgesic panaris*.

Systolic murmur, apical, in mitral regurgitation

JAMES HOPE, English physician, 1801-1841, described an apical systolic murmur sometimes heard in cases of mitral regurgitation. Reported in 1832. Known as *Hope's murmur*.

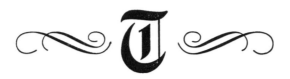

Tabardillo, first description of

FRANCISCO BRAVO, Spanish physician in Mexico, 152?-15??, was the first to describe tabardillo, Spanish or Mexican typhus. Published in 1570. Bravo's book was the first medical book published in the New World.

Tabes dorsalis, classic description of

GUILLAUME BENJAMIN AMAND DUCHENNE DE BOULOGNE, French neurologist, 1806-1875, gave the first classic description of tabes dorsalis. Recorded in 1858 and 1859. Known as *Duchenne's disease.*

Tabes dorsalis, first adequate account of

SIGISMUND EDUARD LOEWENHARDT, German physician, 1796-1875, is credited with giving the first recorded important description of tabes dorsalis. Published in 1817.

Tabes dorsalis, gastric crises of; early description

GEORGES DELAMARRE, French physician, 1831-18??, described the gastric crises of tabes dorsalis. Recorded in 1866.

Tabes dorsalis, joint symptoms in; early description

THOMAS CLIFFORD ALLBUTT, English physician, 1836-1925, described the joint symptoms associated with locomotor ataxia. Published in 1869.

Tabes dorsalis, lightning pains in; first reference

JEAN MARTIN CHARCOT, French neurologist, 1825-1893, with ABEL BOUCHARD, gave the first description of the lightning pains in tabes dorsalis. Recorded in 1866.

Tabes dorsalis, Romberg's sign in

MORITZ HEINRICH ROMBERG, German neurologist, 1795-1873, observed, in 1840, that patients with tabes dorsalis cannot remain standing steady if their eyes are shut and the feet are close together. Published in 1846.

Tabes dorsalis, syphilitic nature of

JEAN ALFRED FOURNIER, French syphilologist, 1832-1914, proposed the view that tabes dorsalis is caused by syphilis. The view was opposed for a time. Recorded in 1876.

Tabes, peripheral and central nervous system forms of

JOSEPH JULES DEJERINE, French neurologist, 1849-1917, is credited with differentiating peripheral tabes from tabes of the central nervous system. Recorded in 1889.

Tabetic arthropathy, original description of

. . . See under *Neurogenic arthropathy.*

Tachycardia, paroxysmal auricular

. . . See under *Auricular paroxysmal tachycardia.*

Tactile nerve endings in submucosa of mouth and tongue

FRIEDRICH SIEGMUND MERKEL, German anatomist, 1845-1919, described tactile corpuscles in the submucous layer of the mouth and tongue, consisting of two flattened epithelial cells containing between the apposed surfaces a biconvex disk which is a continuation of the neurofibrils. Published in 1880. Known as *Merkel's corpuscles* or *disks,* and *tactile disks.*

Tactile nerve endings in tips of fingers and toes

GEORG MEISSNER, German anatomist and physiologist, 1829-1905, with RUDOLPH WAGNER (German physician, 1805-1864), described tactile corpuscles in the dermal papillae of the fingertips and toetips, the external genitalia, the mammae, etc., in 1852. Known as *Wagner's* or *Meissner's corpuscles.*

Taenia echinococcus, experimental infection of dogs with

CARL THEODOR ERNST VON SIE-BOLD, German physician, 1804-1885, was successful in his attempt to infect dogs with *Taenia echinococcus.* Recorded in 1854.

Taenia echinococcus, first accurate description of

KARL GEORG FRIEDRICH RUDOLF LEUCKART, German physician, 1823-1898, gave the first full and accurate description of the morphology and the life history of *Taenia echinococcus.* Published between 1863 and 1876.

Taenzer's disease

. . . See under *Keratosis pilaris,* etc.

Talus, fracture of; eponymic description

FRANCIS J. SHEPHERD, English surgeon, 1851-1929, described a type of fracture involving the lateral process of the talus. Published in 1882. Known as *Shepherd's fracture.*

Talus, posterior process of; eponymic description

LUDWIG STIEDA, German anatomist, 1837-1918, described the posterior process of the talus, *circa* 1870. Known as *Stieda's process.*

Tannic acid in treatment of burns, introduction of

EDWARD CLEMENT DAVIDSON, American surgeon, 1894-1933, introduced tannic acid in the treatment of burns. Published in 1925.

Tannic acid-silver nitrate method for treating burns

ADALBERT G. BETTMAN, American physician, 1883-19??, introduced the tannic acid-silver nitrate method of treating burns. Recorded in 1935.

Tapia's syndrome

. . . See under *Palatopharyngolar-yngeal hemiplegia*.

Tar cancer, experimental pro-duction of, in rabbits

KATSUSABURO YAMAGIWA, Japan-ese physician, 1863-1930, with KOKICHI ICHIKAWA, produced ex-perimental cancer in rabbits by painting their ears with tar. Re-corded in 1916.

Tarchanoff's phenomenon

. . . See under *Psychogalvanic reflex*.

Tardieu's ecchymoses

. . . See under *Ecchymoses under pleura in suffocation*.

Tarin's fascia

. . . See under *Fascia dentata or dentate gyrus*.

Tarsal muscles of Müller

HEINRICH MÜLLER, German anat-omist, 1820-1864, described the in-ferior and superior tarsal muscles, in 1858.

Tarsal navicular bone, osteo-chondrosis of

ALBAN KÖHLER, German physi-cian, 1874-1947, described osteo-chondrosis of the tarsal navicular bone, in 1908. Known as *Köhler's disease* and as *Köhler's tarsal scaphoiditis*.

Tawara's node

. . . See under *Atrioventricular node, first description of*.

Taylor's disease

. . . See under *Skin, idiopathic local-ized atrophy of*.

Tay's choroiditis

. . . See under *Choroiditis guttata senilis, eponymic description of*.

Tectospinal tract, eponymic description of

WILHELM LOEWENTHAL, German physician, 1850-1894, described the tectospinal tract, a descending tract of the spinal cord originating in the tectum of the midbrain. Known as *Loewenthal's tract* or *bundle, pre-dorsal bundle*, etc. Date not avail-able.

Teeth, artificial, early refer-ence to making of

JACQUES GUILLEMEAU, French physician, 1550-1613, was the first to record a reference to the making of artificial teeth, in 1594.

Teeth, classification of, into molars, bicuspids, etc.

JOHN HUNTER, Scottish surgeon in England, 1728-1793, classified the teeth into molars, bicuspids, cus-pids, and incisors. Recorded in 1778.

Teeth, false, first casting of models for

PHILIPPE PFAFF, German dentist, 1715-1767, is credited with being first to describe the casting of models for false teeth. Recorded in 1756.

Teeth, first book on, in United States

RICHARD CORTLAND SKINNER, American dentist, 17??-182?, wrote the first book in America on the structure and diseases of the teeth. Published in 1801.

Teeth, first scientific study of

JOHN HUNTER, Scottish surgeon in

England, 1728-1793, is credited by some as being the first to study the teeth in a scientific manner. Published in 1771.

Teeth, malocclusion of, standard classification for

... See under *Malocclusion*.

Teeth, notched, seen in congenital syphilis

JONATHAN HUTCHINSON, English surgeon, 1828-1913, described notched incisor teeth often seen in congenital syphilis. Reported in 1861. Known as *Hutchinson's teeth*.

Teeth, porcelain, first manufacture of

NICOLAS DUBOIS DE CHÉMANT, French dentist, 1753-1824, was the first to manufacture porcelain teeth. He modified the method suggested by HENRI DUCHÂTEAU in 1776, Published in 1788.

Teeth, porcelain, invention of

HENRI DUCHÂTEAU, French apothecary, 1725-1794, is said to have devised a method for the manufacture of artificial porcelain teeth, in 1776.

Teeth, sound-conducting property of

GIOVANNI FILIPPO INGRASSIA, Italian physician and anatomist, 1510-1580, is credited with discovering the sound-conducting property of the teeth. Published in 1603.

Teichmann's crystals

... See under *Hemin crystals in test for blood*.

Telangiectasis, hereditary hemorrhagic—1876

JOHN WICKHAM LEGG, English physician, 1843-1921, gave the earliest recorded account of multiple hereditary telangiectases, in 1876. Known as *Rendu-Osler-Weber disease*.

Telangiectasis, hereditary hemorrhagic—1896

HENRI JULES LOUIS RENDU, French physician, 1844-1902, described hereditary hemorrhagic telangiectasis, in 1896. Known as *Rendu-Osler-Weber disease*.

Telangiectasis, hereditary hemorrhagic—1901

WILLIAM OSLER, Canadian-English physician, 1849-1919, described "a family form of recurring epistaxis associated with multiple telangiectases of the skin and mucous membranes." Published in 1907. Known as *Rendu-Osler-Weber disease*.

Telangiectasis, hereditary hemorrhagic—1907

FREDERICK PARKES WEBER, English physician, 1863-19??, described "multiple hereditary developmental angiomata of the skin and mucous membranes associated with recurring haemorrhages." Recorded in 1907. Known as *Rendu-Osler-Weber disease*.

Telangiectatic warts

... See under *Angiokeratoma, eponymic description of*.

Teleceptor, introduction of term

CHARLES SCOTT SHERRINGTON, English neurophysiologist, 1857-1952, introduced the term *teleceptor*, to describe a receptor of stimuli from distant objects, as in the case of vision. Published in 1906.

Teleroentgenography, introduction of

ALBAN KÖHLER, German physician, 1874-1947, introduced the method of teleroentgenography of the heart in which the plate is placed about seven feet from the x-ray tube, in order to utilize rays which are more nearly parallel. Recorded in 1905.

Telescope, invention of

GALILEO GALILEI, Italian physicist and astronomer, 1564-1642, is credited with inventing the first scientific telescope, in 1609.

Television phenomenon of Schmidt

. . . See under *Schmidt television phenomenon.*

Telolemma, introduction of term

WILLIE KÜHNE, German physiologist and histologist, 1837-1900, is credited with introducing the term *telolemma,* for the outer covering of the sheath of the neuromuscular end organ. Recorded in 1862.

Telophragma; Z band or disk; Krause's membrane; Dobie's line

. . . See under *Intermediate disk of striated muscle,* and under *Striated muscle fiber.*

Temperature, very low, magnetic method of attaining

WILLIAM F. GIAUQUE, American physical chemist, 1895- , devised the magnetic method for attaining very low temperatures, below one degree absolute. Received the Nobel prize in 1949.

Temporal arteritis, first description of

MAX SCHMIDT, American physician, 1898- , was the first to describe temporal arteritis, in 1930.

Temporal bone, canal in, for chorda tympani nerve

PIERRE CHARLES HUGUIER, French surgeon, 1804-1874, described a canal in the temporal bone which serves as a passage for the chorda tympani nerve, in 1834. Known as *Huguier's canal* and *iter chordae anterius.*

Tender points in course of nerve, in neuralgia

FRANÇOIS LOUIS ISIDORE VALLEIX, French physician, 1807-1855, described tender points along the course of nerves in peripheral neuralgias, marking the place of passage through fascia, etc. Published in 1841. Known as *Valleix's points douloureux.*

Tendon reflex, introduction of term

WILHELM H. ERB, German neurologist, 1840-1921, is believed to have introduced the term *tendon reflex,* circa 1875.

Tendon transplantation, first successful

B. F. PARRISH, American surgeon, 184?-19??, was the first to perform a successful tendon transplantation. Recorded in 1892.

Tendon

. . . See also under name of particular tendon, as *Achilles tendon.*

Tenon's capsule

. . . See under *Eye, fibrous sheath of; eponymic description.*

Tenon's space

. . . See under *Eye, lymph space between Tenon's capsule and.*

Tenosynovitis of muscles of thumb

FRITZ DE QUERVAIN, Swiss surgeon, 1868-1940, described tenosynovitis involving the extensor and abductor muscles of the thumb. Recorded in 1895. Known as *Quervain's disease* and *tendovaginitis stenosans.*

Tensor tarsi muscle, early mention of—1689

JOSEPH G. DUVERNEY, French anatomist, 1648-1730, is credited with having noted the tensor tarsi muscle (later described by HORNER) in 1689.

Tensor tarsi muscle, early mention of—1805

JOHANNES C. ROSENMÜLLER, German anatomist, 1771-1820, is said to have noted the tensor tarsi muscle in 1805.

Tensor tarsi muscle, eponymic description of

WILLIAM EDMONDS HORNER, American anatomist, 1793-1853, gave an accurate description of the tensor tarsi muscle (the pars lacrimalis of the orbicularis oculi), in 1824. Known as the *muscle of Horner.*

Teratology of Fallot, eponymic description of

. . . See under *Heart disease, congenital, marked by a teratology.*

Terry's syndrome

. . . See under *Retrolental fibroplasia.*

Test breakfast of Boas

. . . See under *Boas' breakfast.*

Test meal, early form of

CARL A. EWALD, German physician, 1845-1915, with ISMAR ISIDOR BOAS, German gastroenterologist, 1858-1938, devised a test meal consisting of two slices of dry bread taken with about 10 ounces of water. Recorded in 1885.

Test type in eye examination, introduction of

HEINRICH KÜCHLER, German physician, 1811-1873, introduced the use of test type in the examination of visual acuity. Published in 1843.

Test type, Jaeger's, introduction of

EDUARD JAEGER, Austrian ophthalmologist, 1818-1884, introduced a method for testing the acuteness of central vision by means of type of various sizes. Originated in 1854; published in 1860.

Test type, Snellen, introduction of

HERMANN SNELLEN, Dutch ophthalmologist, 1834-1908, devised a set of type of varying sizes for testing the acuteness of central vision. Recorded in 1862.

Testicle, early classic account of

REGNIER DE GRAAF, Dutch anatomist, 1641-1673, gave a classic description of the testicle, in 1668; at the same time he demonstrated the existence of efferent ductules, now known as *graafian vessels.*

Testicle

. . . See also under name of particular part, as *Epididymis.*

Testicular extract, early use of

CHARLES EDOUARD BROWN-SÉQUARD, English physiologist in France, 1817-1894, injected testicular extract into himself and reported beneficial results. Published in 1889. This experiment represents the first use of male sex hormone.

Testis, appendix of

. . . See under *Hydatid of Morgagni.*

Testis, crystals found in epithelial cells of

OTTO LUBARSCH, German pathologist, 1860-1933, described small crystals occurring in the epithelial cells of the testis; they resemble sperm crystals. Published in 1894. Known as *Lubarsch's crystals.*

Testis, interstitial cells of; earliest description

FRANZ VON LEYDIG, German histologist, 1821-1908, is credited with being first to describe the interstitial cells of the testis, believed to secrete the male sex hormone, in 1850. Known as *Leydig cells* and *Gley's cells.*

Testosterone, synthesis of

ADOLF FRIEDRICH JOHANN BUTENANDT, German biochemist, 1903-, was the first to synthesize testosterone, *circa* 1935.

Testosterone

. . . See also under *Male sex hormone, Testicular extract,* etc.

Tetanus antitoxin, first production of

EMIL ADOLF VON BEHRING, German bacteriologist, 1854-1917, with

SHIBASABURO KITASATO (Japanese bacteriologist, 1852-1931), developed effective tetanus antitoxin. Reported in 1890.

Tetanus bacillus, discovery of

ARTHUR NICOLAIER, German physician, 1862-19??, is credited with the discovery of the tetanus bacillus, in 1884. He did not, however, obtain it in pure culture.

Tetanus bacillus, pure culture of

SHIBASABURO KITASATO, Japanese bacteriologist, 1852-1931, cultivated *Clostridium tetani* in pure culture. Recorded in 1889.

Tetanus, early description of—2nd century

ARETAEUS THE CAPPADOCIAN, Greek physician in Rome, *circa* 81-138 A. D., recognized and left a good description of tetanus. Exact date not available.

Tetanus toxoid, first use of, in man

GASTON RAMON, French bacteriologist, 1885-19??, with CHRISTIAN ZOELLER, was first to use tetanus toxoid in man. Recorded in 1933.

Tetanus transmissibility, demonstration of

ANTONIO CARLE, Italian surgeon, 1854-1927, with G. RATTONE, demonstrated the transmissibility of tetanus, in 1884.

Tetanus, treatment of, by injection of carbolic acid

GUIDO BACCELLI, Italian physician, 1832-1916, introduced a method for treating tetanus by injection of carbolic acid. Reported by Baccelli's assistant, PROF. G. GALLI, in 1906.

Tetany, carpal spasm in
. . . See under *Tetany, Trousseau's sign of*.

Tetany, Chvostek's sign of
FRANTISEK CHVOSTEK, Austrian surgeon, 1835-1884, discovered that in a patient with tetany, tapping of the face in front of the ear produces a spasm of the facial muscles. Recorded in 1876.

Tetany, dihydrotachysterol in treatment of
FRIEDRICH HOLTZ, German surgeon, 1898-   , introduced the use of A.T.10 (dihydrotachysterol in the treatment of tetany. Recorded in 1933.

Tetany, experimental production of, in animals
ANTON F. VON EISELBERG, Austrian surgeon, 1860-1939, produced experimental tetany in animals by means of thyroidectomy. Reported in 1892.

Tetany follows removal of parathyroids, proof that
GIULIO VASSALE, Italian physiologist, 1862-1912, with F. GENERALI, demonstrated that removal of the parathyroid glands is followed by tetany and death. Published in 1896.

Tetany, gastric form of
ADOLF KUSSMAUL, German physician, 1822-1902, described gastric tetany, in 1872. He also described convulsions resulting from dilatation of the stomach.

Tetany, increased irritability of motor nerves in
WILHELM HEINRICH ERB, German neurologist, 1840-1921, discovered the increased electric irritability of motor nerves in tetany. Published in 1873. Known as *Erb's sign*.

Tetany, infant, use of calcium salts in
WALTER HARRIS, English physician, 1647-1732, was probably the first to use calcium salts in the treatment of infantile tetany. Recorded in 1689.

Tetany, infantile, first account of
JOHN CLARKE, English physician, 1761-1815, is believed to have been the first to give an adequate account of infantile tetany. Noted in 1815.

Tetany, **introduction of term**
LUCIEN CORVISART, French physician, 1811-1882, introduced the term *tetany*, in the form of *tétanie*. Published in 1852.

Tetany, parathyroid hormone in treatment of
JAMES BERTRAM COLLIP, Canadian physician and biochemist, 1892-   , with DOUGLAS BURROWS LEITCH, introduced the use of parathyroid hormone in the treatment of tetany. Recorded in 1925.

Tetany, spasm of glottis in
GEORGE KELLIE, Scottish physician, 1777-1846, described the spasm of the glottis in tetany. Recorded in 1816.

Tetany, Trousseau's sign of
ARMAND TROUSSEAU, French physician, 1801-1867, demonstrated that compression of the upper arm in tetany results in carpal spasm. Recorded in 1861. Known as *Trousseau's phenomenon* or *sign*.

Tetany, ultraviolet rays in treatment of

KURT HULDSCHINSKY, German physician, 1883-19??, introduced the use of ultraviolet rays in the treatment of tetany. Recorded in 1920.

Tetraethylthiuram disulfide, introduction of

OLUF MARTENSEN-LARSEN, Norwegian physician, 1902-   , is credited with introducing tetraethylthiuram disulfide (also known as "antabuse") in treating the alcohol habit. The drinking of alcohol after the ingestion of "antabuse" causes nausea and other disagreeable reactions. Recorded in 1948.

Tetralogy of Fallot, eponymic description of

ÉTIENNE LOUIS ARTHUR FALLOT, French physician, 1850-1911, described a form of congenital heart disease marked by dextroposition of the aorta, ventricular septal defects, hypertrophy of the right ventricle, and pulmonary stenosis or atresia. Published in 1888.

Tetralogy of Fallot, pre-eponymic description of

THOMAS BEVILL PEACOCK, English physician, 1812-1882, described a congenital anomaly of the heart marked by pulmonic stenosis, interventricular septal defects, hypertrophy of the right ventricle, and dextroposition of the aorta. Recorded in 1858.

Tetronal, introduction of

EUGEN BAUMANN, German physician and biochemist, 1846-1896, described diethylsulfondiethylmethane or tetronal with reference to its physiologic effect, in 1890.

Texas cattle fever, causative organism of

THEOBALD SMITH, American pathologist, 1859-1934, with F. L. KILBORNE, discovered *Pyrosoma bigeminum,* the causative agent of Texas cattle fever, in 1893. They also proved that the disease is transmitted by the cattle tick *Boöphilus bovis.*

Thalamic syndrome, original description of

JOSEPH J. DEJERINE, French neurologist, 1849-1917, with GUSTAVE ROUSSY (French pathologist, 1874-1948), described the thalamic syndrome, marked by superficial hemianesthesia, mild hemiplegia, hemiataxia, astereognosis, etc., in 1906. Known as *Dejerine-Roussy syndrome.*

Thalassemia

. . . See under *Erythroblastic anemia, familial, in Mediterranean peoples.*

Thebesian valves

. . . See under *Coronary valves, eponymic description of.*

Thebesian veins

. . . See under *Venae cordis minimae.*

Theory of electrolytic dissociation, introduction of

SVANTE AUGUST ARRHENIUS, Swedish physicist and chemist, 1859-1927, introduced the theory of electrolytic dissociation, known as *Arrhenius' theory.* Reported in 1887. Arrhenius received the Nobel prize in 1903.

Theory of inheritance of acquired characteristics

JEAN B. P. LAMARCK, French

naturalist, 1744-1820, promulgated a theory which holds that changes in structure of parts during the life of an individual may be transmitted by heredity to the next generation. Announced in 1801.

Theory of need with regard to organs or parts

JEAN B. P. LAMARCK, French naturalist, 1744-1820, developed a *theory of need* which states that new parts or organs are produced when the need for them exists. Reported in 1801.

Theory of use and disuse of body parts

JEAN B. P. LAMARCK, French naturalist, 1744-1820, proposed a theory which states that the development and power of organs and parts are in direct proportion to their utilization. Recorded in 1801.

Thermal changes involved in muscular activity

. . . See under *Muscle contraction, heat production in.*

Thermo-inhibitory mechanism of body

ISAAC OTT, American physiologist, 1847-1916, described the thermo-inhibitory mechanism of the body, in 1887.

Thermometer, Celsius, introduction of

ANDERS CELSIUS, Swedish astronomer, 1701-1744, invented a thermometer with an interval of 100 degrees between the freezing point and the boiling point of water. Introduced in 1742. Known as the *centigrade thermometer.*

Thermometer, Fahrenheit, invention of

GABRIEL DANIEL FAHRENHEIT, German physicist, 1868-1736, invented an alcohol thermometer in 1709 and a mercury thermometer in 1714. The zero point on this mercury thermometer is the temperature Fahrenheit obtained by mixing snow with sal ammoniac. The boiling point of water is at 212 degrees. Known as *Fahrenheit thermometer* and *scale.*

Thermometer, first recorded clinical use of, in diagnosis

SANTORIUS SANCTORIUS, Italian physician, 1561-1636, described the first use of a thermometer in the diagnosis of disease. Recorded in 1626.

Thermometer, introduction of modern clinical

THOMAS CLIFFORD ALLBUTT, English physician, 1836-1925, is credited with introducing the modern clinical thermometer. Recorded in 1870.

Thermometer, Réaumur's, introduction of

RENÉ ANTOINE FERCHAULT DE RÉAUMUR, French physiologist, 1683-1757, invented a thermometer having an interval of 80 degrees between the freezing point and the boiling point of water, the boiling point being set at 80 degrees. Recorded in 1730.

Thermometry, clinical, first significant work on

GEORGE MARTINE, Scottish physician, 1702-1741, is credited with writing the first significant work on clinical thermometry. Published in 1740.

Thiamine, synthesis of

ROBERT RUNNELS WILLIAMS, American biochemist, 1886-19??, with JOSEPH KALMAN CLINE, synthesized thiamine. Published in 1936.

Thiamine

. . . See also under *Vitamin B-1.*

Thinking-type personality, introduction of concept of

CARL GUSTAV JUNG, Swiss psychiatrist, 1875-19??, introduced the concept of a thinking-type personality, the first of four types of personality; it is the type in which attitudes and actions are determined by thought and deliberation, rather than by feeling, sensation, or so-called intuition. Presented *circa* 1908.

Thiosemicarbazone in tuberculosis

. . . See under *Tuberculosis, thiosemicarbazone in treatment of.*

Third circulation, introduction of term

HARVEY WILLIAMS CUSHING, American neurosurgeon, 1869-1939, suggested the term *third circulation* to designate the cerebrospinal fluid system. Recorded in 1926.

Thirst caused by excision of pancreas

. . . See under *Pancreas, excision of,* etc.

Thomas splint for hip

HUGH OWEN THOMAS, English orthopedist, 1834-1891, devised several kinds of splint, including the *Thomas posterior splint,* used in fracture of the femur and in hip joint disease, and the *Thomas knee splint,* which transfers the weight of the body to the ischium and perineum. Published in 1875.

Thomsen's disease

. . . See under *Myotonia congenita.*

Thomson's fascia

. . . See under *Inguinal ring, external, yellow fibers of.*

Thoracic duct in animals, discovery of

BARTOLOMMEO EUSTACHIUS, Italian anatomist, 1524-1574, is credited with discovering the thoracic duct in animals. Reported in 1552. The record of this finding and of others remained in obscurity for about two centuries.

Thoracic duct in dog, discovery of

JEAN PECQUET, French anatomist, 1622-1674, is credited with the discovery of the thoracic duct in the dog. Recorded in 1651. Known as *Pecquet's duct.*

Thoracic duct in man, discovery of

THOMAS BARTHOLIN, Danish anatomist, 1616-1680, is credited with the discovery of the thoracic duct in man. Recorded in 1652.

Thoracoplasty, early form of, in chronic empyema

JAKOB AUGUST ESTLANDER, Finnish surgeon, 1831-1881, treated chronic empyema by resecting one or more ribs to allow obliteration of the cavity. Reported in 1879. Called *Estlander's operation.*

Thoracoplasty in the United States

GEORGE R. FOWLER, American surgeon, 1848-1906, treated a case of fibrous growth in the chest by thoracoplasty. Recorded in 1893.

Thoracoplasty, performance of first radical

LUDOLPH BRAUER, German surgeon, 1865-1951, is said to have performed the first radical thoracoplasty. Published in 1908.

Thoracoscope, invention of

HANS CHRISTIAN JACOBAEUS, Swedish surgeon, 1879-1937, used the cystoscope in examining various cavities of the body, especially the endopleural space, and thus invented the thoracoscope. Reported in 1910.

Thoracotomy for empyema, early application of

ERNST G. F. VON KÜSTER, German surgeon, 1839-1930, treated a case of empyema by means of thoracotomy. Recorded in 1889.

Thorax, planes used as landmarks in topography of

. . . See under *Planes used as landmarks*.

Thorium dioxide in radiological technique

MITSUTOMA OKA, Japanese radiologist, 1889-19??, is credited with introducing thorotrast or thorium dioxide in radiological procedures. Recorded in 1929. See also under *Thorotrast*.

Thorium, discovery of

JÖNS JAKOB BERZELIUS, Swedish chemist, 1779-1848, discovered the element thorium in thorite, in 1828.

Thorotrast, first use of, in arteriography

REYNALDO DOS SANTOS, Portuguese surgeon and radiologist, 1880-19??, with J. CALDAS, introduced thorium dioxide or thorotrast in arteriography. Reported in 1931. See also under *Thorium dioxide*.

Thromboangiitis obliterans, early description of—1876

CARL FRIEDLANDER, German pathologist, 1847-1887, is believed to have been first to describe thromboangiitis obliterans ("arteritis obliterans"), in 1876.

Thromboangiitis obliterans, eponymic description of

LEO BUERGER, American physician, 1879-1943, gave a clear description of thromboangiitis obliterans. First published in 1908. Known as *Buerger's disease*.

Thrombopenic purpura, early description of—1735

PAUL GOTTLIEB WERLHOF, German physician, 1699-1767, gave an early description of thrombopenic purpura, also known as *essential thrombopenia, Werlhof's disease*, etc., in 1735.

Thrombopenic purpura, early description of—1915

ALFRED E. FRANK, German physician, 1884-19??, described essential thrombopenia or thrombopenic purpura, in 1915. Known also as *purpura haemorrhagica, pseudo-hemophilia, Werlhof's disease*, etc.

Thrombosis and embolism, first adequate description of

RUDOLF LUDWIG KARL VIRCHOW,

German pathologist, 1821-1902, is credited with giving the first comprehensive description of thrombosis and embolism. Recorded between 1846 and 1853.

Thrush, *Candida albicans* in, discovery of

DAVID GRUBY, French dermatologist, 1810-1898, discovered the organism *Candida albicans* in thrush. Reported in 1842. The organism was discovered earlier and independently by LANGENBECK and BERG. See under *Candida albicans*.

Thrush, early description of

MICHAEL UNDERWOOD, English physician, 1737-1820, described aphthae or thrush, in his *Treatise on the diseases of children*. Published in 1784.

Thrush

. . . See also under *Candida Albicans*.

Thymine, discovery of

ALBRECHT KOSSEL, German physiologist, 1853-1927, with H. STEUDEL, discovered thymine. Recorded in 1900.

Thymol as hookworm vermifuge, introduction of

CAMILLO BOZZOLO, Italian physician, 1845-1920, is believed to have been the first to suggest the use of thymol as vermifuge in ancylostomiasis, in 1879.

Thymus, abscess of, in congenital syphilis

PAUL DU BOIS, French obstetrician, 1795-1871, described multiple foci of necrosis in the thymus of infants with congenital syphilis. Reported in 1850.

Thymus, concentrically striated bodies in

ARTHUR HILL HASSALL, English physician and chemist, 1817-1894, described the small concentrically striated epithelial remains found in the thymus. Recorded in 1846. Known as *Hassall's corpuscles*.

Thymus, early description of

BERENGARIUS OF CAPRI, Italian anatomist, 1480-1550, gave an accurate description of the thymus, in 1522.

Thymus, fatal hypertrophy of

FELIX PLATTER, Swiss physician, 1536-1614, is said to have been the first to record a case of death from hypertrophy of the thymus, in an infant. Published in 1614.

Thyroglossal duct, fetal, original description of

WILHELM HIS, *père*, Swiss anatomist and embryologist, 1831-1904, was first to describe the fetal thyroglossal duct. Published in 1901.

Thyroid artery, deep

. . . See under *Artery, deep thyroid*.

Thyroid deficiency is accompanied by reduced metabolic activity

ADOLF MAGNUS-LEVY, German physiologist in the United States, 1865-1955, established the fact that thyroid deficiency is associated with reduced metabolic activity and that the condition may be relieved by the administration of desiccated thyroid. Published in 1895.

Thyroid extract, early successful use of, in myxedema

GEORGE REDMAYNE MURRAY, English physician, 1865-1939, treated myxedema by hypodermic injections of thyroid extract of a sheep, with "highly successful results." Published in 1891.

Thyroid gland, atrophy of, with myxedema

WILLIAM W. GULL, English physician, 1816-1890, described the condition of myxedema with atrophy of the thyroid gland, in 1874. Known as *Gull's disease.*

Thyroid gland, introduction of name

THOMAS WHARTON, English anatomist, 1610-1673, introduced the term *thyroid gland,* in 1656.

Thyroid gland, organic iodine in

. . . See under *Iodine in thyroid gland.*

Thyroid gland, pyramidal lobe of

PIERRE LALOUETTE, French physician, 1711-1792, described an inconstant third lobe of the thyroid gland, arising usually on the left side. Published in 1743. Known as *Lalouette's pyramid.*

Thyroid gland, transplantation of, in cretinism

ODILON MARC LANNELONGUE, French surgeon, 1840-1911, transplanted the thyroid gland from an animal to a human being, for the relief of cretinism. Recorded in 1890.

Thyroidectomy, experimental, with transplantation

J. MORITZ SCHIFF, German physiologist, 1823-1896, reported, in 1859, experimental thyroidectomies which proved fatal. Later, in 1884, Schiff followed his thyroidectomies with intra-abdominal transplantation of the gland, a procedure which saved the experimental animals.

Thyroidectomy, first recorded

JOSEPH HENRY GREEN, English surgeon, 1791-1863, is credited with performing the first recorded thyroidectomy, on June 13, 1829. Green removed the right lobe of the gland; the patient died 15 days after the operation.

Thyroidectomy for exophthalmic goiter, first performance of

LUDWIG REHN, German surgeon, 1849-1930, performed the first recorded operation for the removal of the thyroid in exophthalmic goiter, in 1880. Recorded in 1884.

Thyroidectomy in treatment of angina pectoris

HERMAN LUDWIG BLUMGART, American physician, 1895-   , with S. A. LEVINE and D. D. BERLIN, treated congestive heart failure and angina pectoris by thyroidectomy. Recorded in 1933.

Thyroidectomy, symptoms following; first record of

PAUL SICK, German surgeon, 18??-19??, is credited with being the first to note and record the symptoms following total thyroidectomy. Published in 1867.

Thyroiditis, chronic or ligneous

BERNHARD MORITZ CARL LUDWIG RIEDEL, German surgeon, 1846-1916, described a form of chronic inflammation of the thyroid, in

1896. Known as *Riedel's disease* or *struma*.

Thyroprivia

. . . See under *Thyroidectomy, symptoms following,* etc.

Thyroxine, chemical structure of

CHARLES ROBERT HARINGTON, English biochemist, 1897-   , determined the molecular structure of thyroxine. Published in 1926.

Thyroxine, crystalline, isolation of

EDWARD CALVIN KENDALL, American physiologist and chemist, 1886-19??, isolated crystalline thyroxine on December 25th, Christmas Day, in 1914.

Thyroxine is a derivative of tyrosine

CHARLES ROBERT HARINGTON, English biochemist, 1897-   , demonstrated that thyroxine is a derivative of tyrosine. Published in 1926.

Thyroxine, synthesis of

CHARLES ROBERT HARINGTON, English biochemist, 1897-   , with GEORGE BARGER, synthesized thyroxine. Recorded in 1927.

Tibial tuberosity, painful lesions of—1903

ROBERT BAYLEY OSGOOD, American orthopedic surgeon, 1873-19??, described painful lesions of the tibial tuberosity in children and adolescents. Recorded in 1903. Known as *Osgood-Schlatter disease* and *osteochondrosis of tuberosity of tibia.*

Tibial tuberosity, painful lesions of—1903

CARL SCHLATTER, Swiss surgeon,

1864-1934, described the painful lesions of the tibial tuberosity previously reported by R. B. OSGOOD. Published in 1903. Known as *Osgood-Schlatter disease.*

Tick responsible for Rocky Mountain spotted fever

JOHN F. ANDERSON, American physician, 1873-19??, described tick fever (spotted fever) of the Rocky Mountains and the tick responsible for it, now called *Dermacentor andersoni,* in 1903.

Tietze's disease

. . . See under *Rib cartilages, non-suppurative swelling of.*

Tigroid bodies

. . . See under *Nerve cells, Nissl bodies of.*

Tinctures, introduction of, into medical use

ARNOLD OF VILLANOVA, French physician and alchemist in Spain, *circa* 1235-1312, is believed to have introduced tinctures and medicated wines into the armamentarium of medicine. Date not available.

Tinea cruris, first description of

FRIEDRICH WILHELM FELIX VON BÄRENSPRUNG, German dermatologist, 1822-1864, gave the first description of tinea cruris, in 1855. Known as *eczema marginatum* and as *Bärensprung's disease.*

Tinea cruris, fungous origin of, first recognition

MARIE G. A. DEVERGIE, French dermatologist, 1798-1879, was the first to recognize and demonstrate the fungous cause of tinea cruris, an epidermomycosis affecting chiefly the inguinocrural region and sometimes the submaxillary or axillary folds. The causative agent is a species of *Epidermophyton.* Described *circa* 1857. Known also as *eczema marginatum, tinea circinata cruris, epidermophytosis cruris, trichophytosis cruris, red flap,* and *jockey-strap itch.*

Tinea imbricata, first description of

GEORGE ALEXANDER TURNER, Scottish physician, 1845-1900, was the first to describe tinea imbricata, a severe form of ringworm occurring in tropical countries. Published in 1869-70. The condition was described later, in 1898, by PATRICK MANSON, Scottish parasitologist, 1844-1922.

Tinea nigra, first description of

PATRICK MANSON, Scottish parasitologist, 1844-1922, was the first to describe tinea nigra, a form of tinea caused by *Cladosporium mansoni* and characterized by blackness of the affected parts. Recorded in 1898. Known as *pityriasis nigra* and *microsporosis nigra.*

Tinea nodosa

. . . See under *Trichorrhexis nodosa.*

Tinea tonsurans, causative agent of

. . . See under *Microsporum audouini.*

Tissue, cultivation of, in vitro

. . . See under *Cultivation of tissue in vitro.*

Tissues produce carbon dioxide and consume oxygen

LAZARO SPALLANZANI, Italian physiologist, 1729-1799, discovered that living tissue consumes oxygen and liberates carbon dioxide. Published posthumously in 1804.

Tobacco mosaic virus, isolation of

WENDELL MEREDITH STANLEY, American biochemist, 1904-   , isolated the virus of tobacco mosaic disease in crystalline form and demonstrated that it is a nucleoprotein. Recorded in 1935.

Tobey-Ayer test

. . . See under *lateral sinus thrombosis, pressure test for.*

Tocograph for recording uterine contractions

SANDOR LORAND, Hungarian gynecologist, 1892-   , invented a tocograph for the purpose of recording uterine contractions through the anterior abdominal wall. Published in 1936. Known as *Lorand's tocograph.*

Toe, big, extension of, on stimulation of sole

. . . See under *Babinski toe reflex or sign.*

Toe, great, normal line of

GEORG HERMANN VON MEYER, Swiss anatomist, 1815-1892, stated that the line of the great toe when extended backward will pass through the center of the heel in the normal foot. This condition is said to prevail if no shoes have ever been worn. Recorded in 1858. Known as *Meyer's line.*

Toes, dorsal flexion of, when dorsum of foot is tapped

KURT MENDEL, German neurologist, 1874-1946, demonstrated that in health percussion of the dorsum of the foot causes dorsal flexion of the second to the fifth toes. In certain disorders, as diseases of the pyramidal tracts, the flexion of the toes is plantar. Recorded in 1904. Known as *dorsocuboidal reflex, cuboidodigital reflex, Mendel's dorsal reflex of the foot, Bechterev-Mendel reflex,* etc.

Tomography, first description of

D. L. BARTELINK, German physician, 1901- , was the first to describe body section roentgenography, known as tomography, laminography, planigraphy, etc., in 1933.

Tongue, cancer of, early report concerning

ALEXANDER READ, English surgeon, 158?-1641, reported a case of lingual cancer, in 1635.

Tongue, glands near tip of, early description of

. . . See under *Glands near tip of tongue.*

Tongue, radical excision of, for carcinoma

EMIL THEODOR KOCHER, Swiss surgeon, 1841-1917, devised and performed an operation for radical excision of the tongue in a case of carcinoma. Recorded in 1880.

Tongue, serous and albuminous glands in back part of

VICTOR VON EBNER, Austrian histologist, 1842-1925, described serous and albuminous glands in the back part of the tongue, communicating with the circumvallate papillae. Published in 1873. Known as *Ebner's glands.*

Tonsillar ring of Waldeyer

. . . See under *Ring of adenoid tissue formed by tonsils,* etc.

Tonsillectomy by blunt dissection, introduction of

GEORGE ERNEST WAUGH, English surgeon, 1875-1940, is credited with introducing the method of blunt dissection for tonsillectomy. Recorded in 1909.

Tonsillectomy in which capsule is also removed

GREENFIELD SLUDER, American laryngologist, 1865-1928, is credited with introducing the method of tonsillectomy in which both the tonsil and its capsule are excised. Recorded in 1911.

Tonsillectomy, reverse guillotine method of

SAMUEL SHORT WHILLIS, English surgeon, 1870-1953, with FREDERICK CHARLES PYBUS, introduced the reverse guillotine method of tonsillectomy, in 1909.

Tonsillotome, introduction of modern

PHILIP SYNG PHYSICK, American surgeon, 1768-1837, invented a tonsillotome which was the precursor of the modern instrument. Recorded in 1828.

Tonsils as portals of entry for infection

ABRAHAM BUSCHKE, German physician, 1868-1943, called attention to the tonsils as portals of entry for infection. Reported in 1894.

Tooth enamel, concentric lines in

MAGNUS GUSTAF RETZIUS, Swedish histologist, 1842-1919, described microscopical concentric lines seen in sections of tooth enamel, denoting successive layers of adamantation or enamel formation. Recorded in 1873. Known as *lines of Retzius*.

Tooth fillings of inorganic materials, reference to

JACQUES GUILLEMEAU, French physician, 1550-1613, is credited with being the first to suggest the use of inorganic material for tooth fillings. Recorded in 1594.

Tooth, nerve of, arsenic paste used to devitalize

. . . See under *Paste for devitalizing nerve of a tooth*.

Topinard's angle

. . . See under *Ophryospinal angle*, etc.

Topinard's line

. . . See under *Line between mental point and glabella*.

Torcular Herophili

. . . See under *Sinuses, confluence of*.

Tornwaldt's bursitis

. . . See under *Pharyngeal bursa, chronic inflammation of*.

Torticollis, division of spinal accessory nerve in

WILLIAM WILLIAMS KEEN, American surgeon, 1837-1932, treated spastic torticollis by division of the spinal accessory nerve and the posterior roots of the upper three spinal nerves. Recorded in 1891.

Torticollis, section of sternocleidomastoid muscle in

GUILLAUME DUPUYTREN, French

surgeon, 1777-1835, was the first to treat torticollis by subcutaneous division of the sternocleidomastoid muscle. Performed on January 16, 1822. Recorded in 1823 and 1839.

Torula histolytica infection in man

JAMES LEAVITT STODDARD, American pathologist, 1889-19??, with ELLIOTT CARR CUTLER, described torulosis in man, due to infection with *Torula histolytica* (*Cryptococcus neoformans*), in 1916.

Tourniquet, block-type

FABRIZ VON HILDEN, German surgeon, 1560-1634, introduced a form tourniquet in which a block of wood was placed under a bandage, *circa* 1605.

Tourniquet, block-type, improved

ETIENNE J. MOREL, French army surgeon, 1648-171?, improved the block-type tourniquet of Hilden by incorporating spring tension. Introduced *circa* 1674.

Tourniquet, early reference to

LORENZ HEISTER, German surgeon, 1683-1758, described several kinds of tourniquet used in his day. Published in 1718.

Tourniquet, rubber, for expelling blood

JOHANNES FRIEDRICH AUGUST VON ESMARCH, German surgeon, 1823-1908, devised a rubber tourniquet or bandage applied to a limb from the distal end upward, in order to express the blood. Recorded in 1869.

Tourniquet, screw-type, introduction of

JEAN LOUIS PETIT, French surgeon,

1674-1750, introduced the screw-type tourniquet. Recorded in 1705.

Toxoid, diphtheria, first preparation of

. . . See under *Diphtheria toxin, modification of, with formaldehyde.*

Toxoplasma, discovery of, by Nicolle

CHARLES JULES HENRI NICOLLE, French bacteriologist, 1866-1936, is credited with discovering a genus of sporozoa, parasitic upon mammals, birds, and man, causing various diseases, as encephalopathy, splenomegaly, etc. Published in 1908.

Toxoplasma in North America, existence of

ALBERT BRUCE SABIN, American bacteriologist, 1906-   , demonstrated the existence of *Toxoplasma* in North America. Reported, with P. K. OLITSKY, in 1937.

Toynbee's corpuscles

. . . See under *Corneal corpuscles.*

Trachea, local application to

HORACE GREEN, American laryngologist, 1802-1866, is credited with being the first to attempt local application of medicinal substances to the trachea. The degree of success attained is questioned by some. Recorded in 1846.

Tracheal tugging as sign of aortic aneurysm

ANTONIO CARDARELLI, Italian physician, 1831-1926, described the sign of tracheal tugging observed in aortic aneurysm. Known as *Cardarelli's sign.* Date not available.

Tracheo-bronchoscopy, development of

CHEVALIER JACKSON, American surgeon, 1865-   , devised techniques and instruments for use in tracheo-bronchoscopy. Early report published in 1907.

Tracheotomy, early successful, for diphtheria

PIERRE FIDÈLE BRETONNEAU, French physician, 1778-1862, is credited with the performance of a successful tracheotomy for diphtheria, on July 1, 1825.

Tracheotomy, early successful, for quinsy

PEDRO VIRGILI, Spanish surgeon, 1699-1776, performed a successful tracheotomy for quinsy, at Cadiz, in 1743.

Tracheotomy, first mention of

ASCLEPIADES OF BITHYNIA, Greek physician, 128-56 B. C., is believed to have been the first to mention tracheotomy. Exact date not available.

Tracheotomy in England, first practice of

GEORGE MARTINE, Scottish physician, 1702-1741, is credited with being the first in Britain to perform tracheotomy in cases of diphtheria. Published in 1730.

Trachoma, cytoplasmic inclusion bodies in

LUDWIG HALBERSTAEDTER, German physician, 1876-19??, with STANISLAS JOSEF MATHIAS VON PROWAZEK (Polish zoologist in Hamburg,

1876-1915), described the inclusion bodies found in the epithelial cells of the conjunctiva, in trachoma. Published in 1907. Known as *Prowazek's bodies, Prowazek-Halberstaedter bodies.*

Trachoma, granular form of, classic description of

CARL FERDINAND VON ARLT, Vienna ophthalmologist, 1812-1887, described a granular form of trachoma, known as *Arlt's trachoma,* in 1854-56.

Trachoma, isolation of *Bacillus granulosis* from

. . . See under *Bacillus granulosis, isolation of,* etc.

Trachoma, recognition of contagiousness of

DOMINIQUE JEAN LARREY, French army surgeon, 1766-1842, is credited with being the first to recognize and point out the contagiousness of trachoma. Recorded in 1802.

Trachoma, virus filtration of

CHARLES JULES HENRI NICOLLE, French physician, 1866-1936, with L. BLAISOT and A. CUÉNOD, reported filtration of the trichoma virus. Published in 1912.

Tractors to draw out inflammation and allay pain

ELISHA PERKINS, American physician, 1741-1799, devised a kind of metallic tractors which were alleged to draw out inflammation and allay pain when drawn over the diseased structure. Exposed as worthless. Reported in 1796. Known as *Perkins' tractors.*

Tractus spinocerebralis dorsalis, description of

. . . See under *Fasciculus cerebellospinalis.*

Transferability of hypersensitiveness by intradermal injection

. . . See under *Hypersensitiveness, local, production of.*

Transfusion of blood, direct, from one animal to another

RICHARD LOWER, English physician, 1631-1691, is credited with being first to transfuse blood directly from one animal to another, in 1665.

Transfusion of blood from animal to human being

JEAN BAPTISTE DENIS, French physician, 16??-1704, performed the first recorded transfusion of blood from an animal, a lamb, to a human being, on June 15, 1667.

Transfusion of blood

. . . See also under *Blood transfusion.*

Transfusion of fluids by way of bone marrow

LEANDRO MAUES TOCANTINS, American physician, 1901-   , demonstrated a method for transfusing fluids by way of the bone marrow. Published in 1940.

Translation of Greek medical terms into Latin, first

The first translation of Greek medical terms into Latin was contained in *De Medicina,* medical manuscripts of AULUS CORNELIUS CELSUS, Roman physician and author, *circa* 53 B.C.-7 A.D., discovered in 1443.

Transplantation of arteries

. . . See under *Arteries can be transplanted*, etc.

**Transposition of viscera,
early report on**

MATTHEW BAILLIE, English physician, 1761-1823, described a case of "remarkable" transposition of the viscera, in a paper published in 1788.

Transpyloric plane or line

CHRISTOPHER ADDISON, English anatomist, 1869-1951, described a horizontal plane or line, at the level of the second lumbar vertebra, at which the pylorus usually lies. Recorded in 1899.

**Transuranium elements, discovery
and creation of**

EDWIN M. McMILLAN, American physicist, 1907-   , with GLENN THEODORE SEABORG, American chemist, 1912-   , discovered and created transuranium elements. Both shared the Nobel prize in chemistry, in 1951.

**Transurethral fulguration of
urinary bladder tumors**

EDWIN BEER, American surgeon, 1876-1938, performed the first transurethral fulguration of neoplasms of the urinary bladder, a procedure which led the way to transurethral surgery of the prostate. Reported in 1910.

**Transverse humeral ligament,
eponymic description of**

CHARLES GORDON BRODIE, Scottish anatomist, 1869-1929, described the transverse humeral ligament. Published in 1892. Known as *Brodie's ligament*.

Traube-Hering waves

. . . See under *Vasoconstrictor center, variations in tone of*.

Traumatic infections, bacterial nature of

ROBERT KOCH, German bacteriologist, 1843-1910, established the fact that traumatic infections are caused by bacteria. Recorded in 1878.

**Traumatic spondylitis, eponymic
description of**

. . . See under *Vertebra, compression fracture of*.

Treatment of

. . . See under name of condition, disease, etc.

Treitz's fossa

. . . See under *Duodenal fossa, inferior*.

Treitz's hernia

. . . See under *Hernia, retroperitoneal, through duodenojejunal fossa*.

Treitz's ligament

. . . See under *Ligament extending from duodenojejunal junction to crus of diaphragm*.

Treitz's muscle

. . . See under *Suspensory muscle of duodenum*.

**Tremor, essential;
Minor's tremor**

LAZAR SALOMOVITCH MINOR, Russian neurologist, 1855-19??, described an essential, familial tremor aggravated by emotion and action, usually beginning in childhood. Date of publication not available. Known as *Minor's tremor*.

Tremor, hysterical and volitional

HENRI JULES LOUIS RENDU, French physician, 1844-1902, described a form of hysterical tremor precipitated or aggravated by volitional movements, in 1888. Known as *Rendu's tremor*.

Tremor in exophthalmic goiter

. . . See under *Exophthalmic goiter, tremor in*.

Trench fever, early description of

JOHN HENRY PORTEUS GRAHAM, English physician, 1878-19??, was the first to report a case of trench fever, under the name of "relapsing febrile illness." Published in 1915.

Trench fever, eponymic description of

HEINRICH WERNER, German physician, 1874-1946, described trench fever, in 1916. Known as *Werner's syndrome*. The condition was described in the same year by WILHELM HIS, JR., (German physician, 1863-1934), and is known also as *Werner-His disease*.

Trench fever, introduction of term

GEORGE HERBERT HUNT, English physician, 1884-1926, with ALLAN COATS RANKIN, introduced the term *trench fever*, in a paper published in 1915.

Trench foot, first description of

DOMINIQUE JEAN LARREY, French army surgeon, 1766-1842, was the first to record the condition known as trench foot. Published in 1812.

Trendelenburg's position on operating table

FRIEDRICH TRENDELENBURG, German surgeon, 1844-1924, introduced the placing of a patient on a tilted operating table with the head at the lower end and the legs hanging over the upper end. Recorded in 1890.

Trendelenburg's test for efficacy of valves in varicose veins

. . . See under *Varicose veins, test for insufficiency of*, etc.

Treponema pallidum from a case of paralytic dementia

HIDEYO NOGUCHI, Japanese bacteriologist in America, 1876-1928, isolated the *Treponema pallidum* from a case of paralytic dementia, proving the relation with syphilis. Recorded in 1913.

Treponema pallidum in pure culture

HIDEYO NOGUCHI, Japanese bacteriologist in America, 1876-1928, obtained the *Treponema pallidum* in a pure culture, in 1911.

Treponema pallidum (Spirochaeta pallida), discovery of

. . . See under *Syphilis, causative agent of*, etc.

Triangle, anatomic, limited by rectus muscle, deep epigastric, and Poupart's ligament

FRANZ CASPAR HESSELBACH, German surgeon and anatomist, 1759-1816, described an anatomic triangle bounded by the border of the rectus abdominis muscle, the medial half of the inguinal ligament, and the deep inferior epigastric vessels. Published in 1806. Known as *Hesselbach's triangle.*

Triangle formed by border of rectus muscle and inguinal fold

PHILIPP JAKOB W. HENKE, German anatomist, 1834-1896, described an anatomical triangle formed by the lateral border of the rectus abdominis muscle and the inguinal fold. Reported in 1878. Known as *Henke's triangle.*

Triangle formed by lines uniting alveolar point with basion and nasion

JULES ASSÉZAT, French anthropologist, 1832-1876, described an anatomical triangle bounded by the lines joining the basion, the nasion, and the alveolar point. Introduced *circa* 1865.

Triangle, lumbar; Petit's triangle

JEAN LOUIS PETIT, French surgeon, 1674-1750, described an anatomical triangle in the lumbar region, bounded by the external oblique muscle, the iliac crest, and the latissimus dorsi muscle. Recorded in his work published in 1774. It is said to have been observed by Petit in 1705.

Triangle of vagina corresponding to trigonum vesicae

KAREL J. PAWLIK, Prague gynecologist, 1849-1914, described an anatomical triangle on the anterior vaginal wall which corresponds to the trigonum vesicae lieutaudi. Recorded in 1886. Known as *Pawlik's triangle.*

Triangular space above manubrium, between layers of cervical fascia

ALLAN BURNS, Scottish physician and anatomist, 1781-1813, described the triangular space just above the manubrium and between the layers of the deep cervical fascia, which transmits the anterior jugular vein. Reported in 1811.

Tribromethanol, experimental use of

FRITZ EICHHOLTZ, German physician, 1889-19??, experimented with the use of tribomethanol as a rectal anesthetic. Recorded in 1927.

Tribromethanol, first clinical use of

OTTO BUTZENGEIGER, German physician, 1885-19??, is credited with the first clinical use of avertin. He reported his findings in 1927.

Tribromethanol, first suggestion of

RICHARD WILLSTÄTTER, German biochemist, 1872-19??, was probably the first to suggest the use of tribromethanol as an anesthetic, in 1923.

Tribromethanol, intravenous use of

MARTIN KIRSCHNER, German physician, 1879-1942, used tribromethanol intravenously. Recorded in 1929.

Trichina spiralis, discovery of

JAMES PAGET, English surgeon, 1814-1899, is credited with the discovery of *Trichina spiralis* while he was still a student. It is said that he took specimens to RICHARD

OWEN (English physician, 1804-1892) who described the organisms in 1834.

Trichinella spiralis, discovery of, in the hog

JOSEPH LEIDY, American physician, 1823-1891, is credited with discovering *Trichinella spiralis* in a hog. Recorded in 1846.

Trichiniasis, muscular and intestinal forms of

FRIEDRICH ALBERT ZENKER, German pathologist, 1825-1898, was the first to describe the intestinal and muscular forms of trichiniasis, in 1860.

Trichiniasis, eosinophilia in—1897

WILLIAM SYDNEY THAYER, American physician, 1864-1932, described the occurrence of eosinophilia in trichiniasis. Published in 1897.

Trichiniasis, eosinophilia in—1898

THOMAS RICHARDSON BROWN, American physician, 1872-19??, demonstrated the presence of eosinophilia in trichiniasis. Recorded in 1898.

Trichlorethylene, discovery of

E. FISCHER, German chemist, 1829-189?, is credited with discovering trichlorethylene. Published in 1864.

Trichlorethylene in clinical use

CECIL STRIKER, American anesthesiologist, 1897-   , with S. GOLDBLATT, I. S. WARM, and D. E. JACKSON, reported the results of clinical experience with 300 cases of trichlorethylene analgesia and anesthesia. Recorded in 1935.

Trichlorethylene, introduction of

KARL BERNHARD LEHMAN, German physician and pharmacologist, 1858-1940, introduced the use of trichlorethylene, *circa* 1911.

Trichomonas vaginalis, early description of

ALFRED DONNÉ, French physician, 1801-1878, described the parasite *Trichomonas vaginalis* in 1836. Donné believed that the organism is the cause of gonorrhea.

Trichomonas vaginalis in urine of a man, demonstration of

KINNOSUKE MIURA, Japanese physician, 1864-19??, demonstrated the presence of the *Trichomonas vaginalis* in the voided urine of a male. Recorded in 1894.

Trichophyton ectothrix, first description of

DAVID GRUBY, French dermatologist, 1810-1898, is credited with being the first to describe *trichophyton ectothrix,* the causative agent of sycosis barbae. Recorded in 1842.

Trichophyton tonsurans, discovery of

DAVID GRUBY, French dermatologist, 1810-1898, discovered *Trichophyton tonsurans* in ringworm of the scalp. Recorded in 1844.

Trichophytosis cruris, fungous origin of

... See under *Tinea cruris, fungous origin of.*

Trichorrhexis nodosa, early description of

FRANCIS VALENTINE PAXTON,

English physician, 1840-1924, described trichorrhexis nodosa (tinea nodosa), a condition in which swellings are formed along the shafts of the hairs. Published in 1869.

Tricuspid valve, introduction of term

ERASISTRATUS, Greek anatomist and physician, *circa* 300-250 B. C., described and named the tricuspid valve of the heart. Exact date not available.

Tricuspid valve, ring of fibrocartilage serving as attachment for

ALBRECHT VON HALLER, Swiss physiologist and anatomist, 1708-1777, described the circle or ring of fibrocartilage to which the tricuspid valve is attached. Reported *circa* 1747. Known as *circulus callosus halleri.*

Trigeminal nerve, connecting filaments of

HEINRICH AUGUST WRISBERG, German anatomist, 1739-1808, described delicate fibers connecting the motor and the sensory roots of the trigeminal nerve. Published in 1764. Known as *Wrisberg's lines.*

Trigeminal neuralgia, eponymic description of

JOHN FOTHERGILL, English physician, 1712-1780, recorded a description of trigeminal neuralgia under the title "On a painful affection of the face." Published in 1776. Known as *Fothergill's disease.*

Trigeminal neuralgia, excision of semilunar ganglion in, by temporal approach

VICTOR ALEXANDER HADEN HORS-LEY, English surgeon, 1857-1916, with J. TAYLOR and W. S. COLEMAN, devised a temporal approach in the excision of the semilunar ganglion for trigeminal neuralgia. Published in 1891.

Trigeminal neuralgia, first reliable account of

JOHANNES MICHAEL FEHR, German physician, 1610-1688, with ELIAS SCHMIDT, described trigeminal neuralgia in a eulogy of Dr. JOHANNES LAURENTIUS BAUSCH, who died of the condition in 1665. Published in 1671.

Trigeminal neuralgia, injection of alcohol in semilunar ganglion for relief of

JOSEPH LOUIS IRÉNEE JEAN ABADIE, French surgeon, 1873-19??, injected alcohol in the semilunar ganglion for the relief of trigeminal neuralgia. Recorded in 1902.

Trigeminal neuralgia, intracranial neurectomy for relief of

FRANK HARTLEY, American surgeon, 1856-1913, was the first to use intracranial neurectomy (of the second and third divisions of the trigeminal nerve) in the treatment of trigeminal neuralgia. Published in 1892.

Trigeminal neuralgia, intracranial neurotomy for relief of

CHARLES HARRISON FRAZIER, American neurologist, 1870-1936, with WILLIAM GIBSON SPILLER, American neurologist, 1863-1940, introduced an operation for the relief of trigeminal neuralgia by intracranial division of the sensory root of the trigeminal nerve. Recorded in 1902.

Trigeminal neuralgia, trigeminal tractotomy for relief of

CARL OLOF SJÖQVIST, Swedish neurosurgeon, 1901-   , treated trigeminal neuralgia by division of the tractus spinalis nervi trigemini. Recorded in 1937.

Trigeminal neuralgia

... See also under *Semilunar ganglion*.

Trigone of bladder, eponymic description of

JOSEPH LIEUTAUD, French physician, 1703-1780, was the first to give a clear description of the trigone of the urinary bladder, in 1742. Known as *trigone of Lieutaud*.

Trigone of bladder, posterior bar of

LOUIS AUGUSTE MERCIER, French urologist, 1811-1882, described the transverse ridge extending between the openings of the ureters on the inner surface of the bladder, forming the posterior boundary of the trigone, in 1854. Known as *Mercier's bar*.

Trihexyphenidyl in treatment of parkinsonism

... See under *Parkinsonism, trihexyphenidyl in*, etc.

Trimethylene

... See under *Cyclopropane*.

Trional, introduction of

EUGEN BAUMANN, German physician and biochemist, 1846-1896, described sulfonethylmethane or trional in 1890.

Trochlear nerves, discovery of

ALESSANDRO ACHILLINI, Italian anatomist, 1463-1512, is believed to be the discoverer of the trochlear nerves. Exact date not available.

Tromexan, introduction of

Z. REINIŠ, Swiss physician, 19??-   , with MIRKO KUBIK, introduced tromexan as an anticoagulant. Published in 1948.

Tropical diseases, first classic text on

PATRICK MANSON, Scottish parasitologist, 1844-1922, wrote a manual of tropical diseases which is considered the first complete text of its kind. Published in 1898. Manson is regarded as the founder of tropical medicine.

Tropism in animals, early observations on

JACQUES LOEB, American biologist, 1859-1924, studied the effect of sunlight stimuli on the orientation of animal cells and structures, comparing the results with the reaction of plants. Recorded in 1890.

Tropism in plants, early observation on

ANDREW KNIGHT, English horticulturist, 1758-1838, is credited with performing the first organized experiments on the effect of various stimuli on the direction of growth of plants, *circa* 1802.

Trousseau's disease

... See under *Hemochromatosis, first description of*.

Trousseau's sign

... See under *Tetany, Trousseau's sign of*.

Truss for inguinal hernia, early invention of

BERNARD DE GORDON, French physician, *circa* 1245-1320, devised a truss, "an iron brace of semicircular shape provided with a little tongue," about 1300.

Truss for inguinal hernia, early invention of

NICOLAUS DE BLÉGNY, French physician, 1652-1722, invented a truss for inguinal hernia, in 1676.

Trypan blue in treatment of trypanosomiasis

... See under *Trypanosomiasis.*

Trypan red in treatment of trypanosomiasis

... See under *Trypanosomiasis.*

Trypanosoma cruzi, discovery of

CARLOS CHAGAS, Brazilian physician, 1879-1934, is credited with the discovery of *Trypanosoma cruzi,* the causative agent of Brazilian or American trypanosomiasis, in 1909. The organism is transmitted by reduviid bugs.

Trypanosoma evansi

... See under *Surra, trypanosomes in.*

Trypanosoma gambiense in spinal fluid, discovery of

... See under *Sleeping sickness, African,* etc.

Trypanosoma gambiense, introduction of name

JOSEPH EVERETT DUTTON, English physician, 1877-1905, introduced the term *Trypanosoma gambiense,* to describe the organism he saw in the blood of a patient of DR. ROBERT MICHAEL FORDE, in Gambia. Recorded in 1902.

Trypanosoma rhodesiense, discovery of

JOHN WILLIAM WATSON STEPHENS, English physician, 1865-19??, with HAROLD BENJAMIN FANTHAM, discovered *Trypanosoma rhodesiense,* the causative agent of kaodzera, a form of sleeping sickness prevalent in Rhodesia. Recorded in 1910.

Trypanosome, introduction of term

DAVID GRUBY, French dermatologist, 1810-1898, introduced the term *trypanosome,* in 1843, after discovering the flagellated organism in the frog. The term is based on the Greek *trypao* (bore) and *soma* (body).

Trypanosomes, blood agar for cultivation of—1904

WARD J. MACNEAL, American pathologist, 1881-1946, with FREDERICK GEORGE NOVY, American bacteriologist, 1864-19??, compounded a nutrient blood agar for the cultivation of trypanosomes. Recorded in 1904. Known as *Novy-MacNeal agar* or *medium.*

Trypanosomes in blood of horses

... See under *Surra, trypanosomes in.*

Trypanosomes in human blood

GUSTAVE NEPVEU, French physician, 1841-1903, was the first to observe trypanosomes in human blood, in Algeria. Published in 1891.

Trypanosomiasis, African, first English description of

JOHN ATKINS, English naval surgeon, 1685-1757, was the first to describe African trypanosomiasis or sleeping sickness in the English language. Published in 1734.

Trypanosomiasis, African

. . . See also under *Sleeping sickness.*

Trypanosomiasis, arsenic in treatment of

. . . See under *Nagana.*

Trypanosomiasis, atoxyl in treatment of

HAROLD WOLFERSTAN THOMAS, English physician, 18??-19??, with ANTON BREINL, demonstrated that sodium arsanilate (*atoxyl*) was more effective in treating trypanosomiasis than inorganic arsenic. Published in 1905.

Trypanosomiasis, Brazilian or American

CARLOS CHAGAS, Brazilian physician, 1879-1934, discovered *Trypanosoma cruzi,* the causative agent of Brazilian or American trypanosomiasis, in 1909. The organism is transmitted by reduviid bugs. The condition is known as *Chagas' disease.*

Trypanosomiasis, human, first recognition of

JOSEPH EVERETT DUTTON, English physician, 1877-1905, was the first to recognize human trypanosomiasis in a patient of ROBERT MICHAEL FORDE. Recorded in 1902. He named the organism *Trypanosoma gambiense.*

Trypanosomiasis, suramin in treatment of

LUDWIG HAENDEL, German physician, 1869-1939, with KARL WILHELM JOETTEN, introduced germa-

nin (*suramin, naphuride, Bayer 205,* etc.) in the treatment of trypanosomiasis. Recorded in 1920.

Trypanosomiasis, trypan blue in treatment of

MAURICE NICOLLE, French physician, 1862-1936, with FÉLIX MESNIL, introduced the use of trypan blue in the treatment of trypanosomiasis. Published in 1906.

Trypanosomiasis, trypan red in treatment of

PAUL EHRLICH, German bacteriologist and pathologist, 1854-1915, introduced the use of trypan red in the treatment of trypanosomiasis. Recorded in 1907. Ehrlich dealt with experimental trypanosomiasis only.

Trypanosomiasis, tryparsamide in treatment of

LOUISE PEARCE, American physician, 1886-19??, introduced the use of tryparsamide in the treatment of trypanosomiasis. Recorded in 1921.

Trypanosomiasis

. . . See also under *Tsetse fly.*

Tryparsamide, preparation of

WALTER ABRAHAM JACOBS, American chemist, 1883-19??, is credited with the preparation of tryparsamide, used in treating neurosyphilis and sleeping sickness. Reported in 1919.

Trypsin, discovery of

ALEXANDER YAKOVLEVICH DANILEWSKI, Russian physiologist, 1838-1914, is credited with being the first to recognize trypsin in the pancreatic juice. Recorded in 1862.

Trypsin, isolation of

WILHELM FRIEDRICH (WILLY)

KÜHNE, German physiologist, 1837-1900, isolated trypsin, in 1874.

Tryptophan is by-product of pancreatic digestion, demonstration that

CLAUDE BERNARD, French physiologist, 1813-1878, showed that tryptophan is not a constituent of pancreatic juice but a by-product of pancreatic digestion. Reported in 1856.

Tryptophan, isolation of

FREDERICK G. HOPKINS, English biochemist, 1861-1947, isolated tryptophan, as a by-product of tryptic digestion, in 1901.

Tsetse fly, early description of

DAVID LIVINGSTONE, Scottish explorer and physician, 1813-1873, gave a good description of the tsetse fly and of the disease its bite produces in cattle. Published in 1857.

Tsetse fly is vector of trypanosomiasis

DAVID BRUCE, English pathologist and bacteriologist, 1855-1931, with D. N. NABARRO, studied sleeping sickness in Africa, where they were sent by the Royal Society, and demonstrated that the tsetse fly was the vector of trypanosomiasis. They also showed that sleeping sickness and Gambia fever were different stages of the same disease. Reports published 1903-19.

Tubal pregnancy, early description of

FRANÇOIS MAURICEAU, French obstetrician, 1637-1709, described tubal pregnancy. Recorded in 1668.

Tubal pregnancy, first successful operation for

ROBERT LAWSON TAIT, English surgeon and gynecologist, 1845-1899, is credited with being the first to operate successfully for ruptured tubal pregnancy. Recorded in 1883.

Tube for intestinal drainage having double channel

. . . See under *Intestinal drainage tube.*

Tube, gastrointestinal nasal

. . . See under *Gastrointestinal nasal tube, invention of.*

Tubercle bacilli, bovine, in man

. . . See under *Bovine tubercle bacilli in man.*

Tubercle bacilli, human and bovine, differentiation between

THEOBALD SMITH, American pathologist, 1859-1934, is credited with making the first clear differentiation between the human and the bovine types of tubercle bacillus. Recorded in 1898.

Tubercle bacillus, discovery of

ROBERT KOCH, German bacteriologist, 1843-1910, discovered the tubercle bacillus, *Mycobacterium tuberculosis,* in 1882. Known as *Koch's bacillus.*

Tubercle, description of

GASPARD LAURENT BAYLE, French physician, 1774-1816, described the identity and structure of the tubercle of tuberculosis, in 1803.

Tubercle, giant cells of tuberculous

THEODOR LANGHANS, German anatomist and pathologist in Switzerland, 1839-1915, described the giant cells found in tuberculous tubercles. Published in 1867.

Tubercle, intervenous, of heart

RICHARD LOWER, English physician, 1631-1691, described a tubercle or ridge (not always distinct) on the inner surface of the right atrium between the openings of the two venae cavae. Lower believed that the structure directs the flow of the blood toward the atrioventricular opening. Published in 1669. Known as *Lower's tubercle*.

Tubercle of Morgagni

. . . See under *Olfactory bulb,* etc.

Tubercle on lingual surface of molar teeth

. . . See under *Cusp, fifth,* etc.

Tubercle, scalene, on upper surface of first rib

. . . See under *Scalene tubercle on upper surface of first rib.*

Tubercle, well-developed, on sixth cervical vertebra

. . . See under *Carotid tubercle.*

Tubercles in semilunar valves of aorta and pulmonary arteries

. . . See under *Corpora arantii.*

Tuberculin conjunctival test, introduction of

LEON CHARLES ALBERT CALMETTE, French bacteriologist, 1863-1933, introduced a tuberculin conjunctival test, in 1907. Known as *Calmette's test* or *reaction.*

Tuberculin, introduction of

ROBERT KOCH, German bacteriologist, 1843-1910, introduced tuberculin as an agent in treating tuber-culosis. While it was not effective in treatment, tuberculin proved very useful as a diagnostic material. Recorded in 1890.

Tuberculin test by application to abrasion of skin

CLEMENS PETER PIRQUET VON CESENATICO, Austrian pediatrician, 1874-1929, developed a tuberculin test in which the test material is applied to a superficial abrasion of the skin. Recorded in 1907. Known as *Pirquet's test.*

Tuberculin test, intradermal, introduction of

CHARLES MANTOUX, French physician, 1877-1947, introduced the intradermal test for tuberculosis by means of tuberculin. Recorded in 1908. Known as *Mantoux's test.*

Tuberculosis among ancient Egyptians

GRAFTON ELLIOT SMITH, English physician, 1871-1937, and MARC ARMAND RUFFER (English physician, 1859-1917) demonstrated that tuberculosis existed among the ancient Egyptians, by describing a mummy of 1000 B.C. bearing unmistakable evidence of Pott's disease. Published in 1910.

Tuberculosis, development of preventive vaccine for

LEON C. A. CALMETTE, French bacteriologist, 1863-1933, with CAMILLE GUERIN, developed a preventive vaccine for tuberculosis consisting of living cultures of bovine tubercle bacilli whose virulence has been reduced by growth on glycerinated ox bile. Reported in 1927.

Tuberculosis, human and bovine, differentiation between

ROBERT KOCH, German bacteriologist, 1843-1910, is credited with differentiating between human and bovine tuberculosis, in 1900.

Tuberculosis in cattle, experimental production of

THEODOR ALBRECHT EDWIN KLEBS, German bacteriologist, 1834-1913, was the first to produce tuberculosis in cattle, by feeding them infected milk. Published in 1873.

Tuberculosis in children born of tuberculous parents

GEORGES KUSS, French physician, 1867-1936, demonstrated that the children of tuberculous parents are not born with tuberculosis but are likely to be affected later. Reported in 1898.

Tuberculosis in children, primary lesion of

JOSEPH PARROT, French physician, 1829-1883, was first to describe the primary lesion of pulmonary tuberculosis in children, in 1876. It was described later by ANTON GHON (Ghon's primary focus).

Tuberculosis in children, primary lesion of

ANTON GHON, Austrian pathologist, 1866-1936, described the development of primary tuberculosis in children, recognizing the difference between the lesions of the first infection and those resulting from reinfection, and pointed out the primary lesion of pulmonary tuberculosis in children, seen as a "bean-shaped shadow" on roentgeno-

grams. Reported in 1912. Known as the *Ghon tubercle*.

Tuberculosis in children, primary lesion of, plus satellite lymph nodes

GEORGES KUSS, French physician, 1867-1936, did fundamental research in tuberculosis of children and described a complex lesion composed of the primary lesion or Ghon tubercle plus involved satellite lymph nodes. These are known as the *primary complex, Kuss-Ghon focus,* or *Ghon complex*. Reported in 1898.

Tuberculosis in infants, gastric lavage in diagnosis of

. . . See under *Gastric lavage*.

Tuberculosis in rabbits, experimental

JULIUS FRIEDRICH COHNHEIM, German pathologist, 1839-1884, succeeded in producing experimental tuberculosis in rabbits, in 1877.

Tuberculosis indurativa, description of

. . . See under *Erythema induratum*.

Tuberculosis, isoniazid in treatment of

EDWARD HEINRICH ROBITZEK, American physician, 1912-   , with I. J. SELIKOFF and G. G. ORNSTEIN, introduced isoniazid in the treatment of tuberculosis. Published in 1952.

Tuberculosis, lobectomy in treatment of

SAMUEL OSCAR FREEDLANDER, American surgeon, 1893-   , performed the first lobectomy in the treatment of pulmonary tuberculosis. The era of lung resection for tuberculosis began at this time. Recorded in 1935.

Tuberculosis, miliary, first reference to

. . . See under *Miliary tuberculosis*.

Tuberculosis, nodular and infiltrating forms of

MATTHEW BAILLIE, English physician, 1761-1823, was first to differentiate between the nodular and the infiltrating types of pulmonary tuberculosis. Published in 1793.

Tuberculosis of joints, early description of

RICHARD WISEMAN, English military surgeon, 1622-1676, was the first to give a clear description of tuberculosis of joints, which he called *tumor albus*. Recorded in 1676.

Tuberculosis of spine, early description of

JEAN P. DAVID, French physician, 1737-1784, gave an accurate description of tuberculosis of the spine. Published in 1779.

Tuberculosis of spine, early description of

PERCIVALL POTT, English surgeon, 1714-1788, described a form of spinal curvature which is now known to have been caused by tuberculosis of the spine. It is believed, however, that Pott did not recognize the nature of the disease. His report, in 1779, dealt with "Remarks on that kind of palsy of the lower limbs, which is frequently found to accompany curvature of the spine." Known now as *Pott's disease*.

Tuberculosis, para-aminosalicylic acid in treatment of

JÖRGEN LEHMAN, Swedish physician, 1898- , discovered that para-aminosalicylic acid inhibits the growth of the tubercle bacillus, and introduced the drug in the treatment of tuberculosis. Recorded in 1946.

Tuberculosis, pneumoperitoneum in treatment of

LUDWIG VAJDA, German physician, 18??-19??, introduced the use of artificial pneumoperitoneum in the treatment of pulmonary tuberculosis. Published in 1933.

Tuberculosis, pneumoperitoneum with phrenicotomy in

ANDREW LADISLAUS BANYAI, American physician, 1893-19??, introduced the combined method of artificial pneumoperitoneum and phrenicotomy in the treatment of pulmonary tuberculosis. Published in 1934. The method of pneumoperitoneum enjoyed only temporary popularity.

Tuberculosis, pneumothorax in

. . . See under *Pneumothorax*.

Tuberculosis, pulmonary, correlation of, with tuberculosis of other organs

GASPARD LAURENT BAYLE, French physician, 1774-1816, was instrumental in correlating pulmonary tuberculosis with tuberculosis of other organs. His book on pulmonary tuberculosis was published in 1810.

Tuberculosis, salt restriction in treatment of

ERNST FERDINAND SAUERBRUCH, German surgeon, 1875-1951, with MAX BERNHARD GERSON and A. HERRMANNSDORFER, devised a salt-restricted diet in the treatment of tuberculosis. Published in 1926. Known as *Gerson-Sauerbruch-Herrmannsdorfer diet*.

Tuberculosis, sanocrysin in treatment of

HOLGER MØLLGAARD, Swedish physician, 1885-19??, is credited with the introduction of sanocrysin, a thiosulfate of sodium and gold, in the treatment of tuberculosis. Recorded in 1925.

Tuberculosis, suggestion of bacterial nature of

BENJAMIN MARTEN, English physician, 1700-1782, proposed a theory of tuberculosis, especially pulmonary tuberculosis, based on the assumption that the causative agent is a microorganism. Published in 1720, 162 years before Koch's discovery of the tubercle bacillus in 1882.

Tuberculosis, thiosemicarbazone in treatment of

GERHARD DOMAGK, German pharmacologist, 1895- , with R. BEHNISCH, F. MIETZSCH, and H. SCHMIDT, introduced thiosemicarbazone in the treatment of tuberculosis. Recorded in 1946.

Tuberculosis, transmissibility of, by inoculation

JEAN ANTOINE VILLEMIN, French physician, 1827-1892, demonstrated, by inoculating rabbits and guinea pigs with tuberculous material, that tuberculosis is transmissible. Recorded in 1868.

Tuberculosis, transmission of, by cow's milk

PHILIPP FRIEDRICH HERMANN KLENCKE, German physician, 1813-1881, demonstrated that tuberculosis may be transmitted to man by cow's milk. Published in 1846.

Tuberculous arthritis, multiple, eponymic description of

ANTONIN PONCET, French surgeon, 1849-1913, described tuberculous rheumatism or tuberculous arthritis affecting several joints, in 1897. Known as *Poncet's disease*.

Tuberculous inflammation of head of a bone, especially of tibia

BENJAMIN C. BRODIE, English surgeon, 1783-1862, described a tuberculous abscess or inflammation of the head of the tibia. Recorded in 1832. Known as *Brodie's abscess*. The name was later applied to a tuberculous abscess occurring at the end of any bone.

Tuberculous inflammation of serous membranes, early account of

LUIGI MARIA CONCATO, Italian physician, 1825-1882, gave an excellent description of tuberculous inflammation of serous membranes. Published in 1881.

Tuberculous meningitis in children

ROBERT WHYTT, Scottish physician, 1714-1766, is credited with giving the first account of the course of tuberculous meningitis in children. Published in 1768.

Tuberculous sinuses, bismuth paste in diagnosis and treatment of

. . . See under *Bismuth paste.*

Tuberculous skin disease, first use of radium in

HENRI ALEXANDRE DANLOS, French dermatologist, 1844-1912, with P. BLOCH, used radium in the treatment of tuberculous disease of the skin, in 1901.

Tuberculous spondylitis of neck

JOHANN NEPOMUK RUST, German physician, 1755-1840, described tuberculosis of the cervical vertebrae, in 1834. Known as *Rust's disease.*

Tuberculous sputum, fragments in

. . . See under *Spengler's fragments.*

Tuberculous sputum, non-acid-fast granules in

HANS CHRISTIAN R. MUCH, German physician, 1880-1932, described non-acid-fast, Gram-positive granules found in the sputum of tuberculous patients. They are regarded as modified tubercle bacilli. Published in 1907. Known as *Much's granules.*

Tuberculum auriculae; Darwin's tubercle

CHARLES R. DARWIN, English naturalist, 1809-1882, described a small projection sometimes found on the edge of the helix. It is considered by some as evidence of the simian ancestry of the human species. Exact date not available.

Tuberculum cinereum; Rolando's tubercle

LUIGI ROLANDO, Italian anatomist, 1773-1831, described the club-shaped portion of the posterior part of the lateral funiculus of the medulla oblongata. Recorded in 1809.

Tuberous sclerosis of brain

. . . See under *Brain,* etc.

Tuberous subchorional hematoma, description of

CARL BREUS, Austrian obstetrician, 1852-1914, described a highly nodular blood mole consisting of a tuberous subchorional hematoma of the decidua, in 1892. Known as *hematomole* and as *Breus's mole.*

Tularemia, discovery of causative agent of

CHARLES WILLARD CHAPIN, American bacteriologist, 1877-19??, with GEORGE W. McCOY, isolated the causative agent of tularemia, in 1912. They named it *Bacterium tularense,* in allusion to Tulare County California, where many of the infected squirrels were observed.

Tularemia, finding of organism in sputum in a case of

LEROY HENDRICK SLOAN, American physician, 1892-   , with A. S. FREEDBERG and J. C. EHRLICH, demonstrated the causative organism of tularemia in the sputum of a patient. Recorded in 1936.

Tularemia, first observation of, in squirrels

GEORGE WALTER McCOY, American public health administrator, 1876-1952, was the first to describe tularemia, "a plague-like disease of rodents," in California ground squirrels, in 1911.

Tularemia, introduction of name

EDWARD FRANCIS, American physician and bacteriologist, 1872-19??, introduced the name *tularemia,* in allusion to Tulare County, California, because the affected squirrels originally studied were taken from Tulare. Recorded in 1919.

Tularemia, isolation of causative agent of, from man

WILLIAM BUCHANAN WHERRY, American bacteriologist, 1875-19??, with BENJAMIN HARRISON LAMB, was the first to isolate *Pasteurella tularensis* from a case of tularemia in man. Published in 1914.

Tularemia, Japanese form of; Ohara's disease

HACHIRO OHARA, Japanese physician, 1897-   , described a disease occurring in Japan which is considered to be identical with tularemia. Recorded in 1930. Known also as *yato byo.*

Tularemia, naming of bacterium of

GEORGE WALTER MCCOY, American public health administrator, 1876-1952, attached the term *tularense* to the name of the organism causing tularemia, because the squirrels originally studied were obtained from Tulare, California. Introduced *circa* 1919.

Tumor albus

. . . See under *Tuberculosis of joints,* etc.

Tumor of urinary bladder, resection of, by abdominal route

. . . See under *Urinary bladder tumor,* etc.

Tumors, classification of, as to malignancy

ALBERT C. BRODERS, American pathologist, 1885-19??, classified tumors into four groups with regard to malignancy, on the basis of the undifferentiated state of the cells. Reported *circa* 1920.

Tumors of uterus, differentiation between benign and malignant

. . . See under *Uterine tumors,* etc.

Tumors utilize glucose by glycolysis, discovery that

OTTO HEINRICH WARBURG, German biochemist, 1883-19??, discovered that malignant tumors utilize glucose by glycolysis, in the presence or absence of oxygen. Published in 1926.

Tumors

. . . See also under *Cancer,* and under name of particular type of tumor, as *Epithelioma.*

Türck's trachoma

. . . See under *Laryngitis sicca.*

Turner's cerate

. . . See under *Ointment of calamine.*

Turner's syndrome, eponymic description of

HENRY HUBERT TURNER, American physician, 1892-   , described a syndrome of infantilism marked by retarded sexual development, low posterior hair line, webbing of the neck, etc. Published in 1938.

Twilight sleep, introduction of

RICHARD VON STEINBÜCHEL, German obstetrician, 1861-19??, introduced the hypodermic injection of morphine and scopolamine in the management of labor. Recorded in 1902. Known as twilight sleep.

Tympanic antrum, eponymic description of

ANTONIO MARIA VALSALVA, Italian anatomist, 1666-1723, described the tympanic antrum, an air space in the mastoid portion of the temporal bone communicating with the mastoid cells and with the tympanum. Recorded in 1704. Known as *Valsalva's antrum*.

Tympanic membrane, first pictures of

ADAM POLITZER, Austrian otologist, 1835-1920, was the first to obtain pictures of the tympanic membrane by direct illumination. Recorded in 1865.

Tympanic membrane, flaccid portion of

HENRY JONES SHRAPNELL, English anatomist, 1761-1841, was first to describe the flaccid portion of the eardrum, in 1832. Known as *pars flaccida* and *Shrapnell's membrane*.

Tympanic membrane, Prussak's fibers of

ALEXANDER PRUSSAK, Russian otologist, 1839-1907, described fibers in the tympanic membrane extending from the lateral process of the malleus to the tympanic notch. Recorded in 1876. Known as *Prussak's fibers*.

Tympanic nerve, early description of—1818

LUDWIG LEVIN JACOBSON, Danish anatomist, 1783-1843, described the tympanic nerve, in 1818. Known as *Jacobson's nerve*.

Tympanic plexus, eponymic description of

LUDWIG LEVIN JACOBSON, Danish anatomist, 1783-1843, described the tympanic plexus, a plexus of nerves which supplies the tympanum. Reported in 1818. Known as *Jacobson's plexus*.

Tympanic sulcus, notch at upper border of

AUGUSTUS QUIRINUS RIVINUS, German anatomist and botanist, 1652-1723, described a notch between the greater and lesser tympanic spines, covered by Shrapnell's membrane. Recorded in 1691. Known as *incisura tympanica* and *Rivinus' notch*. It is said that Rivinus first observed the notch in 1680.

Tyndallization, introduction of

. . . See under *Fractional sterilization*.

Typhoid bacillus, discovery of

KARL JOSEPH EBERTH, German pathologist, 1835-1926, discovered the typhoid bacillus, in 1880. The organism is known as *Eberthella typhosa* and *Salmonella typhosa*.

Typhoid bacillus in gallbladder, demonstration of

BERNHARD ANTON, German physician, 1845-19??, with GUSTAV FÜTTERER (German bacteriologist, 1854-1922), demonstrated the presence of typhoid bacilli in the gallbladder of patients. Published in 1888.

Typhoid bacillus, pure cultures of

GEORG T. A. GAFFKY, German

bacteriologist, 1850-1918, was the first to grow pure cultures of the typhoid bacillus, *circa* 1884.

Typhoid fever and typhus, early differentiation of—1836

WILLIAM WOOD GERHARD, American physician, 1809-1872, differentiated between typhoid fever and typhus by observing cases during an epidemic in which both diseases were prevalent. Reported in 1836.

Typhoid fever and typhus, early differentiation of—1849

WILLIAM JENNER, English physician, 1815-1898, is credited with differentiating typhoid fever from typhus, in 1849.

Typhoid fever, cold bath treatment of

ERNST BRAND, German physician, 1827-1897, introduced the cold bath treatment of typhoid fever. Recorded in 1861.

Typhoid fever, contagiousness of; early demonstration

WILLIAM BUDD, English physician, 1811-1880, demonstrated that typhoid fever was spread by contagion. Recorded in 1873.

Typhoid fever, first description of

THOMAS WILLIS, English anatomist and physician, 1621-1675, was the first to give a good account of typhoid fever, in 1643.

Typhoid fever, inoculation against

ALMROTH EDWARD WRIGHT, English pathologist and bacteriologist, 1861-1947, was the first to develop a typhoid vaccine made of killed typhoid bacilli. Recorded in 1896.

Typhoid fever, inoculation against

FREDERICK FULLER RUSSELL, American physician, 1870-19??, investigated the effect of anti-typhoid vaccination in the United States Army and demonstrated the value of such inoculation. Recorded in 1910.

Typhoid fever, introduction of term

PIERRE CHARLES ALEXANDRE LOUIS, French physician, 1787-1872, introduced the term *typhoid fever,* in 1829.

Typhoid fever is a water-borne infection

WILLIAM BUDD, English physician, 1811-1880, advocated the theory that typhoid fever is a water-borne infection. Recorded in 1873.

Typhoid fever is caused by typhoid bacillus, proof that

GEORG T. A. GAFFKY, German bacteriologist, 1850-1918, proved, in 1884, that *Bacillus typhosus* is the cause of typhoid fever.

Typhoid fever, rose spots in

PIERRE CHARLES ALEXANDRE LOUIS, French physician, 1787-1872, described the characteristic rose spots of typhoid fever, in 1829.

Typhoid fever, spread of, by contamination with ejecta

WILLIAM BUDD, English physician, 1811-1880, demonstrated that typhoid fever can be spread by contamination with ejecta from patients. Recorded in 1873.

Typhoid fever, surgical complications of

WILLIAM WILLIAMS KEEN, American surgeon, 1837-1932, described surgical complications of typhoid fever, in 1898.

Typhoid fever, test for

GEORGES FERNAND ISIDOR WIDAL, French physician, 1862-1929, with ARTHUR SICARD, discovered specific agglutinins in the blood of typhoid fever patients and on the basis of this developed a test for the diagnosis of typhoid. Recorded in 1896. Known as the *Widal test*.

Typhoid fever vaccination

... See under *Typhoid fever, inoculation against*.

Typhus, causative agent of; first isolation

HENRIQUE DA ROCHA - LIMA, French physician in Germany, 1879-19??, was the first to isolate the causative organism of typhus. Recorded in 1916. He named the agent *Rickettsia prowazeki*, in honor of HOWARD TAYLOR RICKETTS and STANISLAS JOSEF MATHIAS VON PROWAZEK, both of whom died of typhus.

Typhus, chloromycetin in treatment of

JOSEPH EDWIN SMADEL, American pharmacologist, 1907- , with ELIZABETH JACKSON, introduced the use of chloramphenicol in the treatment of typhus fever. Published in 1947.

Typhus, early description of

GEROLAMO CARDANO, Italian physician, 1501-1576, gave the first clear account of typhus fever, in a book which pointed out 72 errors in the medical practice of his day. Published in 1536.

Typhus endemic in southeastern United States

KENNETH FULLER MAXCY, American physician, 1889-19??, described a form of typhus fever endemic in the southeastern portion of the United States. Published in 1926.

Typhus, first authentic account of

GIROLAMO FRACASTORO, Italian pathologist, 1483-1553, gave the first authentic account of typhus, in 1546.

Typhus, Mexican or Spanish; tabardillo

FRANCISCO BRAVO, Spanish physician in Mexico, 152?-15??, was the first to describe tabardillo, Spanish or Mexican typhus. Published in 1570. Bravo's book was the first medical book published in the New World.

Typhus, para-aminobenzoic acid in treatment of

ANDREW YEOMANS, American physician, 1907- , with J. C. SNYDER, E. S. MURRAY, C. J. D. ZARAFONETIS, and R. S. ECKE, studied the therapeutic effect of para-aminobenzoic acid in the treatment of louse-borne typhus fever. Published in 1944.

Typhus, pediculosis in transmission of

TOBIAS COBER, German physician, 1570-1628, noted the prevalence of lice in the army during epidemics of typhus. Recorded in 1606.

Typhus, pediculosis in transmission of

CHARLES JULES HENRI NICOLLE, French bacteriologist, 1866-1936, demonstrated that typhus can be transmitted by the body louse *Pediculus corporis*. First published in 1910-11.

Typhus, recrudescent; Brill's disease

NATHAN EDWIN BRILL, American physician, 1860-1925, was the first to describe a recrudescence of mild typhus among immigrants from eastern Europe some years after the initial attack. Recorded in 1910. Known as *sporadic typhus, Brill's disease,* and *recrudescent typhus.*

Typhus, scrub, preparation of vaccine for

FORREST FULTON, English bacteriologist, 19??- , with L. JOYNER, cultivated the causative agent of scrub fever (*Rickettsia tsutsugamushi*) in the lungs of rodents and prepared a vaccine for the disease. Published in 1945.

Typhus transmitted to monkeys and guinea pigs

CHARLES JULES HENRI NICOLLE, French bacteriologist, 1866-1936, produced typhus in monkeys and guinea pigs by injection of blood from affected subjects. Recorded in 1910-11. Nicolle received the Nobel prize in 1928.

Typhus, Tunisian, first description of

ALFRED CONOR, French physician, 1870-19??, with A. BRUCH, gave the first description of boutonneuse fever, *fièvre boutonneuse,* a form of typhus prevalent in Tunisia. Recorded in 1910.

Typhus vaccine

. . . See under *Typhus, scrub.*

Typhus, Weil-Felix agglutination test for

EDMUND WEIL, Austrian physician, 1880-1922, with ARTHUR FELIX, Austrian physician, 1887-19??, developed an agglutination test for typhus fever in which Proteus X bacteria are treated with the patient's serum. Recorded in 1916.

Typhus-like fever, bacillus found in

HARRY PLOTZ, American physician and bacteriologist, 1890-1947, discovered a bacillus in typhus-like fevers which he thought was the cause of the disease. Published in 1914. Known as *Plotz's bacillus.*

Tyrosine in urine, in acute yellow atrophy of liver

FRIEDRICH T. VON FRERICHS, German pathologist, 1819-1885, discovered the presence of tyrosine in the urine of patients having acute yellow atrophy of the liver. Reported in 1854.

Tyrosine, synthesis of

EMIL ERLENMEYER, German chemist, 1825-1909, synthesized tyrosine in 1883.

Tyrothricin, discovery of

RENÉ JULES DUBOS, French bacteriologist in the United States, 1901- , discovered tyrothricin, an antibiotic substance isolated from the soil bacillus *Bacillus brevis,* in 1939.

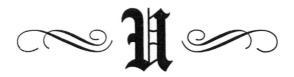

Ulcer, acute vulvar, eponymic description of

BENJAMIN LIPSCHÜTZ, Austrian dermatologist, 1878-1931, described a rapidly spreading non-venereal ulcer of the vulva, believed to be caused by *Bacillus crassis*. Published in 1918. Known as *Lipschütz ulcer*.

Ulcer, gastric, early description of

... See under *Gastric ulcer*.

Ulcer, peptic, experimental production of, in the dog

FRANK CHARLES MANN, American physiologist and surgeon, 1887-19??, with CARL S. WILLIAMSON, produced experimental peptic ulcers in dogs. Published in 1923. Called *Mann-Williamson ulcer*.

Ulerythema ophryogenes

... See under *Keratosis pilaris*, etc.

Ultraviolet rays, early use of

NIELS RYBERG FINSEN, Danish physician, 1860-1904, demonstrated the value of ultraviolet rays, in 1896. Finsen is considered the founder of modern phototherapy; he received the Nobel prize in 1903.

Ultraviolet rays in surgical tuberculosis

AUGUSTE ROLLIER, Swiss physician, 1874-19??, introduced the use of ultraviolet rays in the treatment of surgical tuberculosis, in 1903.

Ultraviolet rays in treatment of rickets

KURT HULDSCHINSKY, German physician, 1883-19??, reported the use of ultraviolet rays in the treatment of rickets. Published in 1919.

Ultraviolet rays

... See also under *Tetany, ultraviolet rays in treatment of*.

Umbilical cord, mucoid connective tissue of

THOMAS WHARTON, English anatomist, 1610-1673, described the soft connective tissue which forms the matrix of the umbilical cord, in 1650. Known as *Wharton's jelly*.

Umbilical cord, strangulation by, early report of

FRANÇOIS MAURICEAU, French obstetrician, 1637-1709, reported a case of strangulation by the umbilical cord. Recorded in 1668.

***Uncinaria americana,* discovery of**

CHARLES WARDELL STILES, American bacteriologist and parasitologist, 1867-1941, discovered *Uncinaria americana*, later called

Necator americanus. Recorded in 1902.

Uncinate process, eponymic description of

JOHANN FRIEDRICH BLUMENBACH, German anthropologist, 1752-1840, described the uncinate process of the cranium, in 1786. Known as *Blumenbach's process.*

Unconscious mind, introduction of concept of

SIGMUND FREUD, Austrian psychiatrist, 1856-1939, with JOSEF BREUER (Austrian psychiatrist, 1842-1925), introduced the concept of the unconscious mind, in 1893.

Underwood's disease

. . . See under *Sclerema neonatorum.*

Undulant fever

. . . See under *Malta fever.*

Unipolar leads in electro-cardiography

FRANK NORMAN WILSON, American physician, 1890-1952, with F. D. JOHNSTON, A. G. MACLEOD, and P. S. BARKER, introduced unipolar leads in electrocardiography, using an electrode connected to the limb electrodes as zero potential. Recorded in 1934.

Unit of wavelength, introduction of

. . . See under *Angstrom unit of wavelength.*

Unna's disease

. . . See under *Seborrheic eczema of Unna.*

Unverricht's disease

. . . See under *Epilepsy, familial myoclonus.*

Uranium radioactivity, discovery of

. . . See under *Radioactivity of uranium.*

Urea concentration test, introduction of

HUGH MACLEAN, English pathologist, 1879-19??, with OWEN LAMBERT VAUGHAN DE WESSELOW, introduced a urea concentration test for kidney function. Recorded in 1920.

Urea, discovery of, in urine

HILAIRE MARIE ROUELLE, French pharmacologist, 1718-1779, discovered urea in the urine. Recorded in 1773.

Urea excretion in urine

JEAN BAPTISTE JOSEPH DIEUDONNÉ BOUSSINGAULT, French physician and physiological chemist, 1802-1887, demonstrated the excretion of urea in the urine. Recorded *circa* 1839.

Urea excretion index; McLean's formula

FRANKLIN CHAMBERS MCLEAN, American physiologist, 1888-19??, devised a formula for determining the urea index, which is a modification of AMBARD's formula. Recorded in 1914. Known as *McLean's formula* or *index.*

Urea, synthesis of—1828

FRIEDRICH WÖHLER, German chemist, 1800-1882, is credited with synthesizing urea in 1828. This was the first synthesis of an organic compound from inorganic constituents.

Urease, crystallization of

JAMES BATCHELLER SUMNER,

American chemist, 1887-1955, is credited with the crystallization of the enzyme urease. Published in 1926. Sumner was the first to crystallize enzymes; received Nobel prize in 1946.

Ureters, implantation of, into rectum, in extrophy of bladder

BENGT LUDWIG BERGENHEM, Swedish surgeon, 1898- , devised an operation for the relief of extrophy of the urinary bladder by implanting the ureters into the rectum. Date not available.

Ureters, ridge extending between openings of

. . . See under *Trigone of bladder, posterior bar of*.

Urethane in treatment of leukemia

. . . See under *Leukemia, urethane in treatment of*.

Urethra, female, cancer of; first record

MARIE ANNE VICTOIRE BOIVIN (*née* GILLAIN), French surgeon, 1773-1841, with ANTOINE DUGÈS (French surgeon, 1798-1838), recorded a case of cancer of the female urethra. Published in 1833.

Urethra, lacunas of; lacunas of Morgagni

GIOVANNI BATTISTA MORGAGNI, Italian anatomist and pathologist, 1682-1771, described the lacunas of the urethra, consisting of depressions or follicles which are especially numerous in the bulbar region. Recorded *circa* 1717.

Urethra, valve in fossa navicularis of

ALPHONSE F. M. GUERIN, French surgeon, 1816-1895, described a fold of mucous membrane sometimes found in the roof of the fossa navicularis of the urethra. Reported in 1864. Known as *Guerin's valve* or *fold*.

Urethral sounds, French scale for measuring

JOSEPH FRANÇOIS BENOIT CHARRIÈRE, French surgeon and instrument maker, 1803-1876, devised a scale for measuring the size of urethral sounds and catheters in which consecutive numbers differ by $\frac{1}{3}$ mm. in diameter. Recorded *circa* 1850.

Uric acid, isolation of, from urine

KARL WILHELM SCHEELE, Swedish chemist, 1742-1786, is credited with being the first to isolate uric acid from urine, in 1776.

Urinary bladder tumor, excision of, by abdominal route

CHRISTIAN ALBERT THEODOR BILLROTH, Austrian surgeon, 1829-1894, was the first to excise a urinary bladder tumor through the abdomen. Reported in 1875.

Urinary bladder tumors, transurethral fulguration of

. . . See under *Transurethral fulguration*.

Urinary bladder

. . . See also under *Bladder*.

Urinary calculi, composition of

WILLIAM HYDE WOLLASTON, English physician and physicist, 1766-1828, demonstrated that renal calculi consist of calcium phosphate, magnesium ammonium phosphate, calcium oxalate, or uric acid, or a mixture of these. Recorded in 1797.

Urine, alkaline tide of, first description of

JOHN BERESFORD LEATHES, English biochemist, 1864-19??, was the first to describe the alkaline tide of the urine. Published in 1919.

Urine formation, filtration and reabsorption theory of

KARL FRIEDRICH W. LUDWIG, German physiologist, 1816-1895, proposed a theory of urine formation which holds that the kidney glomeruli filter a dilute protein-free urine which is concentrated by resorption of water while passing through the tubules. Published in 1843. Known as *Ludwig's filtration theory*.

Urine formation

... See also under *Renal function*.

Urine, gravimetric test of

JEAN BAPTISTE VAN HELMONT, Belgian physiologist and chemist, 1577-1644, is credited with introducing gravimetric determinations in urinalysis. Recorded posthumously in 1648.

Urine, method of obtaining, from each kidney separately

MALCOLM LA SALLE HARRIS, American surgeon, 1862-1936, developed a method for obtaining urine from each kidney separately by using a double cathether. Reported in 1898. Known as *Harris's segregator*.

Uriniferous tubule, Schachowa's portion of

SERAPHINA SCHACHOWA, Russian histologist in Switzerland, 1830-1905, described a portion of the uriniferous tubule between the loop of Henle and the proximal convolution. Published in 1876. Known as *Schachowa's spiral tubule*.

Uriniferous tubule, U-shaped turn in

FRIEDRICH G. J. HENLE, German anatomist, 1809-1885, described a looped, U-shaped portion of the uriniferous tubules in the kidney. Observed *circa* 1839; reported in 1861. Known as *Henle's loop*.

Uriniferous tubules, discovery of

LORENZO BELLINI, Italian anatomist, 1643-1704, described the uriniferous tubules in 1662. Known as *Bellini's tubules*.

Urobilin in intestinal contents, discovery of

MAX JAFFE, German biochemist, 1841-1911, is credited with finding urobilin in intestinal contents, in 1870. Published in 1871.

Urobilin in urine, discovery of

MAX JAFFE, German biochemist, 1841-1911, discovered urobilin in the urine, in 1866. Reported in 1868.

Urogastrone, description of

ANDREW CONWAY IVY, American physiologist, 1893-   , described urogastrone, a substance found in urine which inhibits secretion and motility of the stomach, *circa* 1925.

Urology, founder of

FRANCISCO DIAZ, Spanish surgeon, 1550-16??, wrote the first treatise on the diseases of the kidney, bladder, and urethra, and is considered the founder of urology. Published in 1588.

Urology, local anesthesia in, introduction of

FESSENDEN NOTT OTIS, American urologist, 1825-1900, is credited with being first to use local anesthesia in urology. Reported in 1884.

Urology

. . . See also under names of particular parts, as *Kidney, Bladder,* etc.

Uroselectan, introduction of

ALEXANDER VON LICHTENBERG, German urologist, 1880-19??, with MOSES SWICK, introduced uroselectan in radiography. Recorded in 1929.

Urotropin

. . . See under *Methenamine, introduction of.*

Urticaria papulosa, description of

THOMAS BATEMAN, English physician, 1778-1821, was the first to give a good description of urticaria papulosa, in 1816.

Urticaria pigmentosa, eponymic description of

EDWARD NETTLESHIP, English ophthalmologist and dermatologist, 1845-1913, described a form of urticaria which leaves permanent pigmented stains. It occurs in infants. Published in 1869. Known as *Nettleship's disease.*

Uterine cancer, early classic description of

ADAM ELIAS VON SIEBOLD, German obstetrician, 1775-1826, gave a classic description of cancer of the uterus, in 1824.

Uterine fibroids, enucleation of, by vaginal route

VINCENT CZERNY, German surgeon, 1842-1916, introduced an operation for the enucleation of uterine fibroids by the vaginal route, in 1881.

Uterine fibromyoma, first excision of

GILMAN KIMBALL, American surgeon, 1804-1892, is credited with performing the first successful abdominal hysteromyomectomy, on Sept. 1, 1853. Recorded in 1855.

Uterine mucosa, epithelial depressions in

WILLIAM FETHERSTON MONTGOMERY, Irish obstetrician, 1797-1859, described epithelial depressions in the uterine mucosa, said to be the dilated canals of the tubular glands. Published in 1837. Known as *Montgomery's cups.*

Uterine tubes, eponymic description of

GABRIEL FALLOPIUS, Italian anatomist, 1523-1562, gave a classic description of the human oviducts, in 1561. The tubes were described less adequately, but earlier, by GALEN, SORANUS, and others. Known as the *fallopian tubes.*

Uterine tubes, inflation patency test for

ISIDOR CLINTON RUBIN, American gynecologist, 1883-19??, devised a method for testing the patency of the uterine tubes by intrauterine inflation with oxygen or carbon dioxide. Recorded in 1920. Known as the *Rubin test.*

Uterine tumors, differentiation between benign and malignant

JAMES HENRY BENNETT, English obstetrician, 1816-1891, was the first to differentiate between benign and malignant tumors of the uterus. Reported in 1845.

Uterosacral ligament

. . . See under *Mackenrodt's ligament.*

Uterus and ovaries, first successful excision of

EUGÈNE KOEBERLÉ, French surgeon, 1828-1915, performed the first successful excision of the uterus and the ovaries, in a case of tumor. Recorded in 1863.

Uterus, atrophy of, in prolonged lactation

RICHARD FROMMEL, German gynecologist, 1854-1912, described atrophy of the uterus sometimes observed in cases of prolonged lactation. Recorded in 1882. Known as *Frommel's disease.*

Uterus, cervical ganglion of

ROBERT LEE, Scottish gynecologist and obstetrician in England, 1793-1877, described the cervical nerve ganglion of the uterus, in 1841. Known as *Lee's ganglion.*

Uterus, contraction ring of, during labor

LUDWIG BANDL, German obstetrician, 1842-1892, described a ring-shaped thickening of the uterus just above the internal os observed during labor. Recorded in 1876. The ring marks the lower border of the contractile portion of the uterus. Known as *Bandl's ring.*

Uterus, excision of, for prolapse; first description

BERENGARIUS OF CAPRI, Italian anatomist, 1480-1550, gave the first accurate description of an operation for the removal of the uterus in a case of prolapse. Recorded in 1522.

Uterus, operation for displacement of, by shortening of round ligaments

WILLIAM ALEXANDER, English surgeon, 1844-1919, devised an operation for the correction of prolapsus and backward displacement of the uterus by extraperitoneal shortening of the round ligaments. Recorded in 1884. An earlier report was published in 1882.

Uterus, operation for retroversion of, by shortening round ligaments

JAMES ALEXANDER ADAMS, Scottish surgeon, 1857-1930, devised an operation for the correction of retroversion of the uterus by shortening of the round ligaments. Report published in 1882.

Uterus, operation for retroversion of, by Webster and Baldy

JOHN MONTGOMERY BALDY, American gynecologist, 1860-1934, devised an operation for the suspension of the uterus in which the round ligaments are brought forward through an incision in the broad ligament and sutured to the posterior surface of the uterus. Recorded in 1903. A similar operation was described by J. C. WEBSTER in 1901. Known as the *Baldy-Webster operation.*

Uterus, peritoneal folds of, seen after delivery

JAMES MATTHEWS DUNCAN, Scottish gynecologist, 1826-1890, described folds of loose peritoneum covering the uterus, observed immediately after the expulsion of the fetus. Recorded in 1854. Known as *Duncan's folds*.

Uterus, retroversion of; early description

WILLIAM HUNTER, Scottish surgeon and obstetrician, 1718-1783, is credited with being the first to describe retroversion of the uterus, in 1771.

Uterus, softening of lower segment of, in pregnancy

ALFRED HEGAR, German gynecologist, 1830-1914, described a softening of the lower segment of the uterus in the early stages of pregnancy. Reported in 1884. Known as *Hegar's sign*.

Uveoparotid fever, eponymic description of

CHRISTIAN F. HEERFORDT, Danish ophthalmologist, 1871-19??, described uveoparotid fever in 1909. Known as *Heerfordt's disease*.

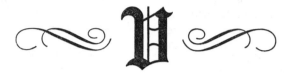

Vaccination for smallpox, introduction of

EDWARD JENNER, English physician, 1749-1823, recognized that immunity for smallpox may be produced by the relatively mild condition of cowpox, a realization which led to his development of smallpox vaccine from cowpox virus. Reported in 1798.

Vaccination for

. . . See also under name of particular disease, as *Typhoid fever*.

Vaccinia, Paschen bodies in

. . . See under *Paschen bodies*.

Vaccinia virus, medium for cultivation, without tissue culture

HUGH BETHUNE MAITLAND, Canadian bacteriologist in England, 1895-   , with MARY C. MAITLAND, developed a medium for the cultivation of vaccinia virus without tissue culture. It contains chicken kidney and serum. Published in 1928.

Vagina, artificial, formation of, from loop of intestine

JAMES FAIRCHILD BALDWIN, American gynecologist, 1850-1936, devised an operation for the formation of an artificial vagina by interposing a loop of intestine between the rectum and the urinary bladder. Reported in 1904.

Vagina, excision of, operation for

ROBERT VON OLSHAUSEN, German gynecologist and obstetrician, 1835-1915, introduced an operation for the excision of the vagina. Reported in 1895.

Vagina, plastic reconstruction of

ALWIN KARL MACKENRODT, German gynecologist, 1859-1925, devised an operation for the plastic reconstruction of the vagina. Published in 1896.

Vagina, popularization of name

GABRIEL FALLOPIUS, Italian anatomist, 1523-1562, is credited with popularizing the term *vagina*, which was used earlier by ORIBASIUS, CELSUS, and others. Reported in his work published in 1561.

Vaginal folds bounding Pawlik's triangle

KAREL J. PAWLIK, Prague gynecologist, 1849-1914, described two folds or columns on the anterior vaginal wall which form the lateral boundaries of Pawlik's triangle and serve as guides to the openings of the ureters. Recorded in 1886. Known as *Pawlik's folds*.

Vaginal hysterectomy, first authentic record of

GIACOMO BERENGARIO DA CARPI, Italian surgeon, 1470-1550, described two cases of vaginal hysterectomy, one performed by his father (n. d.) and the other by himself, in 1507. Recorded in 1521.

Vaginal ovariotomy, first recorded

THEODORE GAILLARD THOMAS, American surgeon, 1832-1903, is credited with performing the first recorded vaginal ovariotomy. Published in 1870.

Vaginal speculum, duckbill, introduction of

JAMES MARION SIMS, American surgeon, 1813-1883, introduced a "duckbill" vaginal speculum. Recorded in 1866. Known as *Sims' speculum*.

Vagotomy in treatment of gastric and duodenal ulcers

. . . See under *Peptic ulcer, vagotomy in treatment of*.

Vagotonus, introduction of concept of

HANS EPPINGER, German physician, 1879-19??, with LEO HESS, German physician, 1879-19??, introduced the theory of a physiological balance between the two branches of the autonomic nervous system. An increase in the parasympathetic tonus was termed *vagotonus*, while an imbalance in favor of the sympathetic system was named *sympatheticotonus*. Recorded in 1910.

Vagus and glossopharyngeal nerves, ascending roots of

MIHALY LENHOSSEK, Hungarian anatomist, 1863-1937, described the ascending roots of the vagus and glossopharyngeal nerves. Recorded in 1894. Known as the *bundle of Lenhossek*.

Vagus, auricular branch of; original description

FRIEDRICH ARNOLD, German anatomist, 1803-1890, was the first to describe the auricular branch of the vagus. Recorded in 1838. Known as *Arnold's nerve*.

Vagus, early description of

MARINOS (or MARINUS), Roman physician and anatomist, *circa* 40-110 A. D., described the vagus nerves, about 65 A. D. Marinos referred to the vagus as the sixth nerve.

Vagus escape, phenomenon of

EDUARD FRIEDRICH WILHELM WEBER, German physiologist, 1806-1871, with his brother ERNST HEINRICH WEBER, German physiologist, 1795-1878, discovered that if the inhibitory effect of the vagus upon the heart is exerted long enough, the heart "escapes" and begins to beat again. Recorded in 1845.

Vagus in relation to heart beat

. . . See under *Heart beat, slowing of*, etc.

Vagus in relation to respiration, study of

JULIEN J. C. LEGALLOIS, French physician, 1770-1814, studied the relation of the vagus nerve to respiration and demonstrated that bilateral section may produce bronchopneumonia. Published in 1812.

Vagus, inhibitory effect of

EDUARD FRIEDRICH WILHELM WEBER, German physiologist, 1806-1871, with his brother ERNST HEINRICH WEBER, German physiologist, 1795-1878, discovered the inhibitory effect of the vagus upon the heart. Recorded in 1845.

Vagus, introduction of term

DOMENICO DE MARCHETTI, Italian anatomist, 1626-1688, is credited with the introduction of the term *vagus,* about 1655.

Vagus stimulation liberates acetylcholine-like substance

OTTO LOEWI, German pharmacologist in the United States, 1873-19??, demonstrated that stimulation of the vagus nerve results in the liberation of a substance identical with acetylcholine which affects the rate of the heart beat. Recorded in 1921.

Valence, observations leading to concept of—1852

EDWARD FRANKLAND, English chemist, 1825-1899, made fundamental observations on the formation of chemical compounds which formed the foundation of the theory of valence. Reported in 1852.

Valleix's points douloureux

. . . See under *Tender points in course of nerve, in neuralgia.*

Valsalva's antrum

. . . See under *Tympanic antrum, enopymic description of.*

Valsalva's maneuver in otitis media

ANTONIO MARIA VALSALVA, Italian anatomist, 1666-1723, described a maneuver whereby the discharge in otitis media is made to appear in the auditory canal. Recorded in 1704.

Valsuani's disease

. . . See under *Pernicious anemia, progressive, in pregnant women.*

Valves of veins, first description of

GIOVANNI BATTISTA CANANO, Italian anatomist, 1515-1579, is credited with the first description of the valves of the veins. Recorded *circa* 1541.

Valves of

. . . See also under name of structure or organ involved.

Valvula venae cavae, first description of

BARTOLOMMEO EUSTACHIUS, Italian anatomist, 1524-1574, described the semilunar valve in the right atrium, in 1563.

Valvulae conniventes, introduction of term

THOMAS THEODOR KERCKRING, German physician and anatomist in Holland, 1640-1693, described the transverse mucous folds of the small intestine and named them *valvulae conniventes,* in 1670. The structures were described earlier, *circa* 1561, by FALLOPIUS.

Valvular disease, chronic, operation for

THEODORE TUFFIER, French surgeon, 1857-1929, is credited with performing the first successful experimental operation in the treatment of chronic valvular heart disease. Recorded in 1914.

**Valvular vegetation, first
description of**

GIOVANNI MARIA LANCISI, Italian
physician, 1654-1720, is credited
with being the first to describe
valvular vegetation. Recorded in
1707.

**Van den Bergh test for
bile pigments**

. . . See under *Bile pigments,* etc.

**Varicella gangrenosa, first
description of**

JONATHAN HUTCHINSON, English
physician, 1828-1913, gave the first
description of varicella gangrenosa
(dermatitis gangrenosa infantum),
in 1882.

Varicella

. . . See also under *Chickenpox.*

**Varicose veins, dextrose
in treatment of**

GABOR NOBL, Austrian surgeon,
1864-1938, was first to use dextrose
by injection in the treatment of
varicose veins. Published in 1926.

**Varicose veins, early
operation for**

BENJAMIN COLLINS BRODIE, English surgeon, 1783-1862, is believed
to have been the first to treat varicose veins by surgical means. Early
operation performed in 1814.

**Varicose veins, injection
treatment of**

PAUL LINSER, German surgeon,
1871-19??, introduced the use of
injections in the treatment of varicose veins. Recorded in 1916.

**Varicose veins, ligation in
treatment of**

FRIEDRICH TRENDELENBURG, Ger-

man surgeon, 1844-1924, ligated
the great saphenous vein in treating
varicosities in the leg. Recorded in
1890.

**Varicose veins, quinine-
urethane in treatment of**

JACQUES M. GÉNÉVRIER, French
surgeon, 1890-19??, is said to have
been first to use quinine-urethane
in the treatment of varicose veins.
Recorded in 1921.

**Varicose veins, sodium chloride
in treatment of**

KARL LINSER, German surgeon,
1885-19??, was first to use sodium
chloride by injection in the treatment of varicose veins. Recorded
in 1925.

**Varicose veins, sodium mor-
rhuate in treatment of**

WILLIAM MORRIS COOPER, American surgeon, 1894-   , introduced
the use of sodium morrhuate by injection in the treatment of varicose
veins. He combined the injection
with preliminary ligation. Published in 1934.

**Varicose veins, sodium salicylate
in treatment of**

JEAN ATHANASE SICARD, French
physician, 1872-1929, with J.
PARAF and J. LERMOYEZ, introduced the use of sodium salicylate
by injection in the treatment of
varicose veins. Recorded in 1922.

**Varicose veins, test for in-
sufficiency of valves in**

BENJAMIN COLLINS BRODIE, English surgeon, 1783-1862, devised a
test for the efficacy of the valves in
cases of varicose veins. Recorded
in 1846. In 1890, the test was de-

scribed by FRIEDRICH TRENDELEN-BURG with whose name it became associated. Known as *Trendelenburg's test.*

Variola, Paschen bodies in
. . . See under *Paschen bodies.*

Variolation, first record of
HEINRICH VOLLGNAD, German physician, 1634-1682, is believed to have performed the first recorded variolation. Published in 1671.

Variolation
. . . See also under *Smallpox vaccination.*

Vascular spasm in extremities, especially in digits
MAURICE RAYNAUD, French physician, 1834-1881, described the phenomenon of recurring vascular spasm in the extremities, especially in the fingers or toes. Published in 1862. Known as *Raynaud's disease, phenomenon,* or *syndrome.*

Vasoconstrictor center, variations in tone of
LUDWIG TRAUBE, German physician, 1818-1876, was first to describe the rhythmic variations in the tone of the vasoconstrictor center. Published in 1865. Known as *Traube-Hering waves.*

Vasoconstrictor fibers originate in lateral horn
WALTER HOLBROOK GASKELL, English physiologist, 1847-1914, demonstrated that the efferent vasoconstrictor nerves originate in the lateral horns of the spinal cord. Published in 1883.

Vasodilatation caused by stimulation of posterior nerve roots
SALOMON STRICKER, German path-

ologist, 1834-1898, discovered that stimulation of the posterior nerve roots results in vasodilatation. Recorded in 1876.

Vasomotor disturbances, periarterial sympathectomy in
. . . See under *Periarterial sympathectomy.*

Vasomotor mechanism, regulation of
AUGUST KROGH, Danish physiologist, 1874-1949, discovered the regulation of the vasomotor mechanism of small vessels. Reported in 1919.

Vasomotor nerves, early description of—1727
FRANÇOIS POURFOUR DU PETIT, French physician and physiologist, 1664-1741, is said to have described the vasomotor nerves in 1727.

Vasomotor nerves, early description of—1858
CLAUDE BERNARD, French physiologist, 1813-1878, described vasodilator and vasoconstrictor nerves, in 1858.

Vasomotor reflexes, discovery of—1866
ELIE DE CYON, Russian physiologist, 1843-1912, with KARL FRIEDRICH W. LUDWIG, German physiologist, 1816-1895, studied and reported the vasomotor reflexes, in 1866.

Vasomotor rhinitis, early recognition of
JULES HIPPOLYTE CLOQUET, French physician, 1787-1840, described vasomotor rhinitis. Recorded in 1821.

Vaso-oscillator bed

. . . See under *Bed, seesawing, for cardiovascular and peripheral vascular disease.*

Vasovagal syncope, original description of

THOMAS LEWIS, English cardiologist, 1881-1945, described a condition caused by hypersensitivity of the carotid sinus and marked by pallor, loss of consciousness, fall of blood pressure, etc. Published in 1932. Known also as *carotid sinus syndrome.*

Vater-Pacini corpuscles

. . . See under *Pacini's corpuscles.*

Vein, basal cerebral, eponymic description of

FRIEDRICH CHRISTIAN ROSENTHAL, German anatomist, 1780-1829, described the vena basalis, the basal cerebral vein which empties into the internal cerebral vein. Date not available. Known as *Rosenthal's vein.*

Vein, emissary, passing through foramen of Vesalius

ANDREAS VESALIUS, Belgian anatomist, 1514-1564, described the emissary vein which passes through the foramen of Vesalius. Recorded in 1543. Known as *Vesalius'* or *vesalian vein.*

Vein, oblique, of Marshall

JOHN MARSHALL, English surgeon and anatomist, 1818-1891, described a small vein extending from the left atrium to the sinus coronarius. Published in 1850.

Veins, common cardinal, description of

. . . See under *Common cardinal veins.*

Veins extending from mesentery to vena cava

ANDERS ADOLF RETZIUS, Swedish anatomist, 1796-1860, described veins which form anastomoses between the veins of the intestine and the inferior vena cava. Recorded *circa* 1830. Known as *Retzius' veins* or *retroperitoneal veins.*

Veins of diploe, early description of

GILBERT BRESCHET, French anatomist, 1784-1845, gave the first good description of the veins of the diploe, in 1819. Known as *Breschet's veins.*

Velocity of blood flow, instrument for measuring

JAN DOGIEL, Russian physiologist, 1830-1905, devised an instrument for measuring the velocity of the blood stream. Recorded in 1867. Known as a *stromuhr.* See also under *Blood flow.*

Velpeau's bandage

. . . See under *Bandage for support of arm in fracture of clavicle.*

***Velum palati,* origin of term**

GABRIEL FALLOPIUS, Italian anatomist, 1523-1562, is credited with having originated the term *velum palati,* for the soft palate, *circa* 1552. It was at this time that Fallopius differentiated between the soft palate and the hard palate, both of which were previously described as the *diaphragma oris.*

Vena cava, valve of

. . . See under *Valvula venae cavae, first description of.*

Vena obliqua atrii sinistri (marshalli)

. . . See under *Vein, oblique, of Marshall.*

Venae cordis minimae, eponymic description of

ADAM CHRISTIAN THEBESIUS, German physician, 1686-1732, described small veins originating in the myocardium and opening into the cavities of the heart. Published in 1708. Known as *Thebesian veins.*

Venereal lymphogranuloma, first satisfactory description of

JOSEPH NICOLAS, French physician, 1868-19??, with J. DURAND and MAURICE FAVRE, gave the first comprehensive description of venereal lymphogranuloma. Recorded in 1913. Known as the *fourth venereal disease, Nicolas-Durand-Favre disease,* and *Frei's disease,* the last in allusion to W. S. FREI, who developed a test for the disease.

Venereal lymphogranuloma, specific test for

WILHELM S. FREI, German dermatologist, 1885-1943, devised a specific test for venereal lymphogranuloma, in 1925. The test consists of an intradermal injection of antigen prepared from material containing the causative virus. The test is known as the *Frei test;* the disease, as *Frei's disease.*

Venereal lymphogranuloma

. . . See also under *Lymphogranuloma venereum.*

Venomous snakes of India, description of

. . . See under *Snakes, venomous,* etc.

Ventilation, artificial, in ships, mines, etc.

STEPHEN HALES, English physiologist and clergyman, 1677-1761, invented a ventilator which introduced artificial ventilation in ships, mines, etc., *circa* 1741.

Ventral hernia, original research in

. . . See under *Abdominal hernia.*

Ventricle, fifth, early description of

. . . See under *Cavum septi pellucidi.*

Ventricle, lateral, first operation on, for drainage

WILLIAM DETMOID, American surgeon, 1808-1894, is believed to have performed the first recorded operation in which the lateral ventricle was opened for drainage of a brain abscess, in 1850.

Ventricle, left, first accurate description of

RAYMOND VIEUSSENS, French anatomist, 1641-1715, was the first to give an accurate description of the structure of the left ventricle of the heart. Published in 1705.

Ventricle of Arantius, early description of

. . . See under *Cavum septi pellucidi.*

Ventricle of brain, fourth, lateral openings of

HUBERT VON LUSCHKA, German anatomist, 1820-1875, described lateral openings in the fourth ventricle of the brain by means of which the ventricle communicates with the subarachnoid space. Recorded *circa* 1863. Known as *foramens of Luschka* or *Luschka's foramen*.

Ventricles, communication between, abnormal

HENRI LOUIS ROGER, French physician, 1809-1891, described an abnormal congenital opening between the ventricles of the heart. Published in 1879. Known as *Roger's disease* or *maladie de Roger*.

Ventricles of brain, communication between

ALEXANDER MONRO *secundus,* Scottish anatomist, 1733-1817, discovered that the lateral ventricles of the human brain communicate with each other. Recorded in 1783.

Ventricles of brain, discovery of air in

WILLIAM HENRY LUCKETT, American surgeon, 1872-19??, discovered the presence of air in the ventricles of the brain, a finding which is said to have given WALTER EDWARD DANDY the idea for ventriculography. Recorded in 1913.

Ventricles of brain, early successful tapping of

WILLIAM WILLIAMS KEEN, American surgeon, 1837-1932, successfully tapped the ventricles of the brain, in 1889.

Ventricular fibrillation, experimental production of

JOHN ALEXANDER MACWILLIAM, Aberdeen physician, 1857-1937, demonstrated that ventricular fibrillation can be produced by injection of poisons into the blood stream. Reported in 1887.

Ventricular fibrillation, sudden death from

JOHN ALEXANDER MACWILLIAM, Aberdeen physician, 1857-1937, gave the first description of a case of sudden death from ventricular fibrillation. Published in 1889.

Ventricular gradient, introduction of term

FRANK NORMAN WILSON, American physician, 1890-1952, introduced the term *ventricular gradient* in electrocardiography, in 1938.

Ventriculography, introduction of

WALTER EDWARD DANDY, Baltimore neurosurgeon, 1886-1946, is credited with the introduction of ventriculography, in 1918.

Ventriculus laryngis morgagni

. . . See under *Morgagni's ventricle of larynx.*

Verheyen's stars

. . . See under *Kidney, stellate veins of.*

Vermiform appendix, first description of

BERENGARIUS OF CAPRI, Italian anatomist, 1480-1550, is believed to have been the first to describe the vermiform appendix, in 1521.

Vernal conjunctivitis, first description of

EDWIN THEODOR SAEMISCH, German ophthalmologist, 1833-1909, was the first to describe vernal conjunctivitis, in 1876.

Verneuil's bursitis or disease

. . . See under *Syphilitic bursitis.*

Veronal, introduction of

. . . See under *Barbital, introduction of.*

Verrucae necrogenicae

. . . See under *Dissecting-room warts.*

Verruga peruana, causative agent of

A. L. BARTON, Peruvian physician, 1874-19??, described the causative organism of verruga peruana, now known as *Bartonella bacilliformis,* in 1909.

Verruga peruana, original description of

TOMAS SALAZAR, Peruvian physician, 1830-1917, described verruga peruana, the nodular cutaneous stage of Carrión's disease. Published in 1858.

Version, spontaneous, in transverse presentation

JOHN CUPPAGE DOUGLAS, Irish obstetrician, 1777-1850, described cases of spontaneous version, a phenomenon sometimes observed in transverse presentations. Recorded in 1815.

Version

. . . See also under *Podalic version,* etc.

Vertebra, compression fracture of

HERMANN KÜMMELL, German surgeon, 1852-1937, described a type of traumatic spondylitis usually coming on a few weeks after an injury and characterized by pain in the spine, intercostal neuralgia, gibbosity, etc. Recorded in 1891. Known as *Kümmell's disease.*

Vertebra, Schmorl's nodule of

CHRISTIAN GEORG SCHMORL, German pathologist, 1861-1932, described a nodule seen on a vertebra and said by some to be due to herniation of the nucleus pulposus of the intervertebral disk into the softened substance of the vertebra. Published in 1926. Known as *Schmorl's nodule.*

Vertebrae, necrosis of epiphyses of

HOLGER WERFEL SCHEUERMANN, Danish orthopedist, 1877-19??, described a condition marked by necrosis of the epiphyses of the vertebrae. Published in 1921. Known as *Scheuermann's disease.*

Vertigo in relation to semicircular canals

MARIE J. P. FLOURENS, French physiologist, 1794-1867, demonstrated the relation of the semicircular canals to vertigo, in 1828.

Vertigo, paralyzing, description of

FELIX GERLIER, Swiss physician, 1840-1914, described an endemic disease occurring in Switzerland marked by vertigo, paralysis, etc. Reported in 1887. Known as *Gerlier's disease, paralyzing vertigo,* etc.

Vesalius' foramen

. . . See under *Foramen of Vesalius at base of skull.*

Vesalius' ligament

. . . See under *Inguinal ligament, early description of.*

Vesalius' vein

. . . See under *Vein, emissary, passing through foramen of Vesalius.*

Vesical trigone

. . . See under *Trigone of urinary bladder.*

Vesicles formed by shaking together oil and albuminous fluid

FERDINAND MORITZ ASCHERSON, German physician, 1798-1879, described the vesicles which form when oil and an albuminous liquid are shaken together. Reported in 1831.

Vesico-vaginal fistula, early successful treatment of—1838

JOHN PETER METTAUER, American surgeon, 1787-1875, operated successfully for vesico-vaginal fistula in August 1838. Recorded in 1840.

Vesico-vaginal fistula, early successful treatment of—1839

GEORGE HAYWARD, American surgeon, 1791-1863, operated successfully for vesico-vaginal fistula in 1839. Recorded in 1839.

Vesico-vaginal fistula, Sims' operation for

JAMES MARION SIMS, American surgeon, 1813-1883, introduced the Sims operation for the correction of vesico-vaginal fistula, in 1852.

Vesiculography, introduction of

HUGH HAMPTON YOUNG, Baltimore urologist, 1870-1945, described x-ray studies of the seminal vesicles and vasa deferentia after urethroscopic injection of the ejaculatory ducts with thorium, in 1921.

Vestibular glands, major, discovery of

CASPAR BARTHOLIN, Danish anatomist, 1655-1738, discovered the major vestibular glands, one on each side of the vaginal orifice. Reported in 1675. Known as *Bartholin's glands, Duverney's glands,* and *Tiedmann's glands.*

Vi antigens, first description of

ARTHUR FELIX, English microbiologist, 1887-19??, with R. MARGARET PITT, gave the first description of Vi antigens, antigens contained in the sheath of a bacterium, in a paper titled "A new antigen of B. typhosus." Published in 1934.

Vibration massage in treatment of nervous disorders

. . . See under *Nerve vibration.*

Vibrio cholerae, discovery of

. . . See under *Cholera, discovery of causative organism of.*

Vibrio comma, discovery of

. . . See under *Cholera, discovery of causative organism of.*

Vibrio proteus, isolation of

DITTMAR FINKLER, German bacteriologist, 1852-1912, with J. PRIOR, isolated the *Vibrio proteus* from stools of patients affected with acute gastroenteritis, in 1884.

Vibrio tyrogenus, description of

THEODOR K. A. DENEKE, German bacteriologist, 1860-19??, described the *Vibrio tyrogenus,* known also as *Deneke's spirillum.* Recorded *circa* 1905.

Vibrion septique, discovery of

LOUIS PASTEUR, French scientist and bacteriologist, 1822-1895, with

JULES F. JOUBERT, discovered the *Vibrion septique* (*Clostridium septique*), in 1877. This organism was the first pathogenic anaerobe to be identified.

Vicq d'Azyr's bundle
. . . See under *Mammillothalamic tract,* etc.

Vidal's disease
. . . See under *Lichen chronicus simplex.*

Vidian artery
. . . See under *Internal maxillary artery.*

Vidian canal
. . . See under *Pterygoid canal.*

Vidian nerve
. . . See under *Nerve of pterygoid canal.*

Vieussens' annulus
. . . See under *Annulus ovalis.*

Vieussens, ansa of
. . . See under *Ansa subclavia,* etc.

Vincent's infection or angina, eponymic description of
JEAN HYACINTHE VINCENT, French bacteriologist, 1862-1950, described a necrotizing ulcerative infection of the gums, tonsils, etc., caused by fusiform bacilli. Recorded in 1898. Known also as *Plaut-Vincent's disease.*

Vincent's infection or angina, pre-eponymic description of
HUGO KARL PLAUT, German physician, 1858-1928, described a necrotizing ulcerative membranous infection, mainly of the tonsils, considered identical with Vincent's infection. Recorded in 1894. Known as *Plaut's angina, Plaut-Vincent's disease,* etc.

Viper venom, early treatise on
FELICE FONTANA, Italian physiologist, 1720-1805, did important experimental work on viper venom. Treatise published in 1767.

Virchow-Robin spaces
. . . See under *Artery, spaces in external coat of.*

Virus B, isolation of
ALBERT BRUCE SABIN, American bacteriologist, 1906-   , with ARTHUR M. WRIGHT, isolated the B virus from the central nervous system of a person who died of ascending myelitis following a bite by a monkey. Recorded in 1934.

Virus, filtrable, as cause of disease in animals
PAUL FROSCH, German physician, 1860-1928, with FRIEDRICH A. J. LOEFLER, German bacteriologist, 1852-1915, showed a filtrable virus to be the cause of foot and mouth disease in animals. Recorded in 1897.

Virus hemagglutination, discovery of
GEORGE KEBLE HIRST, American physician, 1909-   , is credited with discovering the phenomenon of virus hemagglutination, the agglutination of red blood cells by certain viruses. Published in 1941.

Viscera, transposition of, early report on
. . . See under *Transposition of viscera.*

Visceral arches in vertebrates
KARL BOGISLAUS REICHERT, Ger-

man anatomist, 1811-1883, was the first to describe the visceral arches in vertebrate animals. The cartilage of the second pharyngeal arch is known as *Reichert's cartilage*. Recorded in 1837.

Vision, test type for determining acuteness of

. . . See under *Test type*.

Visual association area in parastriate region

SALOMON E. HENSCHEN, Swedish pathologist, 1847-1930, was first to suggest the existence of a visual association area in the parastriate region. Reported in 1919.

Visual purple, discovery of—1851

HEINRICH MÜLLER, German anatomist, 1820-1864, is credited with discovering visual purple, in 1851.

Visual purple, discovery of—1876

FRANZ CHRISTIAN BOLL, German physiologist, 1849-1879, discovered visual purple in the rods of the retina, in 1876.

Visual purple is bleached by light, observation that

FRANZ CHRISTIAN BOLL, German physiologist, 1849-1879, discovered that visual purple is bleached by the action of light. Published in 1877.

Visual purple, isolation of, from retina

WILHELM FRIEDRICH (WILLY) KÜHNE, German physiologist, 1837-1900, is credited with isolating visual purple from the retina, in 1877.

Visual receptive area in region of calcarine fissure

SALOMON E. HENSCHEN, Swedish pathologist, 1847-1930, is credited with being first to suggest the existence of a cortical visual receptive area in the region of the calcarine fissure of the occipital lobe. Reported in 1918.

Vital statistics, first book on

. . . See under *Medical statistics, pioneer in*.

Vitallium cup arthroplasty of hip

MARIUS NYGAARD SMITH-PETERSEN, American surgeon, 1886-1953, introduced the use of a vitallium cap or cup in arthroplasty of the hip. Recorded in 1939.

Vitallium, introduction of, in surgery

CHARLES SCOTT VENABLE, American surgeon, 1877-19??, with W. STUCK and A. BEACH, introduced the metal vitallium in surgery. Vitallium is an alloy of cobalt, chromium, and molybdenum. Recorded in 1937.

Vitamin A and vitamin D, separation of

HARRY STEENBOCK, American physiologist and biochemist, 1886-19??, with M. SELL and M. VAN R. BUELL, succeeded in separating vitamin A from vitamin D, in 1921.

Vitamin A, discovery of

ELMER VERNER McCOLLUM, American biochemist, 1879-19??, with MARGUERITE DAVIS, reported the need of the body for certain "lipins" in the diet during period of growth, thereby demonstrating the presence in certain foods of a "fat-soluble A," later to be known as vitamin A. Published in 1913.

Vitamin A, isolation of crystalline

HARRY NICHOLLS HOLMES, American biochemist, 1879-19??, with RUTH E. CORBET, reported the isolation of a "crystalline vitamin A concentration," in 1937.

Vitamin B-1, isolation of

BAREND C. P. JANSEN, Dutch physiological chemist, 1884-19??, with WILLEM F. DONATH (Dutch physician and biochemist, 1889-19??), isolated vitamin B-1 in 1926. Reported in 1927.

Vitamin B-1, recognition of

CASIMIR FUNK, American biochemist, 1884-19??, recognized the existence of an anti-polyneuritis factor in rice polishings, a substance which later became known as vitamin B-1. Recorded in 1911-12.

Vitamin B-2, chemical formula of

. . . See under *Riboflavin, chemical structure of.*

Vitamin B-3, discovery of

ROBERT RUNNELS WILLIAMS, American biochemist, 1886-19??, with ROBERT E. WATERMAN, discovered vitamin B-3, in 1928.

Vitamin B-5, discovery of

HENRY WULF, English biochemist, 1877-1944, with C. W. CARTER and R. A. PETERS, discovered vitamin B-5, a factor necessary to maintain weight in pigeons and growth in rats. Recorded in 1930.

Vitamin B-12, crystallization of

EDWARD LAWRENCE RICKES, American biochemist, 1912- , with N. G. BRINK, F. R. KONIUSZY, T. R. WOOD, and K. FOLKERS, crystallized vitamin B-12. Published in 1948.

Vitamin B-12, microbiological assay of

MARY SHAW SHORB, American biochemist, 1907- , devised a microbiological assay for vitamin B-12. Published in 1948.

Vitamin C, isolation of

ALBERT SZENT-GYÖRGYI, Hungarian biochemist, 1893- , is credited with isolating vitamin C. Recorded in 1928.

Vitamin C, recognition of

JACK CECIL DRUMMOND, English biochemist, 1891-1952, recognized the existence of vitamin C, in 1919.

Vitamin C, synthesis of

TADEUS REICHSTEIN, Polish chemist and physiologist in Switzerland, 1897- , with A. GRÜSSNER and R. OPPENAUER, synthesized vitamin C. Recorded in 1933.

Vitamin C, synthesis of

WALTER NORMAN HAWORTH, English chemist, 1883-1949, synthesized vitamin C or ascorbic acid, in 1933. Received Nobel prize in 1937.

Vitamin D, isolation of crystalline

FREDERIC ANDERTON ASKEW, English biochemist, 189?- , with R. B. BOURDILLON, H. M. BRUCE, R. K. CALLOW, J. ST. L. PHILPOT, and T. A. WEBSTER, prepared crystalline vitamin D, in 1932.

Vitamin D milk, introduction of

HARRY STEENBOCK, American physiologist and biochemist, 1886-19??, is credited with inventing vitamin D milk. Introduced *circa* 1925.

Vitamin D, recognition of

EDWARD MELLANBY, English physiologist, 1884-19??, is credited with the recognition of the anti-rachitic factor or vitamin D, in 1918.

Vitamin D, synthesis of, by irradiation of sterols

HARRY STEENBOCK, American physiologist and biochemist, 1886-19??, is credited with the synthesis of vitamin D by the irradiation of sterols. Recorded in 1924.

Vitamin D-2, isolation of crystalline

ROBERT BENEDICT BOURDILLON, English biochemist, 1889-19??, with H. M. BRUCE, C. FISCHMANN, R. G. C. JENKINS, and T. A. WEBSTER, isolated crystalline vitamin D-2 (calciferol) from irradiated ergosterol. Recorded in 1931.

Vitamin E, discovery of, in wheat germ

HERBERT M. EVANS, American physician, 1882-19??, discovered the presence of vitamin E in wheat germ. Reported, with K. S. BISHOP, in 1922.

Vitamin E, isolation of, from wheat germ oil

HERBERT M. EVANS, American physician, 1882-19??, isolated vitamin E (alpha-tocopherol) from wheat germ oil. Reported, with O. H. EMERSON and GLADYS A. EMERSON, in 1936.

Vitamin E, synthesis of

PAUL KARRER, Swiss chemist, 1889-19??, with H. FRITZSCHE, B. H. RINGIER, and H. SALOMON, synthesized vitamin E, alpha-tocopherol, in 1938.

Vitamin, early concept of

N. LUNIN, Swiss physiologist, 1852-19??, experimented with synthetic milk and demonstrated that chemically pure foods lack some unknown substance and cannot sustain life. Published in 1881.

Vitamin F, discovery of

GEORGE OSWALD BURR, American biochemist, 1896-   , with MILDRED M. BURR, showed the need of the organism for certain unsaturated fatty acids, i.e., vitamin F. Published in 1930.

Vitamin F, discovery of

HERBERT M. EVANS, American physician, 1882-19??, is credited with discovering vitamin F (linoleic, linolenic, and arachidonic acids), in 1934.

Vitamin, introduction of term

CASIMIR FUNK, Polish chemist, 1884-19??, introduced the term *vitamine,* in 1912, on the assumption that the substances were amines. Later, when it was discovered that they were not amines, the term was changed to *vitamin.*

Vitamin, introduction of term

JACK CECIL DRUMMOND, English biochemist, 1891-1952, suggested the omission of the letter e from the then current form *vitamine*. This was accepted in 1920.

Vitamin K in hemorrhagic disease

HUGH ROLAND BUTT, American physician, 1910-   , with ALBERT MARKLEY SNELL (American physician, 1896-   ), used vitamin K and bile in treating the hemorrhagic diathesis in cases of jaundice. Published in 1938.

Vitamin K, isolation of—1939

HENRIK DAM, Danish-American biochemist, 1895-   , isolated vitamin K from alfalfa, in 1939. The vitamin was isolated independently in the same year by R. W. McKEE and his associates.

Vitamin K-1, synthesis of—1939

LOUIS FREDERICK FIESER, American biochemist, 1899-19??, is credited with synthesizing vitamin K-1, in 1939.

Vitamin K-1, synthesis of—1939

STEFAN ANSBACHER, German-American biochemist, 1905-   , is said to have synthesized vitamin K-1. Reported in 1939.

Vitamin K-2, chemical structure of

STEPHEN BENNETT BINKLEY, American biochemist, 1910-   , with R. W. McKEE, S. A. THAYER, and E. A. DOISY, determined the structural formula of vitamin K-2. Published in 1940.

Vitamin P (citrin), discovery of

STEPHAN RUSZNYÁK, Hungarian physician, 1891-19??, with ALBERT SZENT - GYÖRGYI (Hungarian biochemist, 1893-19??), discovered

vitamin P or citrin. Recorded in 1936.

Vitamin P, isolation of, from lemon peel

CECIL Z. WAWRA, American scientist, 1908-   , with J. LEYDEN WEBB, isolated hesperidin chalcone, vitamin P, from lemon peel. Reported in 1942.

Vitamins, early recognition of

FREDERICK G. HOPKINS, English biochemist, 1861-1947, is credited with being the first to appreciate the significance of accessory food factors, i.e., vitamins, in the diet. Recorded in 1906.

Vitamins, fat-soluble, early concept of

WILHELM OTTO STEPP, German biochemist, 1882-19??, demonstrated that chemically pure fats lack some vital factor, thus in effect discovering the existence of fat-soluble vitamins. Published in 1909.

Vitamins K-1 and K-2, isolation of

RALPH WENDELL McKEE, American biochemist, 1912-   , with S. B. BINKLEY, D. W. MacCORQUODALE, S. A. THAYER, and E. A. DOISY, isolated the vitamins K-1 and K-2. Recorded in 1939.

Vitreous, artificial, operation for

PHILIP HENRY MULES, English ophthalmologist, 1843-1905, devised an operation in which the eyeball is eviscerated and an artificial vitreous is inserted. Recorded in 1885. Known as *Mules' operation*.

Vitreous humor, inflammation of, marked by presence of star-shaped bodies

... See under *Astral hyalitis*.

Vitriol buttons for checking hemorrhage

CHARLES GABRIEL LE CLERC, French surgeon, 1644-1698, used vitriol buttons to stop hemorrhage. Recorded in 1695.

Vivisection, introduction of, in the teaching of physiology

JOHN CALL DALTON, American physiologist, 1825-1889, was the first to illustrate his lectures on physiology with vivisection experiments. In defense of his methods against the opposition, he wrote a book, *The Experimental Method in Medical Science*, published in 1882.

Vocal cord, cartilaginous nodule in

HUBERT VON LUSCHKA, German anatomist, 1820-1875, described a small cartilaginous nodule in the anterior part of the vocal cord. Published in 1873. Known as *Luschka's cartilage*.

Vocal cords, cadaveric position of

CARL ADOLPH CHRISTIAN JACOB GERHARDT, German laryngologist, 1833-1902, introduced the term *cadaveric position*, to describe the vocal cord or cords in the position of total paralysis. Recorded in 1872.

Vocal cords, paralysis of; early recognition

CARL ADOLPH CHRISTIAN JACOB GERHARDT, German laryngologist, 1833-1902, made important contributions to the diagnosis of paralysis of the vocal cords. Published in 1863.

Vogt's syndrome or disease

... See under *Corpus striatum syndrome*.

Volkmann's canals

... See under *Bone, canals in, for blood vessels*.

Volkmann's contracture

. . . See under *Contracture of muscles due to injury or pressure*.

Voltolini's disease

... See under *Ear, internal, acute inflammation of*.

Volumetric analysis, development of

JOSEPH L. GAY-LUSSAC, French chemist and physicist, 1778-1850, is believed to have introduced the method of volumetric analysis, *circa* 1815.

Volvulus, first recorded operation for

ADOLF FREDRIK LINSTEDT, Swedish surgeon, 1847-1915, with JOHAN ANTON WALDENSTRÖM, Swedish physician, 1839-1879, performed the first recorded operation for volvulus, in 1878.

Volvulus, first successful operation for, in England

HENRY EDWARD CLARK, English surgeon, 1845-1909, is credited with performing the first successful operation for the treatment of volvulus in Britain, on February 20, 1883.

Vomeronasal organ, eponymic description of

LUDWIG LEVIN JACOBSON, Danish anatomist, 1783-1843, described a rudimentary (in man) canal above the vomeronasal cartilage opening in the side of the nasal septum. Reported in 1809. Known as *organ of Jacobson.*

Vomiting, physiology and mechanism of, early description

FRANÇOIS MAGENDIE, French physiologist, 1783-1855, gave a clear description of the mechanism and physiology of vomiting, in 1813.

Vomiting sickness of Jamaica, cause of

HENRY HAROLD SCOTT, English physician, 1874-19??, discovered that the vomiting sickness of Jamaica is caused by the consumption of the fruit of the ackee tree. Recorded in 1916.

Von Hippel's disease

. . . See under *Retina, angiomatosis of,* etc.

Von Recklinghausen's disease

. . . See under *Neurofibromatosis.*

Voronoff's operation

. . . See under *Rejuvenation by means of testicular transplants.*

Vulpian atrophy

. . . See under *Muscular atrophy of scapulohumeral region.*

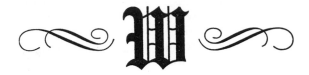

Wachendorf's membrane, eponymic description of

EBERHARD JACOB VON WACHEN-DORF, Dutch anatomist, 1703-1758, described a thin membrane filling in the pupil in the fetus up to the sixth or seventh month. Recorded in 1754.

Wagner's corpuscles; Meissner's corpuscles

GEORG MEISSNER, German anatomist and physiologist, 1829-1905, with RUDOLPH WAGNER, German physician, 1805-1864, described tactile corpuscles in the dermal papillae of the fingertips and toetips, the external genitalia, the mammae, etc. Recorded in 1852.

Wagner's disease, eponymic description of

ERNST LEBERECHT WAGNER, German pathologist, 1829-1888, was the first to describe colloid milium, a yellowish papule in the chorium of the skin undergoing colloid degeneration. Published in 1866.

Waldeyer's epithelium, eponymic description of

HEINRICH WILHELM GOTTFRIED WALDEYER-HARTZ, German anatomist, 1836-1921, described the germinal epithelium, in 1870.

Waldeyer's fossa, eponymic description of

HEINRICH WILHELM GOTTFRIED WALDEYER-HARTZ, German anatomist, 1836-1921, described the two duodenal fossae with reference to hernia. Recorded in 1868. Considered as one, the fossae are known as *Waldeyer's fossa.*

Waldeyer's line, eponymic description of

HEINRICH WILHELM GOTTFRIED WALDEYER-HARTZ, German anatomist, 1836-1921, described the line which forms the boundary of the insertion of the mesovarium in the ovary, at the hilus. Recorded in 1870.

Waldeyer's tonsillar ring

. . . See under *Ring of adenoid tissue formed by tonsils etc.*

Wallerian law of degeneration

AUGUSTUS VOLNEY WALLER, English physiologist, 1816-1870, demonstrated that a nerve fiber can survive only when it maintains continuity with its cell body. Recorded in 1850.

Walther's ganglion; ganglion impar

AUGUSTIN FRIEDRICH WALTHER,

German anatomist, 1688-1746, described a ganglion located on the anterior surface of the coccyx, near the tip. Recorded *circa* 1722.

Wangensteen's tube or apparatus

. . . See under *Intestinal distention, apparatus for decompression of.*

Wardrop's operation, original description of

JAMES WARDROP, English surgeon, 1782-1869, was the first to use distal ligation in treating aneurysm of the carotid artery. Recorded in 1827.

Warts, causative agent of, is filtrable

GIUSEPPE CIUFFO, Italian physician, 1872-1942, demonstrated that what he considered the etiological agent of the common wart was filtrable. Recorded in 1907.

Watch crystal eyeshield, invention of

FRANK BULLER, Canadian ophthalmologist, 1844-1905, invented an eyeshield consisting essentially of a watch crystal set in a frame of adhesive tape. It was used to protect the sound eye from being infected by the discharge from the affected eye. Recorded in 1874.

Watch spring method of treating aneurysm

. . . See under *Aneurysm, treatment of, by insertion of a watch spring.*

Water bag for sterilizing water in camps or in the field

WILLIAM JOHN L. LYSTER, U. S. Army physician, 1869-1947, devised an apparatus, consisting of a rubber-lined canvas bag provided with faucets, for sterilizing water in the field by means of calcium hypochlorite. Reported in 1917. Known as *Lyster bag*.

Water closet, invention of

JOHN HARINGTON, English author, 1561-1612, is credited with inventing the first functional water closet in which the excreta were disposed of by a stream of water. Recorded in 1596.

Water immersion for microscope lens

GIOVANNI BATTISTA AMICI, Italian physicist and astronomer, 1784-1863, is believed to have originated the method of water immersion for the improved achromatic lenses of the compound microscope of his day. Recorded in 1818.

Water purification in field, practical method for

CARL ROGER DARNALL, American Army medical officer, 1868-1941, developed a practical method for purifying water in the field, for troops, by means of sodium hypochlorite. Reported in April, 1908. Known as *Darnall's method*.

Water-hammer pulse in aortic insufficiency

DOMINIC JOHN CORRIGAN, Irish physician, 1802-1880, introduced the term *water-hammer* to describe the pulse in aortic insufficiency. Recorded in 1832. Also known as *Corrigan pulse*.

Waterhouse-Friderichsen syndrome

. . . See under *Meningitis, meningococcus, fulminating type of.*

Wax-plate method of reconstruction in embryology

GUSTAV JACOB BORN, German embryologist, 1851-1900, invented the so-called wax-plate reconstruction method used in embryology. Reported in 1896.

"We think in words," introduction of axiom

... See under *Words,* etc.

Weather in its relation to pain

... See under *Pain and weather, relation between.*

Webbed fingers, operation for correction of

... See under *Syndactylism.*

Weber's paralysis

... See under *Hemiplegia, alternate, involving oculomotor nerve, etc.;* also, *Hemiplegia, alternate, early description of—1856*

Wegner's disease

... See under *Osteochondritic epiphysial separation in congenital syphilis.*

Weichselbaum's coccus

... See under *Meningococcus,* etc.

Weigert's method or stain

... See under *Myelin sheath stain by Weigert.*

Weil-Felix agglutination test for typhus

... See under *Typhus, Weil-Felix agglutination test for.*

Weil's disease, causative agent of

... See under *Leptospira icterohaemorrhagiae, discovery of.*

Weil's disease, eponymic description of

ADOLF WEIL, German physician, 1848-1916, gave a classic description of leptospiral jaundice (leptospirosis icterohemorrhagica), in 1886. Known also as spirochetal jaundice.

Weil's disease, pre-eponymic description of

JEFFERY ALLEN MARSTON, English physician, 1831-1911, described leptospiral jaundice some 23 years before ADOLF WEIL. Recorded in 1863.

Weismann's theory

... See under *Acquired characteristics, theory of non-inheritance of.*

Welch bacillus

... See under *Bacillus aerogenes capsulatus.*

Well-leg countertraction method for treating fracture of femur

ROGER ANDERSON, American orthopedic surgeon, 1891-19??, introduced a new method for treating fracture of the femur by means of a well-leg countertraction apparatus. Reported in 1932. Called *Anderson method* or *splint.*

Wells's facies

... See under *Ovarian disease, facial expression in.*

Werdnig-Hoffman syndrome

... See under *Muscular atrophy, hereditary familial spinal,* etc.

Werner's syndrome; Werner-His disease

... See under *Trench fever, eponymic description of.*

Wernicke-Mann palsy or paralysis

. . . See under *Hemiplegia, spastic, of extremities*, etc.

Wernicke's aphasia

. . . See under *Sensory aphasia, eponymic description of.*

Wernicke's disease

. . . See under *Acute superior hemorrhagic polioencephalitis.*

Westphal's nucleus

. . . See under *Nucleus beneath aqueduct of Sylvius.*

Wharton's duct

. . . See under *Submaxillary gland duct.*

Wharton's jelly

. . . See under *Umbilical cord, mucoid connective tissue of.*

Whistle for determining hearing ability of high tones

Francis Galton, English geneticist, 1822-1911, invented a whistle to determine the upper limit of hearing ability with regard to high frequency tones. Known as *Galton's whistle*. The whistle was provided with a screw adjustment by which the pitch could be varied. Exact date not available.

White bands in layer of large pyramidal cells of cerebral cortex

Jules G. F. Baillarger, French neurologist, 1809-1890, described the white bands found in the layer of the large pyramidal cells of the cerebral cortex. Reported in 1840.

White's disease

. . . See under *Keratosis follicularis, eponymic description of.*

Whitfield's ointment

. . . See under *Ointment of benzoic and salicylic acids.*

Whitmore's disease

. . . See under *Melioidosis, eponymic description of.*

Whole-wheat flour, introduction of

. . . See under *Graham flour.*

Whooping cough, causative agent of

. . . See under *Hemophilus pertussis.*

Whooping cough, first description of

Guillaume de Baillou, French physician, 1538-1616, was the first to record an account of whooping cough, under the name of *tussis quintana*, in 1578. Published in 1640.

***Whooping cough*, introduction of term**

Thomas Sydenham, English physician, 1624-1689, is credited with introducing the term *whooping cough*, in 1675.

Whooping cough

. . . See also under *Pertussis.*

Whytt's reflex

. . . See under *Pupillary contraction in response to light.*

Widal test

. . . See under *Typhoid fever, test for.*

Willebrand's disease

. . . See under *Pseudohemophilia, hereditary.*

Wilms's tumor

. . . See under *Embryonal carcino-sarcoma of kidney.*

Wilson's disease

. . . See under *Dermatitis exfoliativa, eponymic description of.*

Wilson's (Kinnier) disease

. . . See under *Progressive lenticular degeneration.*

Winckel's disease

. . . See under *Hemoglobinuria, epidemic,* etc.

Winking, absence or infrequency of, in goiter

CARL STELLWAG VON CARION, Austrian ophthalmologist, 1823-1904, noted the infrequency or absence of winking in exophthalmic goiter, associated with a widening of the palpebral opening. Recorded in 1869. Known as *Stellwag's sign.*

Winslow's pancreas

. . . See under *Pancreas, lesser.*

Winslow's stars

. . . See under *Choroid, whorls of capillary vessels of.*

Wire saw, invention of, for cutting bone

LEONARDO GIGLI, Italian surgeon and gynecologist, 1863-1908, invented a saw consisting essentially of a wire provided with saw teeth. Gigli devised the saw for his operation of pubiotomy but it was later used for many other types of bone section. Reported in 1894. Known as *Gigli's saw.*

Wire splint in fracture of mandible

EDWARD HARTLEY ANGLE, American orthodontist, 1855-1930, designed a wire splint for use in securing the lower teeth to the upper in fracture of the mandible. Date not available.

Wires or nails for passing through bone in treating fractures

MARTIN KIRSCHNER, German surgeon, 1879-1942, devised wires or nails for passing through bone in treating fractures. Recorded in 1909. Known as *Kirschner's wires.*

Wolffian body

. . . See under *Mesonephros, eponymic description of.*

Wolffian cyst

. . . See under *Broad ligament of uterus, cyst of.*

Wolffian duct

. . . See under *Mesonephros, duct of.*

Wolffian ridge

. . . See under *Mesonephric ridge.*

Wolffian tubules

. . . See under *Mesonephros, functional tubules of.*

Wolfring's glands

. . . See under *Eyelid, posterior tarsal glands of.*

Woman physician, first, in America

ELIZABETH BLACKWELL, 1821-1910, was the first woman to receive a medical degree in America, in 1849.

Wool skein test for color vision, introduction of

ALARIK FRITHIOF HOLMGREN,

Swedish physiologist, 1831-1897, introduced the use of wool skeins of various colors, to be sorted by the patient, in testing color vision. Reported in 1874.

Woolner's tip

. . . See under *Ear, helical apex of*.

Word blindness, classic description of

RUDOLF BERLIN, German ophthalmologist, 1833-1897, gave an excellent description of word blindness, in 1887. He also suggested the term *dyslexia*.

Word blindness, introduction of term

ADOLF KUSSMAUL, German physician, 1822-1902, introduced the term *word blindness*, to describe aphasia. Recorded in 1877.

"Words, we think in," introduction of axiom

HENRY CHARLTON BASTIAN, English neurologist, 1837-1915, wrote an important treatise on aphasia and proposed the axiom "We think in words." Recorded in 1869.

Wormian bones

. . . See under *Skull sutures, small bones in*.

Worms, intestinal, early book on

. . . See under *Intestinal worms*.

Wright's stain for blood cells

JAMES HOMER WRIGHT, American pathologist, 1869-1928, devised several stains of which the most popular is the mixture of eosin and methylene blue, used for the differential staining of blood cells and for the staining of malarial parasites. Recorded in 1902.

Wrisberg's cartilage

. . . See under *Larynx, cuneiform cartilage of*.

Wrisberg's corpuscles

. . . See under *Larynx, cuneiform cartilage of*.

Wrisberg's ganglion

. . . See under *Cardiac ganglion, eponymic description of*.

Wrisberg's ligament

. . . See under *Ligament of lateral meniscus*.

Wrisberg's lines

. . . See under *Trigeminal nerve, connecting filaments of*.

Wrisberg's nerve

. . . See under *Nerve, medial cutaneous, of arm*.

Wrisberg's pars intermedia

. . . See under *Nerve, intermedius, of Wrisberg*.

Wrist deformity caused by distortion of radius

OTTO WILHELM MADELUNG, German surgeon, 1846-1926, described a deformity of the wrist caused by a distortion of the lower end of the radius and by ulnar displacement. Recorded in 1878. Known as *Madelung's deformity*.

Wrist drop in lead poisoning

. . . See under *Lead poisoning, paralysis of fingers and wrist in*.

Wuchereria bancrofti, eponymic description of

JOSEPH BANCROFT, English physician, 1836-1894, discovered the white threadlike worms which by obstructing the lymphatic circulation cause elephantiasis and similar disorders, in 1877. Recorded in 1877 and 1878.

Wuchereria bancrofti is transmitted by *Culex* mosquito

PATRICK MANSON, English physician, 1844-1922, demonstrated that the organism causing filarial elephantiasis in man (*Wuchereria bancrofti*) is transmitted by *Culex* mosquitoes. Recorded in 1877.

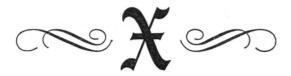

Xanthoma, eponymic description of

PIERRE FRANÇOIS OLIVE RAYER, French dermatologist, 1793-1867, gave the first description of xanthoma and named it so, in 1826. Known also as *Rayer's disease.*

Xanthoma multiplex, early description of

PIERRE FRANÇOIS OLIVE RAYER, French dermatologist, 1793-1867, was probably the first to describe xanthoma multiplex. Published in 1826.

Xanthomatosis of Niemann-Pick

ALBERT NIEMANN, German physician, 1880-1921, described a form of xanthomatosis, in 1914. The same condition was described more fully in 1926 by LUDWIG PICK, German pediatrician, 1868-19??. Known as *Niemann-Pick disease.*

Xanthomatosis

... See also under *Craniohypophysial xanthomatosis.*

Xenon, discovery of—1898

WILLIAM RAMSAY, English scientist, 1852-1916, with M. W. TRAVERS, discovered xenon ("the stranger") in 1898.

Xenopsylla cheopis as vector of plague

MASAKI OGATA, Japanese physician, 1864-1919, demonstrated that the flea *Xenopsylla cheopis* is a vector of bubonic plague. Recorded in 1897.

Xenopus toad test

... See under *Pregnancy, Xenopus toad test for.*

Xeroderma pigmentosum, eponymic description of

MORITZ KAPOSI, Hungarian dermatologist, 1837-1902, described xeroderma pigmentosum, a disease marked by brown spots and ulcers of the skin, telangiectasis, and atrophy of cutaneous and muscular tissues. Recorded in 1882. Known as *Kaposi's disease, atrophoderma pigmentosum,* and *melanosis lenticularis progressiva.*

X-ray cinematography, first showing of

JOHN MACINTYRE, Scottish physician, 1857-1928, is credited with being the first to produce x-ray motion pictures. Recorded in 1897.

X-ray kymography, introduction of

PLEIKART STUMPF, German roentgenologist, 1888-19??, devised an apparatus for recording the movements of a structure made visible by x-rays. Recorded in 1928 and 1931.

X-ray report, first clinical

JOHN COX, Canadian physicist, 1851-1923, with ROBERT CHARLES KIRKPATRICK, Canadian surgeon, 1863-1897, gave the first clinical x-ray report of a case in which the "new photography" was used. It involved a patient with a bullet in the leg. Recorded in 1896.

X-ray stereoscope, introduction of

ELIHU THOMSON, American physicist, 1853-1937, invented the first practical roentgen stereoscope, in 1896.

X-ray therapy, deep, introduction of

GEORG CLEMENS PERTHES, German surgeon, 1869-1927, is credited with being the first to use deep x-ray therapy. Reported in a study of the effect of roentgen rays on epithelial tissue and carcinoma, in 1903.

X-ray tube of tungsten filament and anode, invention of

WILLIAM DAVID COOLIDGE, American scientist, 1873-19??, invented an x-ray tube having a high vacuum, hot tungsten cathode, and a massive tungsten anode. Reported in 1913. Called *Coolidge tube*.

X-rays, effect of, on production of antibodies

LUDVIG HEKTOEN, American pathologist, 1863-1951, demonstrated that x-rays slow or check the production of antibodies. Recorded in 1915.

X-rays in diagnosis of pregnancy, first use of

LARS EDLING, German roentgenologist, 1878-19??, is credited with the earliest use of x-rays in the diagnosis of pregnancy. Published in 1911.

X-rays in leukemia, first use of

NICHOLAS SENN, American surgeon, 1844-1908, is credited with being the first to use x-rays in the treatment of leukemia. Recorded in 1903.

X-rays, inhibitory effect of, on neoplastic growth

GEORG CLEMENS PERTHES, German surgeon, 1869-1927, noted the inhibitory effect of x-rays on neoplasms, especially on carcinoma. Reported in 1903.

X-rays

. . . See also under *Roentgen rays*.

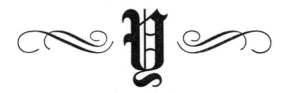

Yato byo; Ohara's disease
HACHIRO OHARA, Japanese physician, 1897-   , described a disease occurring in Japan which is considered to be identical with tularemia. Recorded in 1930.

Yatren, introduction of, in treating amebiasis
PETER MÜHLENS, German physician, 1874-1943, introduced yatren (chiniofon) in the treatment of chronic amebic dysentery. Published in 1921.

Yaws, differentiation of, from syphilis
WILLEM PISO (GUILLAUME LE POIS), Dutch naturalist, 1611-1678, is credited with being first to distinguish between yaws and syphilis. Recorded in 1648.

Yaws, establishment of etiological agent of
ALDO CASTELLANI, Italian pathologist, 1878-19??, was the first to demonstrate *Treponema pertenue* as the causative agent of yaws. Reported in 1905.

Yaws, flies in transmission of
EDWARD NATHANIEL BANCROFT, English physician, 17??-18??, recorded his observations on the transmission of yaws by flies. Published in 1769.

Yeast, autolyzed, in pernicious anemia of tropics
LUCY WILLS, English physician, 18??-19??, demonstrated that autolyzed yeast is effective in treating pernicious anemia of the tropics. Reported, in a survey of dietetic and hygienic conditions of women in Bombay, in 1930.

Yeast cell, discovery of
CHARLES CAGNIARD-LATOUR, French biologist, 1777-1859, discovered the true nature of yeast by recognizing that it is composed of living cells. Observed in 1836; published in 1838. At about the same time, and independently of Cagniard-Latour, THEODOR SCHWANN also discovered the yeast cell. Published in 1837.

Yeast cell plasma, discovery of
. . . See under *Zymase expressed from dried yeast.*

Yellow fever, control of, in Panama Canal zone
WILLIAM CRAWFORD GORGAS, American Army surgeon, 1854-1920, directed the control of the antimalaria and anti-yellow fever campaign in Panama during the

construction of the Panama Canal. In charge from 1904-13.

Yellow fever, convalescent serum in

EMILE MARCHOUX, French physician, 1862-1943, with E. SALIMBENI and P. L. SIMOND, made use of convalescent serum of yellow fever patients in prophylaxis and treatment. Published in 1903.

Yellow fever, eradication of, from Cuba

WILLIAM CRAWFORD GORGAS, American Army surgeon, 1854-1920, went to Cuba in 1901 and introduced methods of sanitation which in about 3 months practically eliminated yellow fever from Havana. Published in 1909.

Yellow fever, etiology of

WALTER REED, American Army surgeon, 1851-1902, with JAMES CARROLL (American Army medical officer, 1854-1907), ARISTIDE AGRAMONTE Y SIMONI (Cuban parasitologist, 1868-1931), and JESSE WILLIAM LAZEAR (American physician, 1866-1900), studied the etiology of yellow fever and reported that the disease is caused by a filtrable virus which is transmitted to man by the mosquito *Aëdes aegypti*. Recorded in 1901.

Yellow fever, fall of pulse rate with rise of temperature in

JEAN C. FAGET, French physician, 1818-1884, observed that in yellow fever the pulse rate decreases while the temperature rises or remains at the same level. Reported in 1875. Called *Faget's sign*.

Yellow fever, first definite description of

JEAN BAPTISTE DU TERTRE, French priest, 1614-1684, was the first to give a clear description of yellow fever in his account of the outbreaks at Guadeloupe and St. Kitts in 1635, 1640, and 1648. Recorded in 1667.

Yellow fever, incubation period of

HENRY ROSE CARTER, American public health officer, 1852-1925, determined the incubation period of yellow fever, a finding which influenced the work of WALTER REED later on. Recorded in 1900.

Yellow fever, introduction of term

GRIFFITH HUGHES, English naturalist, 171?-1779, is believed to have been the first to use the term *yellow fever,* in his work *Natural History of Barbadoes*. Published in 1750.

Yellow fever, mosquito in transmission of—1848

JOSIAH CLARK NOTT, American physician, 1804-1873, is credited with being the first to suggest that the mosquito was responsible for the transmission of yellow fever. Recorded in 1848.

Yellow fever, mosquito in transmission of—1881

CARLOS JUAN FINLAY, Cuban physician, 1833-1915, was the first to suggest that the mosquito carried the infection of yellow fever from one person to another. Recorded in 1881-2.

Yellow fever, mosquito in transmission of—1900

WALTER REED, American Army

surgeon, 1851-1902, with JAMES CARROLL (1854-1907), ARISTIDE AGRAMONTE Y SIMONI (1868-1931), and JESSE WILLIAM LAZEAR (1866-1900), provided definite proof that the causative organism of yellow fever is transmitted to man by the mosquito *Aëdes aegypti*. Published in 1900. J. W. LAZEAR died of yellow fever during the investigation.

Yellow fever, mouse test for

MAX THEILER, South African physician and bacteriologist, 1899-, developed a test for the diagnosis of yellow fever which is based on the susceptibility of white mice to the intracerebral inoculation of the virus. Recorded in 1930. Known as the *intracerebral protection test*.

Yellow fever, Philadelphia epidemic of

MATHEW CAREY, Philadelphia physician, 1760-1839, gave a clear description of the Philadelphia yellow fever epidemic of 1793. Recorded in 1793. He also gave an evaluation of the efficacy of the several forms of treatment.

Yellow fever, prophylactic serum for

WILLIAM ALFRED SAWYER, American epidemiologist, 1884-19??, with S. F. KITCHEN and W. D. M. LLOYD, developed an immune serum for prophylactic use against yellow fever. Published in 1932.

Yellow fever, transmission of, to monkeys

ADRIAN STOKES, Nigerian physician, 1887-1927, with J. H. BAUER and N. P. HUDSON, experimentally transmitted yellow fever to *Macaca rhesus*. Recorded in 1928. Stokes died of yellow fever during the investigation.

Yellow fever vaccine

EDWARD HINDLE, English physician, 189?-, prepared the first known prophylactic vaccine against yellow fever. Recorded in 1928.

Yellow fever vaccine by Theiler

MAX THEILER, South African physician and bacteriologist, 1899-19??, developed two vaccines against yellow fever, *circa* 1937. Received the Nobel prize in 1951.

Yellow fever virus, cultivation of, in vitro

WRAY DEVERE MARR LLOYD, American physician, 189?-1936, with M. THEILER and N. I. RICCI, modified the virulence of yellow fever virus by cultivating it in organic tissues in vitro. Published in 1936.

Yolk-sac method of cultivating rickettsiae

... See under *Rickettsiae, yolk-sac method of cultivating*.

Young's rule of dosage

... See under *Children, dosage of medicine for*.

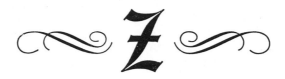

Zaufal's sign of congenital syphilis

EMANUEL ZAUFAL, Austrian rhinologist and otologist, 1833-1910, described the condition known as saddle nose, and pointed out that when this is associated with alopecia it may be considered pathognomonic of congenital syphilis. Recorded *circa* 1875.

Ziehen-Oppenheim disease; torsion spasm

GEORG THEODOR ZIEHEN, German psychiatrist, 1862-1924, described torsion spasm or dystonia musculorum deformans. Published January 16, 1911. On October 1 of the same year, the condition was also reported by HERMANN OPPENHEIM, German neurologist, 1858-1919.

Zinc chloride disinfectant solution

WILLIAM BURNETT, Scottish surgeon, 1779-1861, compounded a disenfectant solution composed chiefly of zinc chloride. A variation of the original formula contained a small amount of ferrous chloride. Reported in 1857.

Zinc insulin, introduction of

ROBERT BEWS KERR, Canadian scientist, 1908-   , with C. H. BEST, W. R. CAMPBELL, and A. A. FLETCHER, suggested the combination of insulin with zinc, to slow down the rate of absorption. Recorded in 1936.

Zinc, introduction of term

PARACELSUS (AUREOLUS THEOPHRASTUS BOMBASTUS VON HOHENHEIM), Swiss physician, 1493-1541, is credited with introducing the term *zinc,* in the form of *zinken, circa* 1525.

Zinc Oxide paste; Lassar's paste

OSKAR LASSAR, German dermatologist, 1849-1908, introduced zinc oxide paste for the treatment of eczema. Published in English in 1889.

Zinn's central artery

. . . See under *Retina, central artery of.*

Zinn's ligament

. . . See under *Ligament, annular, of recti muscles of eye.*

Zonular spaces; canals of Petit

FRANÇOIS POURFOUR DU PETIT, French physician and physiologist, 1664-1741, described spaces which surround the capsule or periphery of the crystalline lens. Recorded *circa* 1715.

Zonule of Zinn, eponymic description of

JOHANN GOTTFRIED ZINN, German anatomist, 1727-1759, described a fibrous ring part of which forms the suspensory ligament of the crystalline lens. Recorded in 1755. Known also as *ciliary zonule* and *zone of Zinn.*

Zuckerkandl's bodies; aortic paraganglia

EMIL ZUCKERKANDL, Austrian anatomist, 1849-1910, described chromaffin bodies situated along the course of the aorta and associated with the sympathetic ganglia. Recorded *circa* 1880.

Zuckerkandl's convolution, eponymic description of

EMIL ZUCKERKANDL, Austrian anatomist, 1849-1910, described the gray substance covering the under surface of the rostrum of the corpus callosum, *circa* 1895. Known also as *gyrus subcallosus.*

Zuckerkandl's tubercle; pharyngeal tonsil

EMIL ZUCKERKANDL, Austrian anatomist, 1849-1910, described the pharyngeal tonsil, *circa* 1882.

Zymase expressed from dried yeast

HANS BUCHNER, German bacteriologist, 1850-1902, described zymase expressed from dried yeast. Known as *yeast cell plasma* and *Buchner's zymase.* Date not available.

Zymogen, introduction of term

RUDOLF PETER HEINRICH HEIDENHAIN, German physiologist, 1834-1897, introduced the term *zymogen,* about 1876. It means, literally, "ferment generator."

Zymogens, early recognition of

RUDOLF PETER HEINRICH HEIDENHAIN, German physiologist, 1834-1897, demonstrated that the cells of the pancreas do not contain formed enzymes but do contain substances which are converted into enzymes on coming in contact with co-enzymes. To such precursors of enzymes he applied the term *zymogens.* Recorded *circa* 1876.